GENERAL MEDICINE PRACTICE HANDBOOK

VOLUME 2

SPECIALIZED CARE, PROCEDURES, AND PRACTICAL COMPETENCIES IN GENERAL MEDICINE

Dr. Kashieca Yap

ALLIED HEALTH PRESS

General Medicine Practice Handbook

Volume 2: Specialized Care, Procedures, and Practical Competencies in General Medicine

Author: **Dr. Kashieca Yap**

Allied Health Press
4164 Lakeshore Road
Burlington ON L7L 1A4
Canada
www.alliedhealthpress.com
Email: orders@arclereducation.com

ISBN: 978-1-77956-857-1

ABOUT THE AUTHOR

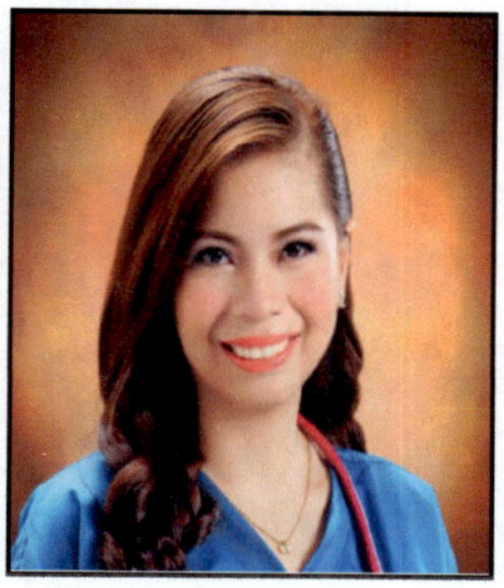

Kashieca Yap, M.D., is a devoted medical doctor and medical writer. She currently works as a general practice physician in a rural town, where she handles adult and pediatric cases, infectious diseases, and chronic medical conditions. Kashieca also lectures on mental health, clinical pharmacology, physiology, and psychiatry and is an enthusiastic researcher and medical writer. She obtained her medical degree from Cebu Doctor's University College of Medicine and further developed her clinical skills at a large public hospital. Alongside her professional endeavors, Kashieca dedicates her time to volunteering at NGOs and medical missions, reaching out to people in geographically isolated areas. Her unwavering passion for medicine and her strong desire to serve people is a testament to her compassion and skill as a healthcare professional.

Brief Table of Contents

Chapter Openers

A list of Chapter Outline is presented providing a brief Introduction to what will be covered in the chapter.

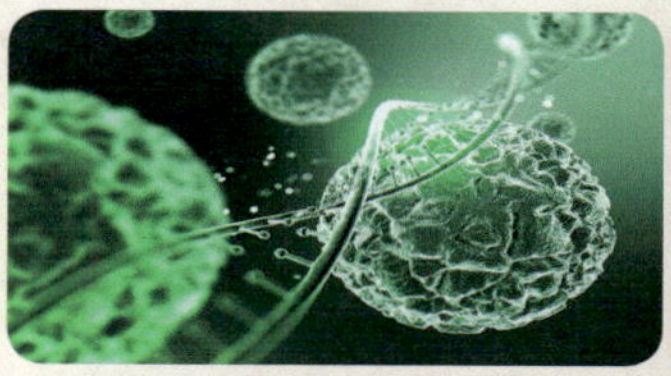

Introduction

Often referred to as the science of life, biology is a broad field of study aimed at comprehending the several kinds of life on Earth, from tiny creatures to sophisticated multicellular entities. Comprising several subfields, including molecular biology, ecology, and evolutionary biology, each of which advances our knowledge of living systems, this field clarifies the mechanisms controlling life events, including development, reproduction, and interaction with the surroundings, which is the central goal of biology. Moreover, biology fills in the void between the natural sciences and medicine by offering a necessary understanding of health, illness, and the interactions between organisms and their environments. Dealing with urgent global issues such as climate change, biodiversity loss, and new diseases depends on an awareness of these complex biological interactions, therefore highlighting the critical part biology plays in modern civilization. Fundamentally, biology explores and tests ideas about the living world using the scientific method. Through methodical observation and experimentation,

LEARNING OBJECTIVES

After studying this chapter, you will be able to:

1. Discuss the scientific method in biology;
2. Explain the cell theory;
3. Discuss the genetics and heredity;
4. Evolution and natural selection;
5. Focus on ecology and ecosystems;
6. Learn about human biology;
7. Evaluate the plant biology;
8. Explain the microbiology;
9. Focus on current trends in biology.

1.1. The Scientific Method in Biology

Learning Outcome

1. Describe the steps of the scientific method;
2. Focus on hypothesis formation;
3. Learn about experimental design.

Learning Outcomes

The beginning of each section of every chapter contains a set of Learning Outcomes that inform students of concepts they should understand. These outcomes help students understand what they should be able to do if they have mastered the material in that section.

Test Your Knowledge

Throughout each chapter, Test Your Knowledge cues you to note which topics have been covered and to self-test your understanding of the material presented.

Test Your Knowledge

1. Explain why correlation does not imply causation in scientific experiments.
2. How does the scientific method help reduce the influence of personal opinions in research?

Chapter Summary

The Summary Section appear at the end of each chapter and summarize main concepts covered throughout the chapter. These points provide key concepts in an engaging and meaningful way.

Summary

The investigation of biological principles highlights the importance of a comprehensive view of life by reflecting the intricate interactions that occur within living systems. The complexity of biology goes beyond individual species or systems, as this essay highlights; it also includes the interactions that mold ecosystems and affect biodiversity. Researchers can conduct in-depth analyses of metabolomic data using sophisticated technologies like MetaboAnalyst, which offer insights into the molecular mechanisms underlying these interactions. As demonstrated by the developments in MetaboAnalyst, for example, the integration of diverse omics data promotes a thorough understanding of metabolic pathways and helps identify important biological markers necessary for research on development and disease (Chong et al., 2018). Additionally, the phenomenon of ecological invasions is a key component of biological research and a vital field of study. The introduction of non-native species into unfamiliar habitats has significant ramifications and calls for multidisciplinary management strategies. Examining the origins and effects of these biological incursions, invasion science has become a crucial field that highlights the need to comprehend ecological dynamics and community interactions. As interest in biological invasions increases, new findings are emerging that put conventional ecological theories and practices to the test. The importance of incorporating various scientific viewpoints is shown by this developing discipline, which also highlights how invasive species shape ecosystems and advances our knowledge of ecological resilience (David et al., 2013). When taken as a whole, these discoveries from invasion science and metabolomics highlight the value of multidisciplinary biology research. Fostering cross-disciplinary collaboration and utilizing technological breakthroughs to improve our comprehension of intricate biological interactions are crucial as we look to the future of biological research. In addition to deepening our understanding of the complexities of life, this method lays the groundwork for tackling urgent environmental issues. Future studies can ensure the continued relevance of biology in a world that is constantly changing by acknowledging the interconnection of biological systems and opening the door to creative solutions that support sustainability and biodiversity conservation. We might imagine a thorough comprehension of life that serves both academia and society at large through ongoing investigation and integration of scientific knowledge.

Knowledge Assessment

The chapter includes material designed to review and reinforce each content. It includes Critical Thinking Questions to help test of your understanding of information presented in the chapter and Short answer Questions to review your understanding of the key concepts presented in the chapter.

Critical Thinking Questions

1. **Who is known as the "Father of Modern Biology"?**
   a. Aristotle
   b. Charles Darwin
   c. Gregor Mendel
   d. Louis Pasteur
2. **What is the basic unit of life?**
   a. Atom
   b. Molecule
   c. Cell
   d. Organism
3. **Which branch of biology studies the interaction of organisms with their environment?**
   a. Genetics
   b. Ecology
   c. Physiology
   d. Botany
4. **Which macromolecule is the main source of energy for living organisms?**
   a. Proteins
   b. Lipids
   c. Carbohydrates
   d. Nucleic acids
5. **DNA is primarily responsible for which function in living organisms?**
   a. Energy production
   b. Protein synthesis
   c. Storing genetic information
   d. Regulating body temperature

Short Answer Questions

1. What is biology, and why is it important to study biology?
2. What are the three main domains of life, and how are they different from one another?
3. Define homeostasis and give an example of how it works in living organisms.
4. What is the cell theory, and why is it fundamental to biology?
5. How do autotrophs and heterotrophs differ in the way they obtain energy?
6. What is the scientific method, and how is it applied in biological research?
7. Discuss how biology helps address global challenges such as climate change, disease, and food security.
8. Explain the levels of biological organization from the smallest unit to the largest. Provide examples at each level.
9. Describe the relationship between structure and function in biology, giving specific examples from cells or organs.
10. How has the discovery of genetics shaped our understanding of inheritance and variation among organisms?

Supplementary Materials

Key Terms: A list of key terms is given for quick reference

KEY TERMS FROM THIS CHAPTER

Annotation enrichment analysis	Biological structure	Cell
Cell theory	Cellular structure	Ecology
Ecosystems	Genetics	Human biology
Microbiology	Natural selection	Organism
Plant biology		

Further Resources: Recommendations for additional readings, websites, and multimedia resources.

References

1. Argelaguet, R., Velten, B., Arnol, D., Dietrich, S., Zenz, T., Marioni, J. C., Buettner, F., et al. (2018). Multi-omics factor analysis—A framework for unsupervised integration of multi-omics data sets. *Molecular Systems Biology, 14*. https://doi.org/10.15252/msb.20178124.
2. Bacher, S., Blackburn, T. M., Essl, F., & Genovesi, P. (2017). *Socio-Economic Impact Classification of Alien Taxa (SEICAT)*. https://core.ac.uk/download/286567949.pdf (accessed on 8th March 2025).
3. Barnett, R., Brace, S., Cucchi, T., & Dobney, K. (2013). *Divergent Evolutionary Processes Associated with Colonization of Offshore Islands*. https://core.ac.uk/download/20664364.pdf (accessed on 8th March 2025).

Detailed Table of Contents

CHAPTER 3

Psychiatry in General Practice 71

CHAPTER 4

Dermatology for Physicians 107

CHAPTER 5

Allergy and Immunology 143

CHAPTER 6

Environmental and Occupational Medicine 179

CHAPTER 7

Emergency Medicine in General Practice 211

LIST OF FIGURES

PREFACE

Aging populations, chronic disease exacerbation, and diversity of patient presentation have all significantly amplified the practice of the general physician. No longer are primary care providers (PCPs) merely acute disease physicians, but are being increasingly challenged to deal with multifactorial disease across the life cycle. This transformation of healthcare means that general practitioners (GPs) must be competent and assertive in a wide range of areas—from the management of older patients with polypharmacy concerns to psychiatric presentations and interpretation of dermatological findings. The ability to deliver holistic, primary-level treatment has now become crucial to preventing specialist referral and continuity of care.

At the same time, societal changes and increasing recognition of special health needs—ranging from women's health needs to illnesses on the job—have placed broader expectations on generalists. Practitioners must not only possess core clinical proficiency but also procedural expertise and adequate documentation protocols. With shifting diagnostic technology and treatment modalities, updated knowledge must be maintained not only to be clinically effective but also medico-legally safe and patient-trusting. Doctors must continue to be competent at interpreting investigations, performing minor procedures, and handling emergencies and yet continue to deliver person-centered care.

General Medicine Practice Handbook – Volume 2 attempts to fill this need for a longer and more practical handbook to meet the needs of daily practice of primary and generalist physicians. This volume is a continuation of the first one, with further elaborate treatment of systems, conditions, and competencies central to today's general practice. The book weaves together clinical synopses and focused procedural guidance to serve both experienced practitioners and those continuing to develop their first-line care skills. It aims to enhance readiness in managing real practice medical scenarios, with usable strategies that can be used in various care settings.

Chapter 1 provides an overview of important issues in geriatric medicine, such as the multifactorial etiology of aging and the management of multimorbidity, frailty, functional impairment, and drug considerations in late life. It features strategies for comprehensive geriatric assessment (CGA), prevention of falls, and cognitive assessment to facilitate physicians in managing the complex requirements of elderly patients.

Chapter 2 discusses women's health in general medicine with a focus on preventive screening, reproductive and hormonal complaints, and care of gynecologic conditions within the primary care setting. The chapter also outlines the generalist's role in pregnancy care, menopause management, and gender-specific control of risk factors for chronic disease.

Chapter 3 explains primary care psychiatry in describing usual presentations such as depression, anxiety, substance use disorders (SUDs), and somatization. The material highlights recognition, initial management, risk assessment, and referral criteria with useful algorithms and communication tips within time-limited consultations.

Chapter 4 covers dermatologic conditions commonly seen in general practice and diagnostic pointers for distinguishing between rashes, nodules, infections, and inflammatory skin disorders. It offers guidance on visual assessment, dermoscopy basics, initial treatment approaches, and referral or biopsy red flags.

Chapter 5 addresses allergy and immunology, including such subjects as the identification of allergic reactions, reading allergy tests, the management of anaphylaxis, and treating chronic immunological conditions such as asthma and autoimmune disease. The chapter addresses emergency measures and the generalist role in the management of long-term disease.

Chapter 6 covers environmental and occupational medicine, helping clinicians detect work-related exposure, toxin-related syndrome, and illness patterns of environmental stressors. History-taking for occupational hazards, preventive interventions, and reporting requirements are covered, enabling physicians to deal with this very often neglected area.

Chapter 7 includes emergency medicine practice that is applicable within the general context, with systematic management of emergent conditions such as acute chest pain, respiratory failure, seizures, trauma management, and first-responder maneuvers. Early stabilization, use of emergency drugs, triage practice, and escalation to advanced care are given special emphasis.

Chapter 8 is a step-by-step procedural skills guide to intravenous (IV) access, lumbar puncture, electrocardiogram (ECG) interpretation, arterial blood gas (ABG) analysis, and thoracocentesis. Step-by-step instructions, clear images, and safety checklists are provided to facilitate competency in the accomplishment of these procedures safely and confidently.

Chapter 9 provides generalist critical care principles, including early recognition of deteriorating patients, titrating oxygen therapy, sepsis protocols, and ventilator essentials. The material educates the importance of prompt intervention and is used to instruct when to activate intensive care teams, which is applicable for practicing in rural or resource-limited settings.

Chapter 10 concludes general practice medicine in pain treatment. Topics include classification of pain, multimodal analgesia, opioid stewardship, and management of chronic non-cancer pain. Safe prescribing is emphasized, along with a patient communication strategy and choice for referral for interventional or psychological therapy.

Chapter 11 is devoted to clinical documentation and medical records with a focus on timely, accurate, and legally accurate record-keeping. Best practices are outlined for SOAP notes, discharge summaries, referral letters, and computerized record management. Patient confidentiality, effective communication through written notes, and addressing medico-legal requirements are stressed.

This book is intended for a general readership of medical doctors practicing generalist practice. General practitioners, family doctors, and internal medicine specialists will also find this book helpful in guiding their day-to-day clinical decisions. It is also a useful tool for junior doctors, residents, and final-year medical students preparing for independent practice. It is an added resource for nurse practitioners and physician assistants who practice in general medicine roles.

GERIATRIC MEDICINE

1

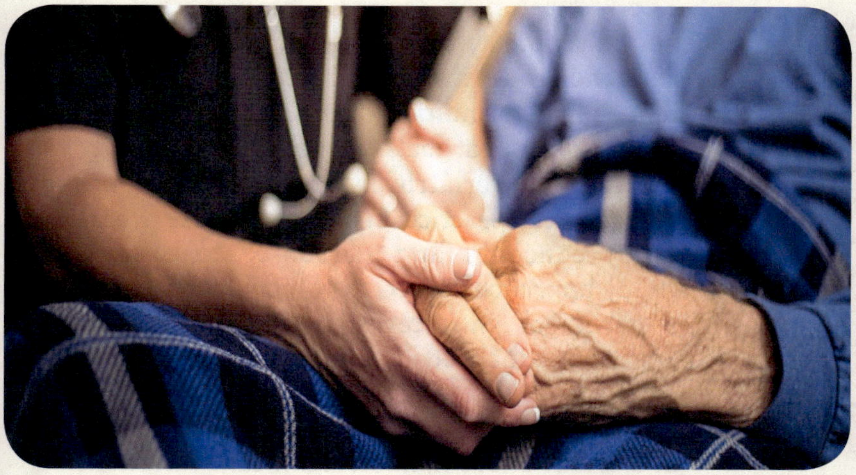

Introduction

The field of geriatric medicine is increasingly recognized as playing a significant role in the management of the complex healthcare needs of the elderly. As the population lives longer, the prevalence of chronic disease and comorbidities in the elderly adds to the growing need for specialized medical care. Geriatric medicine is not only interested in the treatment of disease but also in optimizing overall quality of life in older adults through comprehensive assessment and targeted interventions. This holistic approach treats the physical, psychological, and social dimensions of aging, which brings with it improved control of health. By the emphasis on multidisciplinary care teams, geriatric medicine is committed to addressing the complex problems of the older patient to provide improved overall health outcomes and greater patient satisfaction. In addition to addressing the immediate health needs of the patient, geriatric medicine also recognizes the potential for assistive technologies to improve the health and well-being of aging citizens. Technologies aimed at ambient assisted living (AAL)

LEARNING OBJECTIVES

After studying this chapter, you will be able to:

1. Understand common health issues in the elderly;
2. Discuss geriatric assessment;
3. Describe pharmacological considerations;
4. Focus on non-pharmacological interventions in geriatric medicine;
5. Explain palliative and end-of-life care;
6. Deal with challenges in geriatric medicine.

and age-friendly environments play a pivotal role in improving autonomy and the quality of life among elderly citizens. In addition to easing everyday functioning, they facilitate the capacity of caregivers to provide care. Due to the continuous advancement of care practices and medical devices, technology's role in geriatric care cannot be overstated. Both policymakers and researchers have noted the vast socio-economic consequences of these changes and emphasized the necessity of formulating solutions that can fit the unique needs and resources of future elderly populations. In the process, geriatric medicine seeks to provide a framework that embraces the benefits and challenges of aging. Beyond this, information on the relationship between cost and healthcare complexity is also imperative in geriatric medicine. Older adults will have with them an intricate set of health issues complicating their treatment histories that directly affect the quality and cost of their healthcare services. As cited in current literature, care management can bring significant improvement to patients' outcomes while concurrently reducing overall healthcare expenditure. This is of particular relevance given the current increased burden on healthcare systems worldwide. By addressing challenges such as patient vulnerability and the interaction of multiple chronic conditions, geriatric medicine can optimize care efficiency. Not only do these interventions benefit individual patients, but they also contribute to the sustainability of healthcare systems, necessitating urgency to create innovative solutions for dealing with the mounting pressure of an aging population (Berry-Millett & Bodenheimer, 2009; Eberhardt et al., 2009).

Definition and Scope of Geriatric Medicine

Geriatric medicine encompasses the overall healthcare of older adults. Predominantly classified as an internal medicine subspecialty, geriatric medicine deals with the diagnosis, treatment, management, and prevention of diseases associated with aging. With populations aged 65 and above growing worldwide, the complexity of geriatric care has exponentially increased, necessitating a multidisciplinary approach. Geriatricians are trained to address the physical, psychological, and social complexities of aging, including the treatment of chronic diseases, cognitive impairment, and promotion of functional independence.

The extensive scope emphasizes a multidisciplinary approach to health among the geriatric group, in which treatment balances a range of comorbidities in combination with the patient's personal goals and beliefs. Significantly, the field of geriatric medicine involves not only clinical practice but also long-term care (LTC) concerns and person-centered care (PCC) approaches. LTC development registers a paradigm shift towards services in line with individualized needs and preferences of older people and a strengthening of cultural background in care provision. An international LTC profile sheds light on significant variations in financing, ownership, and regulation between nations that influence the character of services provided within nations (Siegel et al., 2019). Through adoptive international models for care delivery, geriatric medicine can enhance its own practice of high-quality care provision to better respond to evolving requirements of aging populations while not compromising cultural and contextual diversity. Moreover, one of the issues with geriatric medicine is polypharmacy, or the employment of multiple medications at once which has a propensity to create deleterious effects.

This is a very prevalent practice among elderly patients who, most times, have various chronic illnesses to be treated with medication (Sharma et al., 2016). The complexity of management of polypharmacy calls for evidence-based evaluation strategies and standardized approaches to deprescribing, where medications are gradually weaned out when the harms outweigh the benefits. The development of evidence-based practices and guidelines towards maximizing medication management is critical for improved patient outcomes in geriatric medicine. Hence, ongoing improvement in drug-related definitions and interventions in polypharmacy is a vital element in the entire spectrum of geriatric medicine (Figure 1.1).

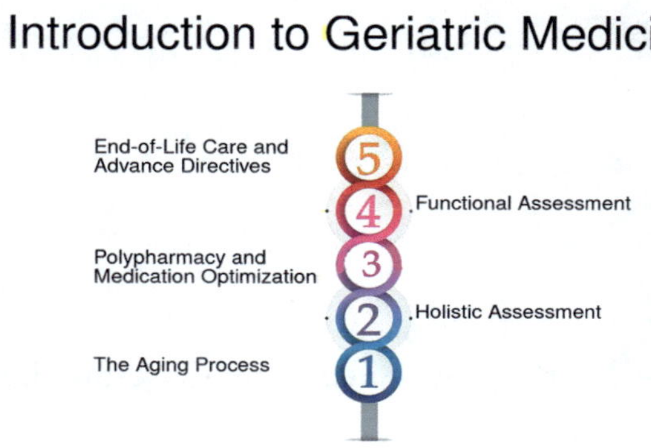

Figure 1.1. The specialty that addresses the health and aging of older adults.

Source: https://fastercapital.co/i/Geriatric-medicine--The-Specialty-that-Addresses-the-Health-and-Aging-of-Older-Adults--Introduction-to-Geriatric-Medicine.webp.

Importance of Specialized Care for Older Adults

With the growing population of the older generation, geriatric care becomes increasingly obvious. Older individuals have very characteristic health problems that require treatment using specialized interventions and approaches.

General practitioners, while competent in managing a variety of diseases, may lack geriatric-oriented knowledge concerning the care of the elderly. Such a need makes the existence of healthcare specialists educated specifically in the nuances of aging all the more vital. Specialized treatment has a tendency to address complex medical conditions, chronic diseases, and the psychosocial aspects that are part of elderly adults' health. By prioritizing geriatric medicine, we can improve outcomes in health and enhance the quality of life for the population, allowing them to receive all of the holistic treatment to which they are entitled. Considering the reality that specialized training has a direct impact on the quality of care provided, caregiver training models need to be created and refined.

Standardized training programs can be developed to equip caregivers with evidence-based practices specific to geriatric care. Educating them creates an educated workforce qualified to manage all aspects of care for older adults, from medical procedures to counseling. In particular, the implementation of curricula following paid in-home caregiver standards, as noted, would enhance professionalism and efficacy of in-home services (The Stern Center for Evidence-Based Policy, 2015). Through this specialized training, home caregivers would not only learn basic skills but also meet the increasing demand for quality care as the aging population continues to expand.

In addition, establishing a tiered educational route for geriatric home caregivers is a double-edged sword. It meets the increasing demands of older adults who require assistance with activities of daily living and, at the same time, constructs an adequate workforce in the private home care sector. By standardizing caregiver training and providing ongoing education, we can ensure caregivers are adequately trained to manage the complexity of geriatric care. This initiative will eventually translate into a more professional and compassionate approach to caregiving, addressing the complex needs of older adults while supporting caregivers' career advancement (Longhurst et al., 2015). By assigning particular training in geriatric medicine top priority, society enhances the quality of care for older people, elevating their dignity and well-being in the process (Figure 1.2).

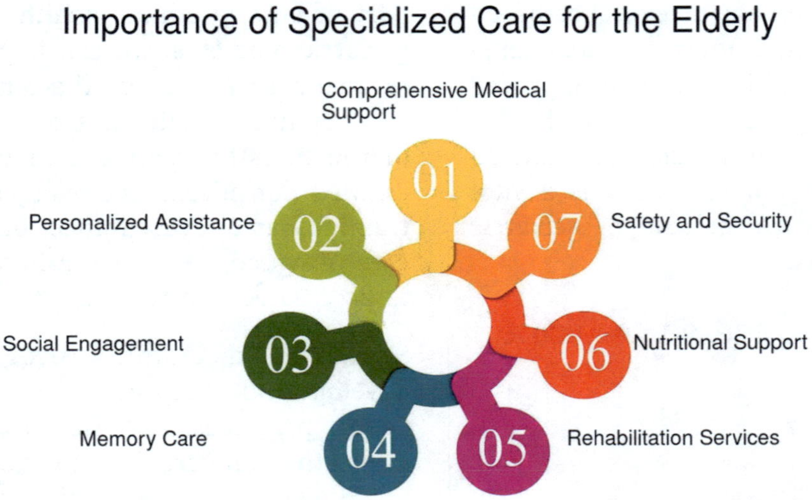

Figure 1.2. Importance of specialized care for the elderly.

Source: https://fastercapital.co/i/Geriatric-Care-Center--Importance-of-Specialized-Care-for-the-Elderly.webp.

Overview of the Aging Population and Its Implications

An aging population is a key demographic shift poised to reverberate throughout various segments of society, particularly in healthcare. With the advancement of medical science and technology, life expectancy has increased, and the proportion of older citizens in the population has been rising. According to estimates, the population of 65 and over will represent an ever-larger share of society by the year 2030, raising grave questions about whether healthcare systems currently in place will be able to meet their unique needs. This demographic change is not just about numbers; it means that healthcare workers need to change services so that they respond to a population whose health issues are complex, ranging from chronic disease and dementia to impaired cognition. Therefore, geriatric medicine will be a compulsory subject as well as a challenging frontier for health professionals to tackle the multifaceted issues of aged patients. Significantly, the impact of an aging population is not merely on healthcare delivery but also has economic and policy implications. An aging population means increased medical care needs that exert pressure on existing healthcare resources and infrastructure. Moreover, the increasing costs of aging population demand stringent policymaking. Experience has proven how strongly implementing evidence-based policy focusing on prevention and care coordination with a strong focus on older people's health outcomes can be effective. Patient self-management support and palliative care, for instance, must be enhanced in a bid to ease the healthcare burden at the expense of enhancing the quality of life among aging adults. The resulting imperative for strategic initiatives that foster interdisciplinary cooperation is vital to ensure the continued viability and effectiveness of geriatric medicine in an evolving healthcare landscape, as underscored in current literature. Addressing the specific demands of the elderly requires optimal comprehension and incorporation of comprehensive geriatric assessments (CGAs) into practice. These assessments inform individualized health profiles of older patients, more accurately predicting morbidity and mortality than traditional measures. They also target important domains, such as frailty, social support, and nutrition, as robust determinants of health outcomes. Despite their proven benefit, however, a minority of oncogeriatric patients are actually given this important evaluation before surgical interventions. In regard to bridging this gap, medical student training will be crucial, with a focus on equipping the best possible expertise to perform sufficient evaluations and exams within clinical settings. Building the geriatric cornerstone for future healthcare providers will further improve care provision as this population continues to increase and needs specialized facilities and resources, as stated by Lampugnane (2017) and The Stern Center for Evidence-Based Policy (2015).

1.1. Common Health Issues in the Elderly

Learning Outcome

1. Discuss chronic diseases prevalent in older adults;
2. Focus on mental health challenges, including dementia and depression;
3. Explain mobility and physical health concerns.

Because the population of elderly individuals is growing, it is important to recognize and act upon the most common health issues that they face. A main issue is the increase in the incidence of chronic diseases such as hypertension, diabetes, and arthritis. Such conditions not only risk the quality of life of the elderly but also lead to an increased demand for medical treatment. In particular, hypertension is typically asymptomatic but may cause severe complications, such as stroke and heart disease. Management of such long-term diseases requires careful vigilance over the quirky physiological changes that occur with aging. Consequently, clinical practitioners must adopt widespread strategies in the form of medication management, lifestyle modification, and continuous monitoring to ensure maximum benefit to aged patients in terms of health. The complexity in their treatment points to the need for geriatric medicine training and education in specialty care for healthcare professionals and the importance of individualized care plans. Cognitive impairment is also among the leading health issues of the elderly, with dementia and Alzheimer's being increasingly prevalent. These cognitive impairments not only affect the directly involved individuals but also place a big physical and emotional burden on family members and caregivers. Detection and early intervention are crucial in managing such conditions because they can enhance available cognitive functioning and retard disease onset. Geriatric assessments are essential in the diagnosis of cognitive disorders related to aging, but the application is affected by the shortness of time for use by healthcare professionals. As stated, the application of geriatric assessments based on relevant cognitive areas holds the promise of detecting risks and modifying interventions accordingly to enhance the quality of life of cognitively impaired elderly patients (Lampugnale, 2017). There are also several other complications that may occur among the elderly, such as mental illness like depression and anxiety. These have a tendency to go undiagnosed and untreated, but can significantly lower the quality of life and result in poor health. Geriatric medicine practitioners need to be vigilant for screening of mental health status because, unlike other populations, they may present differently and even masquerade or complicate physical health conditions. Mental health is not only pharmacologic but also includes psychosocial measures as well to encourage social interaction and support. Growing sensitivity to older people's psychological needs highlights the worth of an interdisciplinary model of care that integrates mental health into total health care planning (Mallia & Fiorini, 2003). Through favoring a system that allows for open conversation about mental concerns, health care practitioners are better able to deal with emotional and psychological issues of older people.

1.1.1. Chronic Diseases Prevalent in Older Adults

Chronic diseases are a common problem in geriatric medicine, particularly with the ageing population, and are responsible for increased disease incidence, such as hypertension, diabetes, and arthritis. The conditions have a negative impact on quality of life by causing functional impairment and increased health needs. For instance, hypertension is a common diagnosis in elderly individuals often with the additional presence of other chronic diseases. The management of hypertension is also rendered difficult by the presence of comorbid conditions, and close control of medicines is needed to prevent polypharmacy—a prevalent condition in this population. A review highlights that polypharmacy, particularly in cancer patients with advanced age, arises because of several reasons, including the management of adverse drug reactions (ADRs) and comorbid diseases (Shrestha et al., 2019).

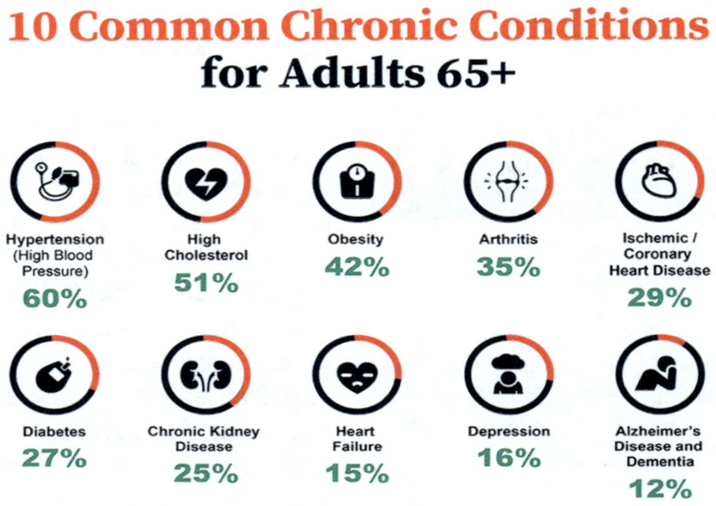

Figure 1.3. Ten common chronic conditions for adults above 65.

Source: https://assets-us-01.kc-usercontent.com/ffacfe7d-10b6-0083-2632-604077fd4eca/597cb13e-449a-4b4d-937e-8914d859640f/Ten_Common_Chronic_Conditions2.png.

It emphasizes the requirement for an integrated approach for managing the special challenges of chronic diseases with polypharmacy in the elderly. Diabetes mellitus is a chronic disease commonly found in elderly people that strongly influences their general health and well-being. It is connected with a number of complications such as cardiovascular disease, neuropathy, and retinopathy. The comorbidity of diabetes with other chronic conditions deteriorates health conditions in the elderly and places them on a downward spiral of health. In addition, the elderly are also likely to require treatment with personalized management protocols depending on their own drug response and nutritional requirements. Research indicates the variability in the control of hypertension, with African American older adults having higher rates of hypertension and being prescribed a greater number of anti-hypertensive medications but not achieving satisfactory blood pressure regulation (Allman et al., 2015). The findings underscore the importance of individualized healthcare interventions that consider race, gender, and comorbidities to effectively treat diabetes and its complications in older adults. Arthritis is another pervasive chronic condition of the old, and it also poses significant challenges to independence and mobility. Osteoarthritis and rheumatoid arthritis pain and stiffness cause impairment of function and activity and secondary conditions like obesity and depression. The interaction between arthritis and comorbidities generates a complex care situation in geriatrics that necessitates multidisciplinary care that focuses on pain management and facilitating physical function. Effective management principles must be applied to provide mobility and overall quality of life in older patients with arthritis. Clinicians also must be vigilant towards the risk of polypharmacy when treating such patients so that they do not expose them to unjustified medication that aggravates existing disease states. Care for chronic disease in the elderly, as a rule, must be complex and individualized to cover a variety of care components to achieve maximal health gain (Figure 1.3).

1.1.2. Mental Health Challenges, Including Dementia and Depression

With increasing age, various mental diseases face the elderly, with dementia and depression ranking as the two most important diseases in geriatric practice. Dementia or progressive decline of intellectual functioning in the elderly is an enormous challenge not only for the patients themselves but also for their caregivers. Caregiving burdens have been found to lead to increased stress, emotional strain, and even mental decline for carers, which calls for their needs to be addressed in a holistic way. It has been found through research that older carers, being typically underrepresented in studies and policy discussions, have specific stressors that overlay their own mental health concerns. By gaining an understanding of these dynamics, the healthcare professionals are better able to create more effective interventions involving both the older patient with dementia and their caregivers, highlighting the importance of developing strategies of resilience and coping techniques in this group (Henwood et al., 2017) (Figure 1.4).

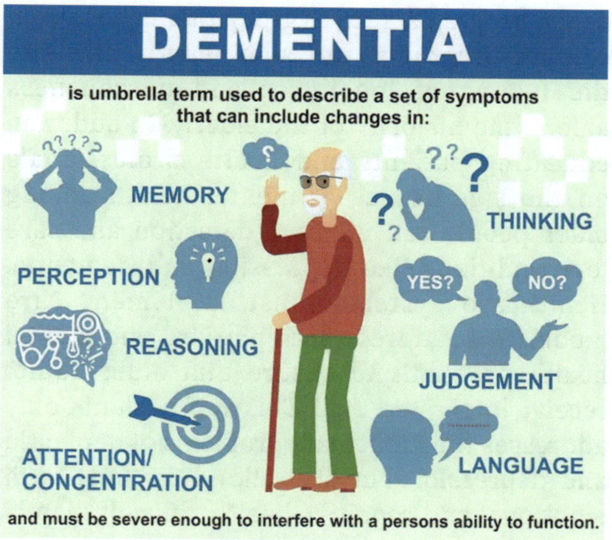

Figure 1.4. Dementia symptoms.

Source: https://www.careinsurance.com/upload_master/media/dementia-symptoms.webp.

Depression is also common in older adults, often found together with chronic physical illness and cognitive impairment, making clinical detection and treatment difficult. Of special concern is the interconnection between depression and dementia because depressive symptoms can aggravate cognitive functioning further, producing a cycle of worsening mental and physical health. The challenges lie in adequately screening for depressive disorders among older adults, especially those with cognitive impairment. The National Academy of Neuropsychology has identified routine cognitive testing and the early detection of mental illnesses in geriatrics, specifically the care of comorbidities (Perry et al., 2018). Beyond enhancing the quality of care, this multi-dimensional process enhances the overall health outcomes, validating the necessity for individualized screening tools that consider the affective and cognitive dimensions of the aging population. In addition, it is important to create a climate that facilitates mental well-being among the elderly, with a focus on preventive geriatric care. The incorporation of mental health programs, such as group therapy or social contact programs, can significantly alleviate the feeling of loneliness and nervousness among the majority of the elderly. In addition, educating patients and health professionals on the significance of mental health among older people can improve detection and care for conditions like depression and dementia. Healthcare systems must implement care models that address both physical and mental health problems to ensure that older adults receive integrated, PCC. This approach not only addresses the immediate problems of dementia and depression but also allows for long-term emotional and cognitive health, thus ultimately enhancing quality of life in older populations (Figure 1.5).

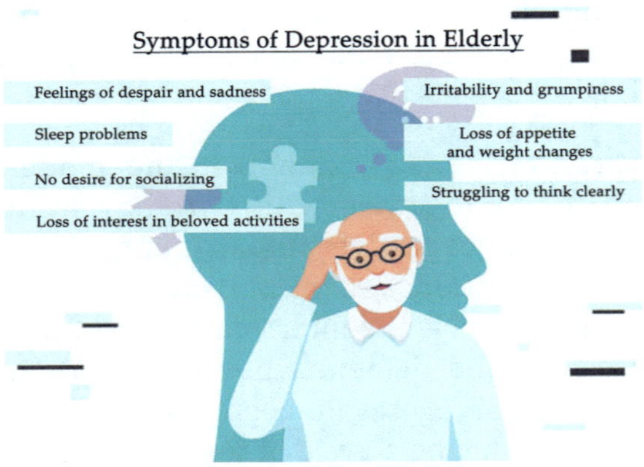

Figure 1.5. Symptoms of depression in the elderly.

Source: https://ezcareclinic.io/wp-content/uploads/2022/10/Depression-in-elderly-Symptoms-Causes-Treatment-support-image2.jpg.

1.1.3. Mobility and Physical Health Concerns

With such a growing scope of Geriatric Medicine, mobility and physical complaint-related matters still remain paramount in managing the elderly population efficiently. Elderly individuals are normally plagued with a range of mobility problems that arise from musculoskeletal and neurological illnesses, apart from general frailty. Such illnesses have tremendous repercussions on their ability to perform simple activities of daily living, thereby affecting their quality of life as a whole. Research verifies that mobility has to be maintained, since this plays an essential role in independence and well-being. A properly entrenched medical school curriculum with comprehensive geriatric training will equip future healthcare providers with the suitable expertise to mitigate these mobility impairments. Interventions like those at Dalhousie University emphasize the importance of valuing the particular needs of older patients, and there is the potential for a reduction in mobility-related illness in this age range (Mallery et al., 2003). Along with considerations for mobility, physical health among older individuals also includes assessment of multimorbidity, social support, and diet. CGAs are key to an understanding of the multi-determined nature of these determinants. Research emphasizes the need to integrate geriatric assessments, especially in treating conditions such as cancer, which disproportionately impact older patients. Although they are acknowledged as important, most health professionals find it difficult to integrate these assessments into their workload because of time pressures and workload demands. Hence, education programs for geriatric assessment can bring more clarity to optimizing physical health so that geriatric patients receive proper intervention that is targeted to their mobility and health-related issues (Lampugnane, 2017). Lastly, finding answers to mobility in elderly people involves not only medical interventions but also community-based interventions aimed at optimizing mobility in the activities of daily living. Interventions for promoting exercise, balance, and social interaction can prove to be of tremendous benefit when developed through interprofessional education programs. For instance, coordination among geriatricians, physical therapists, and occupational therapists can help create a multidimensional support system for older adults. Multidisciplinary approaches are likely to have improved mobility outcomes with therapeutically focused interventions of a specialized nature in order to optimize musculoskeletal strength and global physical functioning. As frailty and concomitant mobility issues rise further in elderly populations, health education and community mobilization efforts will have to be coordinated if they are to address the pressing imperatives of geriatric medicine (Mallery et al., 2003; Lampugnale, 2017) (Figure 1.6).

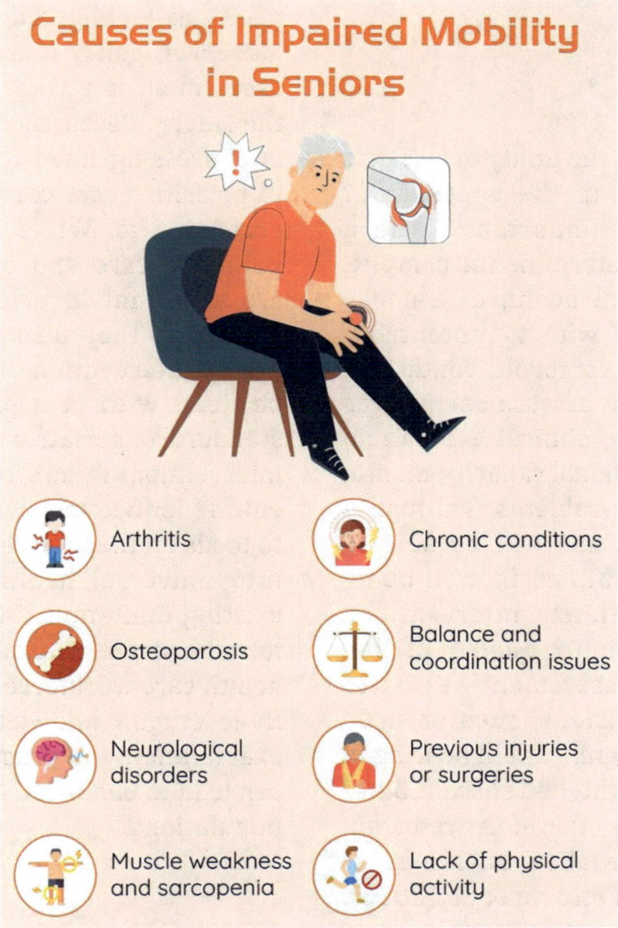

Figure 1.6. Causes of impaired mobility in seniors.

Source: https://ghost-cms.s3.ap-south-1.amazonaws.com/2025/03/Causes-of-Impaired-Mobility-in-Seniors_the-wellness-corner.jpg.

Test Your Knowledge

1. What are the most common chronic diseases affecting older adults?
2. How can early detection of dementia and other cognitive disorders improve the management and care of elderly individual?
3. What are the primary risk factors for depression in older adults?

1.2. Geriatric Assessment

Learning Outcome

1. Understand the comprehensive geriatric assessment process;
2. Describe tools and methods used in assessment;
3. Explain the importance of individualized care plans.

With an ageing population, the utility of geriatric assessment is enhanced in the specialty of geriatric medicine. It is important to do a complete assessment to determine the complex care and multidimensional health care needs of the older individual, who is potentially presenting with multiple comorbid conditions and complex care needs. The assessment involves extensive medical history, clinical evaluation, and evaluation of the functional capacity, mental status, and psychosocial problems. Through a systemic approach, clinicians will be able to identify even slight alterations in well-being and health, facilitating timely interventions that optimize older patients' quality of life. Furthermore, geriatric assessment serves to guide the treatment decisions, such as drug management, which are significant in bearing in mind the older adults' heightened susceptibility to ADRs and interactions, therefore reducing the likelihood of the negative outcomes of inapt prescribing, as per Petrovic et al. (2016). Implementation of geriatric assessment tools and strategies can significantly help improve patient outcomes. Assessment tools for medications, for instance, play a crucial role in minimizing the risks of polypharmacy that are normally associated with older adults. Implicit and explicit principles of inappropriate prescribing direct professionals in managing the challenges of personalized treatment, taking care of dosing, compliance, and potential drug-drug interactions. Interdisciplinary collaboration between health care professionals is also critical in implementing these strategies. Through cooperation between doctors, pharmacists, and nurses, geriatric assessments can be undertaken more widely and thoroughly. This not only allows the process of pharmaceutical care but also is in keeping with the general philosophies of geriatric practice, which are centered around holistic care tailored to each geriatric patient's individualized needs, as highlighted by Petrovic et al. (2016). Moreover, policy reasoning regarding geriatric assessment is pivotal in advancing the care of the elderly. Research evidence reveals that there is a pressing need for evidence-based policy to prioritize care coordination and prevention, according to. While a few domains, such as palliative care and patient self-management, are abundant in evidence to prioritize their centrality, they also reveal a gigantic gap in policy intervention. These inequities need to be dealt with at a priority level in order to standardize geriatric assessment and resultant interventions in care, but make it accessible to all elderly individuals. Future initiatives will need to focus on the integration of these assessments into universal health care systems, beyond existing limitations, while also bringing to the fore the pivotal role of family caregivers and the health care workforce in providing quality care. By leveraging knowledge gained from geriatric examination, the practice of geriatric medicine can lead to enhanced health outcomes for older populations.

1.2.1. Comprehensive Geriatric Assessment (CGA) Process

The comprehensive geriatric assessment (CGA) process is a multi-dimensional, inter-disciplinary assessment instrument whose aim is to evaluate the medical, psychological, and functional capacity of elderly persons. This multi-faceted approach is more extensive than routine medical assessments since it taps more than one domain, such as cognitive function, physical status, social context, and mood. The utility of this assessment is particularly evident when applied to the treatment of complicated health states, when one condition will necessarily have concomitant comorbidities. Of specific interest, in oncogeriatric patients, the worldwide application of this assessment can help tailor treatment regimens that deal with both cancer-related concerns and the geriatric patients' medical status in general (Lampugnale, 2017). By clearly defining risk and enhancing interprofessional collaboration among healthcare professionals, CGAs enhance clinical decision-making, ensuring that certain older adults' evolving needs are tackled in an optimal way. Despite the clear benefits of the CGA process, its deployment continues to be bedeviled by barriers to out-and-out adoption. Time constraints in healthcare environments are an overarching obstacle, with healthcare professionals frequently being unable to fit thorough assessments into their busy schedules. Indeed, studies have shown that numerous oncogeriatric patients undergo insufficient assessments, even when they are recognized by healthcare workers (Lampugnale, 2017). In addition, staff training and familiarity with the areas of assessment could make implementation even more challenging. Interventions in education among medical students and professionals are thus called for to mitigate such challenges. This education would highlight the most predictive areas of measurement for postoperative complications, equipping future clinicians with the competencies necessary to perform effective geriatric assessments and ultimately leading to improved patient outcomes. Findings based on CGAs can not only be useful in the treatment of individual patients but also in shaping healthcare policies in the elderly. The need for preventive interventions and care coordination has been emphasized again and again through research, particularly against the backdrop of future population dynamics in the aging population. The healthcare systems can better contribute towards improved health outcomes in older adults through a coordinated integration of assessment findings and evidence-based policies. By stimulating an interprofessional setting involving the family caregivers and patient self-management, CGAs will be in a position to make meaningful impacts beyond clinical settings. As populations grow old, it is critical that the medical community recognizes the potential of comprehensive assessments to inform policy, enhance service delivery, and ultimately improve the quality of care provided to our aging population (Figure 1.7).

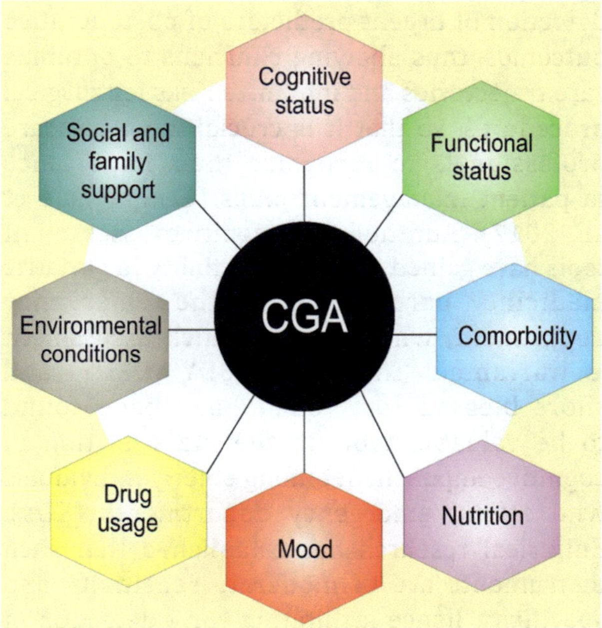

Figure 1.7. Comprehensive geriatric assessment (CGA): An organized evaluation method to provide a multidisciplinary assessment of and care for the elderly.

Source: https://www.researchgate.net/publication/346542805/figure/fig2/AS:11431281211610800@1702468437731/Comprehensive-geriatric-assessment-CGA-is-an-organized-evaluation-method-to-provide-a.tif.

1.2.2. Tools and Methods Used in Assessment

Geriatric patient evaluation demands specialized equipment and protocols specific to addressing the complexities of aging. Central to this evaluation is the CGA, encompassing physical status, mental status, social circumstances, and functional ability. This holistic approach not only facilitates individually directed treatment of patients but also optimizes the validity of treatment plans by analyzing each patient's individual circumstance in depth. For instance, for oncogeriatrics, a thorough pre-surgical geriatric assessment turns into a necessity to tailor surgical procedures to the personal needs and desires of the older patients. It aids in the detection of urgent predictors of postoperative outcomes, thus allowing clinicians to optimize care trajectories and minimize risks for surgical procedures, so that it is crucial for healthcare professionals to recognize their importance in patient management plans (Lampugnale et al., 2017). Additionally, cognitive assessment tools have gained increased visibility in geriatric medicine, particularly in the emergency department, where such a quick assessment is warranted. The Ottawa 3DY (O3DY) and short blessed test (SBT) have been found to be valuable tools in the identification of cognitive impairment among elderly individuals who attend emergency departments (EDs). Empirical research has established that such instruments are of moderate sensitivity and specificity, hence facilitating early detection of cognitive impairment that significantly impacts patient management and outcome. By using such standardized assessment tools, clinicians can more effectively triage interventions among elderly patients, therefore improving the quality of care. Further, being aware of the inter-rater reliability of such tests is crucial since consistent application by clinicians can ensure reproducible and stable findings in cognitive screening (Barbic et al., 2018). Besides cognitive and comprehensive tests, there are many other methods utilized to effectively evaluate geriatric patients. These are functional assessments, such as the ability of older adults to perform activities of daily living, and tools like the Frailty Index or the Geriatric Depression Scale, which are meant to assess physiological and psychological domains relevant to care of the elderly. The use of these varied evaluation tools is an effort to address the multicategory nature of aging so that clinicians can provide comprehensive, patient-centered care. Evidently, the integration of these diverse assessment instruments enhances the general level of comprehension of the unique requirements of individual geriatric patients and facilitates improved clinical decision-making. Eventually, geriatric medicine depends on the effective use of assessment tools to enhance health outcomes and the quality of life for older adults as they confront the vicissitudes of aging (Lampugnale, 2017) (Figure 1.8).

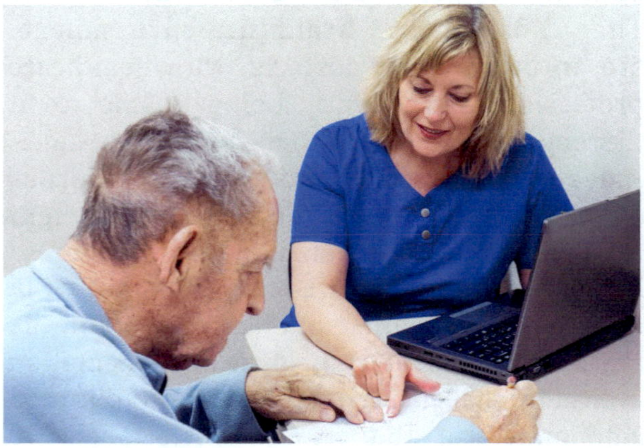

Figure 1.8. Cognitive assessment for seniors.

Source: https://floridaseniorconsulting.com/wp-content/uploads/2024/10/cognitive-assessment-for-seniors-1.jpg.

1.2.3. Importance of Individualized Care Plans

In the specialty of geriatric medicine, specific care plans cannot be bypassed. As older people have their own specific physical, emotional, and cognitive problems, such specific plans play a vital role in addressing their respective needs. Individualized care plans aid in general planning, which allows medical personnel to consider various aspects such as the individual's medical history, personal choices, and social status. This tailored approach enhances patient satisfaction and engagement, as elderly patients are more respected and understood within their care environment. Moreover, it enhances better inter-professional team coordination, ultimately leading to healthier results and improved quality of life among the elderly (Figure 1.9).

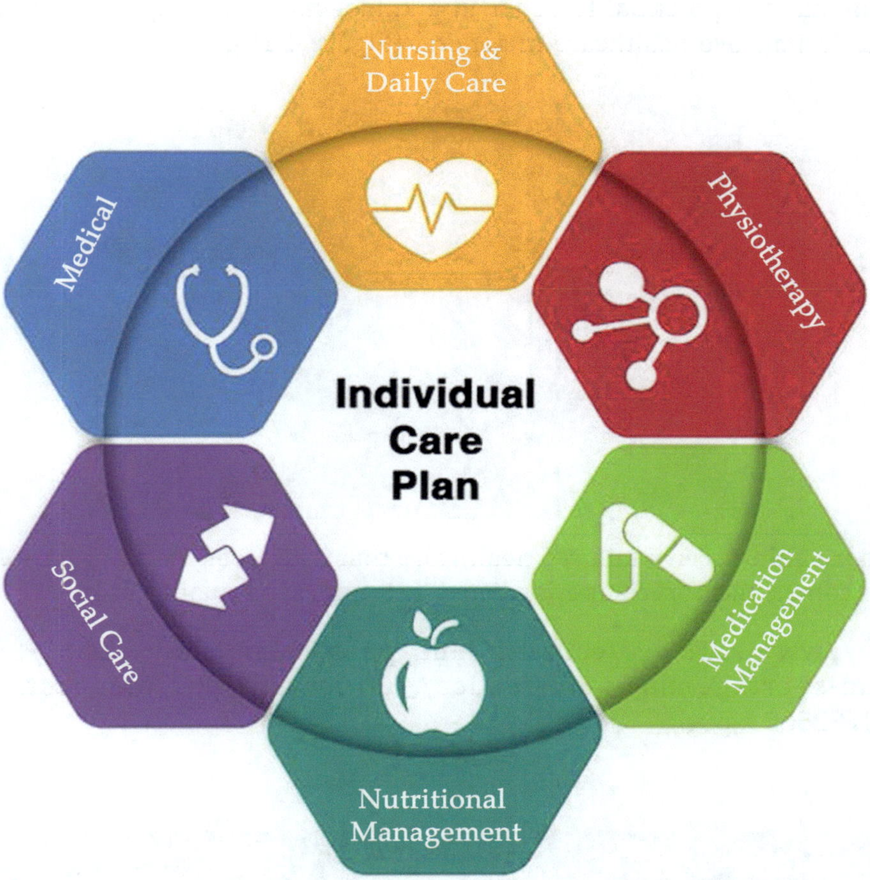

Figure 1.9. Individualized care plan.

Source: https://www.pinecaregroup.com/wp-content/uploads/2019/04/Individualized-Care-Plan.jpg.

Individualized care plans are also a key framework for promoting resident-focused care within institutional environments. In nursing homes, for instance, the implementation of tailored approaches can significantly alter the dynamics of resident interactions and care delivery. As suggested by research of a 2008 interdisciplinary panel, the barriers to the effective application of individualized care often stem from insufficient nurse engagement in culture change efforts and deficient training in resident-oriented care (Kantor et al., 2009). By prioritizing individualized plans, healthcare organizations are able to confront these shortcomings systematically and provide nurses and caregivers with the expertise needed for a more patient-focused setting for older residents. Such initiatives not only align with best geriatric practice but also aim to create a culture shift in support of highlighting the unique needs of each resident. The impact of individualized care plans extends throughout the facilities, as demonstrated in pilot initiatives encouraging resident-centered care through regulatory surveys. These examples illustrate the potential benefit of coordinating care practice with compliance, both in terms of the quality of care delivered and the residents' experience (David et al., 2010). These types of initiatives promote a positive orientation, where the emphasis is on identifying and meeting individualized requirements and not merely conforming to standard processes. Through highlighting the value of patient-specific methods in the spectrum of care, geriatric medicine has the potential to usher in a kinder model in respect to the individuality of older groups and to improve healthcare in general (Figure 1.10).

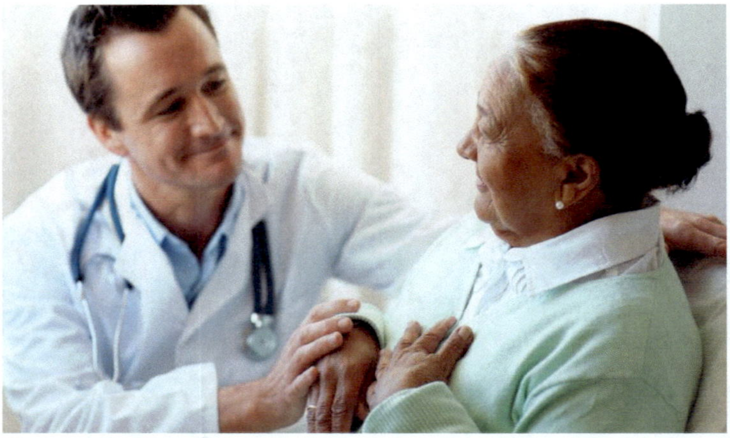

Figure 1.10. Older adults receive tailored healthcare that addresses their unique needs, promoting better health outcomes, increased independence, and improved quality of life.

Source: https://www.rand.org/content/rand/pubs/commentary/2012/08/addressing-the-geriatrician-shortage-may-help-reduce/_jcr_content/par/blogpost.crop.888x522.cm.jpeg/1720736825659.jpeg.

Test Your Knowledge

1. What is the role of a comprehensive geriatric assessment (CGA) in evaluating the overall health of older adults?
2. Why is it critical to develop individualized care plans based on the results of a geriatric assessment?

1.3. Pharmacological Considerations

Learning Outcome

1. Discuss the phenomenon of polypharmacy the realm of geriatric medicine;
2. Understand age-related changes in drug metabolism;
3. Focus on strategies for safe medication management.

In the field of geriatric medicine, drug factors are most relevant due to the multifactorial interaction between aging, multiple comorbidities, and polypharmacy. Pharmacokinetic and pharmacodynamic changes are typical in geriatric patients that influence drug efficacy and safety profile. These changes may include decreased kidney and liver function, alteration in body composition, and variation in receptor sensitivity with an increase in potential vulnerability to ADRs (Petrovic et al., 2012). Thus, clinicians must take extra caution when dealing with the medication of older patients, ensuring that dosing regimens are optimized to meet the specific needs of these patients. Clinical tools such as the Beers Criteria and the STOPP/START criteria can be used by clinicians in identifying potentially inappropriate drugs and therapeutic regimen optimization for the ultimate purpose of enhancing patient safety (PS) and quality of care. The prevalence of ADRs in elderly patients is high, making it paramount for cautious monitoring and assessment of medication dosing regimens. The use of the GerontoNet ADR Risk Score, one of the primary prevention methods for ADRs, is instrumental in enabling doctors to recognize high-risk patients (Petrovic et al., 2012). Identification of such high-risk patients enables caregivers to implement targeted interventions aimed at reducing medication-related complications. These preventive practices can include rigorous review of medications, alterations in prescribed regimens, and augmented patient education regarding the importance of adherence and ADR identification. Furthermore, interdisciplinary teamwork, especially involving clinical pharmacists, is crucial in the facilitation of medication safety since they bring specialist expertise into drug-related assessment and management of geriatric patients' needs. In addition to the individual-level interventions, systemic measures on prescribing practices also reduce negative outcomes in older people. Systems of care in healthcare require robust communication pathways between PCPs and specialists to provide care continuity and due adjustment of medicines as the patient transitions from one healthcare setting to another. CGAs are types of programs that can provide an overall view of the health status of an older patient, revealing nuances that must be handled meticulously with drug therapy (Petrovic et al., 2012). Moreover, electronic prescribing systems can enhance safety by real-time flagging of likely drug interactions and contraindications. Encouraging a culture of safety and prudence in prescribing practice not only improves the quality of prescribed medication but is also critical to achieving enhanced health outcomes among older people in the community and in clinical practice.

1.3.1. Polypharmacy and Its Risks

Polypharmacy, or the concurrent prescription of numerous drugs, is a prominent issue in the specialty of geriatric medicine. It is ubiquitous in older populations, especially those with comorbid conditions, and most often rationalized by the treatment of the complexity of multiple health issues. The consequences of polypharmacy are profound and complex. Elderly patients tend to develop ADRs, drug-drug interactions, and increased hospitalization rates, which in turn complicate their health. These complications decrease the overall quality of life, thus presenting a vicious cycle of medical therapy that could potentially aggravate their condition.

Hence, healthcare professionals should take note of the impact of polypharmacy and seek possible mitigants since they play an integral role in maximizing the outcome of therapy in the elderly population. In addition, recent literature has noted the intricate interaction between polypharmacy and geriatric oncology, with the result that elderly cancer patients have a higher risk of adverse drug outcomes. Polypharmacy in such patients generally occurs as a result of treatment for cancer, comorbidity, and side effects of chemotherapy. While clinical pharmacists by default play a pivotal role in resolving such issues in developed health care systems by tradition, their role is short of expectation in the majority of resource-poor contexts. A harmoniously coordinated plan using the services of pharmacists can be absolutely pivotal in determining and managing the risk of polypharmacy in elderly cancer patients. Such an intervention is even more necessary, keeping in mind that many existing studies lack the comprehensive approach to polypharmacy as a predictor for bad outcomes in geriatric oncology, reflecting on a lack in the existing clinical model (Shrestha et al., 2019). The need for standardized approaches to the assessment and control of polypharmacy becomes increasingly evident for geriatric therapy. Well-established medication review practices must be employed since variations in definition and measurement instruments can potentially lead to non-uniform estimations of polypharmacy's impact. At the center of this conflict is the deprescribing process, which aims to decrease medications with greater drawbacks than benefits. Although numerous processes exist for identifying candidates for deprescribing, their evaluation within the geriatric oncology patient population remains limited. By developing open protocols for medication reviews, healthcare professionals are able to tackle issues of polypharmacy more effectively as a matter of urgency while simultaneously improving the overall health of the elderly. In general, the use of standardized interventions will be critical in addressing polypharmacy by ensuring elderly patients have access to the safest and most effective therapeutic regimens possible (Sharma et al., 2016) (Figure 1.11).

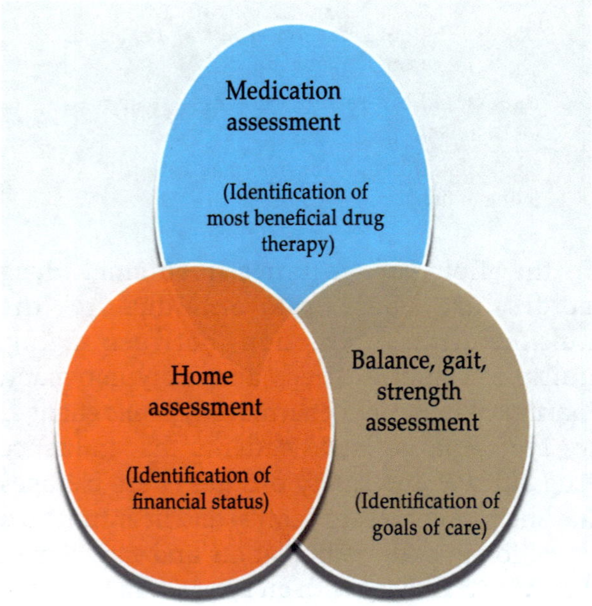

Figure 1.11. Management plans for polypharmacy.

Source: https://www.mdpi.com/geriatrics/geriatrics-07-00097/article_deploy/html/images/geriatrics-07-00097-g003.png.

1.3.2. Age-Related Changes in Drug Metabolism

As one grows older, there are tremendous physiological alterations that have tremendous effects on the pharmacokinetics of drugs, with unique challenges to geriatric practice. Drug pharmacokinetics—absorption, distribution, metabolism, and excretion—will generally be altered in older people because of decreased liver and renal function, body composition changes, and variation in enzymatic activity. This diminished organ function leads to decreased drug clearance rates, which can result in prolonged drug action and increased risk for ADRs. Notably, elderly individuals tend to have multiple drugs, particularly for the management of chronic illnesses, and therefore an increased risk of drug-drug interactions and reduced therapeutic outcomes. It is extremely crucial to understand these changes following aging to tailor drug therapy for minimizing risks and maximizing therapeutic benefit in this high-risk group. The practice of polypharmacy—defined as the simultaneous use of several drugs—magnifies drug metabolism problems in geriatric patients. This often occurs, particularly with patient groups experiencing complex health conditions, such as those with cancer and comorbidities. With such patients, polypharmacy can result from additive cancer treatment effects, toxicities of anti-neoplastic agents, and medications for comorbidities. The interrelated character of these treatments requires careful monitoring in order to avoid possible drug interactions that can further complicate patients' care. A major concern occurs when the implications of polypharmacy among older adults are neglected by healthcare providers, which commonly results in the misuse of drug regimens. Shrestha et al. (2019) emphasize the most important task of clinical pharmacists in rectifying polypharmacy issues through reviewing prescriptions and making personalized recommendations according to the unique needs of patients. As a solution to counteract the dangers of drug metabolism impairment in older populations, healthcare systems must ensure priority for the CGAs. CGAs permit an exhaustive review of the clinical condition of an elderly patient, in which some pharmacological requirements are recognized while remaining cognizant of their unique physiological alterations. This combined methodology can ensure better medication management through focus on drug therapy optimization and prevention of ADRs. Secondly, enhancing the education and training of healthcare professionals in the field of geriatric pharmacology will help increase sensitivity to the complex process of drug metabolism in elderly individuals. Effective strategies, such as the implementation of electronic health records (EHRs) that warn of possible pharmacological interactions and collaboration among multidisciplinary teams, can lead to safer prescribing behaviors and fewer ADR events. As Petrovic et al. (2012) posit, such interventions are essential for ensuring that the elderly receive effective, safe, and individualized pharmacotherapy based on their evolving health status (Figure 1.12).

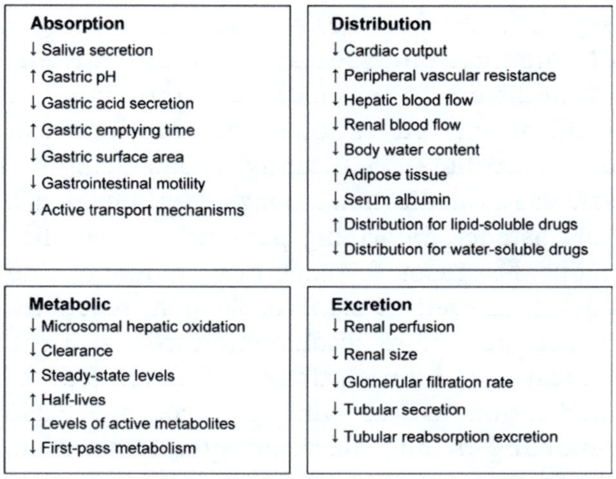

Figure 1.12. Age-related changes in pharmacokinetics.

Source: https://www.researchgate.net/publication/304356937/figure/fig2/AS:11431281256254099@1719513501683/Age-related-changes-in-pharmacokinetics.jpg.

1.3.3. Strategies for Safe Medication Management

Best medication management in geriatric care is necessary since the drug needs of geriatric patients are complex. The patient becomes susceptible to polypharmacy with advancing age, which exposes them to drug interactions and ADRs. One easy approach is to implement extensive medication reviews, where the treatment team goes through all the drugs prescribed and evaluates their appropriateness and redundancies. Such reviews can help identify unnecessary medications, which would enable providers to streamline treatments and adapt treatment plans to the individual patient's requirements. In addition, ensuring open communication between healthcare teams of physicians, nurses, and pharmacists can ensure a unified approach towards medication management. When all concerned are informed of a patient's medication regimen, the risk of errors reduces, and improved overall patient outcomes ensue, particularly in those who are experiencing frail health and are in danger of medication-associated complications. In addition to meticulous monitoring of medications, educational interventions can also contribute significantly to enhancing the safe use of medication among older individuals. For instance, informing patients and families about the reason for each drug, potential side effects, as well as signs of adverse reactions, makes them more accountable care providers. Educational interventions can deter fear of medication use as well as encourage early reporting of any alarming symptoms. Also, the integration of pharmacists in the learning process can be particularly helpful as they will have up-to-date information about drug-to-drug interactions and patient-specific outcomes, especially with complex medication regimens. By integrating pharmacists within the multidisciplinary team, healthcare professionals can employ their expertise to create more effective and safer medication regimens that target geriatric patients specifically, thereby addressing challenges posed by polypharmacy and improving overall quality of care (Shrestha et al., 2019). Another effective strategy for safe drug management is the application of protocols to support continuous monitoring of drug safety and effectiveness. They can be in the form of continuous follow-up, technology utilization such as EHRs and prescription monitoring systems. Geriatric fracture programs have been noted to have positive outcomes in pain management of fragility fractures, demonstrating the role of protocols in improving pain management and potentially decreasing opioid dependency. Here, multidisciplinary care integrated with diversified pain management techniques, like acetaminophen and fascia iliaca compartment blocks, can further be used to promote patient comfort and reduce opioid usage. By utilizing such multifaceted systems, healthcare professionals can categorically assess and modify medication in a way that limits side effects, all the while targeting the specific medical requirements of the geriatric patient population (Casey et al., 2017) (Figure 1.13).

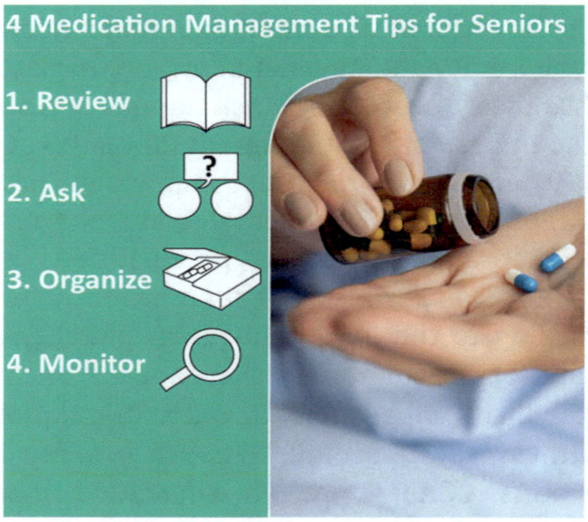

Figure 1.13. Medication management tips for seniors.

Source: https://littlenursinghome.com/wp-content/uploads/2021/03/may-blog.jpg.

Test Your Knowledge

1. What are the primary risks associated with polypharmacy in older adults?
2. How do age-related physiological changes (e.g., alterations in liver and kidney function) affect the pharmacokinetics of medications in elderly individuals?
3. What are some best practices for ensuring safe medication management in geriatric patients?

1.4. Non-Pharmacological Interventions

Learning Outcome

1. Explain the role of physical therapy and rehabilitation in geriatric medicine;
2. Understand the importance of nutrition and dietary management;
3. Discuss how engagement in social activities influences the mental health of older adults.

The growing emphasis on non-pharmacological interventions in geriatric medicine highlights their significance for maximizing the care of the elderly. There has traditionally been a conventional overreliance on pharmacological interventions that are oblivious to other methods that could address the complex needs of this age group effectively. Non-pharmacological interventions involve different strategies like CBT, complementary therapies, and educational interventions for maximizing patient outcomes. A systematic review has shown that these interventions are very effective in addressing chronic pain among older adults, giving strategies that restrict the use of drugs, which are associated with the risks of dependence or toxic side effects. The literature review indicates that even though pharmacological approaches are superior, there is sufficient evidence to suggest that these other approaches are worth studying and their integration into regular clinical practice (Schofield & Reid, 2006). Apart from pain management, non-pharmacological approaches have been found to assist patients suffering from dementia, as far as their behavioral and psychological symptoms are concerned. Systematic review of randomized controlled trials has demonstrated that person-centered interventions such as family carer training and psychological counseling can significantly impact the outcomes for community-dwelling people with dementia. Not only do such interventions empower carers, but they also improve the quality of life for older people with troublesome symptoms. The effectiveness of such non-medicinal interventions highlights the need for health practitioners to mutually develop techniques that react to the individualized triggers of signs in addition to creating an empowering environment. Integrating these interventions not only optimizes care plans but also decodes the burden on families and health systems, demonstrating their invaluable place in geriatric medicine (Braun et al., 2018). Moreover, implementation of non-pharmacologic interventions involves a modification of professional culture in geriatric care. As a rule, professional training of healthcare workers tends to be focused on pharmacologic therapies, without taking into account the exploration of other methods. However, evidence shows that non-pharmacologic interventions encourage serious reconsideration of clinical training and interprofessional practice. For instance, nurses and occupational therapists can potentially play a leading role in discussing these interventions, but there is poor integrated communication of the complexity of behavioral and psychological symptoms among professionals. To close this gap in knowledge, further research must elucidate the most effective aspects of complex non-pharmacologic interventions so that practicing healthcare professionals get the information and resources they need to implement these strategies (Schofield & Reid, 2006; Braun et al., 2018).

1.4.1. Role of Physical Therapy and Rehabilitation

The role of physical rehabilitation and therapy in geriatric medicine is multifaceted and essential to enhancing the quality of life in the elderly. As individuals age, they are more likely to suffer from decreased physical function, which diminishes their ability to perform tasks of daily living independently. Physical therapy not only restores patients to mobility but also enhances strength, balance, and overall physical health.

This proactive rehabilitation fosters an active lifestyle, preventing comorbidities that are commonly associated with aging. Facilitating improvement over physical disabilities and fostering resilience, rehabilitative programs can significantly improve patients' physical and psychological condition, enabling them to exert greater control over their lives. Such a need emphasizes the pivotal position physical therapists hold on the multidisciplinary team treating geriatric patients. Despite the perceived benefits of rehabilitation, obstacles exist to delivering effective physical therapy to the elderly. Research on the experiences of the elderly indicated that effective communication between health workers and the elderly is important, as time pressures typically deter effective contact between the elderly and health workers (Atwal et al., 2007). This communication breakdown can lead to unmet rehabilitation needs as well as a lack of information regarding the roles of various allied health practitioners who are treating them. With the changing face of healthcare towards more patient-centered practices, it is important that these gaps be filled by making available the right information regarding the rehabilitation process to older patients. By open communication, health care providers would be able to better individualize interventions in response to the specific needs of older patients in such a way that total rehabilitation effectiveness is enhanced. Furthermore, integration of the services of rehabilitation into geriatric medicine should be prioritized so that there is no regression to random residual care, which has been lamented in previous nursing practice (Nolan et al., 1997). As has been shown through the study of the past, the possibility of nursing and rehabilitation careers cannot be defined by acute settings but must extend to ongoing care for seniors recovering in the home. Expansion of the presence of physical therapy in LTC models can counteract powerlessness among patients and caregivers as well. Continuing education and training of health professionals, as well as further fostering interdisciplinary collaboration, can serve to ensure that rehabilitation services remain integral to geriatric practice. As we are able to promote this awareness of the possibility for physical therapy to reconceptualize the lives of older persons through an integrated whole-person paradigm, we can produce an environment conducive to healing, as well as dignity and meaning in aging (Figure 1.14).

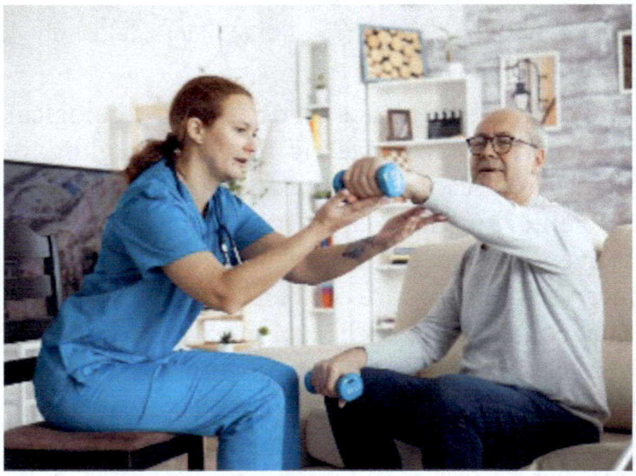

Figure 1.14. Physiotherapist for elderly care.

Source: https://fastrelief.zandupainrelief.com/wp-content/uploads/2023/02/Role-of-Physiotherapy-in-Geriatrics-1.jpg.

1.4.2. Importance of Nutrition and Dietary Management

The role of nutrition in the practice of the elderly cannot be stressed too much, as dietary habits play an important part in the overall health and well-being of the aged. As body age progresses, alterations in physiology require reassessment of nutritional needs, with particular reference to the intake of macronutrients and micronutrients. For instance, older persons have decreased appetite and changed metabolism, which can predispose them to malnutrition and its complications. Therefore, individualized nutritional management is now essential to attain and maintain a maximum state of health without contracting chronic diseases. Given the knowledge of the interconnection between nutrition and health, healthcare policies are now directed more toward integrating evidence-based nutritional principles within models of geriatric care (The Stern Center for Evidence-Based Policy, 2015). Hence, an effective nutritional management plan is a part of the integral practice of comprehensive geriatric medicine. In addition to providing appropriate nutrient consumption, nutrition management in the elderly is intended to avoid conditions that are age-related. The studies highlight the use of some nutrients, such as omega-3 fatty acids, vitamins, and minerals, to counterbalance the effects of conditions like osteoporosis and dementia.

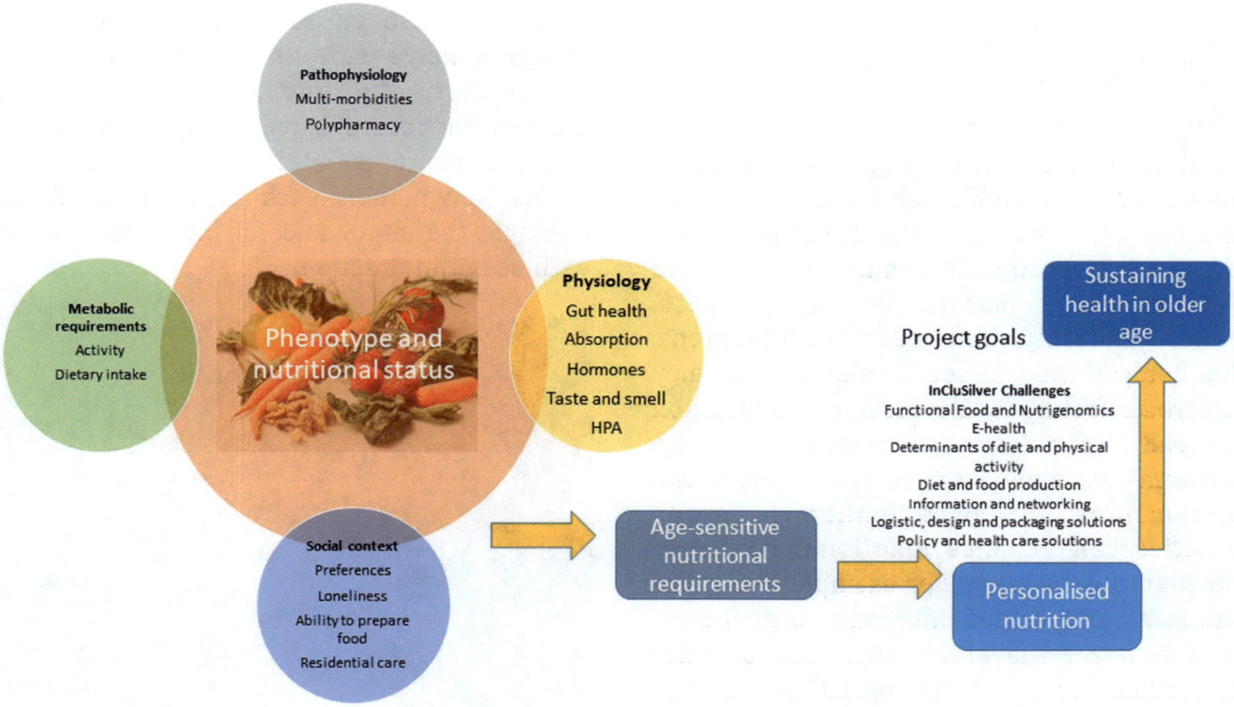

Figure 1.15. Prevalent influences on nutritional requirements in older adults [HPA: hypothalamic-pituitary axis].

Source: https://www.researchgate.net/publication/328520394/figure/fig1/AS:685787700015104@1540515937698/Prevalent-influences-on-nutritional-requirements-in-older-adults-HPA.png.

By promoting fruit, vegetable, and whole-grain eating habits, health professionals are able to promote physical, as well as mental, well-being in older persons. Community-oriented nutrition interventions such as meal schemes and nutrition education have also been found to be useful for reaching older individuals who may be disabled from healthy eating. The initiation of such community initiatives is an indicator of the growing recognition of nutrition's central role in geriatric care (Madeira et al., 2016). In addition, management by diet is not merely what elderly people eat, but understanding one's own values and preferences. Proper care of the elderly involves individualized nutrition approaches that honor cultural roots and individual tastes, encouraging improved adherence to dietary recommendations. An approach that is centered on the individual encourages motivation among the elderly to develop healthy diets. Additionally, involving family caregivers in the nutritional counseling process has been effective in encouraging dietary modifications. As the literature shows, policies that support the facilitation of caregiver support can also help improve the impact of nutrition in enhancing geriatric health (The Stern Center for Evidence-Based Policy, 2015). In conclusion, an understanding of the intricate relationship between nutrition and health is pivotal to optimizing the care of the elderly, highlighting the importance of integrated dietary management in geriatric medicine (Figure 1.15).

1.4.3. Social Engagement and Mental Stimulation

Social engagement has a significant effect on the mental health of older adults, especially on those who have cognitive impairment. As a person ages, social contact may be diminished by a series of factors, including illness, reduced mobility, and loss of companions. This deterioration in social relationships may exacerbate feelings of depression and isolation and lead to a reduction in overall well-being. Research has demonstrated that close social relationships and participation in group activities can enhance emotional resilience and cognitive function. For example, programs with community-based interventions have been found to harvest favorable outcomes for older individuals through fostering companionship and creating a mutually supportive environment.

The two-way nature of social engagement embraces emotional support and cognitive stimulation, which play an important role in maintaining quality of life among seniors. Furthermore, mental stimulation by formal activity forms the cognitive well-being among the elderly. Engaging in mentally stimulating tasks such as puzzle exercises, reading, or even discussion groups can prove useful in maintaining cognitive abilities and even slowing down dementia symptom progression.

Specifically, cognitive stimulation has been known to have long-term psychological impacts, particularly when coupled with effective caregiver training. Livingston et al. (2005) prove that interventions such as cognitive stimulation and behavioral management not only enhance acute cognitive engagement but also improve understanding and management of neuropsychiatric manifestations of dementia patients. These activities provide an opportunity for older individuals to challenge their cognitive abilities while enhancing social interactions. Thus, they are an essential component of comprehensive care in geriatric medicine. Furthermore, the setting in which social interaction occurs is very important to the effectiveness of mental stimulation in older adults. New models, such as green care farms, highlight the importance of integrating nature with social interaction.

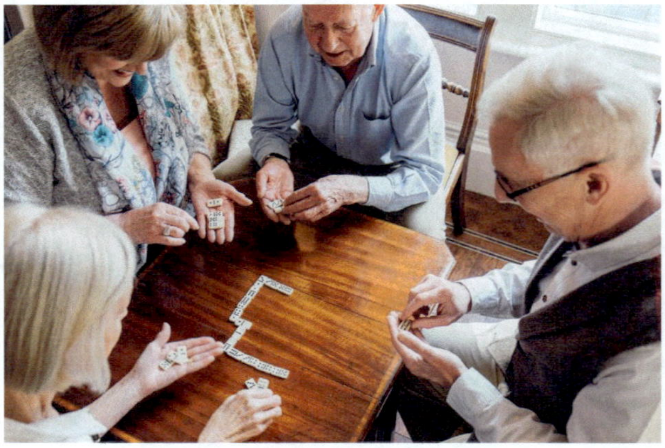

Figure 1.16. Addressing the social needs of older adults.

Source: https://www.mcmasteroptimalaging.org/images/default-source/blog-post-images/unspecified-9.tmb-blogpost.jpeg?Culture=en&sfvrsn=d9ec07d6_8.

These settings facilitate participation in a variety of physical and cognitive activities while also facilitating social relationships among participants. Research indicates that patients suffering from dementia and who are introduced to such dynamic environments have increased physical activity and nutritional intake levels compared to the normal day-care situation. de

Bruin (2009) theorizes that such fluctuation in program structures in the facilities can help preserve cognitive as well as emotional health in the long term, enhancing the quality of life. By facilitating social engagement in motivating environments, geriatric medicine may create multidirectional approaches that optimize the physical as well as mental health of the elderly and thereby address the multifaceted needs of this group (Figure 1.16).

Test Your Knowledge

1. What is the role of physical therapy in improving mobility, strength, and balance in older adults?
2. How does proper nutrition impact the health and well-being of older adults?
3. How do social engagement and mental stimulation contribute to the cognitive health and emotional well-being of elderly individuals?

1.5. Palliative and End-of-Life Care

Learning Outcome

1. Explain the principles of palliative care in geriatrics;
2. Focus on advanced care planning (ACP) and decision-making;
3. Understand support for families and caregivers in geriatric care.

The integration of end-of-life and palliative care in geriatric medicine is the doorway to addressing the diverse needs of an aging population. Throughout life, individuals cannot help but come across advanced stages of disease that will have a profound effect on their quality of life. Palliative care emphasizes a person-centered strategy, not only pain management, but psychological and social as well. It is meant to improve the overall well-being of patients, as well as their families, in order to provide decisions for preferences in treatment and care objectives. Importantly, research has revealed that enhancing support towards palliative care can promote a gentler healthcare encounter for older adults suffering from serious illnesses. This has been substantiated in a study that evidenced a strong correlation between patient satisfaction and effective preference communication regarding good care (Morton et al., 2015). This also suggests a key role for palliative care in geriatric care. Moreover, the uniquely difficult case of elderly patients in LTC facilities supports the need to integrate palliative care into existing systems. The majority of the elderly reside in nursing homes or long-term care assisted living facilities, environments in which they can lose both mental and physical function. The quality of life in such environments is often compromised by a lack of individualized care plans that take into account the emotional and psychological issues of the residents. Research has noted a discernible gap in the literature surrounding palliative care in long-term care facilities, an area that is significant as geriatric care needs become increasingly complex (Szczepura et al., 2008). By focusing on enhancing quality in palliative care, it is feasible to enhance both physical comfort and emotional well-being among older adults, thereby facilitating a dignified end-of-life experience. Key to the successful implementation of palliative care is training and enabling healthcare practitioners who are attending to geriatric patients. Appropriate delivery of palliative and end-of-life care requires that practitioners possess a thorough understanding of the complexities of delivering care to the elderly. In addition, interprofessional practice among nurses, physicians, social workers, and therapists is paramount. By promoting a team-oriented model, healthcare providers can optimally resolve the complex issues of their patients, offering a cohesive strategy that encompasses comfort and dignity. Investment in this team-based model could improve care coordination, resulting in improved outcomes for older persons with serious illness. As researchers and policymakers battle for progress in this area, it is certain that robust palliative care systems will be required to confront the evolving demands of the aging population (The Stern Center for Evidence-Based Policy, 2015).

1.5.1. Principles of Palliative Care in Geriatrics

Palliative care guidelines are essential in the field of geriatrics since they underscore symptom management from pain and discomfort associated with terminal diseases among the elderly. Physical comfort is not the only concern; but psychological, social, and even spiritual needs must be measured. Such a multidimensional assessment guarantees comprehensive care for elderly patients based on their specific cases. By prioritizing quality of life, palliative care allows for a respectful life in the face of advanced age or terminal illness. As populations age, these ideas become increasingly vital to integrate into geriatric medicine, relating medical care to the patients' values and choices. Despite the evident benefits, there remain obstacles to integrating palliative care and geriatric medicine. Most of the healthcare practitioners know little about the other discipline's contributions, resulting in patient care gaps. Inadequate communication and a lack of common practices also contribute to difficulties in effective teamwork. This is achieved through continuous education and building strong collaborative frameworks. According to multi-country research, it was discovered that creating interdisciplinary conversation and collaboration can significantly enhance patient outcomes among this group of individuals. Therefore, it is critical to support these communications and experiences to bridge gaps in the quality of palliative care for older people and thereby improve the well-being and health of this vulnerable group (Dale et al., 2016). Moreover, furthering the promotion of the inclusion of palliative care principles in geriatric training programs is necessary for future healthcare providers. Establishing academic chairs for palliative care in geriatrics would promote education and research at this critical juncture. Training geriatricians in fundamental skills of palliative care will improve their ability to practice with serious symptoms and communicate better with patients and families. Furthermore, awareness of the ethical issues that are common in end-of-life care discussions is required to provide empathetic and knowledgeable care. Through the integration of these principles into the core of geriatric education, the healthcare profession will be equipped to offer older adults the assistance they require as they experience severe illness, contributing to improved healthcare experience and results for an increasingly aging population (Albers et al., 2016) (Figure 1.17).

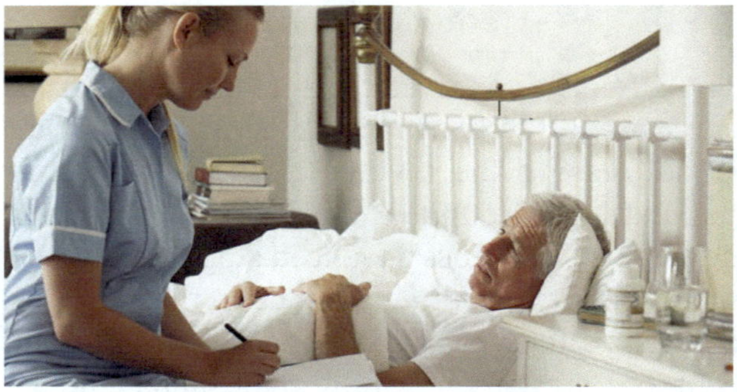

Figure 1.17. Palliative care.

Source: https://papayacare.com/wp-content/uploads/2023/09/Palliative-Care-for-Seniors-papaya-care.jpg.

1.5.2. Advanced Care Planning (ACP) and Decision-Making

Effective advanced care planning (ACP) and decision-making are paramount to the geriatric medicine practice, especially because older individuals have multidimensional and chronic health conditions. ACP includes discussion with patients and caregivers about patients values, desires, and expectations of future medical care. This assists in preparing healthcare providers with the information required to modify treatment plans that value the choice of their elderly patients. Above all, particularly in cases where patients have progressive conditions such as dementia, having a well-formulated plan can lead to more logical end-of-life care, which is especially important for maintaining the dignity and comfort of patients during their terminal illness. Most patients do not engage in ACP, thereby leaving patient desires unknown or unmet, which underscores the need for taking initiative in geriatric care facilities. In dementia, ACP is more critical since cognitive impairment can interfere with a patient in making his/her wishes known as the disease progresses.

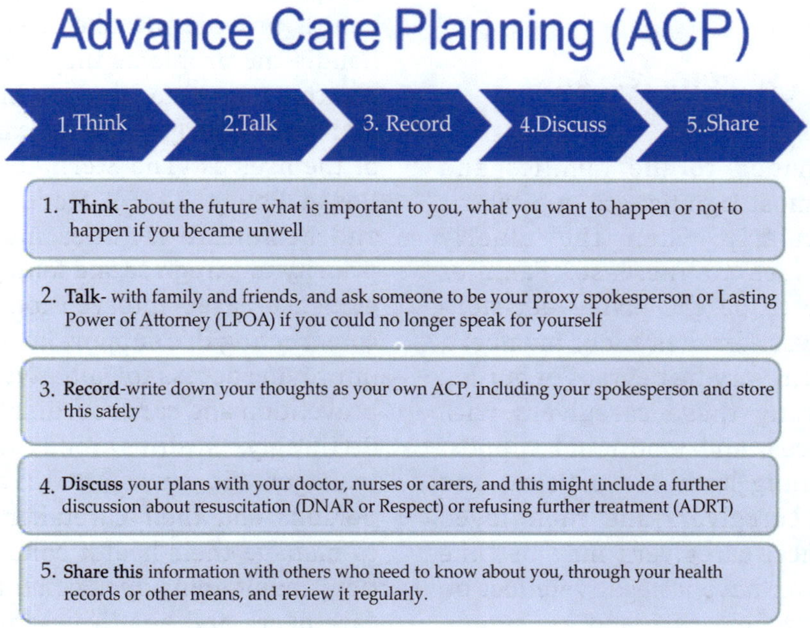

Figure 1.18. Advanced care planning (ACP)

Source: https://www.goldstandardsframework.org.uk/cd-content/uploads/images/newimages/ACP%20Table.png.

Perhaps the greatest challenge in dealing with dementia is being in a position to accurately foresee the needs of the patient in the progression of the disease over time, particularly in the terminal phase. Research indicates significant challenges to delivering appropriate palliative care to individuals with dementia, primarily regarding prognostication and communication challenges (Birch & Draper, 2008). Furthermore, difficulties in accessing specialist palliative care services are a significant issue, which can heighten suffering and lower quality of life. Thus, medical practitioners must enable not only discussions about advance directives but also enable means to implement these plans when the disease advances. Last but not least, systematic mapping of research findings into health policy shows increasing appreciation for the role of ACP in geriatric care. Despite the clear benefits that accrue from front-end planning—e.g., improved patient self-management and enhanced care coordination—translation of research into practice through policy has been inconsistent (The Stern Center for Evidence-Based Policy, 2015). To illustrate, aligning healthcare systems with palliative care values, such as necessary resources and training, could profoundly impact older adults' end-of-life experiences. Promoting overall strategies that are both beneficial to the family as well as the patient in terms of education and resource allocation can create a more empathetic health care setting. In this way, it is easier to navigate the complexities of ACP effectively, thereby enhancing the general quality of care being provided to the elderly (Figure 1.18).

1.5.3. Support for Families and Caregivers

The support provided to the families and caregivers is of utmost significance in geriatric medicine, particularly when the elderly population continues to increase. Families typically continue to be the prime decision-makers and caregivers for their older members, which might result in varying degrees of burden and stress. Assisting these caregivers with education, resources, and emotional support is key to maintaining both the physical and mental health of caregivers and their loved ones. In its absence, caregivers may become burnt out, which can have a negative effect on their capacity to provide care and assistance. Application of systematic programs that inform families about effective caregiving practices and services that are accessible to them can improve such problems, as well as the general quality of life of the elderly persons and their caregivers. This is also assisted by the use of thorough assessments, which play a big role in assisting families and caregivers. Geriatric evaluations, despite being largely underutilized, have proven to identify the distinct needs of older persons, which is critical for developing customized care plans. These assessments, which include measurements of physical health, mental health, and social support, are necessary for identifying the specific areas in which caregivers can use assistance or counseling. Research indicates that an active strategy to geriatric assessment can stratify risk and improve outcomes. By ensuring that caregivers are given information about the complexities of their loved ones' conditions, health providers make it easier for them to handle the problems they are confronted with, creating a condition under which both caregivers and frail elderly patients can make the most of themselves (The Stern Center for Evidence-Based Policy, 2015). Moreover, policymakers and healthcare facilities must accord utmost priority to caregiver and family support through evidence-based interventions. Suggestions for constructing this support involve, among others, improving access to palliative care and utilizing prevention and care coordination interventions. Strikingly, studies focus on patient self-management, an aspect that empowers older persons and their caretakers with the ability to manage their health condition. At the same time, maintaining open communication between caretakers and health practitioners allows for information and resource exchange in favor of successful caretaker management. With the progress in the area of geriatric medicine, such policies being addressed not only improve the healthcare system but also acknowledge the vital role caregivers have in the interprofessional care of old patients, eventually leading to better health outcomes (The Stern Center for Evidence-Based Policy, 2015).

Test Your Knowledge

1. What are the core principles of palliative care in geriatric medicine?
2. How can healthcare providers facilitate advanced care planning for elderly patients?

1.6. Challenges in Geriatric Medicine

Learning Outcome

1. Discuss the barriers to accessing healthcare for older adults;
2. Explain the importance of training and education for healthcare providers for geriatric medicine;
3. Focus on ethical considerations in geriatric care.

The increasing prevalence of polypharmacy among elderly patients is a significant problem in the practice of geriatrics. Because older patients usually have multiple chronic diseases, they often take more than one drug, leading to complex treatment programs. This risk elevation for polypharmacy can lead to ADRs, drug interactions, and overall drug mismanagement, particularly in resource-constrained settings. Research indicates that, in older cancer patients, polypharmacy is further exacerbated by anticancer and comorbidity drugs administered to them, thus bringing about a great demand for intervention. Intervention by clinical pharmacists in such cases has been identified as critical, as they can audit the medication regimens and recommend alternatives that help minimize risks associated with polypharmacy. The underlying issues in drug management bring to the fore the necessity of interprofessional interventions in elderly patients' care, that is, the complexities of drug requirements for the elderly patients (Shrestha et al., 2019). In addition to the needs of medication management, the incidence of geriatric injury poses further challenges to health practitioners. The uniqueness of geriatric trauma, involving increased susceptibility to injury, necessitates special attention to delicacies in treatment methods. Statistics reveal that a significant percentage of elderly patients present with various mechanisms of trauma, typically in their own homes. Excessive rates of trauma, like falls and assaults, combined with patients' pre-existing medical status, complicate their treatment and prognosis. Complication rates are especially high due to the combination of physical vulnerability and possible cognitive impairment in this population, which has an impact on recovery and increases mortality rates. Addressing these challenges calls for an interdisciplinary effort that focuses on prevention and reasserts the importance of early intervention and general trauma care in geriatric practice (Chalya et al., 2012). Moreover, the incorporation of comprehensive geriatrics training into medical education is a requirement for improving the management of challenges in geriatric practice. Despite the increasing number of elderly patients, especially in developing nations, medical schools often fail to cover the intricacies of geriatric care, leaving new medical professionals ill-prepared. There needs to be emphasis on specific training regarding geriatric syndromes, such as cognitive impairment and frailty, and the management of polypharmacy and geriatric trauma. Enlarging medical training to encompass these dimensions can ensure a more advanced understanding of the intricacies of working with older adults. With an aging population, equipping future doctors with the skills and knowledge necessary to match will be crucial in overcoming the challenges of geriatric medicine, ensuring ultimately better health for this vulnerable population.

1.6.1. Barriers to Accessing Healthcare for Older Adults

The ability of older people to access healthcare services is greatly hindered by a broad range of barriers, which can significantly impact their overall well-being. Socioeconomic determinants, such as limited resources and ill-fitting insurance protection, often become major impediments among these barriers. Many older persons have fixed incomes, which constrain them from paying for not just routine medical care but also treatments and medications needed. Moreover, myths about health care may deter older individuals from seeking services in a timely manner. For instance, aged individuals may believe their health issues are a result of natural aging and, therefore, may refrain from receiving care, thereby aggravating their conditions. Eradicating these barriers requires a thorough grasp of the distinctive needs of this subpopulation, emphasizing the need for specifically aimed interventions to enhance access to health care specifically tailored for the elderly. Another significant barrier to access to geriatric health care is the lack of specialized geriatric care and expert services. Traditional medical systems are not usually suited to respond to the special needs of geriatric patients, which may lead to intensified health disparities. For instance, the inability to include oral health examination in routine check-ups for general health has effects not just on physical well-being but also on quality of life since oral disease can lead to extensive systemic disease. It was reported that older adults who are frail tend to miss routine dental consultations due to multiple barriers, such as the lack of training of healthcare providers about geriatric oral health (Kossioni et al., 2017). This knowledge deficit serves to underscore the imperative need for educational paradigms for preparing healthcare professionals with geriatric skills specifically to improve health outcomes for older adults. Systemic difficulties in healthcare policy also play a profound role in perpetuating disparities in access to care for older adults. A number of policies in place currently do not effectively facilitate preventative care or coordination of care, and this leaves the elderly with fragmented services that are insufficient to meet their needs. Evidence-based policies that facilitate preventative interventions and effective self-management have been proven to be poorly executed in spite of the capacity to improve health outcomes (The Stern Center for Evidence-Based Policy, 2015). Apart from this, the role of family caregivers is usually taken lightly, but they are also very important in the healthcare process of the elderly. Better policymaking, incorporating the needs of caregivers, promoting citizen activism, and dealing with exceptional challenges facing aging societies will be key to dismantling such barriers and facilitating greater access to healthcare for the elderly (Figure 1.19).

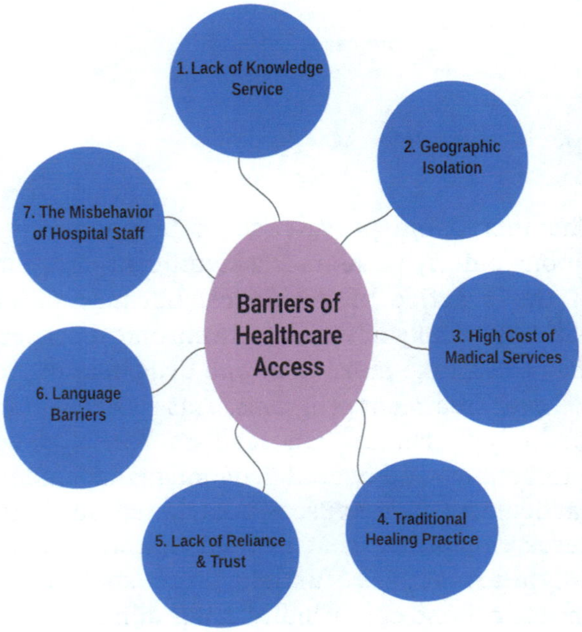

Figure 1.19. Barriers to healthcare access.

Source: https://www.researchgate.net/profile/Md-Sohel-8/publication/373192804/figure/fig1/AS:11431281182216482@1692329024069/Barriers-to-healthcare-access.png.

1.6.2. Training and Education for Healthcare Providers

In the evolving terrain of geriatric medicine, it is necessary that specialty education and training become paramount for healthcare practitioners. With an increasingly aging population, the subtleties of geriatric treatment require that health providers, in addition to basic medical knowledge, possess an understanding of elderly patients' distinctive physiological and psychosocial needs. Evidence-based practice-focused innovative training programs are required to empower healthcare professionals to address such challenges effectively. Research findings can be mapped to policy recommendations through a systematic approach that can guide curriculum design to enhance training programs aimed at improving health outcomes among the elderly. Specifically, such programs should emphasize care coordination and prevention strategies, as recommended by emerging studies identifying fruitful evidence-based policies in these domains. Thus, early and continuous geriatric healthcare education can potentially improve the quality of care for this vulnerable population (Morton et al., 2015). Incorporation of CGAs into healthcare professional training is another essential component for optimizing providers' capability to treat older adults. Despite an overwhelming consensus among geriatricians and surgeons that these assessments are essential, their utilization remains woefully low across clinical practices. Factors contributing to the gap include the slow pace of evaluations, which contradicts the demands of busy clinical work timelines. Therefore, training programs for medical professionals such as Physician Assistants and Medical Students must focus on developing streamlined assessment methods. New advances in educational interventions, including simulation training, have been seen to be very effective in teaching critical assessment skills while giving trainees practical experience in a controlled environment. Through education that emphasizes the significance of these assessments, healthcare practitioners can better identify risks and refine treatment plans for their elderly cancer patients (Lampugnane et al., 2017). Besides, fostering teamwork among geriatricians and other health workers is critical in enhancing the expansion of geriatric education. The complexity of treating chronic conditions and surgery needs in geriatric patients demands multidisciplinary care, where knowledge sharing and teamwork care plans become the central theme. Weaving in joint training modules that allow different specialties to engage with geriatric principles not only enriches the learning process but also increases the shared appreciation of the specialty issues within geriatric medicine. Such collaboration can improve care coordination and better health systems' response to the diverse needs of older persons. With geriatric medicine expansion, incorporating this cooperative learning model will ultimately lead to better outcomes for the elderly and an enhanced healthcare workforce in a position to address future needs.

1.6.3. Ethical Considerations in Geriatric Care

Geriatric practice ethical issues are a priority, particularly as the population gets older. Balancing care requirements against the autonomy of older patients who may present with compromised capacity is one of the key ethical challenges. The health practitioners must make the tough decisions between honoring people's capacity for their own decisions and intervening when incapacity or self-harm is apparent. As the complexities in self-neglect indicate, older persons have an ego associated with self-independence, but service providers cannot differentiate between the inability to care for oneself and refusal to do so. The dilemma poses ethical concerns about safeguarding vulnerable adults from harm and maintaining their autonomy and personal choice (Braye et al., 2011). Finally, geriatric care needs to change so that it serves first and foremost the dignity and desire of older patients, creating an environment conducive to safety and autonomy. Another pressing ethical issue is access to health services for older people. Systematic neglect of older people in most areas, including Tanzania, is likely to mean poor provision of health care, and so there are huge inequities in access and treatment. The old not only have physical and mental issues but also endure social suffering as a result of inadequate resources and respect. Even though the rights of the old to receive free social services and treatment have been recognized by the Tanzania National

Ageing Policy of 2003, most are not informed of these rights, thus escalating their issues. This discrepancy raises ethical challenges of justice and equality in healthcare, as the most vulnerable groups may be deprived of such essential care. The systematic negligence with societal disdain demands advocacy of such policies and practices that actually embrace the rights of older adults in geriatric care (Ngallaba et al., 2016). Besides, the ethical disanalogy to provide humane and culturally sensitive care is pivotal in the practice of geriatric medicine. This includes identification and respect for the personal values, backgrounds, and beliefs of the elderly. Caregivers must be trained to appreciate the historical and social contexts that characterize the lives of their patients, particularly in societies where respect for the elders is traditionally most significant. Sensitive care that is adjusted for the cultural nuances not only enhances compliance with treatment but also builds trust between carers and the elderly patients. In addition, it is crucial to address the issue of elder abuse in caregiving environments. Through greater understanding of elder abuse, there is a need to establish systems that address not just the physical well-being but the emotional and psychological well-being of older individuals so that they are treated with the respect and dignity they deserve (Ngallaba et al., 2016).

Test Your Knowledge

1. What are the most common barriers that older adults face in accessing healthcare services?
2. What are some of the key ethical dilemmas that arise in geriatric care?

SUMMARY

The context of an inquiry into geriatric medicine demonstrates the need for specialized approaches to healthcare for the elderly population. With rising rates of chronic diseases and multimorbidity in the elderly population, healthcare professionals have a duty to adjust their approach to satisfy the unique needs of these patients. The use of CGAs, particularly in oncology, demonstrates a key lack within current medical practice. Although geriatricians and surgeons recognize the utility of evaluating factors like frailty, social support, nutrition, and psychological health, time constraints in clinical practice make their application difficult. Therefore, creating awareness and capacity building in geriatric assessments is essential for enhancing the quality of care in older patients and facilitating them to get the optimal available treatment. Furthermore, the concerns raised by an aging population extend beyond strictly clinical assessments. Effective management of care must consider the complexity of older patients' health issues and balance cost considerations with quality of care. Chronic disease and functional decline among the elderly can mean increased healthcare expenditure, making it essential to employ innovative care models that increase health gains without added expense. Through targeting patient-centered care that considers the patient's values, social conditions, and preferences, the healthcare experience of older adults can be significantly enhanced by providers. These strategies increase patient satisfaction and treatment adherence, which can ultimately lead to better health outcomes among geriatric patients. Lastly, the progression of the specialty of geriatric medicine needs to be on a multi-faceted level with educational programs to prepare future healthcare professionals with the richness of geriatric care. The use of simulation-based educational interventions would be a long way toward improving the level of proficiency of medical students and healthcare workers and facilitating them to conduct effective geriatric assessments. As noted on this topic, having clinicians familiar with prognostic predictors of surgical outcomes and ongoing care management will ultimately improve the treatment environment for oncogeriatric patients. As geriatric oncology as a field continues to develop, filling these gaps in training and streamlining models of care will be crucial to fostering enhanced healthcare delivery and the quality of life for the elderly, so that they may receive empathetic, rational, and sensitive medical care in an increasingly changing healthcare system.

In geriatric care, innovations in the present day and scholarship collaborations become central factors in enhancing the delivery of care to the elderly. The establishment of Leicester Academy for the Study of Ageing (LASA) attests to a commitment to inter-professional research aimed at meeting the total needs of older individuals. This initiative brings together various stakeholders, including health service organizations, universities, and local government agencies, to create an overall strategy for improving health outcomes. By employing applied and translational research, LASA seeks to solve issues such as functional ability, cognitive health, and social determinants of aging in the older individual. Such collaborative research is the greatest demonstration of what academic research collaborations are capable of doing in establishing suitable care strategies for older adults and caregivers based on evidence-based practice guidelines and service delivery (Agarwal et al., 2019). In addition to collaborative research activity, clinical practice in geriatric medicine has been enhanced to better address the problems associated with aging populations. The CGA model has become crucial in the management of frail older patients, where multidisciplinary competencies converge to deliver a good balance of care. In Leicester, the introduction of the CGA in the acute and emergency care environments is a significant achievement in medicine. The system enables the early recognition of frailty as well as the roll-out of appropriate treatment pathways, where patients can be triaged into suitable care settings. Furthermore, the establishment of specialized facilities, such as frail-friendly EDs, should also signify the attempt to improve recovery outcomes and lower hospital-associated complications among older adults (Agarwal et al., 2019). Research in geriatric medicine also extends to historical narratives that make valuable contributions to the field's development. An interview-based study of geriatric care pioneers' histories exposes the professional stories that defined the approach during its initial phases. By analyzing these oral histories, researchers can learn from the challenges and achievements of geriatricians in their early days, particularly in their efforts to raise the profession's intellectual status. This examination of history paints a picture of how cultural diversity among practitioners can influence career development within the field of geriatric medicine. Ultimately, such analysis strengthens the contemporary context of the specialty, driving practice and policy formulation aimed at introducing more respectful and responsive elder care strategies.

KEY TERMS FROM THIS CHAPTER

Adoptive international models	Advanced care planning (ACP)
Adverse drug reactions (ADRs)	Ambient assisted living (AAL)
Blood pressure regulation	CGA process
Comorbid diseases	Coping techniques
Dementia	Depression
Effective management principles	Electronic health records (EHRs)
Emergency departments (EDs)	Geriatric assessments
Geriatric care	Geriatric fracture programs
Geriatric home caregivers	Geriatric medicine,
Health providers	Healthcare providers

CRITICAL THINKING QUESTIONS

1. Which of the following is the most common chronic condition in elderly individuals?

a. Hypertension

b. Diabetes

c. Osteoarthritis

d. Dementia

2. Which of the following is a key component of a comprehensive geriatric assessment (CGA)?

a. Blood pressure measurement

b. Cognitive function assessment

c. Complete blood count (CBC)

d. Chest X-ray

3. Which of the following is a common challenge in prescribing medications for elderly patients?

a. Higher drug metabolism due to aging liver

b. Increased renal clearance of drugs

c. Polypharmacy and drug-drug interactions

d. Reduced sensitivity to medications

4. Which of the following is a primary goal of palliative care for elderly patients?

a. To cure the underlying disease

b. To delay the progression of the disease

c. To improve quality of life and alleviate suffering

d. To prolong life at any cost

5. Which of the following is a significant barrier to providing high-quality care for older adults?

a. Reduced healthcare costs

b. High patient turnover in geriatric clinics

c. Increased access to specialist care

d. Age-related physical and cognitive decline

Short Answer Questions

1. What are the most prevalent chronic diseases in older adults, and how do these conditions impact their physical and mental well-being, especially when coexisting with one another?
2. How does a comprehensive geriatric assessment (CGA) evaluate not only medical but also functional, cognitive, and social aspects of elderly individuals?
3. What are the key considerations when prescribing medications to older adults?
4. How does polypharmacy affect the health outcomes of elderly patients?
5. What role do non-pharmacological interventions, such as physical therapy, nutrition management, and mental stimulation, play in improving the health and quality of life for elderly individuals with chronic conditions?
6. What are the key principles of palliative care in geriatrics, and how do they help improve comfort, dignity, and quality of life for elderly patients nearing the end of life?

Answers to Critical Thinking Questions

1. (a); 2. (b); 3. (c); 4. (c); 5. (d)

REFERENCES

1. Perry, W., Lacritz, L., Roebuck-Spencer, T., Silver, C., Denney, R. L., Meyers, J., McConnel, C. E., Pliskin, N., Adler, D., Alban, C., Bondi, M., Braun, M., Cagigas, X., Daven, M., Drozdick, L., Foster, N. L., Hwang, U., Ivey, L., Iverson, G., Kramer, J., ... Golden, T. (2018). Population Health Solutions for Assessing Cognitive Impairment in Geriatric Patients. *The Clinical neuropsychologist, 32*(7), 1193–1225. https://doi.org/10.1080/13854046.2018.1517503(accessed on 27th June 2025).
2. Agarwal, S., Bankart, J., Bannerjee, J., Bell, D., et al. (2019). *East Midlands Research into Ageing Network (EMRAN) Discussion Paper Series*. https://core.ac.uk/download/228199189.pdf (accessed on 27th June 2025).
3. Madeira, T., Peixoto-Plácido, C., Goulão, B., Mendonça, N., Alarcão, V., Santos, N., de Oliveira, R. M., Yngve, A., Bye, A., Bergland, A., Lopes, C., Nicola, P., Santos, O., & Clara, J. G. (2016). National survey of the Portuguese elderly nutritional status: study protocol. *BMC geriatrics, 16*, 139. https://doi.org/10.1186/s12877-016-0299-x(accessed on 27th June 2025).
4. Albers, G., Froggatt, K., Van den Block, L. *et al.* A qualitative exploration of the collaborative working between palliative care and geriatric medicine: Barriers and facilitators from a European perspective. *BMC Palliat Care* **15**, 47 (2016). https://doi.org/10.1186/s12904-016-0118-3(accessed on 27th June 2025).
5. Allman, R. M., Clay, O. J., Crowther, M., Ford, D., et al. (2015). Race and sex differences in correlates of systolic blood pressure in community-dwelling older adults. https://digitalscholarship.unlv.edu/cgi/viewcontent.cgi?article=1269&context=jhdrp (accessed on 27th June 2025).
6. Atwal, A., Tattersall, K., Murphy, S., Davenport, N., Craik, C., Caldwell, K., & McIntyre, A. (2007). Older adults experiences of rehabilitation in acute health care. *Scandinavian journal of caring sciences, 21*(3), 371–378. https://doi.org/10.1111/j.1471-6712.2007.00469.x(accessed on 27th June 2025).
7. Sharma, M., Loh, K. P., Nightingale, G., Mohile, S. G., & Holmes, H. M. (2016). Polypharmacy and potentially inappropriate medication use in geriatric oncology. *Journal of geriatric oncology, 7*(5), 346–353. https://doi.org/10.1016/j.jgo.2016.07.010(accessed on 27th June 2025).
8. Braun, A., Trivedi, D. P., Dickinson, A., Hamilton, L., Goodman, C., Gage, H., Ashaye, K., Iliffe, S., & Manthorpe, J. (2019). Managing behavioural and psychological symptoms in community dwelling older people with dementia: 2. A systematic review of qualitative studies. *Dementia (London, England), 18*(7-8), 2950–2970. https://doi.org/10.1177/1471301218762856(accessed on 27th June 2025).
9. Siegel EO, Backman A, Cai Y, et al. Understanding Contextual Differences in Residential LTC Provision for Cross-National Research: Identifying Internationally Relevant CDEs. *Gerontol Geriatr Med.* 2019;5:2333721419840591. Published 2019 Jun 27. doi:10.1177/2333721419840591(accessed on 27th June 2025).
10. Barbic, D., Barbic, S. P., Carpenter, C. R., Kemplin, R., et al. (2018). Diagnostic accuracy of the Ottawa 3DY and Short Blessed Test to detect cognitive dysfunction in geriatric patients presenting to the emergency department. https://core.ac.uk/download/212860802.pdf (accessed on 27th June 2025).

11. Berry-Millett, R., & Bodenheimer, T. (2009). Care management of patients with complex health care needs. https://core.ac.uk/download/71346306.pdf (accessed on 27th June 2025).

12. Birch, D., & Draper, J. (2008). A critical literature review exploring the challenges of delivering effective palliative care to older people with dementia in the acute hospital setting. https://core.ac.uk/download/82906952.pdf (accessed on 27th June 2025).

13. Braye, S., Orr, D., & Preston-Shoot, M. (2011). Self-neglect and adult safeguarding: Findings from research. https://core.ac.uk/download/2721774.pdf (accessed on 27th June 2025).

14. Casey, S. D., Hirsch, C. H., Mumma, B. E., Slee, A., et al. (2017). Emergency department pain management following implementation of a geriatric hip fracture program. https://core.ac.uk/download/323071629.pdf (accessed on 27th June 2025).

15. Chalya, P. L., Dass, R. M., Gilyoma, J. M., Mabula, D., et al. (2012). Geriatric injuries among patients attending a regional hospital in Shanyang, Tanzania. https://core.ac.uk/download/pdf/18410878.pdf (accessed on 27th June 2025).

16. Szczepura, Ala, Clay, Diane, Hyde, Julia, Nelson, S. (Sara) and Wild, Deidre (2008) *Models for providing improved care in residential care homes: a thematic literature review.* [Coventry]: [University of Warwick].(accessed on 27th June 2025).

17. Petrovic, M., Somers, A., Onder, G. (2016). Geriatric Pharmacotherapy: Optimisation Through Integrated Approach in the Hospital Setting. In: Stegemann, S. (eds) Developing Drug Products in an Aging Society. AAPS Advances in the Pharmaceutical Sciences Series, vol 26. Springer, Cham. https://doi.org/10.1007/978-3-319-43099-7_33 (accessed on 27th June 2025).

18. de Bruin, S. R. (2009). *Sowing in the Autumn Season: Exploring Benefits of Green Care Farms for Dementia Patients.* https://core.ac.uk/download/pdf/29250250.pdf (accessed on 27th June 2025).

19. Eberhard, Birgid & Fachinger, Uwe & Henke, Klaus-Dirk, 2009. "Better Health and Ambient Assisted Living (AAL) from a global, regional and local economic perspective," MPRA Paper 16210, University Library of Munich, Germany.(accessed on 27th June 2025).

20. Mallia, P. & Fiorini, A.(2003). Rethinking care for the sick elderly. Malta Medical Journal. 2003, Vol.15(1), p. 18-20 https://core.ac.uk/download/46601837.pdf (accessed on 27th June 2025).

21. Mallery, L., Gordon, J., & Freter, S. (2003). A 3 Week Geriatric Education Program for 4th Year Medical Students at Dalhousie University. *Medical education online*, *8*(1), 4342. https://doi.org/10.3402/meo.v8i.4342(accessed on 27th June 2025).

22. Kossioni, A. E., Hajto-Bryk, J., Maggi, S., McKenna, G., Petrovic, M., Roller-Wirnsberger, R. E., Schimmel, M., Tamulaitienè, M., Vanobbergen, J., & Müller, F. (2018). An Expert Opinion from the European College of Gerodontology and the European Geriatric Medicine Society: European Policy Recommendations on Oral Health in Older Adults. *Journal of the American Geriatrics Society*, *66*(3), 609–613. https://doi.org/10.1111/jgs.15191(accessed on 27th June 2025).

23. Henwood, M., Larkin, M., & Milne, A. (2017). Seeing the wood for the trees. Carer related research and knowledge: A scoping review. https://core.ac.uk/download/145186527.pdf (accessed on 27th June 2025).

24. Livingston, G., Johnston, K., Katona, C., Paton, J., Lyketsos, C. G., & Old Age Task Force of the World Federation of Biological Psychiatry (2005). Systematic review of psychological approaches

to the management of neuropsychiatric symptoms of dementia. *The American journal of psychiatry, 162*(11), 1996–2021. https://doi.org/10.1176/appi.ajp.162.11.1996(accessed on 27th June 2025).

25. Kantor, B., Mueller, C., Beck, C., Algase, D., Mitty, E., Rader, J., Anderson, K., et al. (2009). Nurses' involvement in nursing home culture change: Overcoming barriers, advancing opportunities. https://core.ac.uk/download/71353499.pdf (accessed on 27th June 2025).
26. E. Ngallaba, S. , Makerere, D. , Nyanza, E. , Kapesa, A. and Marwa, K. (2016) Common Preventable Health and Social Problems Encountered by Elderly in Shinyanga Region in the Northern Part of Tanzania. *Open Journal of Preventive Medicine,* **6**, 115-123. doi: 10.4236/ojpm.2016.63010.(accessed on 27th June 2025).
27. Shrestha, S., Shrestha, S., & Khanal, S. (2019). Polypharmacy in elderly cancer patients: Challenges and the way clinical pharmacists can contribute in resource-limited settings. *Aging medicine (Milton (N.S.W)), 2*(1), 42–49. https://doi.org/10.1002/agm2.12051(accessed on 27th June 2025).
28. Lampugnale, C. A. (2017). Surgical assessment of the geriatric oncology patient. https://open.bu.edu/bitstream/2144/26707/5/Lampugnale_bu_0017N_13146.pdf (accessed on 27th June 2025).
29. The Stern Center for Evidence-Based Policy (2015). Addressing the health needs of an aging America: New opportunities for evidence-based policy solutions. University of Pittsburgh. https://core.ac.uk/download/75783019.pdf (accessed on 27th June 2025).
30. Nolan, M. (1997). Gerontological nursing: Professional priority or eternal Cinderella? https://core.ac.uk/download/56526.pdf (accessed on 27th June 2025).
31. Petrovic, M., van der Cammen, T., & Onder, G. (2012). Adverse drug reactions in older people: detection and prevention. *Drugs & aging, 29*(6), 453–462. https://doi.org/10.2165/11631760-000000000-00000(accessed on 27th June 2025).
32. Schofield, P. & Reid, D. M. (2006). The assessment and management of pain in older people: A systematic review of the literature. https://core.ac.uk/download/177013.pdf (accessed on 27th June 2025).

WOMEN'S HEALTH IN GENERAL MEDICINE

2

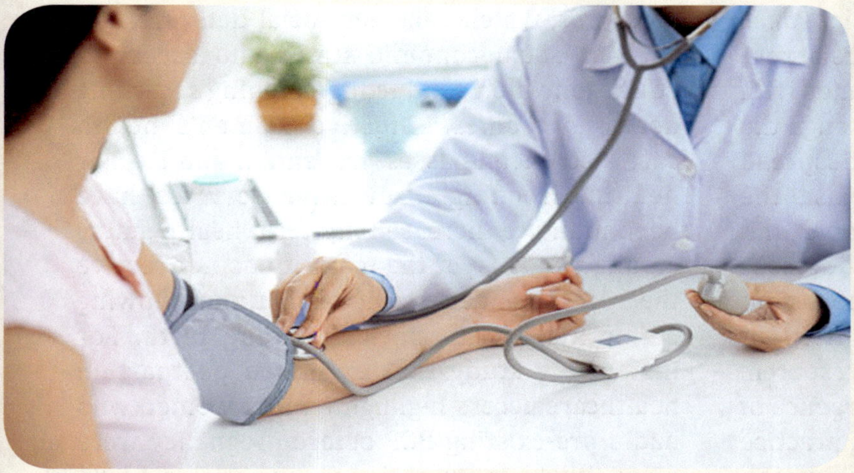

LEARNING OBJECTIVES

After studying this chapter, you will be able to:

1. Understand the historical context of women's health in general medicine;
2. Describe reproductive health;
3. Define maternal health;
4. Discuss chronic conditions in women;
5. Explain how mental health plays a crucial role in the overall well-being of women;
6. Define the role of preventive care in women's health.

Introduction

The study of women's health in general medicine is a strict and complicated task that demands attention of utmost gravity due to its long-term implications for public health. Initial thoughts illustrate that previous inequalities in access to healthcare and outcomes between women and sociocultural factors have been the major forces behind the background of women's health. As an integral part of medical practice, understanding these factors helps health professionals to tailor their approach in order to meet the particular requirements of women patients. Various scholarly works indicate that communication and ethnicity occupy a key position in ensuring quality delivery of care, and this reflects the necessity for interpreters, advocacy, and translation services in general medical practice (Szczepura et al., 2005). Moreover, disease prevalence, reproductive health, psychological status, and socioeconomic status complexities crosscut these variables, instilling the need to push forward fully integrated models that address women's health. Holistic treatment of women's health involves a consideration of the distinct biological and societal determinants that influence their healthcare outcomes. For instance, gender-based health disparities are generally founded on systemically created barriers that affect access to quality care and preventive healthcare services. Medical practice and research have traditionally privileged male groups, thus overlooking the unique health needs of women that span from reproductive health to diseases such as autoimmune diseases that occur predominantly in women. In addition, culturally competent communication is important to improve patient-provider relations, to provide women of different backgrounds with appropriate care (Swainson, 1998). Through the integration of these concerns into widespread medical training and practice, there exists the potential to push forward an equitable and responsive healthcare system that addresses women's needs. Overall, women's health in general medicine is an emergent field of research that calls for continuous research, activism, and policy reform. The convergence of ethnicity, communication, and medical practice underscores the health system navigation complexity for women to access care. There is a strong imperative to eradicate legacy obstacles that constrain equal access to high-quality health services in favor of patient-centered strategies that appreciate cultural and linguistic diversity (Szczepura et al., 2005). As the discussion of women's health continues to evolve, it is imperative that healthcare professionals continue to be vigilant and attuned in practice, dedicated to creating an atmosphere which sees and reacts to the many influences on women's health outcomes.

Definition of Women's Health

Women's health has also been defined to include a broad scope of physical, mental, and social well-being, more than reproductive health. Historically, medical research focused primarily on men's health, ignoring the particular health issues that women face during their lifespan. This has long-term implications; the particular experiences of women—from hormonal changes to pregnancy and menopause—need a specialized care approach. Sufficient understanding of women's health includes the acknowledgment that women's common ailments, such as cardiovascular disease and breast cancer, may be under-researched due to historical discrimination. Secondly, the multifaceted nature of women's health places emphasis on comprehensive healthcare measures, which consider social determinants such as socioeconomic status and access to education when conducting planning regarding health outcomes. Effective women's health care also encompasses prevention and regular health screening. Preventive services have been found to increase long-term health status among women, yet the majority do not receive the recommended services on time following major life events, such as giving birth. For instance, a study that examined postpartum healthcare access highlighted that women who had a pre-existing PCP before pregnancy were more likely to experience preventive visits after delivery; yet, those without a PCP were less likely to pursue health checks that they required in the late postpartum period, and consequently, missed the chance of preventative intervention (Price & Seagrave, 2020). These findings highlight the importance of establishing a reliable health care provider and education about the services offered. The combination of preventive visits with continuity in health can effectively enhance the overall well-being and health trajectory of women across their lifetime. Providing education and person-centered care within women's health practice is required to address the diverse needs of this population. Prenatal policies often do not incorporate detailed educational components, which are fundamental in facilitating women to make adequately informed health decisions (Hanson et al., 2009). As more healthcare professionals realize the importance of patient education as part of quality care, greater emphasis is put on personalized information to meet needs and circumstances. This patient-centered system not only increases participation but also enables women to be offered support suitable to their specific health condition and situation. Through a focus on personalized care and continued communication between patients and health workers, loopholes in the health services can be corrected and the overall health outcomes for women improved. This combined approach is necessary to advance women's health throughout general medicine, ultimately translating into individual and public health results (Figure 2.1).

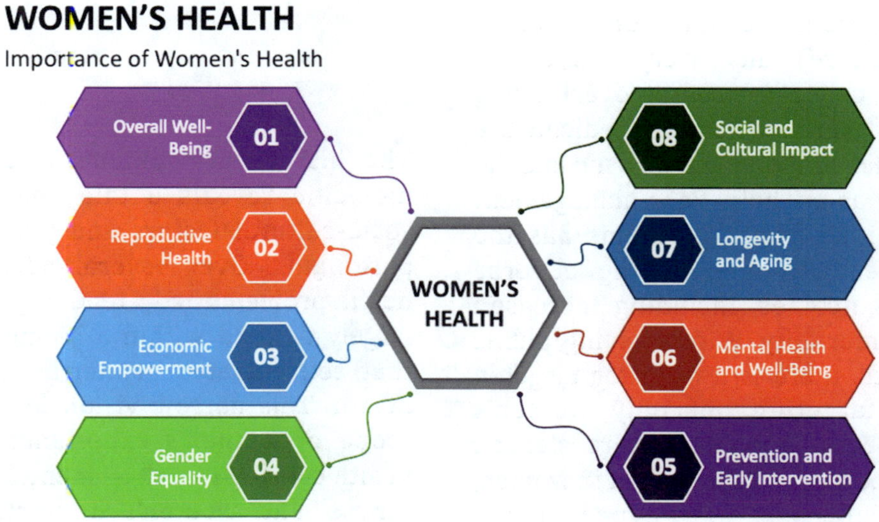

Figure 2.1. Women's health.

Source: https://www.collidu.com/media/catalog/product/img1/b/9/b93b8d81b3fbb922a06d7af0e3ceb34088c6dac511dc2129816c7dcdfc4e0cc9/women-health-slide6.png.

Importance of Women's Health in General Medicine

The significance of women's health to the field of general medicine goes beyond mere statistical inclusion and has a direct influence on clinical outcomes. Women have been underrepresented throughout history in medical studies, leaving enormous knowledge gaps about female-specific health concerns. An awareness of this imbalance is significant, as women's health encompasses a discrete set of physiological, psychological, and social variables that are fundamentally different from those relevant to men. As physicians increasingly see the value of gender-specific strategies, the incorporation of women's health considerations into all aspects of medicine is on the upswing. This transformation not only enhances the standard of care but also allows women the autonomy to be engaged participants in their health care, ultimately resulting in better health outcomes overall, as observed through progressive policies and initiatives dealing with women's health (Avery et al., 2007). Furthermore, women's health also has a direct interaction with social determinants, thus rendering the practice of general medicine even more complicated. Socioeconomic factors, education, and access to healthcare have significant impacts on women's health outcomes, creating disparities that must be addressed. Such determinants affect not only individual health but also the health systems of the population at large. Interventions to these disparities are often interdisciplinary in nature among healthcare workers, policymakers, and community agencies.

For instance, sensitization of injuries related to maternal health, which predominantly occur among women, is crucial in improving overall health outcomes. An integrated method that takes these social factors into account is essential to the process of guaranteeing that women's health concerns are well-represented and treated in medicine and, consequently, promoting healthcare equity (Avery et al., 2007). Ultimately, the consequences of overlooking women's health overall in general medicine are not limited to the individual but also include the broader society as a whole. Poor management of women's unique health problems has the potential to lead to far-reaching adverse public health outcomes, including increased morbidity and mortality. With evolving public health initiatives, there is a need for targeted interventions targeting not only women's reproductive health but also atherosclerotic diseases disproportionately prevalent in women, including osteoporosis and hypertension. Through improving our understanding of these conditions through research and education, the healthcare community can work towards the establishment of effective preventive measures and treatments. Investment in women's health thus not only benefits women's health but also leads to a better healthcare system that can cater to all populations (Avery et al., 2007) (Figure 2.2).

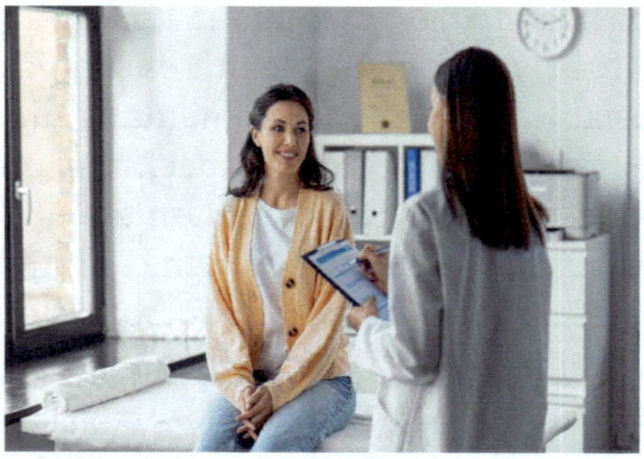

Figure 2.2. A gynecologist assessing a woman's health.

Source: https://medlineplus.gov/images/WomensHealthCheckup_Share.jpg.

2.1. Historical Context

Learning Outcome

1. Focus on the evolution of women's health in medical practice;
2. Discuss key milestones in women's health advocacy;
3. Understand the impact of historical biases on current practices.

The history of women's health in general medicine reveals a tale shaped largely by socio-cultural factors and prevailing medical paradigms. Over several decades, women's health problems had a tendency to be displaced, largely defined within a biomedical paradigm that concentrated primarily on reproductive health. This narrow vision ignored the broad scope of women's experience and women's health concerns, such as mental health, chronic illness, and women's distinctive social and economic issue contexts. With the evolution of medical practice in the 20th century, women's rights movements began questioning these historical accounts by demanding a more holistic concept of health that accounts for the interplay between biological, psychological, and socio-cultural determinants. More and more, this has become necessary to actualize how health professionals can better address the unique needs of women towards a more integrative concept of their healthcare experience. With this shifting environment, significant attention has been given to incorporating marginalized groups into medical practice and education. The establishment of sexual and gender minorities (SGM) as a component of women's health has caught a lot of attention and controversy. Despite acknowledging the importance of SGM perspectives, obstetric anesthesia and other areas of medical education have been slow to include relevant training material. From a survey of North American obstetric anesthesia fellowship programs, while most teachers acknowledge the imperative to train medical professionals in the care of diverse patient populations, there is a gap that is such that only 19% include SGM content within their curricula (Hanson et al., 2009). This discrepancy highlights the urgent necessity for retooling medical education to ensure that future professionals will be appropriately equipped to provide the holistic, inclusive care that considers the dynamism of gender identity and its attendant health considerations. The interface of gender identity and health has similarly been examined critically using sociocultural approaches, particularly in the context of eating disorder issues. Traditional accounts of such conditions only reduced them to mere side effects of societal body image pressures, thus siloing the intricate relationship between gender identity and health. Feminist and socio-cultural frameworks suggest that there is a need for deeper examination of how gender forces shape women's experiences with eating disorders and suggest treatment approaches that integrate these views (Holmes, 2016). By collaborating with women's personal accounts and evaluating existing feminist discourses, researchers have begun illuminating the gaps within traditional treatment frameworks. It is about healthcare systems' need to recognize the multifaceted impacts on women's health, leading to more compassionate and skilled care that is attuned to what they learn from living through it.

2.1.1. Evolution of Women's Health in Medical Practice

The evolution of women's health in the medical practice has undergone tremendous transformations over the past century, with significant influence from social, cultural, and scientific advancements. Medical studies traditionally focused on men's health, with a consequent gender imbalance that did not reflect the unique health concerns of women. This lopsided perspective encouraged a lagging understanding of female-predominant disease, including reproductive disease, which has direct implications for quality of life. With the development of awareness of health disparities, women's health came to be a focal issue of overall medicine, influencing medical curricula and requiring the integration of women's health issues into research agendas. A move away from a paternalistic approach to a patient-oriented approach and of greater awareness of women's autonomy in healthcare decision-making as a significant step toward medical practice equality. Also, the initiation of more comprehensive women's health programs has played a vital role in fighting specific health risks to women, particularly among underserved communities. For example, research records staggering shortfalls in cervical cancer awareness and vaccination within poor and minority communities. One in every seven female patients in the ED had never even heard of human papillomavirus (HPV) and many did not know about the HPV vaccine. Statistics like these show that there must be particular outreach and education that will increase awareness and prevent disparities among these high-risk populations. The ED, often an underserved woman's safety net, is an innovative vehicle through which to deliver health interventions to at-risk individuals, improving the utilization and accessibility of required medical care (Walter et al., 2020). The model of integration involving numerous healthcare providers—e.g., physicians and pharmacists—also enhances women's health care provision by establishing a more integrated health system. Effective communication among physicians, pharmacists, and patients is key to medication plan management, particularly when there is a suggestion for switching to generic drugs that could, unbeknownst, affect compliance with treatment. According to a study, the problem faced in this aspect with a lack of comprehensive information and concerted effort among healthcare practitioners jeopardizes patient outcomes. The evolution of women's health not only encapsulates the need for systemic change but also calls for improved collaboration among healthcare professions. This allows for a collaborative approach that addresses diversified medical complications while empowering women in terms of knowledge and equitable access to care, thus complementing the imperative evolution of women's health in general medicine (Păduraru et al., 2018) (Figure 2.3).

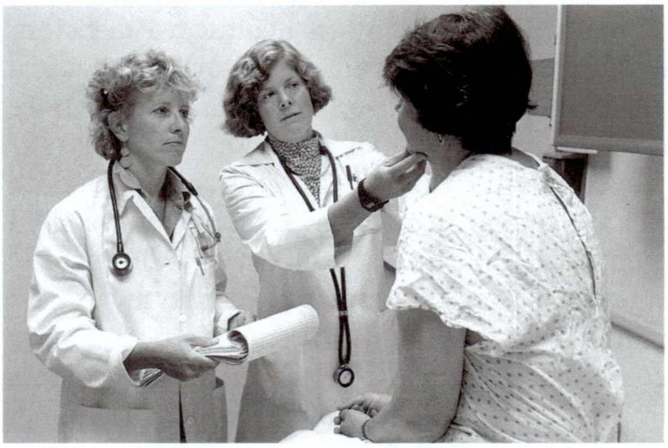

Figure 2.3. Women's health in medical practice has undergone significant transformations over the past century.

Source: https://drivendata-prod-public.s3.amazonaws.com/comp_images/ppfa_tile.jpg.

2.1.2. Key Milestones in Women's Health Advocacy

Women's health advocacy boasts a history of milestones that have actually altered the landscape of women's healthcare. One of these was in the mid-20th century, when gender-specific health issues began making inroads into the health landscape. This was partly because there was greater sensitivity to the inadequacy of studies that targeted fulfilling the unique health needs of women. As women's health activists called for access to clinical trials and medical studies, they opened the door to subsequent reforms that would extend to medical education and practice. Institutions such as the Women's Health Initiative in 1991 were characteristic of this milestone because they provided critical information about the health dangers and interventions of women, hence calling for a more differential policy of women's healthcare. To medical training, summits and collaborative ventures have been as important as creating women's health advocacy. Most notable is the 2015 Sex and Gender Medical Education Summit that provided an interdisciplinary forum to discuss adding sex and gender principles to medical courses. With the involvement of experts and teachers, the summit placed emphasis upon creating a change to better incorporate the notion of health from an understanding that encompasses not only biological but also sociocultural determinants that shape women's health. The outcome was not only a plan for curricular change but also an appeal to action, with 61% of the participants having increased their awareness of gender-specific medicine, illuminating their institutions to the imperative for change in healthcare discussion and delivery systems (Chin et al., 2016). This educational initiative was a vital step towards providing an equalized model of health education. In addition, the women's health movement has also been strongly embedded in broader social justice movements, amplifying the call for equality in healthcare treatment and access. Legislation and policies implemented, such as those created by the No Child Left Behind movement, brought attention to erstwhile disenfranchised communities, such as women who faced systemically established barriers in access to healthcare. This heightened awareness transformed the rhetoric of women's rights by noting the necessity to overcome not only legislative barriers but also social attitudes that prevail regarding women's roles in health care decisions. Women's health activism has been slow to locate and dismantle such barriers, resisting the patriarchal institutions that limit women's entry and dominion in their health care process. The concerted efforts towards improving the provision of healthcare to women better articulate the tenacity and resilience of advocacy action to push for justice and equity (DuBose, 2024) (Figure 2.4).

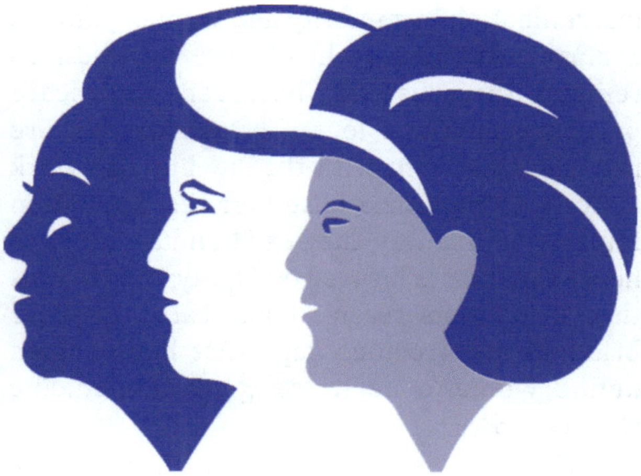

Figure 2.4. Logo for the Women's Health Initiative (WHI).

Source: https://upload.wikimedia.org/wikipedia/commons/thumb/1/1e/Women_logo.png/800px-Women_logo.png.

2.1.3. Impact of Historical Biases on Current Practices

The correct spelling is: The impact of historical bias on current practice in women's health is extreme, and it is communicated both at the structural and interpersonal levels of care. Historical perspectives had a tendency to render women's health concerns secondary to men's concerns, thus establishing systemic bias that remains present in medical literature and clinical practice. This bias impacts the way that medical providers treat women, particularly from minority groups. As recognized by research at UPMC Magee-Women's Hospital, there is a need for physicians to receive diversity training on the intersectionality of race and gender and patient care. By becoming acquainted with these historical backgrounds, which excluded women's health demands, practitioners can progress toward more equitable healthcare solutions that respect the particular lives of women, particularly Women of Color, who navigate double layers of discrimination and prejudice in the clinic environment (Moore, 2020). Health professionals' awareness and control of these biases are imperative to improving women's health outcomes. Culturally competent care-based training provides healthcare professionals with the skills to identify and respond to the disparities that Women of Color experience. Research indicates that the experiences of healthcare professionals affect their ability to know about diversity and, in turn, the quality of care they can provide. Addressing these prejudices not only serves ethical values but also has significant effects on their patients' outcomes. Inability to positively confront these historical biases stands to further extend perpetuating health inequities.

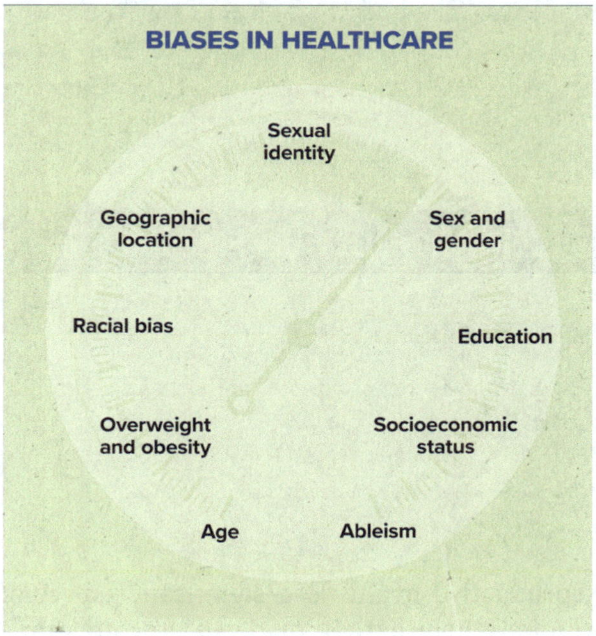

Figure 2.5. Biases in healthcare.

Source: https://i0.wp.com/post.medicalnewstoday.com/wp-content/uploads/sites/3/2021/09/bias-infographic-1168364-in-body-1296-v3-929x1024.png?w=1155&h=3000.

Through mandating diversity training and by fostering a culture of inclusion, institutions like UPMC Magee-Women's Hospital can encourage its staff to be in a better position to meet the multiple needs of their patient populations

(Moore, 2020). Moreover, the implications of customer discrimination in healthcare settings cannot be disregarded. Historical biases extend to institutional practice but extend further to patient engagement with health systems and, as a result, the quality of care provided for women. Research suggests that discrimination is both gender- and race-based and impacts minority patients' experiences within healthcare environments adversely. While anti-discrimination laws primarily protect workers from discrimination by their employers, they do very little in an effort to reverse the challenge of discrimination by minority and women patients against customers in healthcare facilities. To remedy these issues, however, healthcare professionals need to use strategies that are not only compliant with the law but also work actively to minimize customer discrimination impacts. In this way, they can build a culture of healthcare that is focused on equity and ensures that all patients receive equal care, therefore bridging the previous gaps that have helped define women's health in general medicine (Figure 2.5).

Test Your Knowledge

1. How has the understanding and treatment of women's health evolved over time within medical practice?
2. What have been some of the most significant milestones in the history of women's health advocacy?

2.2. Reproductive Health

Learning Outcome

1. Explain the importance of reproductive health services;
2. Discuss common reproductive health issues;
3. Deal with access to contraception and family planning.

Reproductive health is a significant aspect of women's health that involves a wide range of issues, from reproductive coercion to relationship abuse to the delivery of healthcare services. Recent studies have portrayed staggering numbers wherein approximately 12% of high school girls who were sexually active reported exposure to reproductive coercion, and another 17% reported physical or sexual teen dating violence. These factors not only restrict the entry of young women to necessary reproductive health care but also contribute to unstable sexual health behaviors. Care-seeking behavior study in the experiences demonstrates the necessity for healthcare providers to incorporate screenings for relationship abuse and reproductive coercion into routine care. This way, practitioners are likely to provide a more care-oriented healthcare culture that places prime importance on the safety and well-being of young women, thus leading to improved outcomes in reproductive health. Moreover, the issue of coercion and partner violence extends beyond the direct physical harm; it overlaps with more universal health policies that unintentionally continue to support these cycles of abuse. Research has indicated that reproductive coercion relationships could be linked with partners that are significantly older or have more numbers of sexual partners, which in turn can increase vulnerabilities. Surprisingly, both females who suffered from reproductive coercion and adolescent dating violence were found to have higher probabilities of being in serious relationships with significantly older partners, which might increase their risk of further abuse and harmful sexual health outcomes. Hence, it is essential to encourage comprehensive health education and resources that recognize these disparate dynamics. Reproductive coercion needs to be tackled well, not only with clinical care but also with systems-level reform in how adolescent relationships are understood and treated through healthcare systems. In addition, public policy addressing substance use during pregnancy has been shaped by more ingrained societal attitudes, particularly surrounding abortion. There is proof of an alarming trend where policies are being influenced more by an anti-abortion agenda than by concern for the health of women and their babies. It may discourage previous conversations about alcohol consumption during pregnancy, thereby causing negative health impacts. Steer clear of the acceptance of abortion as a healthy choice among women who abuse drugs is proof of broader societal stigma and can result in appropriate healthcare intervention. It is crucial that policymakers place equal emphasis on evidence-based practices that minimize risks to reproductive health, irrespective of the prejudices of presently dominant social standards. This could make the situation in which women's health is taken into account in its entirety possible, making access to support systems accessible to women in reproductive health.

2.2.1. Importance of Reproductive Health Services

Reproductive health care is also important because it contributes to enhancing women's health as it entails a wide range of health provisions that are used in addressing physical, social, and emotional well-being. The services incorporated include family planning, maternal healthcare, sexually transmitted infections (STIs) testing, and reproductive education. Reproductive health services help enable women to make educated choices regarding their reproductive lives, thus enhancing children's and mother's health. Proper care for women decreases the risks of pregnancy and delivery dramatically. This preventive approach is required in curtailing maternal mortality rates and maximizing neonatal well-being, which are important when dealing with high-risk populations. Unfortunately, obstacles such as restrictive policies create a turnaround that denies access to these services, depriving essential healthcare opportunities that generally determine the long-term patterns of health in women and their families. The role of reproductive health services also includes countering social determinants of women's health outcomes. Evidence is available that states that proper education and access to reproductive health services can empower women, and through this, they will make improved choices and have control over their bodies. Particularly, if women are confident to delay giving birth, they can make decisions about their life and income, and in turn enjoy improved health for themselves and their children. By improving women's nutritional status and reducing the generators of domestic violence, reproductive health services provide an enabling environment conducive to healthier pregnancies. The targeting of such psychosocial determinants is particularly critical in third-world countries, where limited access to reproductive health care is directly linked to high prematurity and maternal morbidity levels (Afulani et al., 2017). Comprehensive reproductive health services, therefore, constitute an imperative priority in the pursuit of equitable health outcomes. Secondly, the intersection of reproductive health services with public policy cannot be overstressed. Policymaking with reproductive health incorporated can create dramatic changes in standards of health at the public level. For instance, safely ensuring access to abortion services, along with prenatal and postnatal care, becomes vital in controlling unwanted pregnancy and reducing the stigma associated with reproductive decisions. However, as noted in more recent research, there are some state policies motivated by agendas of lower-priority public health, producing divergence from evidence-based practices (Roberts, 2019). Their impact can be adverse, inclined to perpetuate cycles of poor health outcomes for women and children. Therefore, advocating for policies favoring evidence-based reproductive health care is critical in combating such unwanted trends and creating a health-oriented agenda for women's health in mainstream medicine (Figure 2.6).

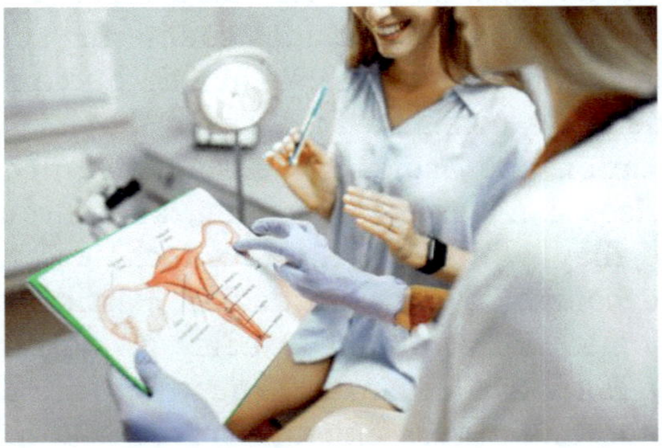

Figure 2.6. Educating women on reproductive health.

Source: https://www.hrmagazine.co.uk/media/2yehzjyl/women-health.jpeg?width=525&height=350&bgcolor=White&v=1d942223e56af90.

2.2.2. Common Reproductive Health Issues

Reproductive health issues encompass a wide range of conditions that significantly affect women's health across different populations. Of these, unwanted pregnancy and STIs are endemic issues that necessitate evidence-based public health solutions. Unwanted pregnancy can result from inadequate access to contraception methods, sexual illiteracy, or inadequate use of available services. The effects can extend far beyond individual health, influencing socioeconomic status, education, and overall quality of life. STIs are a serious public health problem as well, with young women being particularly vulnerable based on biology and social circumstance. Resolution of the issues will require several simultaneous efforts that include expanding access to health care, sex education, and community-based prevention and health literacy programs. One final key component of reproductive health involves the role of relationship dynamics on women's health status. The two terms of reproductive coercion and relationship abuse highlight how intimate partner violence can directly impact reproductive decision-making and health. Studies have indicated that young women with reproductive coercion, in which coercion may appear as force to use a specific contraceptive or become pregnant, often experience significant barriers to accessing reproductive health care. For instance, research has established that relationship abuse is linked to a higher risk for risky sex, which in turn raises the risk for STIs and unplanned pregnancy. Among sexually active adolescents, having an understanding of such dynamics is important; peer support and knowledge about resources can allow young women to reach the proper care and make appropriate decisions about their reproductive health (Hill et al., 2019). Moreover, drug use while pregnant continues to be a reproductive health controversy, as it has an enormous effect on the health outcomes of the mother and fetus. State alcohol-use-during-pregnancy policies have been described in recent literature as having more of an anti-abortion agenda and less to do with public health concerns. This shift affects health practice, in which a recommendation for abortion after exposure to alcohol during pregnancy is no longer widely acknowledged. Such policy frameworks can discourage women from seeking early prenatal care, which is most important to avoid substance-related harm during pregnancy. Thus, public health interventions must shift to highlight evidence-based practices that improve maternal health in the absence of the stigma surrounding reproductive choice, thereby reducing the incidence of alcohol-related pregnancy complications (Roberts, 2019) (Figure 2.7).

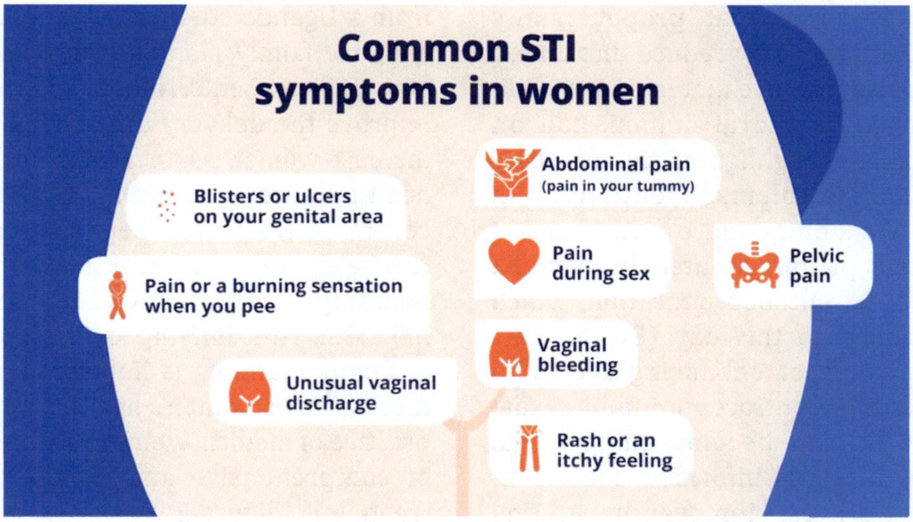

Figure 2.7. Common STI symptoms in women.

Source: https://res.cloudinary.com/zava-www-uk/image/upload/c_fill/q_70/a_exif,f_auto,e_sharpen:100,c_thumb,w_720,h_405/v1641554053/uk/services-and-products/sexual-health/sti-test-kits/content-pages/sti-symptoms-in-women/sus6mgjk2niaeerneygs.jpg.

2.2.3. Access to Contraception and Family Planning

Family planning and contraception availability is a critical element of women's health that allows women to make informed reproductive choices and attain general health. In societies worldwide, access to such vital services is denied on socio-economic grounds, geographic locations, and cultural stigmatization.

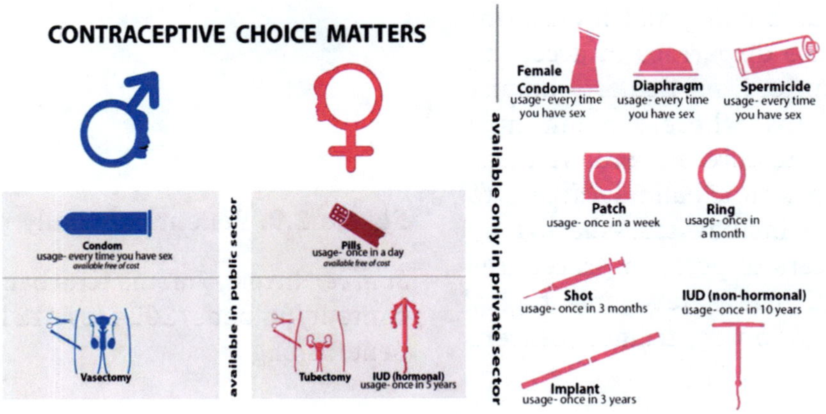

Figure 2.8. Access to contraception.

Source: https://cdn.slidesharecdn.com/ss_thumbnails/access-to-contraceptionpfi-160318041946-thumbnail.jpg?width=640&height=640&fit=bounds.

Evidence has revealed that proper family planning programs not only reduce unplanned pregnancy, but also improve maternal and child health outcomes. The Royal Commission on Human Relationships highlighted the necessity to address such problems, mentioning in particular the availability and effectiveness of the existing family planning centers in Australia and responsible parenthood education, which remains a problem to this day (Evatt et al., 1977). The outcome of enhancing access to education regarding contraception and sexual health is that women become empowered, enabling them to make informed choices in their reproductive lives. Moreover, integrating family planning services in the course of regular medical care is essential for enhancing women's health (Figure 2.8). Effective family planning activities can alleviate the medical, social, and psychological loads faced by women regarding unwanted pregnancy. The findings suggest a necessity for proper training in contraceptive techniques among healthcare providers to effectively counsel women (Evatt et al., 1977). Improved training and sensitization of medical staff can lead to effective support mechanisms for women, enabling them to better manage reproductive health issues. Closing these gaps by way of additional training and investment can eventually reduce disparities in access to family planning services, particularly among disadvantaged groups where women may face double barriers to care. In rural settings, innovative approaches to expanding access to contraception could include task-sharing by trained clinical officers to perform procedures like tubal ligation. The safety and highly acceptable tubal ligation by trained officers from a Uganda study showed a model that can enhance family planning services in resource-poor environments. Not only do these strategies improve the delivery of services, but they also increase women's satisfaction with reproductive health choices. Examining different models of contraceptive access, better service to women can be delivered by health systems, ultimately resulting in reproductive autonomy and equity in health. This unifying focus on the availability of family planning is important in the current discussion of women's health across the general practice of medicine, emphasizing an imperative of comprehensive and inclusive options for treatment (Figure 2.9).

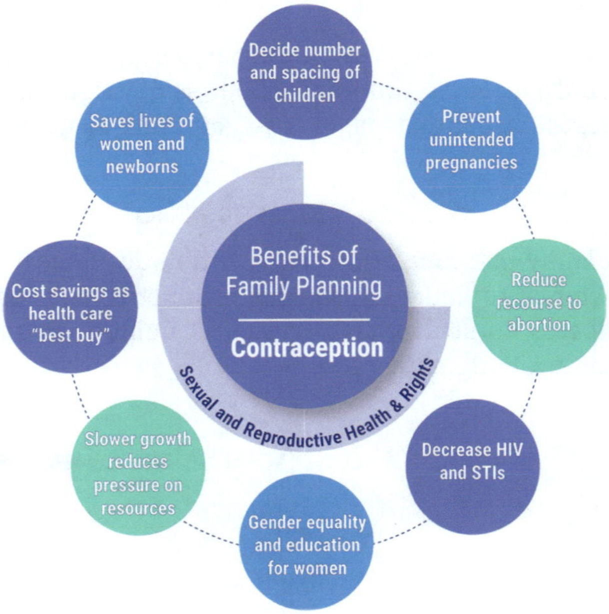

Figure 2.9. Benefits of family planning.

Source: https://media.tciurbanhealth.org/wp-content/uploads/2024/07/12110147/circles-benefits.png.

Test Your Knowledge

1. Why is access to comprehensive reproductive health care vital for women's physical, emotional, and economic well-being throughout different stages of life?
2. What are the most common reproductive health conditions affecting women?

2.3. Maternal Health

Learning Outcome

1. Understand prenatal care and its significance;
2. Discuss complications during pregnancy and childbirth;
3. Focus on postpartum care and mental health.

Maternal health is a significant component of women's general health in general medicine, with immediate impact on short-term and long-term health status in both mothers and their children. Delivery of effective prenatal care (PNC) is a fundamental requirement in the fulfillment of the personal needs of expectant women. Literature in opposition to existing PNC recommendations reports such to be marred with contradictions in the education and counseling components provided to pregnant mothers. Successful prenatal education is not only necessary in educating women on their health but also in empowering them to make intelligent choices on their care. Empowerment positions women as active participants in managing their health, having a sense of agency, which is central to their health as a whole. Addressing the peculiar needs and bridging research gaps remains vital in developing guidelines that actually prioritize maternal health, and thereby promoting families' and communities' health as a whole (Hanson et al., 2009). Premature sickness is a critical area in maternal health since prematurity, which is the leading cause of mortality among children aged five and below worldwide, is a significant challenge. In order to solve the issue of prematurity, one needs an approach that is multidimensional, with consideration of clinical and sociocultural determinants behind the trend. Women's empowerment has been viewed as crucial in minimizing the risk of premature births. Indicators of this are improved access to health care, increased decision-making power on reproductive health, and a reduction in domestic violence. These factors allow better maternal nutrition, enhance pregnancy spacing, and ultimately lead to better pregnancy outcomes. Although there is not much direct evidence showing empowerment's relationship to a reduction in prematurity rates, the indirect gains from empowering women illustrate the necessity to give women's health programs priority in mainstream medicine (Afulaniet al., 2017). Incorporating maternal health issues into a broad perspective of women's health within general medicine not only highlights the complexity at play but also underscores interventions aimed at specific areas as most important. Stakeholders must place the highest priority on research that examines women's empowerment as the lead determinant in realizing better maternal health. Such efforts can drive policy reforms and improve access to services that address women's needs. This integrative approach to women's health can lead to a better understanding of the interconnection between social, economic, and health determinants of maternal health. Identification and attention to these connected factors can help the medical field develop a more integrative approach that enhances the health and autonomy of women and is also advantageous for families and communities (Hanson et al., 2009; Afulani et al., 2017).

2.3.1. Prenatal Care and Its Significance

The importance of prenatal care to the health of women is of high magnitude since it forms a basis for normal infant and maternal outcomes as well as pregnancies. Prenatal visits for check-ups in low-risk pregnancy visits allow physicians to monitor the physical as well as emotional health of pregnant mothers and detect early complications that can occur, which can be controlled. The proactive approach is critical in controlling risks associated with giving birth. For instance, studies indicate that early vaginal deliveries are less likely to lead to higher maternal morbidities, compromised quality of life, particularly among primiparas compared to women with vaginal delivery (Mousavi et al., 2013). Thus, PNC can significantly assist in curtailing unwarranted surgical interventions, facilitate healthier delivery processes, ultimately culminating in improved maternal health and satisfaction. Besides addressing physical health, prenatal care can also play a major part in addressing the mental aspect of pregnancy. The majority of women experience mental illness during this time, ranging from anxiety, depression or even postpartum distress.

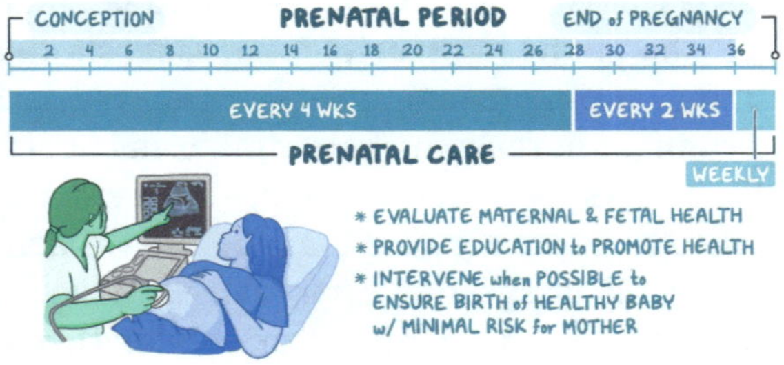

Figure 2.10. Prenatal care.

Source: https://www.osmosis.org/_next/image?url=https%3A%2F%2Fd16qt3wv6xm098.cloudfront.net%2FdGX20zPGSW23qsccDIBvKHQKTS6SIZ9f%2F_.jpg&w=3840&q=75.

For example, a study of Saudi Arabian young mothers indicated a prevalence of psychological distress of 35.2%, showing an immediate need for appropriate mental health screenings during pregnancy (Amr et al., 2011). Incorporating mental health screenings within prenatal care can assist in identifying at-risk women and intervening accordingly. This dual focus on mental and physical health ensures that women receive holistic care, significantly enhancing both their pregnancy experience and ability to cope with the changes and challenges thereof. Moreover, effective prenatal care offers an educational platform that can equip pregnant women with the information they need concerning pregnancy, birth, and post-childbirth care. Health practitioners can provide advice regarding diet, exercise, and lifestyles that produce healthier outcomes for the mother and child (Figure 2.10). Educating women on warning signs of potential complications and the importance of early medical care can be an essential element to salvage risks of adolescent pregnancies or those complicated by antecedent concomitant health factors like gestational diabetes (Amr et al., 2011). Thus, prenatal care is not just a sequence of medical visits but an essential aspect of integrated maternal health to empower women to be the masters of their reproductive health and well-being during pregnancy (Figure 2.11).

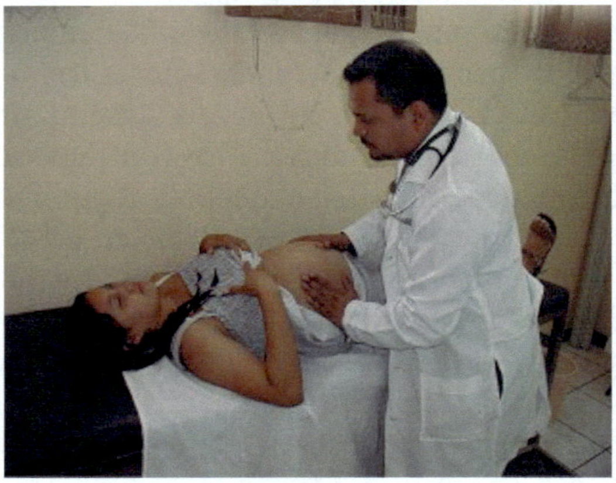

Figure 2.11. A doctor performs a prenatal exam.

Source: https://upload.wikimedia.org/wikipedia/commons/b/be/Hoact21.jpg.

2.3.2. Complications During Pregnancy and Childbirth

Pregnancy and child complications are a significant concern in women's health that both impact maternal and fetal outcomes. Complications can be brought about by numerous diverse causes, such as pre-existing disease, economic status, and mental health. For instance, a teenage pregnancy is likely to have a high risk of physical health complications and postpartum psychiatric disorders. One of the studies conducted in Al Ahsa, Saudi Arabia, revealed 35.2% of young mothers with signs of psychological distress and risk factors of low family income, husband's poor support, and gestational diabetes. The findings highlight the necessity of careful screening and perinatal care interventions focused on overcoming not only physical but also psychological and social aspects of maternal health before, during, and after pregnancy (Amr et al., 2011). The. Another pressing concern is the rise in the rate of cesarean deliveries that has been attributed to some maternal morbidities. It has been established through research, a woman's quality of life would be adversely affected by cesarean deliveries, particularly for first-time mothers (primiparas). A study from Shahroud, Iran, compared outcomes related to the quality of life of women who had cesarean and vaginal deliveries.

Results showed that primiparas with cesarean births scored lower for physical, psychological, and social quality of life in comparison to those who gave birth through vaginal delivery. The extreme variance in results highlights the relevance of meticulous consideration of delivery method, particularly for low-risk pregnancies, with emphasis on informed consent and collaborative decision-making between the healthcare providers and expectant women (Mousavi et al., 2013). Furthermore, complications during childbirth extend from immediate physical well-being issues to include long-term psychological and emotional effects. The traumatic nature of birth, often intensified by unplanned medical interventions like emergency cesareans, can lead to extreme psychological trauma, post-traumatic stress disorder (PTSD) for new mothers as well. The trend speaks to the multifaceted nature of childbirth and support systems that enable emotional healing alongside physical healing. Accompanying postpartum care, such as mental health screening and supportive counseling, is crucial to enable holistic recovery and address the unique needs of women at this vulnerable period. Prioritizing physical and mental well-being in perinatal care has the potential to enable the healthcare professionals to initiate better long-term outcomes for mothers and infants (Figure 2.12).

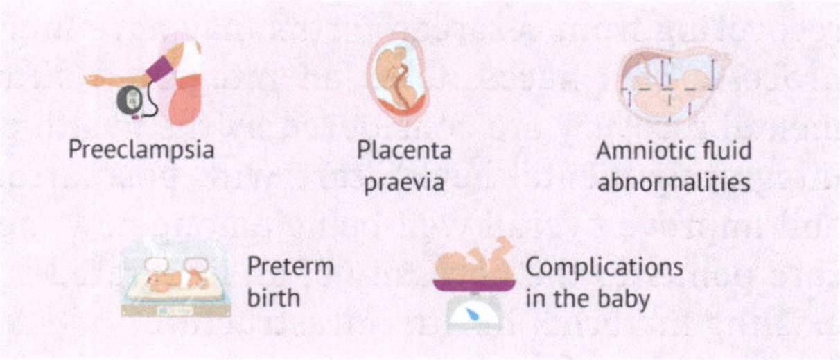

Figure 2.12. Examples of possible complications during pregnancy.

Source: https://www.invitra.com/en/wp-content/uploads/2014/04/complications-during-pregnancy-1536x653.png.

2.3.3. Postpartum Care and Mental Health

Postpartum is a crucial phase that requires serious attention in women's health, particularly with reference to mental health. Women, after having given birth, experience drastic physical and psychological transformations, which could eventually lead to a range of psychological problems. Studies have consistently found that postpartum psychological distress is prevalent and affects approximately 35.2% of new mothers, particularly in certain groups. Risk factors, including low income at home, partner's support, and medical conditions , including gestational diabetes are significant predictors of postpartum distress (Amr et al., 2011). Early intervention and detection will be critical since the risk factors must be determined and interventions that are suitable can lead to improved health outcomes for infants and mothers. Integration of routine mental health screening into postpartum care can allow for early treatment and support and therefore lead to better maternal and child health. Other than psychological distress, the mode of delivery can also influence postpartum mental health status. Research has proven that women who undergo cesarean sections can have their quality of life decreased when compared with women who deliver vaginally. In one of the experiments that examined women who gave birth by cesarean, the women with cesarean births had lower physical, psychological, and social quality of life scores at eight weeks following childbirth (Mousavi et al., 2013). The implication of this is quite drastic: women recovering from cesarean births may have more emotional challenges to get through the recovery process. This necessitates an integrated strategy of postpartum care where the physical and mental recovery are considered by the health providers in line with the mode of delivery. Through integrating mental health care with postpartum care, healthcare systems can enhance resilience and improve overall well-being among new mothers. Also, the intricate interaction of postpartum care points to the necessity of an integrated strategy that includes mental health interventions in existing maternal health infrastructure.

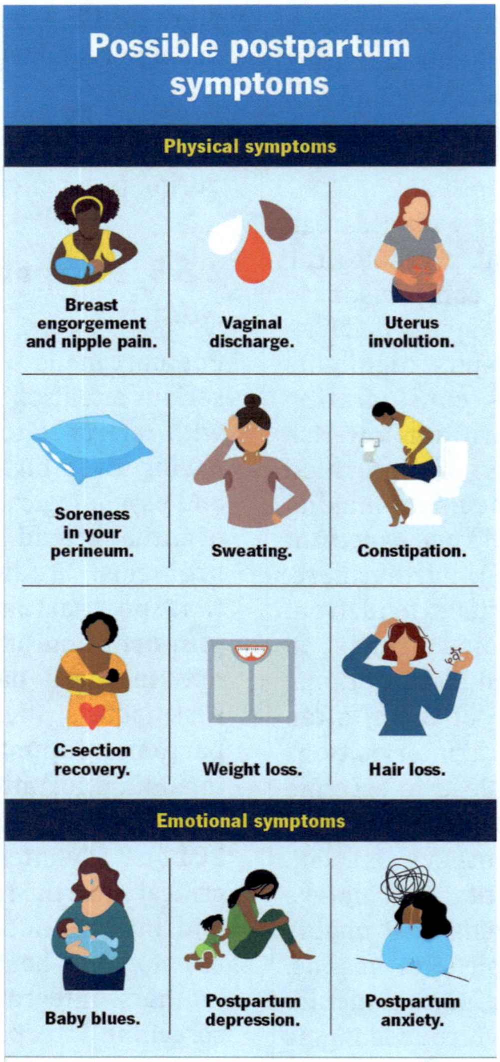

Figure 2.13. Possible postpartum symptoms to care.

Source: https://my.clevelandclinic.org/-/scassets/images/org/health/articles/postpartum.

Training and sensitization on symptom and sign awareness of postpartum mental health disorders can empower women and families. Creating environments that are conducive and supportive, where mental health is discussed regularly can encourage women to seek services when needed. In addition, consideration of sociocultural variables, such as family and partner participation, can be instrumental in personalizing support services for new mothers (Amr et al., 2011). Ultimately, better postpartum care requires the combined effort of healthcare professionals, families, and communities to place mental health as a priority of equal importance as physical health on women's healthcare agendas. By doing this, society can create healthier generations and reduce the long-term effects of undiagnosed postpartum mental disorders (Figure 2.13).

Test Your Knowledge

1. Why is regular prenatal care essential for both maternal and fetal health?
2. What are some of the most common complications that can arise during pregnancy and childbirth?

2.4. Chronic Conditions

Learning Outcome

1. Understand the prevalence of chronic diseases in women;
2. Discuss gender differences in disease presentation and treatment;
3. Explain the importance of tailored management strategies.

Chronic diseases are a great threat to the field of women's health and manifest in many forms, like hormonal disorders, autoimmune conditions, and syndromes of chronic pain. Chronic pelvic pain (CPP) is among the most debilitating chronic diseases. It has been defined as pain lasting more than three to six months. CPP may be extremely debilitating for the quality of life of a woman by hindering everyday activities and good health. The etiology of CPP is multifactorial, comprising both structural pathologies, such as endometriosis, and idiopathic. Current scientific wisdom emphasizes that an integrated model is required in therapy, encompassing not just the medical line but also lifestyle modifications and psychosocial guidance. The integrated model not just addresses the bodily symptoms of the disease but also the psychosomatic burdens usually entailed in chronic pain syndromes (Ball & Khan, 2020). Furthermore, the intersection of chronic disease and social determinants of health further complicates the case of women's health more complicated. Economic disparity is also a central element in a woman's ability to seek care and manage chronic conditions appropriately. In major urban cities such as Los Angeles, homelessness exacerbates health threats, particularly for women with chronic disease. The chronic stress of homelessness, along with limited healthcare access, creates a perfect storm that fast-tracks the prevalence of health problems. Research has established that homeless individuals experience higher rates of death and chronic disease due to the interaction of environmental determinants and limited access to care. As such, interventions into women's health must consider an awareness of these broader structural determinants in order to build effective health interventions (Kuhn et al., 2020). Additionally, the prevention of chronic diseases in women's health necessitates gender-specific public health interventions and research. Much of what is present data about chronic conditions does not accurately reflect the unique physiological and psychosocial processes affecting women differently than men. Such illnesses as rheumatoid arthritis and fibromyalgia, which disproportionately affect women, necessitate gender-specific treatments regarding hormonal alteration and social stigmatization. It is critical to promote increased funding of women's health research, as well as priority access policies supporting comprehensive care for the involved groups. Lastly, the creation of more efficacious treatment protocols through increased understanding of how chronic illness generally engages with women's health can result in healthier outcomes for women from various demographics and socioeconomic statuses (Ball & Khan, 2020) (Figure 2.14).

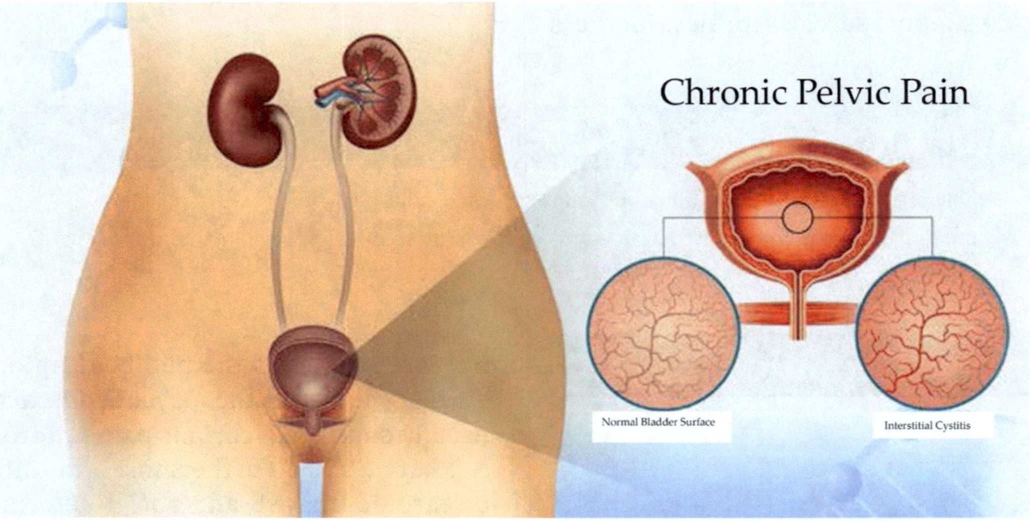

Figure 2.14. Illustration of chronic pelvic pain.

Source: https://drdhanshreegynaec.com/images/services/chronic-pelvic-pain.jpg.

2.4.1. Prevalence of Chronic Diseases in Women

The prevalence of chronic diseases among women is a significant public health concern in which consideration should be given consideration in general practice. Women disproportionately develop diseases such as diabetes, hypertension, and cardiovascular disease, and they are particularly affected as years pass. Studies indicate that women are more likely than men to develop several chronic conditions at the same time, often referred to as multimorbidity, whose management and treatment become more complicated. The outcomes of such chronic ailments extend beyond the physical health of women to influence mental well-being and the capability to take part in life. With the health of women changing over time, it is imperative to have an understanding of these estimates of prevalence in framing healthcare services and developing targeted prevention measures using women's own experience and needs within a clinical environment. Addressing the problem of chronic disease in women entails understanding the social determinants and economic drivers of health inequity. Disadvantaged women are subjected to higher risk factors for chronic disease, which are normally linked to socioeconomic position, access to healthcare, and determinants of health. These inequities may lead to delayed diagnosis, uncontrolled disease, and poorer outcomes, perpetuating a cycle of chronic disease that affects women's quality of life. Interventions and health policy must include consideration of these, with a view to bridging gaps in access to care as well as promoting educational interventions that empower women to make their health choices. Additionally, placing community-based resources on the health agenda can serve to enhance women's health outcomes, reiterating the importance of integrative healthcare provision. The working role of healthcare providers is still at the center for tackling chronic diseases prevalent in women. Coordination of care must be efficient, especially when patients experience multimorbidity. Clinicians must make prioritization of thorough examination that will tackle the diverse and complex interplays of these chronic conditions. Moreover, they must facilitate open communication and collaborative decision-making with patients such that care is compatible with women's personal and social contexts. By enhancing the strategies for diagnosis, treatment, and management of chronic disease, practitioners can enhance women's health outcomes. With continuous progress in research, institutions such as the International Council on Women's Health Issues (ICOWHI) advocate for more emphasis on women's health, since they again call for collaboration in research, education, and policy to promote women's health globally (Almirall et al., 2013). These are the areas that need to be tackled because they directly affect the future health of women in society (Almirall & Fortin, 2013).

2.4.2. Gender Differences in Disease Presentation and Treatment

Gender variation in the presentation of disease is significant in the practice of women's health, particularly in general medical practice. Research indicates that biological, psychological, and sociocultural determinants influence the way diseases present themselves in women compared to men. For instance, coronary heart disease (CHD) tends to manifest symptoms that are relatively different between the two genders. Women may present with atypical symptoms, such as dyspnea or anxiety-based presentations, instead of the typical chest pain with CHD in men. Such variability complicates diagnosis and management, indicating the importance of adopting a gender-sensitive approach to clinical care. By discerning and addressing these differences, healthcare professionals are better positioned to individualize their practice, leading to improved results and patient satisfaction among women patients, as supported by personalized medicine goals advocated in contemporary medical literature (Gemmati et al., 2019). In diagnostic tests as well, there are also gender differences pertaining to treatment protocols and drug responsiveness. For instance, women are more likely to report symptoms typical of anxiety disorders in circumstances that might overlap with bodily distress. Studies revealed that women were more prone to complaining of heart flutter and dizziness than men, thereby demonstrating the extent to which psychological processes can obscure the clinical presentation of underlying illness. Also, the prescription of antianxiety or antidepressant medication is more likely in women who present with symptoms of CHD, demonstrating the manner in which treatment models might inadvertently exclude the possibility of cardiovascular disease for female patients. This requires treatment protocols to be reassessed to include these gender-specific responses so that they might be better managed (Carmin et al., 2008). Not only is the importance of gender differences transcendent in presentation and treatment strategies, but it also emphasizes the necessity of an integrative medical science approach. Trends towards the application of gender medicine can help to bridge gaps in what has been established with respect to the contribution of sex and gender to outcomes along life's stages. A concentration on multidisciplinary questions integrating biological markers with psychosocial activities has the potential to transform healthcare practice. This dynamic approach, addressing prevention of disease and enhanced prognosis, encourages equally effective and equitable care for every patient as well. Therefore, with the practice of medicine proceeding further in the direction of personalized approaches, gender differences are still a fundamental principle toward enhancing women's health in general medicine, eventually leading to parity in healthcare delivery (Gemmati et al., 2019) (Figure 2.15).

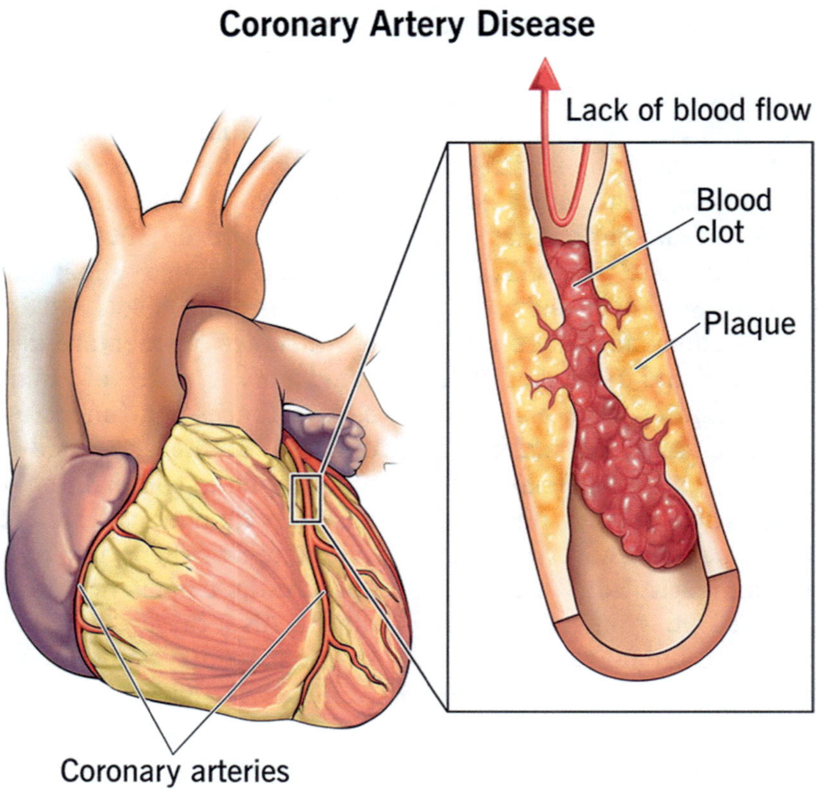

Figure 2.15. Coronary heart disease (CHD)

Source: https://my.clevelandclinic.org/-/scassets/images/org/health/articles/16898-coronary-artery-disease.

2.4.3. Importance of Tailored Management Strategies

The need for gender-specific management approaches in women's health is reflected by the addition of gender-specific variables to practice. The traditional approach has a tendency to overlook how unique combinations of biological and psychosocial variables occur in women. This oversight can lead to less-than-optimal prevention and treatment strategies that fail to recognize the nuances of female health. By incorporating gender medicine, which emphasizes the significance of both biological sex and sociocultural gender, clinicians are able to create individualized care plans with these in mind. Putting sex/gender first in clinical assessment and treatment guidelines allows clinicians to more effectively identify risk to health and optimize therapeutic intervention and, ultimately, enhance outcomes in female patients. Such a paradigm shift is necessary to construct a more integrated, individualized concept of women's health that is congruent with the changing needs of today's diverse populations (Gemmati et al., 2019). Management approaches tailored to the individualized needs of individual categories of women have also proven particularly valuable in addressing lifestyle-related health challenges. For instance, recent investigations of an Internet-delivered physical activity intervention for sedentary Latinas revealed stunning physical activity increases when the intervention was individually tailored and culturally adapted to participants' needs. This study demonstrated that women in a tailored intervention reported large physical activity gains compared with a control group and illustrated the merit of culturally sensitive approaches to health promotion (Bock et al., 2016). The effectiveness of such individualized strategies affirms the premise that management plans, with synchronization in the specific cultural and social contexts of women, can lead to significant health behavior and outcome enhancements, marking the necessity of tailoring healthcare services. The impacts of individualized management extend beyond the physical plane, incorporating psychological and social issues that affect women's experiences of healthcare. For example, responding to mental health needs through a needs-based approach can deconstruct barriers that tend to limit women's access to care. By recognizing the unique stressors that women may face, such as caregiving responsibilities or societal stress, physicians can create more effective support systems and interventions. These initiatives not only empower women but also contribute to an improved healthcare model that values and respects their diversity. The acceptance of personalized management practices in women's health therefore becomes not just a medical requirement but also an ethical imperative, fostering overall well-being and equal access to the care of all women and, in turn, furthering the larger goals of medicine in general (Gemmati et al., 2019).

Test Your Knowledge

1. What are the most common chronic diseases affecting women?
2. How do certain chronic diseases, like cardiovascular disease or depression, present differently in women compared to men?
3. Why is it essential to develop and implement chronic disease management plans that are specifically tailored to women's unique physiological, hormonal, and psychosocial needs?

2.5. Mental Health

Learning Outcome

1. Describe common mental health issues affecting women;
2. Explain societal factors influencing women's mental health;
3. Understand the importance of mental health screenings in general practice.

Mental well-being is a critical aspect of the overall health of women, particularly when they transition to various phases of life. Interpersonal violence, including physical and verbal abuse, significantly impacts the mental outcomes of women's health. Research indicates that most women, particularly post-menopausal women, experience any degree of abuse, leading to compromised physical and mental functioning over time. The psychological toll of such incidents can be anxiety, depression, and overall decreased quality of life. It requires consciousness to eliminate these in the backdrop of women's health, as well as proactive measures by medical professionals to identify and treat such individuals. Clinicians must be capable of recognizing the signs of abuse and its mental effects, utilizing interventions that foster recovery and motivate healthy mental health in survivors (Cannell et al., 2015). As women's health in general medicine continues to evolve, the inclusion of mental health services becomes increasingly important, especially with marginalized groups. The SGM needs must be met in this case, as the groups tend to suffer specific mental health problems combined with institutional biases and a lack of inclusive healthcare policy. While there has been acknowledgment of the aforementioned disparities, a staggering disparity remains in the curriculum materials presented to healthcare professionals regarding SGM health issues, of which mental health is prominent. Scholarship indicates that program directors are more amenable to having more integrated training in SGM health within medical curricula, but are impeded by barriers such as perceived lack of need. This mismatch not only impacts education for future healthcare providers but also provides mental health courses for SGM patients, who are stigmatized and misunderstood in clinical settings (Hanson et al., 2009). Given the interconnectedness of mental and other aspects of women's health, holistic solutions have to be developed to facilitate global care. Having the ability to recognize the multi-factorial determinants of mental health, such as socio-economic status, culture, and access to healthcare, enables one to better comprehend what women are up against. General medicine must put a high value on women's mental health assessments and treatments. Secondarily, developing an open discussion culture regarding mental health can encourage vulnerable women to seek assistance without threatening their self-respect or respect from others. This not only enhances individual health but also community resilience, with the ultimate goal being improved overall health in women from a variety of environments. With the management of physical and mental health together, the practice of general medicine can be a transformative force in women's health (Cannell et al., 2015).

2.5.1. Common Mental Health Issues Affecting Women

The female psychological profile is marked by its own particular set of difficulties, which are most commonly based on society and gender-related issues. Widespread diseases such as depression and anxiety are heavy burdens for women, and many studies have determined that women are two times more likely than men to be impacted by mood disorders. These mental illnesses can be compounded by illnesses such as reproductive health episodes, including premenstrual syndrome (PMS), pregnancy, and menopause, which can trigger or aggravate depressive illness. Also, the presence of trauma, including domestic violence and rape, may validate a cycle of declining mental health among women. The necessity of addressing such issues is highlighted through historical reviews, e.g., the Royal Commission on Human Relationships, whereby priority was highlighted in determining the intersection of gender, mental health, and family structures of support, hence the call for required public discourse and policy adaptation towards women's mental health (Evatt et al., 1977). Notably, the complexities of eating disorders also provide a dismal perspective on women's mental health issues. Anorexia and bulimia, for instance, are not simply personal issues; they are strongly influenced by sociocultural contexts that affect gender identity and body perceptions. Feminist accounts provide significant commentary on such issues, grounded in the argument that societal construction of femininity establishes the norms to which women feel compelled to aspire, leading to self-destructive tendencies. Research indicates that women with such histories are likely to find their treatment pathways influenced—or dissuaded—by prevailing biomedical models that dismiss the sociocultural dimensions of their experiences. Encouraging women to speak about these dynamics has been found to enrich and empower therapeutic interventions, turning treatment into an experience of empowerment and self-definition (Holmes, 2016). Moreover, the stigma of mental illnesses gives an extra complicated level of challenge to women when they want help. Social culture makes people enforce vulnerability and strength standards, and most women are socialized to conceal their suffering. Stigma has the chance to lead to symptom magnification and prolonged suffering indirectly by minimizing mental illnesses and avoiding professional help. Initiatives via mental health awareness campaigns and education programs focused on breaking these stigmas are essential to establishing enabling environments in which open discussion is encouraged. Additionally, additional training for healthcare providers in reading these gender-specific illnesses can become a crucial measure in the promotion of early detection and treatment. With women's mental wellbeing now very much at the forefront of the global health agenda, it is essential that policy makers heed these complexities in a bid to implement an even more inclusive and effective healthcare system tailored to women's unique needs (Evatt et al., 1977) (Figure 2.16).

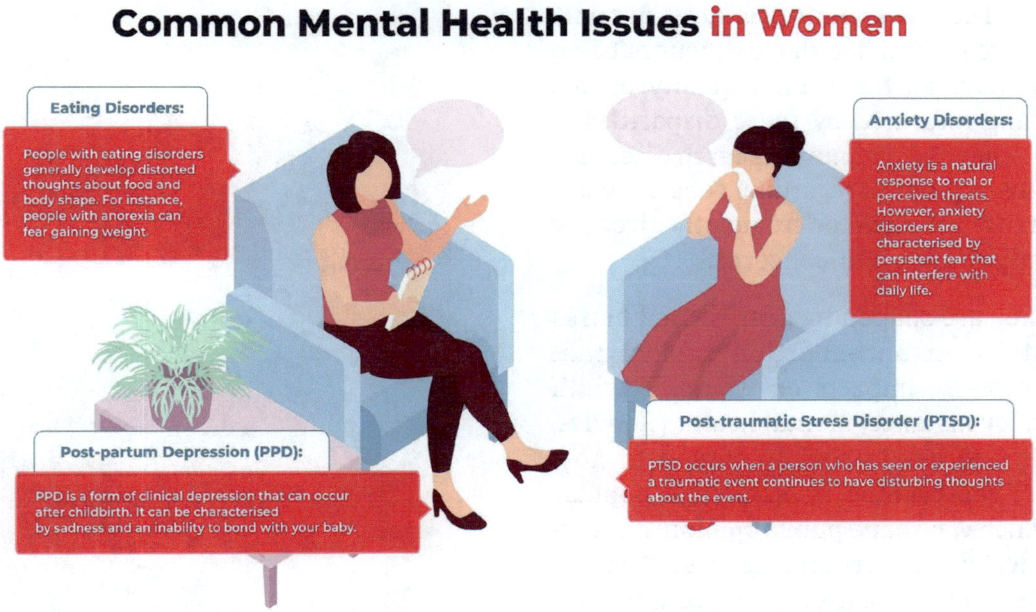

Figure 2.16. Common mental health issues in women.

Source: https://ik.imagekit.io/d7t01fhx21/Ovum_Hospitals/Blogs/Women's%20mental%20health%20common%20issues%20and%20how%20to%20get%20help-01.jpg?updatedAt=1734592538570.

2.5.2. Societal Factors Influencing Women's Mental Health

The intricate play of societal factors has a marked influence on women's mental health, with gender roles and cultural norms at the fore. Societal norms around caregiving roles for women can lead to increased tension and anxiety in balancing more than one role at a time such as work, family, and societal expectations. These pressures will further women's mental diseases such as depression and anxiety, thus making it challenging for them to access necessary mental health care. Furthermore, stigma within society can bar women from receiving assistance, leading to a cycle of pain and isolation. Organizations like the ICOWHI advocate for the empowerment of women through education and research, highlighting the urgent need for caring environments that recognize the impact of societal expectations on women's mental well-being (Almirall & Fortin, 2013). Economic disparities introduce additional social determinants of impact on women's mental well-being, at times reinforcing one another. Women, especially those in disadvantaged groups, can regularly encounter barriers to employment, leading to economic insecurity. Since gender discrimination at work is so deeply entrenched, women can earn less than their male colleagues, instilling inadequacy and anxiety. These economic pressures not only limit access to mental health treatment but also have an impact on the overall quality of life. Policymaking informed by these disparities is desperately needed; yet new research discovers that state-level policies regarding substance use and pregnancy are aitch too frequently diverting away from public health concerns.

Instead, they are shaped by deep-seated biases motivated by an anti-abortion agenda that can have adverse impacts on women's health outcomes, for instance, mental health (Roberts, 2019). Also, forces in society extend to how women are represented in media and popular culture, which can shape public opinion and self-concept. Idealized beauty and idealized living, as depicted on various platforms, place immense pressure on women to achieve a standard, posing a likelihood of inducing a feeling of inadequacy or low self-worth. Ubiquitous social media culture exacerbates these, with users constantly comparing and contrasting, leading to negative effects on mental health, for example, anxiety and body image disorders. It is important that society acknowledges the damaging effects of such representations and demands more realistic and representative representations of women. By nurturing tales that affirm and uplift rather than sully women's self-worth, mental illness can be avoided, and so a broader cultural shift toward wellness and resilience in women's health discourse.

2.5.3. Importance of Mental Health Screenings in General Practice

Routine mental health screening is essential to the detection and management of psychological issues in women, who are often at heightened risk after a host of biological and sociocultural influences. Women experience unique challenges of mental health that include the risk of pregnancy and motherhood and can elicit powerful affective responses.

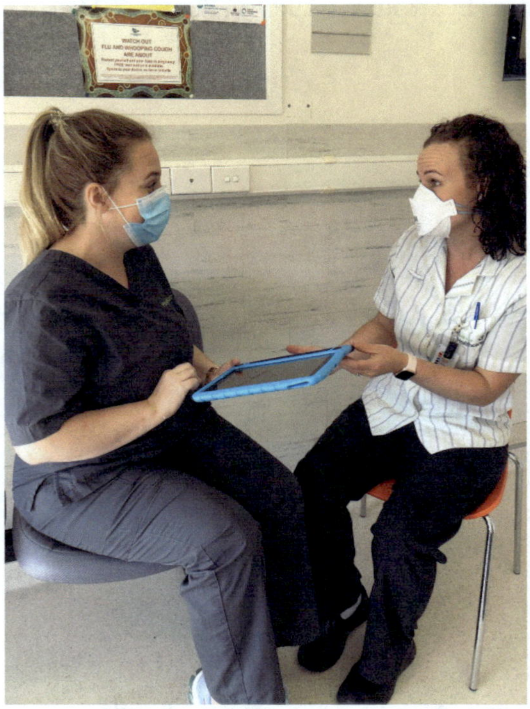

Figure 2.17. Illustration of mental health screening.

Source: https://southwesthealthcare.com.au/wp-content/uploads/IMG_7492-scaled.jpg.

The following are grounds for it being highly essential that physicians adopt routine mental health screening on regular visits. Research indicates that systematic screening is able to uncover underlying conditions that would otherwise be concealed by the patient, allowing interventions to be introduced in good time. Such preventive interventions eventually result in a reduction in the prevalence of mental disorders, enhancement in quality of life, and enhanced overall health outcomes for women, further highlighting the essential role that general practitioners' mental health screenings play as part of women's healthcare. Besides, mental impact can often be amplified at critical life periods, such as pregnancy and postpartum periods. For instance, postpartum periods have been indicated to contain increased rates of depression, and it is documented that a fifth of mothers of preterm infants develop clinically significant depressive symptoms as opposed to 1 in 10 mothers of full-term infants (Bush et al., 2022). These discrepancies reflect the value of targeted screening of certain populations, particularly those with additional stressors. To this end, the addition of mental health screens into primary practice not only assists in identifying at-risk patients but also promotes a preventative model, allowing for the offering of support and resources by healthcare providers. This is also in line with existing guidelines that emphasize the need for integrated care systems to take physical and mental health in combination. Secondly, evidence from more recent studies confirms the benefits of routine mental health screening throughout a woman's lifetime. Effective screenings can lead clinicians to identify trends in signs and symptoms of mental health and support individualized care plans. For example, comprehensive prenatal care policies suggest that women's educational needs be met alongside physical health screening to meet their needs properly (Hanson et al., 2009). Incorporating mental health as part of standard medical practice can enable women to take an active role in their care, which can lead to better long-term health for mothers and families. By early intervention and identification, mental health screening could prevent long-term damage from untreated mental health disorders and increase the quality of care in women's health across general practice (Figure 2.17).

Test Your Knowledge

1. What are the most prevalent mental health disorders among women?
2. How do societal pressures impact women's mental health across different cultures and age groups?
3. Why is it critical for general practitioners and primary care providers to include routine mental health screenings for women?

2.6. Preventive Care

Learning Outcome

1. Understand the fundamentals of recommended screenings and vaccinations for women;
2. Explain the role of lifestyle factors in women's health;
3. Discuss the importance of patient education and awareness.

Preventive care is significant for women's health as a preventative approach to the avoidance of disease and general health. Preventive care in the form of periodic health screenings, immunizations, and lifestyle changes can significantly mitigate threats from common women's health diseases such as cardiovascular disease, diabetes, and cancers. These preventive interventions are particularly crucial during times of life transition, such as pregnancy and postpartum, times of greatest vulnerability to medical suggestion. Prevalence of preventive care should take priority; healthcare providers can foster women's health improvement, reduce healthcare costs from chronic diseases, and facilitate better patient-provider relationships that encourage sustained engagement in health-improving activities. Evidence points towards the importance of having a PCP before pregnancy since women who do have such an arrangement are more apt to receive preventive care postpartum, thereby supporting the continuation of care models that focus on continuity as well as convenience of health services (Price & Seagrave, 2020). In addition, disparities in preventive care access among diverse populations further point toward the complexity of women's health dynamics. Vulnerable populations, for example, those of lower economic status or with minimal health coverage, are typically disenfranchised from receiving timely and appropriate preventive care. Studies on follow-up intervals after abnormal mammograms found that high-volume institutions with high proportions of vulnerable women had longer follow-up periods, contributing to an escalation in advanced-stage diagnoses (Karliner et al., 2019). This finding points towards the urgent need for context-dependent interventions and services that aim at improving access to preventive care services among vulnerable groups. Addressing these disparities through policy interventions, improving healthcare facilities, and targeted outreach can be a major step in increasing early detection and treatment rates, which in turn can improve overall health outcomes for women across various socio-demographic groups.

A successful preventive care program in women's health must also address education and awareness. Education of women regarding the importance of regular screenings, such as Pap smears, mammograms, and bone density tests, can enable them to take charge of their own health. Public information campaigns to promote awareness of the importance of preventive services can enhance levels of participation, especially among the less aware. Furthermore, designing an enabling environment where women are comfortable discussing their health concerns with health workers is critical in dispelling the stigma and fear associated with accessing care. By enhancing patient education and preventive care focus, health systems can develop a culture of active health management, leading to healthier women and minimal rates of preventable illnesses in the long run (Price & Seagrave, 2020).

2.6.1. Recommended Screenings and Vaccinations for Women

Regular screenings and immunizations are integral parts of women's health care, offering preventative care that greatly reduces the risk of serious diseases. Mammograms, for example, are recommended once a year for women aged 40 and above to detect breast cancer at its earliest stage, where treatment is most possible. Similarly, Pap smears should be taken every three years for women starting at age 21, converting to Pap and HPV co-testing every five years after the age of 30. Both tests are significant reasons for identifying precancerous changes and early cancers, ultimately contributing to improved survival rates.

In addition, the HPV vaccine is an advised immunization in preteens and young adults, which is a significant factor in preventing cervical cancer and other HPVs caused by diseases. Implementing routine screening and vaccination schedules can make women healthier by taking the initiative to address their health care providers. These preventive health services are allocated unequally and are disproportionately availed by women in rural areas and migrant women. It has been found through research that rural women are far less likely to receive preventive tests such as mammograms and HPV vaccination than urban women. In particular, outreach initiatives to enhance access among these populations are critical, as the reports show that there are still disparities even after adjustment for sociodemographic variables (Ziller et al., 2019). There is, thus, the need for policy interventions to close these gaps in access to equity in health care so that all women, regardless of the geographic or migratory situation, receive essential screenings and vaccines. This is particularly important in the quest to improve the overall health status of the population and alleviate the disease burden attributable to preventable illnesses in women, particularly those in disadvantaged groups. Furthermore, the association between migration background and access to preventive healthcare services reveals yet another facet of complexity in women's health outcomes. Evidence suggests that individuals with a personal experience of migration are less unlikely to be involved in routine health checks and cancer screening than non-migrants (Hajek et al., 2024). This pattern suggests a potential barrier to effective healthcare access that could be rooted in cultural, language, or system factors. In order to most effectively address these challenges, it is essential to create targeted health education programs that reach women of all backgrounds and instill in them awareness of, and sensitivity to, advised vaccinations and screening tests. By facilitating an open healthcare system, we can make significant progress toward guaranteeing all women achieve maximal benefits of health from preventive care (Figure 2.18).

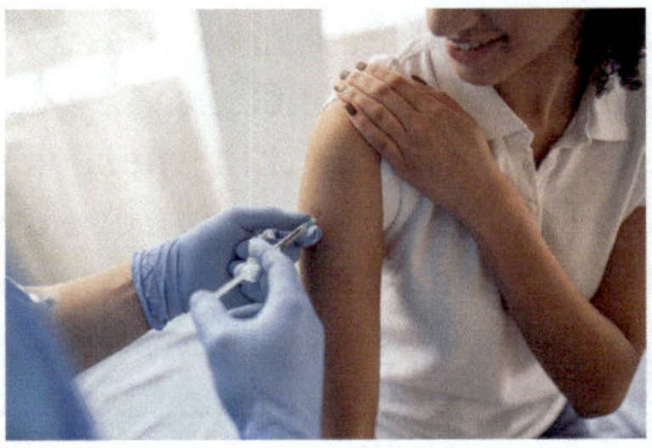

Figure 2.18. HPV vaccination for women.

Source: https://ssbhealthcare.com/wp-content/uploads/2022/09/Untitled-1-1.png.

2.6.2. Role of Lifestyle Factors in Women's Health

Lifestyle contributes importantly to women's health outcomes across the lifespan. Of these factors, diet and physical activity have the greatest significance, and both have direct effects on short- and long-term health. Dietary consumption dictates women's nutrient status, reproductive health, and risk of chronic diseases. For instance, an optimal diet with good intake of vitamins, minerals, and fats can help reduce the complications caused by obesity, diabetes, and cardiovascular disease. Moreover, exercise is also associated with not only physical well-being but also mental health advantages, such as the reduction of anxiety and mood improvement. With the encouragement of healthy habits and lifestyle change, women can get healthier and thereby create a better quality of life for themselves and also reduce future healthcare expenses. The role of prenatal care as part of women's health cannot be ignored, particularly during pregnancy, as lifestyle factors have a determinant impact on fetal outcomes. Group prenatal care models, as proposed by recent findings, offer a novel strategy by making available to women community support and education focused on health management during pregnancy. For example, while a meta-analysis revealed that group prenatal care was not shown to have statistically significant differences in gestational weight gain compared with traditional models, social interaction and shared learning experiences established through group settings have the ability to reinforce motivation and adherence to healthy behaviors for pregnant women (Kominiarek et al., 2019). These group interventions point to the importance of lifestyle choices, in this case, dietary choices and exercise, that then translate into improved fetal and maternal health. Outside of nutrition and prenatal well-being, mental health must be given some consideration in what is being discussed regarding women's health. Changes in lifestyle, such as stress diminishment through mindfulness and regular exercise, have proven effective in diminishing anxiety and depressive symptoms. Furthermore, educational interventions that occur during prenatal care can be helpful in equipping women with coping strategies in dealing with the pressures of motherhood and pregnancy (Hanson et al., 2009). With knowledge of the overlap between mental and physical health, practitioners can tailor their approach to fit the needs of women, making changes to lifestyle a part of comprehensive care. Thus, intervention in lifestyle variables not only increases short-term health outcomes but also achieves longer-term improvements in health among women and their families.

2.6.3. Importance of Patient Education and Awareness

Understanding the complexity of women's health requires a solid basis of patient education and awareness. This is particularly crucial when considering the incidence of disease, which is disproportionately found in women, such as cervical cancer and other forms of interpersonal violence. Educating women regarding their health gives them the power to make informed choices regarding preventive care and treatment. As an illustration, discussions regarding the merit of cervical cancer screening and the HPV vaccine can have a considerable impact on health. With appropriate education, women can be ignorant of available resources and prevention strategies, resulting in greater health disparities. Therefore, clinical education must be shifted to address these areas specifically so that women not only understand the risks that they are undergoing but also learn to avoid them, as stated in existing research on the impact of healthcare disparities on women's health outcomes. Beyond this, learning about the impact of interpersonal violence on women's health is also the important for patient awareness. Research also indicates that physical and psychological consequences of exposure to abuse can persist over time, reducing the quality of life in most women. For instance, it has been discovered that victims of abuse have their physical functioning levels comparable to those of non-abused women who are 20 years older, reflecting the serious effect of such abuse on health (Cannell et al., 2015). This connection emphasizes the need for healthcare professionals to remain vigilant and watchful in recognizing signs of abuse and ensuring that patients get adequate care and support. More patient education programs can not only recognize abuse but also provide a channel for communication about mental health, hence allowing for holistic care for women who may not candidly disclose their experience in the conventional medical setting. Lastly, proper patient education is pivotal for the integration of health services within high-risk groups. Most women, as well as minority and low-income women, have poor health awareness about HPV and its threat (Walter et al., 2020). These individuals are likely to be marginalized when undergoing preventive care and thus more at risk of developing conditions like cervical cancer. Healthcare systems have to capitalize on such opportunities, such as in EDs, to vaccinate these high-risk groups efficiently. By developing a culture of learning within these healthcare facilities, the providers can improve awareness of HPV and enhance vaccination coverage. This forward-thinking approach not only seeks to educate patients but also seeks to dismantle the structural barriers that fuel health disparities and ultimately reap better health outcomes for women across different backgrounds.

Test Your Knowledge

1. What are the key preventive screenings and vaccinations recommended for women at different life stages?
2. How can preventive care be tailored to support women's health during major life transitions?
3. Why is patient education essential in empowering women to make informed decisions about their health?

SUMMARY

The general medicine review of women's health highlights significant gaps and areas for potential improvement in healthcare provision. Systematic critical synthesis of current prenatal care guidelines recognizes an ongoing absence of uniformity in addressing women's educational requirements during prenatal consultation. While the primary function of healthcare is to heal and educate patients, many of the existing guidelines fail to meet comprehensive approaches, giving precedence to the individual needs of women through their medical procedures. As per pointed research, prioritizing the special needs of women in healthcare remains a high agenda, particularly in transforming prenatal care so that enhanced health is the result (Hanson et al., 2009). This emphasis on individualized education reflects not only a broader trend toward patient-focused methods but also buttresses the demand for forward-thinking healthcare policy and procedure. In addition, including diverse populations such as SGM underscores the importance of comprehensive educational systems in medical school programs. The research illustrates that the vast majority of obstetric anesthesia fellowship programs recognize the importance of SGM health education, but that only a few percent have included it in their curricula (Hanson et al., 2009). This breakdown illustrates a broader problem in medical education: the need to prepare healthcare professionals sufficiently for the reality of diverse patient backgrounds. By encouraging more understanding of SGM issues and making education materials inclusive, healthcare systems can strengthen patient-provider relationships and thus ultimately patient outcomes. Prioritizing inclusion in training frameworks will not only benefit marginalized communities but will also ultimately contribute to a higher quality of care in general. Finally, the persistent debate of women's health in mainstream medicine demands a commitment to continuous research and guideline updating that responds to the changing profile of healthcare demands. Practitioners need to keep pace with emerging best practices and new evidence that advance women's health and well-being. Sealing knowledge gaps in existing maternal health stories, such as those , including SGM and other vulnerable groups, will require joint efforts from health care leaders and educators. This will not only enhance the effectiveness of prenatal care but also propel advancement in women's health in general, guiding the medical profession toward a more equitable path in health care delivery. By committing to this integrated strategy, we can more effectively care for women and their families, leading to healthier communities overall.

In women's health practice in general medicine, overwhelming proof comes to light on the victory and hardship of women following surgery and disease diagnosis. One classic study focused on women recovering from fistula repair in Uganda, indicating major gains in both physical and psychosocial health in the first year post-surgery. The research demonstrated the striking improvement in urinary incontinence and overall weakness, along with marked improvement in the quality of overall health. The findings demonstrate the significance of early medical care and its relevance to women's return to society, self-esteem, and general quality of life, amidst some lingering concerns of stigma and self-perception at the one-year follow-up. These longitudinal designs highlight the need for psychosocial care targeted towards recovery, emphasizing that physical symptoms have long-term psychosocial consequences for women (El Ayadi et al., 2019). High on the list of women's health issues is also coronary artery disease (CAD), which continues to go underdiagnosed in women due to the challenge posed by atypical presentations of symptoms. A pioneering trial that employed a blood-based precision medicine test assessed the age/sex/gene expression score (ASGES) to improve detection rates of obstructive CAD in women. Findings from the PRESET Registry indicated that women with low ASGES were significantly less likely to be referred for further cardiac evaluation compared with women with high scores, illustrating a significant clinical management gap in the use of biological markers. This stratification allows physicians to select out women who obviously require more intimate investigation, avoiding all patients being subjected to unnecessary treatments, which can be physically and emotionally taxing. The research also indicated lower incidences of significant adverse cardiac events in women with lower ASGES, affirming the utility of this precision medicine approach in real-world application (El Ayadi et al., 2019). The intersection of these studies illustrates the multiplicity of women's health issues and further emphasizes the need for persistent attention in general medicine. Advances in the treatment of medicine are directly related to improved health status for women through longitudinal studies in physical and psychosocial recuperation. Moreover, the use of sophisticated diagnostic equipment like the ASGES in routine clinical evaluations can significantly enhance the treatment of diseases that are overwhelmingly prevalent among women, such as CAD. As research progresses, study findings need to be shared widely with medical practitioners to ensure that women are given equitable and efficient care in diverse medical environments. Thus, developing a culture that encourages women's health not just fosters personal health but also overall public health.

KEY TERMS FROM THIS CHAPTER

- Autoimmune diseases
- Biological sex
- Chronic disease
- Chronic illness
- Clinical environment
- Clinical settings
- Clinical trials
- Contraception
- Coronary heart disease (CHD)
- Family planning
- Female-specific health
- Gender variation
- General medicine
- Health condition
- Health disparities
- Health issues
- Health outcomes
- Healthcare experience
- Hormonal changes
- HPV vaccine

CRITICAL THINKING QUESTIONS

1. What is a major risk factor for gestational diabetes during pregnancy?

a. Low body weight

b. High physical activity

c. Obesity

d. Smoking

2. Which mental health condition is twice as common in women as in men?

a. Bipolar disorder

b. Depression

c. Schizophrenia

d. ADHD

3. Which of the following strategies is considered a primary preventive measure in women's reproductive health?

a. Chemotherapy

b. Hysterectomy

c. HPV vaccination

d. Hormone replacement therapy

4. Which screening test is recommended for early detection of cervical cancer in women?

a. Pap smear

b. Mammography

c. Colonoscopy

d. Bone density scan

5. What is the primary benefit of preventive healthcare in women?

a. To cure chronic diseases after symptoms appear

b. To increase hospital admissions

c. To avoid any form of medication

d. To detect diseases early and reduce morbidity

Short Answer Questions

1. How does access to comprehensive reproductive health services impact women's autonomy and long-term health outcomes?
2. What are the most critical components of maternal health care, from prenatal to postpartum support, and how do they affect both maternal and infant health outcomes?
3. Why is it important to recognize gender-specific patterns in chronic diseases?
4. What are the most prevalent mental health challenges faced by women?
5. How do chronic physical health issues in women often intersect with mental health conditions?
6. What preventive screenings and vaccinations are most critical at different stages of a woman's life, and how do these measures help detect and reduce the burden of disease?
7. How do modifiable lifestyle factors contribute to the prevention of common women's health issues?
8. How does enhancing health education and literacy among women improve their engagement with healthcare services?

Answers to Critical Thinking Questions

1. (c); 2. (b); 3. (c); 4. (a); 5. (d)

REFERENCES

1. Amr MA, Balaha M, Al Moghannum M. Postpartum Mental Health among Young Women. *Online J Health Allied Scs.* 2011;10(4):6 (accessed on 27th June 2025).
2. Almirall, J., & Fortin, M. (2013). The coexistence of terms to describe the presence of multiple concurrent diseases. https://core.ac.uk/download/pdf/29572312.pdf (accessed on 27th June 2025).
3. Cannell, M. B., Weitlauf, J. C., Garcia, L., Andresen, E. M., Margolis, K. L., & Manini, T. M. (2015). Cross-sectional and longitudinal risk of physical impairment in a cohort of postmenopausal women who experience physical and verbal abuse. *BMC women's health*, *15*, 98. https://doi.org/10.1186/s12905-015-0258-2c(accessed on 27th June 2025).
4. Ball, E., & Khan, K. S. (2020). Recent advances in understanding and managing chronic pelvic pain in women with special consideration to endometriosis. https://core.ac.uk/download/305120038.pdf (accessed on 27th June 2025).
5. El Ayadi, A. M., Barageine, J., Korn, A., Kakaire, O., Turan, J., Obore, S., Byamugisha, J., Lester, F., Nalubwama, H., Mwanje, H., Tripathi, V., & Miller, S. (2019). Trajectories of women's physical and psychosocial health following obstetric fistula repair in Uganda: a longitudinal study. *Tropical medicine & international health : TM & IH*, *24*(1), 53–64. https://doi.org/10.1111/tmi.13178(accessed on 27th June 2025).
6. Holmes, S. (2016). 'Blindness to the obvious'? Treatment experiences and feminist approaches to eating disorders. *Feminism & Psychology*, *26*(4), 464-486. https://doi.org/10.1177/0959353516654503 (Original work published 2016)
7. (accessed on 27th June 2025).
8. Gemmati, D., Varani, K., Bramanti, B., Piva, R., Bonaccorsi, G., Trentini, A., Manfrinato, M. C., Tisato, V., Carè, A., & Bellini, T. (2019). *"Bridging the Gap"* Everything that Could Have Been Avoided If We Had Applied Gender Medicine, Pharmacogenetics and Personalized Medicine in the Gender-Omics and Sex-Omics Era. *International journal of molecular sciences*, *21*(1), 296. https://doi.org/10.3390/ijms21010296(accessed on 27th June 2025).
9. Swainson, N (1998). *Promoting Girls' Education in Africa–The Design and Implementation of Policy Interventions.* ISBN:
10. 1-86192-046-6. https://core.ac.uk/download/pdf/6443151.pdf (accessed on 27th June 2025).
11. Afulani, P. A., Altman, M., Musana, J., & Sudhinaraset, M. (2017). Conceptualizing pathways linking women's empowerment and prematurity in developing countries. *BMC pregnancy and childbirth*, *17*(Suppl 2), 338. https://doi.org/10.1186/s12884-017-1502-6 (accessed on 27th June 2025).
12. Bock, B. C., Dunsiger, S. I., Gans, K. M., Hartman, S. J., et al. (2016). *Pasos Hacia La Salud: A Randomized Controlled Trial of An Internet-Delivered Physical Activity Intervention for Latinas.* https://core.ac.uk/download/323064378.pdf (accessed on 27th June 2025).
13. Bush, N. R., Buss, C., Conradt, E., Cordero, M., et al. (2022). Trajectories of depressive symptoms among mothers of preterm and full-term infants in a national sample. https://core.ac.uk/download/619687522.pdf (accessed on 27th June 2025).

14. Carmin, C. N., Kondos, G. T., Ownby, R. L., Wiegartz, P. S., et al. (2008). Women and non-cardiac chest pain: Gender differences in symptom presentation. https://core.ac.uk/download/51077079.pdf (accessed on 27th June 2025).

15. Eliza L. Chin, Marley Hoggatt, Alyson J. McGregor, Mary K. Rojek, Kimberly Templeton, Robert Casanova, Wendy S. Klein, Virginia M. Miller, and Marjorie Jenkins (2016). Sex and gender in medical education, and proceedings from the 2015 Sex and Gender Education Summit. https://core.ac.uk/download/215481794.pdf (accessed on 27th June 2025).

16. Kuhn, R., Richards, J., Roth, S., & Clair, K. (2020). Homelessness and Public Health in Los Angeles. *UCLA: Campuswide Homelessness Initiative*. Retrieved from https://escholarship.org/uc/item/2gn3x56s(accessed on 27th June 2025).

17. Department of Health (, including: Szczepura, Ala, Johnson, Mark R. D., Gumber, Anil, Jones, Kip, Clay, Diane and Shaw, A.). (2005) *An overview of the research evidence on ethnicity and communication in healthcare.* [Coventry]: [University of Warwick]. (Final report). (accessed on 27th June 2025).

18. Evatt, E., Arnott, F., & Deveson, A.(1977). *Royal Commission on Human Relationships*. https://core.ac.uk/download/pdf/30676707.pdf (accessed on 27th June 2025).

19. DuBose, R. (2024). The road to equity–Have women made adequate progress? https://core.ac.uk/download/641620657.pdf (accessed on 27th June 2025).

20. Păduraru, D. N., Ion, D., Nica, A. E., Coman, F., Coțofană, M., Badiu, D. C., Grigorean, V. T., Bolocan, A., & Andronic, O. (2018). The Switch from Patented Medicine to the Generic One: An Option or a Necessity? *Journal of Mind and Medical Sciences, 5*(2), 230-235.(accessed on 27th June 2025).

21. Hanson, L., VandeVusse, L., Roberts, J., & Forristal, A. (2009). A critical appraisal of guidelines for antenatal care: components of care and priorities in prenatal education. *Journal of midwifery & women's health, 54*(6), 458–468. https://doi.org/10.1016/j.jmwh.2009.08.002(accessed on 27th June 2025).

22. Walter LA, Leader E, Galbraith JW. Human Papillomavirus Awareness, Vaccine Status, and Risk Factors in Female Emergency Patients. *West J Emerg Med*. 2020;21(2):203-208. Published 2020 Feb 24. doi:10.5811/westjem.2019.12.44422(accessed on 27th June 2025).

23. Hajek, A., Kameraj, A., & König, H. H. (2024). Migration background and use of preventive healthcare services: Findings of the German Ageing Survey. https://www.ssoar.info/ssoar/bitstream/document/96534/1/ssoar-bmcph-2024-kameraj_et_al-Migration_background_and_use_of.pdf (accessed on 27th June 2025).

24. Hill, A. L., Jones, K. A., McCauley, H. L., Tancredi, D. J., Silverman, J. G., & Miller, E. (2019). Reproductive Coercion and Relationship Abuse Among Adolescents and Young Women Seeking Care at School Health Centers. *Obstetrics and gynecology, 134*(2), 351–359. https://doi.org/10.1097/AOG.0000000000003374(accessed on 27th June 2025).

25. Ziller E, Lenardson J, Paluso N, Janis J. Preventive Health Service Use among Rural Women. Portland, ME: University of Southern Maine, Muskie School of Public Service, Maine Rural Health Research Center; April, 2019. PB-73. (accessed on 27th June 2025).

26. Karliner, L. S., Kaplan, C., Livaudais-Toman, J., & Kerlikowske, K. (2019). Mammography facilities serving vulnerable women have longer follow-up times. *Health services research, 54 Suppl 1*(Suppl 1), 226–233. https://doi.org/10.1111/1475-6773.13083(accessed on 27th June 2025).

27. Kominiarek, M. A., Lewkowitz, A. K., Carter, E., Fowler, S. A., & Simon, M. (2019). Gestational weight gain and group prenatal care: a systematic review and meta-analysis. *BMC pregnancy and childbirth, 19*(1), 18. https://doi.org/10.1186/s12884-018-2148-8 (accessed on 27th June 2025).

28. Rosemary Avery, Donald Kenkel, Dean R. Lillard and Alan Mathios(2007). Private profits and public health: Does advertising smoking cessation products encourage smokers to quit? Journal of Political Economy https://core.ac.uk/download/pdf/6863938.pdf (accessed on 27th June 2025).

29. Moore, B. J. (2020). The role of diversity training on healthcare professionals' understanding of diversity at UPMC Magee-Women's Hospital. https://core.ac.uk/download/328827292.pdf (accessed on 27th June 2025).

30. Mousavi, S. A., Chaman, R., Khosravi, A., Mortazavi, F., et al. (2013). Quality of life after cesarean and vaginal delivery. https://core.ac.uk/download/52204616.pdf (accessed on 27th June 2025).

31. Price, K., & Seagrave, M. (2020). Women's use of preventive primary care in the late postpartum period. https://core.ac.uk/download/304590488.pdf (accessed on 27th June 2025).

32. Roberts, S. C. M. (2019). The presence and consequences of abortion aversion in scientific research related to alcohol use during pregnancy. https://core.ac.uk/download/323073633.pdf (accessed on 27th June 2025).

PSYCHIATRY IN GENERAL PRACTICE

3

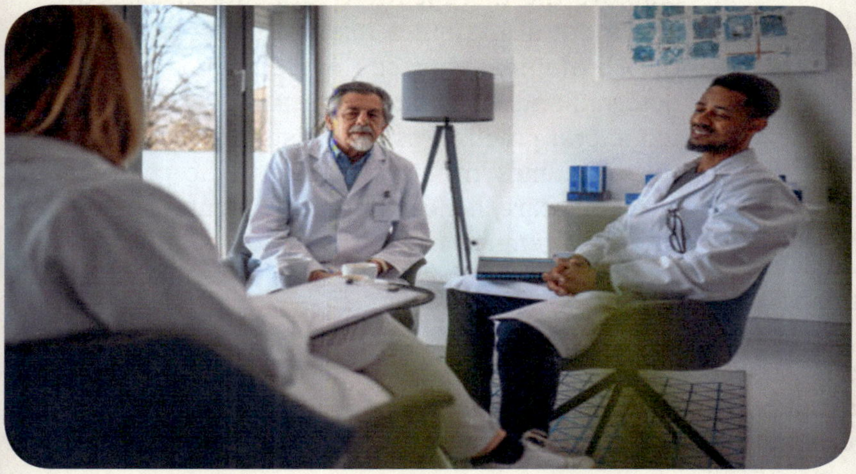

LEARNING OBJECTIVES

After studying this chapter, you will be able to:

1. Understand the historical context of psychiatry;
2. Explain the role of general practitioners in mental health;
3. Describe common mental health disorders in general practice;
4. Discuss diagnostic tools and techniques;
5. Focus on treatment approaches in general practice;
6. Deal with challenges in integrating psychiatry into general practice.

Introduction

General practice psychiatry is a significant intersection of mental health and primary care in which the interwoven dynamics of psychological well-being and physical well-being are addressed. General practitioners (GPs) are often the first point of contact for patients who come in with mental health issues, such as depression and anxiety. Since psychiatric disorders are increasingly taking the forefront of general morbidity causes, good psychiatric assessment becomes even more imperative in general practice. The inclusion of psychiatric principles in general practice not only improves care for patients but also allows for a holistic method of dealing with patients. The convergence makes it easier for early psychiatric disorder identification and timely intervention, eventually leading to improved patient outcomes. From the perspective of specialist knowledge, it is possible today to develop practice guidelines which inform GPs—the cornerstones of community health—how to treat complex psychiatric conditions most effectively and thus maintain the critical role of psychiatry in primary care (Yager et al., 2014). A more in-depth analysis of the history of psychiatry proves how Antoni Kępiński and other psychiatrists have contributed to contemporary thinking regarding mental illness treatment. Kępińskis reflections emphasized the vital role of psychiatry within the broader medical landscape, thereby influencing the integration of psychiatric care into general practice. His insights fostered an understanding that psychiatric problems do not exist in isolation but rather intersect with various physical ailments, aligning with modern biopsychosocial models of healthcare. The relevance of Kępińskis ideas still holds, demonstrating that the philosophical debates he engaged with continue to be relevant within present psychiatric debates. Through evaluation of the evolution of psychiatric thinking in conjunction with current practice, GPs can foster a more sophisticated understanding of mental health issues, eventually enhancing their capacity to deal with such issues effectively within practice (Zawiła-Niedźwiecki, 2016). Besides, psychiatric evaluations enhance GPs' training and skills, equipping them with expertise to assess and treat psychological conditions. With evidence based on sound studies that highlight the benefits of methodical psychiatric examination in first assessments, GPs are better placed to deliver improved patient outcomes using evidence-based guidelines. The utilization of systematic approaches facilitates the detection of how psychiatric conditions manifest in various groups in a way that they can easily be detected and addressed early. Employment of expert consensus and practice guidelines grounded on community opinion, such as what has been taken into account in formulating protocols on psychiatric examination, is essential. This collaborative approach not only strengthens the GP practice but also upholds the status of psychiatry as a core element of general healthcare, emphasizing the value of ongoing debate and research within this evolving specialty (Yager et al., 2014).

Definition of Psychiatry

Psychiatry, a vital field of medicine, is basically concerned with the diagnosis, treatment, and prevention of mental illness. Psychiatry has progressed to address a wide range of psychological illnesses, from depression and anxiety disorders to severe ones like schizophrenia and bipolar disorder. Being a discipline that crosses medical knowledge and psychopathology, psychiatry not only employs the therapeutic treatments discussed above but also applies itself to understanding the biological, psychological, and social determinants of mental illness. As an adjunct to general practice, psychiatrists play a crucial role in identifying such patients who require specialist care, hence integrating mental health into the generic management of healthcare. This synergy is increasingly significant given the growing recognition of mental health as paramount in achieving better health outcomes across populations. Furthermore, the practice of psychiatry is becoming increasingly relevant within general practice, especially as healthcare systems lean towards integrated care models. Broad-based training initiatives have emphasized the importance of developing practitioners who can navigate multiple specialties, including psychiatry, to provide comprehensive patient care. For instance, offering schemes that expose trainees to practice placements in general practice, psychiatry, and pediatrics seeks to provide a balanced model of patient management. Generalist training prepares GPs to be effective in the complex interaction of physical and mental disorders by bridging the gap between specialist care and general health service provision. Within this context, psychiatry is not a distinct field but a core component of routine care, requiring an amalgamation of several healthcare professionals to meet increasingly high demands for mental health treatment (Muddiman et al., 2016). Furthermore, increased interest in mindfulness as an intervention for treatment highlights the evolving nature of psychiatry in routine practice.

Mindfulness therapies, derived from Buddhist philosophies, have become part of mainstream psychiatric practice as efficacious treatments for a variety of mental illness conditions. Research indicates that the addition of mindfulness-based treatments to psychiatric treatments can enhance patient outcomes, illustrating the adaptability of psychiatry in meeting new challenges to health care. However, as the popularity of mindfulness broadens, there is a critical need to review its empirical evidence and clinical effectiveness. Follow-up studies must synthesize evidence, control for bias, and investigate mechanisms to ensure that mindfulness can be effectively integrated into general psychiatric practice. Identification of such advancements emphasizes psychiatry's proactive role in the practice of general psychiatry, so that mental health treatment continues to be adaptive to the changing needs of patients (Van Gordon et al., 2015) (Figure 3.1).

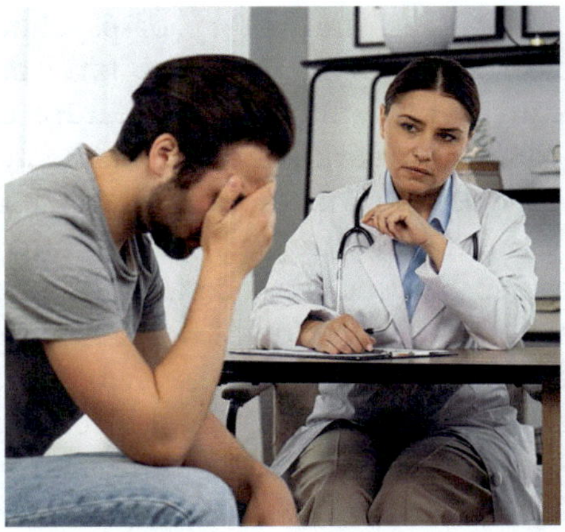

Figure 3.1. A psychiatrist observing a psychiatric patient.

Source: https://suryahospitals.com/speciality/6561e6ee81bdeExpertise---Psychiatry-(Adult).jp.

Importance of Psychiatry in General Practice

The integration of psychiatry into general practice is central to addressing the multifaceted aspects of patient care. GPs are generally the first contact that patients with mental illness will have, but most feel they do not receive adequate training for dealing with such illnesses. As such, primary care centers need to incorporate a more holistic approach encompassing the evaluation and treatment of mental health. The inclusion of psychiatric principles within core examinations encourages physicians to recognize and address psychological issues that complicate physical illnesses. This is particularly important given the results that emphasize the interconnection between physical health and mental well-being. Addressing psychological issues not only improves patient outcomes but can also save secondary care services the agony, which means a healthier healthcare system overall. Secondly, mental illness tends to be stigmatized, and this can go a long way in deterring sufferers from seeking help. Patients usually present with somatic complaints whose underlying psychiatric conditions cannot be easily identified; hence, due to a lack of education, GPs will miss all this crucial information. The role of psychiatry within the general practice is to bridge the gap by promoting a setting in which these issues can be freely addressed. By giving practitioners the training to identify psychiatric signs and refer appropriately, patients are more actively involved in their treatment of mental health. Care models that include collaboration, bringing mental health professionals into primary care, have greater patient satisfaction and improved clinical outcomes. This collaborative relationship enhances the therapeutic relationship between providers and patients and eventually results in integrated care. Apart from improving the individual patient results, integration of psychiatry within general practice can also improve the function of wider public health programs. As mental illness disorders become primary determinants of total morbidity, working together between general practices and psychiatric services can help address key population health trends. This convergence becomes feasible to collect valuable information to utilize in informing community health plans and interventions aimed at early intervention and prevention. Besides, with advances in neuroscience revealing the profound linkage between emotional and intellectual health and illness and disease, learning from research can inform general practice guidelines and treatment strategies. Therefore, both fields have much to benefit from cross-appraisal of knowledge, and an improved-informed healthcare setting that seeks to comprehend and address the full scope of human health and enhance the quality of life for populations' patients (Grey, 2015).

3.1. Historical Context of Psychiatry

Learning Outcome

1. Understand the evolution of psychiatric practices;
2. Discuss key figures in psychiatry;
3. Explain the impact of historical events on psychiatric approaches.

History is closely associated with the evolution of medical practices and mental illness by the general public. Initially, individuals presenting symptoms of mental illness were stigmatized and confined to asylums in deplorable conditions. This began to change during the Enlightenment era with notable thinkers such as Descartes initiating humane treatment and additional depth into mental disorder issues. This explanation not only directed the creation of institutions that would provide care but also led to psychiatric frameworks that sought to explain the complexities of the human mind. Of particular interest, central movements such as the anti-psychiatry movement opposed the conventional medical model, emphasizing the socio-political aspects of mental health care and the value of incorporating personal experience and social context into psychiatric practice, ultimately influencing contemporary psychiatric practice within general practice. In modern psychiatry, one observes an emphasis on integrated models of care that aim at treating mental health within the broader settings of health. This development comes in the form of a paradigm shift from ascriptive institutionalization to community-based care that is centered on patient autonomy and social reintegration. The World Health Organization has identified the need for balanced care systems, highlighting collaboration between various sectors, such as education and social services, for maximizing mental health outcomes. The "balanced care" model offers a powerful model for addressing mental health needs in general practice as it promotes delivery of services in close proximity to the patient's environment. Because this kind of integration is integral since mental health issues in youth first emerge outside of the health system—at school and in community environments—there is a need for comprehensive strategies beyond clinical environments (Mommerency et al., 2011). Moreover, the history of psychiatry is characterized by bringing to the forefront the significance of the influence of culture on the knowledge and treatment of mental health. For instance, variation in mental health practice between nations such as Japan and Italy emphasizes how cultural constructs organize interventions and social representations of mental illness. This heterogeneity of understanding highlights the shortcomings of a one-size-fits-all international psychiatry and necessitates sensitivity to local considerations in developing effective mental health care models. Empirical evidence, for example, from an examination of the influence of modernization in Japan's Meiji and Edo periods, illustrates how cultural models have influenced contemporary psychiatric practice and the evolution of art and community participation as alternative forms of social integration (Bucci, 2014). As psychiatry evolves further, these aspects are imperative to formulating integral treatment paradigms for widespread use.

3.1.1. Evolution of Psychiatric Practices

The evolution of psychiatric care has been significantly impacted by the transition from institutional to community-based care, particularly since the post-war era. In reaction to the Ministry of Health's 1961 decision to close down psychiatric hospitals across the UK, various regions experienced unique paths in reorganizing their structures of mental health care. In Scotland, for instance, hospitals did not fade overnight; instead, they reorganized their procedures to accommodate the changes in attitudes towards mental illness. It was an evolutionary period, where centers of institutions began adopting practices that aimed to enhance patient care, thus contributing to the overall reorganization of psychiatric care. The investigation into Glasgow's psychiatric service during the 1970s illustrates the extent to which profound reliance on underfunded hospitals existed alongside new ideologies of deinstitutionalization, ultimately toward a dynamic evolution and not a fixed position of care (Long, 2016). Within the framework of psychiatric practice, mounting recognition of the interrelation between art and mental health has also shaped the debate about psychiatric care. Performance art, in its characteristically raw exploration of the human condition, poses challenging questions concerning the intersection of physicality, mental illness, and the world's perception of sanity. Kira O'Reilly's experience is a shining example of how institutions grapple with the meaning of showing art that engages with bodily and psychological experience. In her performance 'Wet Cup,' O'Reilly defied institutional safety and health issues in addition to subverting assumptions about normalcy and mental sanity. The meaning attributed to her action illuminates a broader societal issue that pervades the representation of mental illness through the arts, with tension between institutional control and artistic freedom. These reflections also make the meanings of psychiatric practices ambiguous because they become intertwined with cultural representations of the artist's body and mental health (Bartram, 2012).

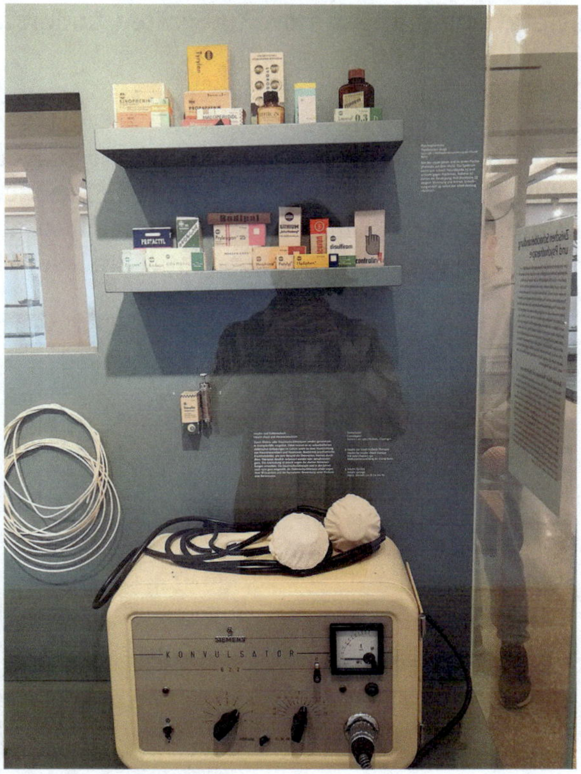

Figure 3.2. Psychiatric medication and an ECT machine, in the Berlin Museum of Medical History.

Source: https://upload.wikimedia.org/wikipedia/commons/thumb/b/bc/Psychiatric_Items.jpg/800px-Psychiatric_Items.jpg.

The history of psychiatric practices mirrors a broader societal shift in the way mental health has been conceptualized differently through the lenses of policy change, becoming more integrated within the community, and cultural reflection. New approaches were created that sought to place patient well-being and community participation over simple management of symptoms within the walls of the institution. These included the establishment of outpatient services and community mental health programs designed to foster support without the stigma of hospitalization. As psychiatric practice itself expanded to incorporate more integrated approaches, concepts of care began to encompass patient agency and active utilization of community resources. The continuous engagement between shifting ideologies, policy changes, and cultural discourses underscores the necessity of a dynamic and adaptive psychiatric practice that is attuned to the complexity of mental health within contemporary society, facilitating a more integrated understanding of human psychological health (Figure 3.2).

3.1.2. Key Figures in Psychiatry

In psychiatry, various key figures have played a significant role in the development of the field and its practice, particularly in general practice. Sigmund Freud, among other pioneers, introduced groundbreaking concepts of psychoanalysis that would essentially redefine the understanding of the human mind as well as mental illnesses.

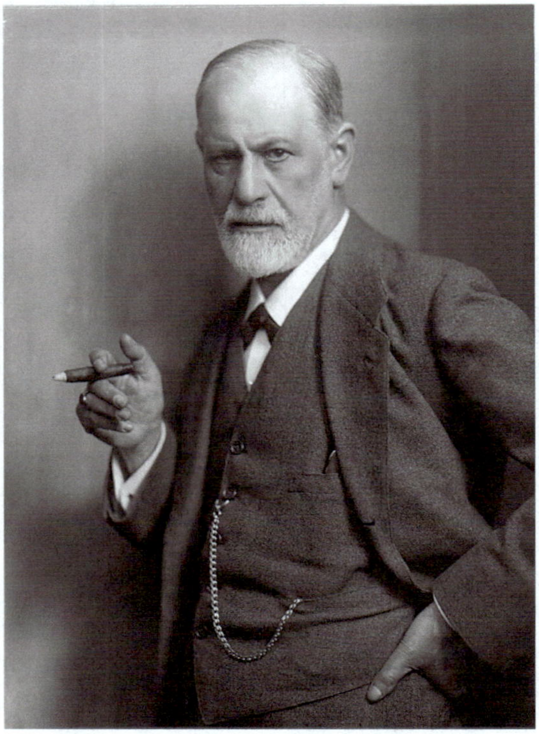

Figure 3.3. Sigmund Freud, an Austrian neurologist and the founder of psychoanalysis.

Source: https://upload.wikimedia.org/wikipedia/commons/thumb/3/36/Sigmund_Freud%2C_by_Max_Halberstadt_%28cropped%29.jpg/800px-Sigmund_Freud%2C_by_Max_Halberstadt_%28cropped%29.jpg.

Freud's work emphasized unconscious processes as well as early childhood effects, creating a foundation that has outlived various advancements in psychotherapy. His concentration on conversation therapy provided the premise for future psychotherapeutic practice, defining the integration of psychiatric practice into general practice. The early theories have had an impact on modern practices such that clinicians are able to unravel the intricate dynamics of mental illness through a therapeutic framework. Thus, knowledge of Freud's contributions helps place in perspective the importance of honoring historical figures in psychiatry when considering the implications of modern practice in general medicine. Another prominent name is Emil Kraepelin, who is regarded as the father of contemporary psychiatry due to his enormous body of work and classification of mental ailments. Kraepelin's scientific approach to classifying psychiatric illnesses according to observable behavior laid down a vital foundation for current diagnostic procedures. His work, in addition to facilitating improved structured understanding of mental illness, also resulted in the development of the Diagnostic and Statistical Manual of Mental Disorders (DSM). Such evidence-based classification indicates the ongoing pertinence of Kraepelin's work in informing GPs. As psychiatric conditions are increasingly integrated into primary practice, understanding these classifications is crucial to making the proper diagnosis and treatment for that patient so that they may be provided with overall care that addresses their unique mental health. The integration of research evidence into psychiatric practice is placed in high relief by contemporary advancements, such as those outlined in psychological therapy services. These services offer a variety of evidence-based therapeutic modalities, but their implementation in clinical practice generally encounters barriers, as highlighted by recent debate over evidence-based practice. In consideration of the complexities of research translation to day-to-day care, it is evident that a broad approach is required to link evidence and usability. Systematic evaluation and integration of feedback into such services enable clinicians to reflect on their practice and adopt new ways toward improved patient outcomes. Such actions resonate with the growing pressure for intervention within general practice and underscore the need for continuous readjustment in the delivery of psychiatric treatment. As these services mature, they not only recognize pioneers in psychiatry but also mature to meet challenges in contemporary times through thoughtful practice and research (Lucock et al., 2005; Kallert et al., 2013) (Figure 3.3).

3.1.3. Impact of Historical Events on Psychiatric Approaches

The evolution of psychiatric techniques has been largely influenced by historical occurrences that rebuilt society's perception and clinical methods. For instance, the major conflicts served as triggers for the progress in the knowledge of psychological trauma, causing new psychiatric techniques to emerge. World War I and World War II brought to light the psychological traumas faced by soldiers, and this prompted the development of psychotherapy and rehabilitation techniques aimed at treating previously untreated psychological diseases. This shift opened the door to a gentler treatment policy toward mental illness, going beyond physical treatments only. Consequently, the integration of psychological elements in clinical practice was called for, and this was a paradigm shift that defined the boundaries and the function of psychiatry within general practice. Also, significant historical events have similarly resulted in changes in the perception of gender and its impact on mental health. The feminist movements of the late 20th century drew attention to the special experiences of women in psychiatric care, illustrating how the interplay between gender exercises a determining influence on psychiatric diagnosis and treatment. Research reveals that traditional psychiatric practice mostly overlooked such gendered issues, thereby generating a vicious cycle of misperception by doctors concerning women's mental illnesses. For example, findings from a Q-methodological study highlighted nine distinct descriptions of women's challenging behavior in secure psychiatric settings, indicating that direct care staff rarely considered gender in their clinical assessments. This highlights the urgent need for the integration of feminist perspectives into psychiatric training and practice as demanded by practitioners in the field, and therefore, to current approaches in women's mental health care (Anderson et al., 2003). Additionally, the writings of pioneering psychiatrists left an indelible imprint on current practice, as is evident from the pages of scholars like Antoni Kępiński. His essays about the intersection of psychiatry and broader philosophical concerns resulted in debates that resonate to this day in arguments about mental health. Pitting Kępińskis ideas against those of contemporary paradigms allows one to map the evolution of psychiatric thinking across the centuries. His emphasis on the psychophysical problems in psychiatry generated a more integrated attention to mental health, recognizing the complexity of human experience. Recognition of the historical roots of psychiatric practice thus not only pays homage to what earlier thinkers have done but enables richer insight into how this is still applicable to practice today, supporting forward progress in the practice of psychiatry within general practice (Zawiła-Niedźwiecki, 2016).

Test Your Knowledge

1. How did the treatment of mental illness evolve from ancient times to the 19th century?
2. Who were some of the key figures in the development of modern psychiatry, and what were their main contributions?

3.2. Role of General Practitioners (GPs) in Mental Health

Learning Outcome

1. Understand the first point of contact for patients;
2. Deal with the integration of mental health assessments;
3. Focus on collaboration with mental health specialists.

The GP's role within mental health is becoming ever more important, given their status as the initial contact for patients. GPs have an exceptional chance to spot mental illness, including depression or anxiety, early on. Their holistic understanding of patients' medical histories and social contexts positions them to note how physical health intersects with mental. But that gatekeeper role is inefficient in the instance of more particular disorders like attention deficit hyperactivity disorder (ADHD). Research has proposed that GPs themselves may at times not be aware of the symptoms, sometimes because of stigmas around the diagnosis of mental illness, or sometimes because of reluctance to refer to mental illness specialists (Tatlow-Golden et al., 2016). Therefore, knowledge development and attitudinal change among GPs are essential to maximize ADHD diagnosis and treatment procedures. In the majority of healthcare systems, GPs are usually accountable for the provision of psychological treatments that are both challenging and offer opportunities for effective mental health interventions. They are in the position to conduct initial assessments and embark on treatment protocols with direct effects on patient outcomes. Nevertheless, the implementation of evidence-based practices within routine clinical practice generally encounters obstacles. For instance, applying the latest research on mental health interventions can be troublesome, particularly when evidence itself might not necessarily fit into everyday practice or the complexities of individual patient demands (Lucock et al., 2005). Therefore, the GPs must utilize their practical experience to bridge the gap between research evidence and practice so that care informed by research is delivered but contextualized within specific situations. Furthermore, integrating mental health services within general practice has far-reaching consequences for healthcare as a whole. Cross-disciplinary practice in this way ensures a setting where various health professionals can share information and techniques.

GPs are able to provide an integrated appreciation of mental health needs by participating in shared care approaches and co-working with psychologists and psychiatrists. But the achievement of this synergy requires continuous training and professional development for GPs so they feel confident to tackle mental health problems proficiently. By enhancing the abilities and expertise of GPs, they can negotiate more successfully the complexities of mental healthcare and thus be pivotal in relieving barriers to access for the vulnerable. These improvements will act to move towards a healthcare system that more effectively prioritizes both mind and body (Figure 3.4).

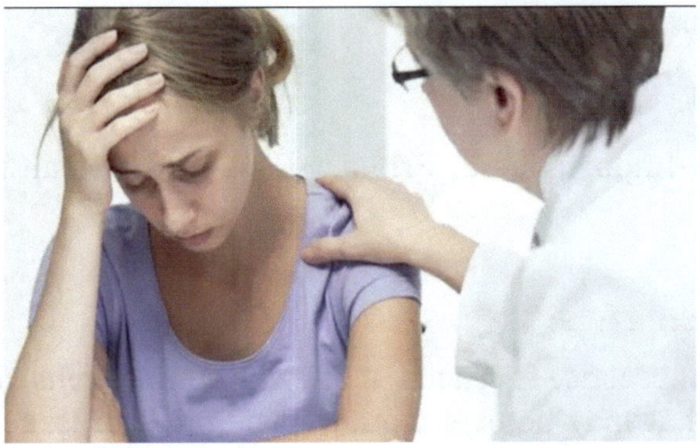

Figure 3.4. A psychiatrist motivating a patient.

Source: https://ichef.bbci.co.uk/ace/ws/640/cpsprodpb/0942/production/_92207320_mentalhealth.jpg.webp.

3.2.1. First Point of Contact for Patients

The role of PCPs as first points of contact with mental health patients is at the core of the practice of psychiatry within general practice. The practitioners usually encounter patients with mental illness symptoms, but frequently remark that they do not feel qualified to adequately manage such complex issues. In reality, many GPs have reported feeling short of confidence in their ability to recognize and deal with mental illness, resulting in lost chances for early intervention. The effects of this deficiency are extensive in that delayed or insufficient response to psychological distress can result in more severe conditions among patients and overwhelmed healthcare systems. To maximize the efficacy of primary care, GP training in mental health assessment and intervention skills is needed, hence enabling them to make more informed decisions and make appropriate referrals for subsequent care. The necessity of smooth communication and collaboration between providers is also emphasized by the inconsistency of needs among patients with mental illness. As the first line of contact, GPs are not just required to treat and diagnose but also to listen and decode the broader social determinants that shape their patients' health. A qualitative study identifies the frustration that bereaved families feel when they observe system failure as they perceive that mental health symptoms have gone undetected, yet it also emphasizes the crucial role played by the GP in picking up on these signs early and responding suitably. Moreover, family members express concern regarding too much reliance on drug therapies, presenting the potential for a more integrated practice through psychosocial measures to be advisable. In bringing patient history, social networks, and family guidance into the decision to treat, GPs can promote more mental health successes and provide supportive settings for individuals who need it. Finally, first contact in psychiatry is not necessarily all about the clinical assessment; it is also about gaining patients' trust and rapport. Mental conditions are extremely stigmatized, and patients can attend their GPs either with fear or anxiety of being judged. Therefore, GPs should employ methods that offer a comfortable situation for patients to express their worries freely. This entails working with patients collaboratively to address their mental health without downplaying their experiences or stereotyping the complexity of their illness. Moreover, increasing access to mental health care and community services is crucial in guiding patients towards integrative care. Such collective effort can bring attention to the central role of PCPs in preventing mental health crises, as emphasized by the need for proactive health education and outreach programs for patients and families to create awareness about available support systems, ultimately leading to better health outcomes in the area of psychiatric care (Romeo et al., 2012; Leavey et al., 2017) (Figure 3.5).

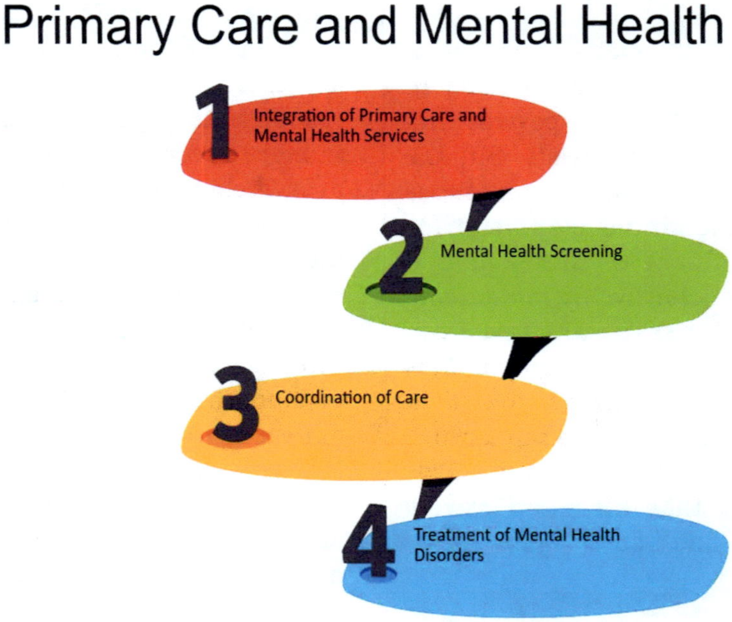

Figure 3.5. Primary care and mental health.

Source: https://fastercapital.co/i/Primary-Care--The-Importance-of-Primary-Care-in-the-Health-Care-Sector--Primary-Care-and-Mental-Health.webp.

3.2.2. Integration of Mental Health Assessments

The integration of mental health screening into general practice is crucial in offering comprehensive care to patients. PCPs can identify mental illnesses that may be overshadowed by medical issues through this practice, hence gaining an overall view of patient health. Despite the recognized importance of mental health screening, PCPs struggle to implement systematic screening due to various reasons. This may result in uneven collection of essential information pertaining to a patient's biopsychosocial status, which is fundamental for efficient case conceptualization and treatment planning. Current research identifies the need for additional training and support in mental health assessment methods among GPs so that valuable information is gathered in an organized manner to guide interventions that maximize outcomes (Meyer & Melchert, 2011). In addition, meeting the specific needs of vulnerable subpopulations, such as schizophrenia patients, is essential in the process of implementing mental health screening. The inclusion of exercise as a beneficial intervention in this context points to the need for individualized screening that takes into account not only psychological issues, but also patients' physical health. GPs must tackle the barriers to the engagement of such populations in physical activity, including mental health screening that takes into account psychological well-being as well as physical health markers. Asking about physical activity and its benefits will enable practitioners to better understand the specific barriers to the attainment of physical activity for those with mental health conditions. This interdisciplinary methodology ensures that mental health assessments lead to practice-planned interventions for the improvement in quality of life as a whole (Vancampfort et al., 2016).

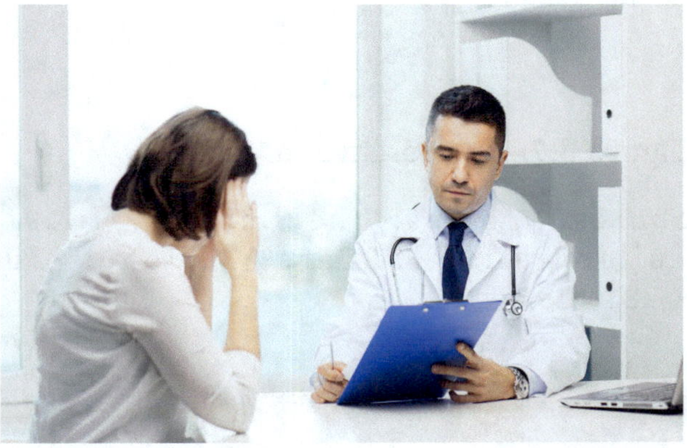

Figure 3.6. Illustration of mental health assessment.

Source: https://www.highfocuscenters.com/wp-content/uploads/2017/04/Does-a-Mental-Health-Assessment-Always-Lead-to-Being-Admitted.jpg.

Efficient application of mental health assessment in general practice rests ultimately on encouraging an interdisciplinary approach. Inter-communication among healthcare practitioners—psychiatrists, psychologists, and physical therapists—enables formulation of merged management plans that take into account mental and physical well-being. This is crucial in effectively treating patients who usually present with complex health conditions. Further, the use of standardized assessment measures and questionnaires can result in the standardized measurement of mental health as well as physical health issues, thereby making the treatment more effective. Through implementing a systematic approach to mental health assessment, GPs ensure all aspects of a patient's health become comprehensive, leading to improved therapeutic outcomes and patient satisfaction when treating psychiatric illness (Meyer & Melchert, 2011; Vancampfort et al., 2016) (Figure 3.6).

3.2.3. Collaboration with Mental Health Specialists

The integration of mental health professionals in general practice is the greatest way to optimize the patients' outcomes, particularly in child and adolescent psychiatry. The GPs could be involved with cases that need psychiatric assessment and treatment, but could not have specific training for this purpose. With coordination with mental health professionals, GPs can participate in holistic models of care that address the complexity of mental health issues. For instance, a study indicated differences between admission diagnoses and collaborative reviews with working diagnoses, calling for multidisciplinary assessment to improve treatment planning and optimize psychopharmacological intervention. This collaborative approach ensures that GPs are capable of proper management of psychiatric drugs and fosters the kind of environment that encourages ongoing education and skill mastery in mental health management (Camilleri et al., 2009). The importance of intense training and ongoing support for GPs cannot be stressed enough, particularly since they usually become the initial contact for adolescents with mental health issues. In the majority of cases,

GPs have to deal with complex psychiatric disorders requiring an advanced understanding of progressive treatments and protocols. Collaboration with mental health professionals not only enhances the GP to effectively diagnose and treat these disorders, but also equips them with a clearer direction on when to refer. The results of the SNAP survey emphasize the significance of having GPs in a position to call upon professional expertise and collaborative opinion, which can play a critical role in the quality of care young patients with emotional and behavioral issues receive. This collaboration ultimately strengthens a more stable trajectory for the mental health of youth (Furnivall et al., 2006). Moreover, having effective communication system between GPs and mental health workers can serve as a prevention strategy against potential misdiagnoses and inappropriate drugs. The need for effective consultation and referral processes is supported by evidence that a high percentage of children who had previously been prescribed antipsychotics had their treatment plan changed following specialist review. This kind of collaboration helps to avoid dangers associated with non-specialist treatment of psychiatric medication and provides enhanced evidence-based practice adherence in general practice. In addition, ongoing contact between mental health workers and GPs ensures a culture of knowledge sharing, ultimately providing better outcomes to adolescents. By prioritizing such multidisciplinary relationships, the general practice of psychiatry can potentially improve its practice and address the mental health epidemic among youths better (Camilleri et al., 2009).

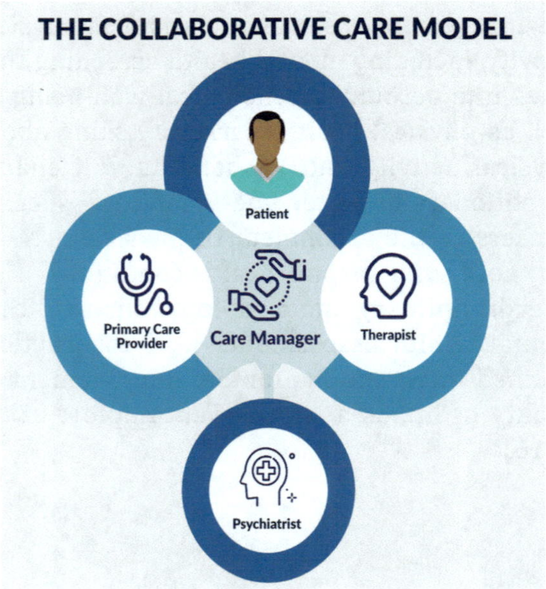

Figure 3.7. Collaborative care model.

Source: https://heal.nih.gov/files/Collaborative%20Care%20Model%20%281%29.png.

Test Your Knowledge

1. Why are general practitioners (GPs) often the first point of contact for patients experiencing mental health issues?
2. How do general practitioners collaborate with mental health specialists, such as psychiatrists or psychologists, to provide comprehensive care for patients?

3.3. Common Mental Health Disorders in General Practice

Learning Outcome

1. Understand depression and anxiety disorders;
2. Describe substance use disorders;
3. Explain stress-related disorders.

Mental illnesses are common in general practice and include a variety of prevalent disorders like anxiety disorders, depression, and bipolar disorders. They greatly affect the daily functioning of the patients as well as the quality of their lives and, therefore, need to be noted and treated in primary care facilities. GPs are most often the initial point of contact for patients with psychological distress and hence they must be equipped to identify and address such issues successfully. As a result of the overlap between mental and physiological health, sensitivity to the nuances of such disorders allows greater patient-centered and effective care and better patient outcomes. In addition, early intervention in a familiar health arena can go a long way towards reducing the impact of such disorders, pinpointing the importance of integrating mental health into models of general practice. A major step to transcending mental health disorders in general practice is recognizing the role of underpinning psychological traits, neuroticism being one that has been powerfully associated with a variety of psychopathologies. The new evidence indicates that neuroticism is a general liability that can cause the emergence and recurrence of common mental disorders, including anxiety and mood disorders (Bentley et al., 2017). These results give a shift in paradigm to treatment, focusing efforts on modifying stable traits instead of managing the expressions of specific disorders alone. By addressing these underlying weaknesses, practitioners can enhance the power and efficacy of psychological treatment, moving the focus towards a more integrated understanding of patient health. This is very much in accordance with new mental health treatment models that focus on early intervention and integrated care in general practice. Another added complication to GPs' challenges in addressing mental health issues is the socio-demographic dynamics at play in the way parents understand weight-related health threats among children that can be reflective of broader psychological challenges. One notable study discovered that high percentages of parents did not consider their obese child's weight to pose a health risk, even though identification of their child's weight status was highly critical in understanding associated health conditions (Park et al., 2013). The gap served as a call for GPs not only to treat existing mental illness, but also to promote education and awareness of the psychological impacts of illnesses as a whole. Through promotion of frank discussions of such issues, clinicians can facilitate families being able to identify and treat psychological risks early, thereby bringing mental health considerations into their general patient care strategies within general practice.

3.3.1. Depression and Anxiety Disorders

The task of integrating Psychiatry into the practice of general physicians is particularly crucial in the scenario of treating increasing rates of Depression and Anxiety Disorders. Mental illness that is comorbid with chronic medical illnesses complicates treatment and management. There is strong evidence to attest that both physical and psychiatric disorders are linked with higher risks of adverse outcomes, including increased mortality and lower care quality. Also, the economic burden of such interconnected illnesses is heavy, impacting health systems and requiring a reorientation of current setups for treating patients. What is required in addressing such complexities is a collaborative effort, with GPs not just having the ability to diagnose symptoms of mental illness but also the capacity to tackle the multifaceted impacts these diseases have on the general state of health outcomes, ultimately serving the interest of the patient's welfare and the effectiveness of health (The Stern Center for Evidence-Based Policy, 2015). Besides, the need for effective prevention and intervention strategies is critical in the management of Depression and Anxiety Disorders, particularly in settings like college universities where young adults are more vulnerable to these disorders (Figure 3.8).

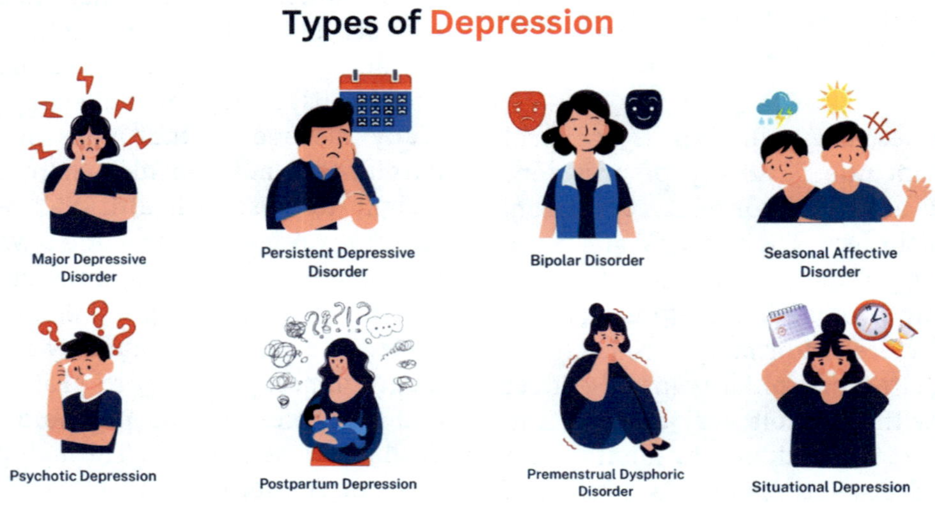

Figure 3.8. Types of depression.

Source: https://relevancerecovery.com/wp-content/uploads/2023/10/httpsrelevancerecovery.comblogwhat-is-grey-area-drinking-2-1024x576.png.

The reason why traditional interventions fall short is that they are too lengthy and too precise, lowering the intervention's accessibility and efficacy. Recent findings in psychological science indicate that cognitive-behavioral prevention programs that aim to be transdiagnostic hold promise in the prevention of the onset of anxiety and depression in high-risk groups. They target healthy adaptive coping skills within a brief intervention period, enhancing not only the short-term coping ability but also long-term resilience. Data from proof-of-concept studies suggest that such interventions, not only are they well-accepted to the participants, but also, they are successful in conveying necessary skills for emotional management, showing a trend towards more effective and more inclusive mental health approaches within general practice (Sauer-Zavala et al., 2017). Incorporating these intervention and prevention models into general practice is a significant possibility to enhance the quality of mental health services. Because of the endemic nature of depression and anxiety, clinicians must adopt a holistic approach that values the interface between physical and mental health. Appropriate training of GPs to recognize early signs of mental illness can result in early interventions and subsequently simplify the burden on patients as well as the health system. Furthermore, by integrating evidence-based treatments focusing on emotional and physical health, medical practitioners can further guarantee a better-balanced and comprehensive model of patient care. These advancements not only enhance patient health but also lay the cornerstone for a more robust and responsive healthcare system, better equipped to meet the varied needs of its population (The Stern Center for Evidence-Based Policy, 2015) (Figure 3.9).

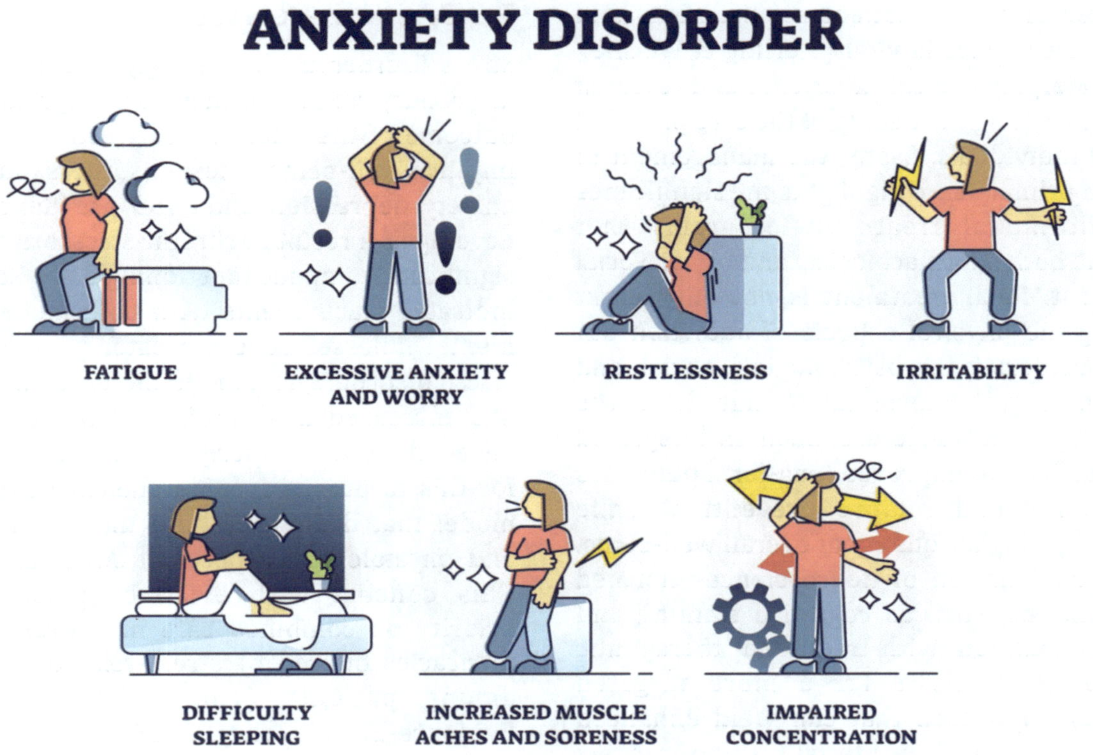

Figure 3.9. Anxiety disorders.

Source: https://relevancerecovery.com/wp-content/uploads/2022/02/Types-of-Anxiety-Disorder-1024x576.png.

3.3.2. Substance Use Disorders (SUDs)

Substance use disorders (SUDs) are serious concerns within the specialty of psychiatry in primary care that require their underlying mechanisms to be understood from a holistic perspective. They are characterized by compulsive drug use and drug-seeking behavior despite the occurrence of negative consequences, which are caused by alterations in brain functioning and structure. Clinicians must recognize that SUDs are not behavioral issues but complex biopsychosocial disorders that necessitate holistic approaches to treatment. The inclusion of knowledge from neuroscience in clinical practice is crucial but usually not addressed. For instance, initiatives such as the Neuroscience Interest Group of the International Society of Addiction Medicine act to cross the bridge between clinical application and addiction neuroscience to encourage the use of cognitive tests and neuroimaging technologies to enhance the efficiency and effectiveness of treatment methods for SUDs (Verdejo-Garcia et al., 2019). Moreover, translating research findings into effective clinical practice is important in maximizing outcomes in SUDs. The establishment of a research-practice integration (RPI) model is one sample collaborative effort that engages various stakeholders, including researchers, clinicians, and patients, in designing and updating treatment protocols. This model invites practitioners to use up-to-date research in informing their clinical practices and adjust treatment options as needed. Case studies are used to show how major research evidence can directly influence the plan of treatment services, such as in adolescent substance abuse, where adapting the intervention to patient requirements and available evidence is vital (Sterling & Weisner, 2006). Merging clinical experience and research is vital in raising the quality of the care provided to SUD individuals. Lastly, the management of SUDs in primary care highlights the significance of multi-modal treatment programs that combine both pharmacological and psychosocial treatment. Ideal treatment is not only about treating the physical aspects of addiction but also considering the psychological, social, and environmental determinants that drive the behavior of substance use. Such an integrated view can lead to improved long-term outcomes in patients and relapse prevention while achieving a higher quality of overall well-being. The amalgamation of neuroscience-informed interventions, such as cognitive training and neuromodulation, with traditional therapeutic interventions allows for a more targeted treatment approach that can yield enhanced results. Facilitating global collaborations between researchers and clinicians to promote evidence-based practices is thus imperative in shaping the future of addiction treatment across general psychiatric practice (Verdejo-Garcia et al., 2019) (Figure 3.10).

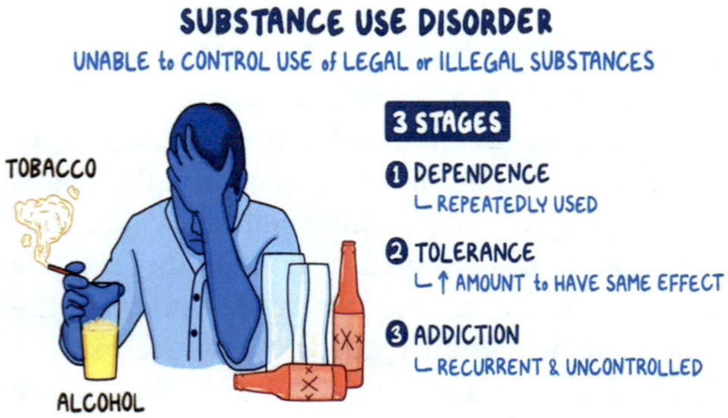

Figure 3.10. Substance use disorder.

Source: https://www.osmosis.org/_next/image?url=https%3A%2F%2Fd16qt3wv6xm098.cloudfront.net%2FnNkHRDLGSi6CFI-9G-1TKT-0Q4qjL8pU%2F_.jpg&w=3840&q=75.

3.3.3. Stress-Related Disorders

Stress disorders are increasingly being recognized as primary conditions in general psychiatry, the outcome of the interplay between mental and physical well-being. These disorders, including anxiety, depression, and PTSD, are identified to develop as a result of chronic stressors and can significantly impede functioning daily. Research indicates that patients with both medical and mental illnesses have a greater prevalence of stress disorders, leading to increased mortality and increased healthcare system burden. To have this issue properly addressed, it is vital for GPs to pursue a comprehensive treatment model that deals with both the psychological and physiological aspects of such conditions. This concurs with evidence placing high priority on combined care in addressing the intricacies offered by stress-related disorders among patients (The Stern Center for Evidence-Based Policy, 2015). Moreover, the role of psychoeducational interventions (PIs) cannot be overstated to prevent and treat stress-related disorders, particularly among vulnerable populations like adolescents. With such high levels of depression and anxiety in this population, evidence-based psychosocial interventions are now essential. Systematic reviews have revealed that PIs can provide simple health information to enhance a better understanding and symptom management. These treatments not only facilitate improved communication and interaction but also bolster mental health outcomes. Family and group interventions and school and web-based approaches have been encouraging with respect to treating the complexities of disorders related to stress, proposing the likelihood of these modalities to be used as first-line or complementary treatment for affected individuals (Jones et al., 2017). The implications of successfully addressing stress-related disease are beyond individual health impact, affecting broader social dynamics. The economic cost of such disorders is generally realized as high costs in lost productivity and greater healthcare utilization. An accurate definition of causative factors for stress-related disease is crucial in designing effective public health interventions aimed at prevention and intervention. Policy makers are invited to give utmost importance to evidence-based treatment approaches targeting self-management assistance to patients, particularly in general practice. With growing awareness of mental health, the integration of stress-related disorder management into routine medical practice can lead to better quality of care and consequently mitigate the cost burden on healthcare systems (The Stern Center for Evidence-Based Policy, 2015) (Figure 3.11).

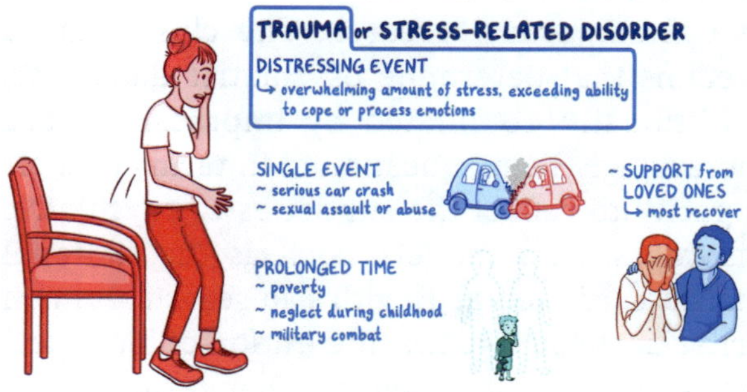

Figure 3.11. Stress-related disorders.

Source: https://d16qt3wv6xm098.cloudfront.net/Ka7_IVZ4QViFUNEwVAY8IR_3Srqz599c/_.jpg.

Test Your Knowledge

1. What are the typical signs and symptoms of depression and anxiety disorders that general practitioners should look for during consultations?
2. What role do general practitioners play in the early identification and management of substance use disorders?
3. How can general practitioners support patients in managing stress-related disorders alongside other physical health conditions?

3.4. Diagnostic Tools and Techniques

Learning Outcome

1. Discuss clinical interviews and assessments;
2. Describe standardized screening tools;
3. Understand the importance of patient history.

The combination of diagnostic instruments and methods in practice psychiatry is necessary to enhance patient outcomes. Among all the methods used, the use of standardized questionnaires and structured interviews has helped assess various psychiatric disorders. The instruments assist professionals to obtain systematic, complete data, facilitating accurate diagnosis. For instance, the use of the autism diagnostic observation schedule (ADOS) has been in the spotlight for its ability to effectively diagnose autism spectrum disorders (ASD) in diverse populations. Specifically, as highlighted by studies, developments in machine learning techniques are optimizing ASD detection, and this may help shorten the diagnostic process while enabling clinicians to be better equipped with differential diagnostic frameworks. These advances underscore the necessity of the adoption of reliable instruments to enhance diagnostic precision in all general practice environments, ultimately translating into enhanced therapeutic interventions. Secondly, the evolving nature of psychiatric diagnosis necessitates an overhaul of traditional approaches against the broader perspective of contemporary research. The classification systems that determine psychiatric diagnoses, traditionally dominated by impressions, are increasingly being questioned in terms of their capacity to reflect the subtleties of psychiatric disorders. New models, such as the National Institute of Mental Health's Research Domain Criteria, encourage the integration of biological assessments with psychological measurements. This has helped to advance the prospects of biomarker identification to simplify diagnostic criteria as well as optimize treatment methods. With these evolving standards being adopted by clinical practitioners, the integration of psychological constructs and biomedical approaches becomes necessary in promoting the practice of psychiatry within general practice environments due to the redefinition of mental health complications (Whyatt & Torres , 2018).

It is also important to consider that the application of diagnostic tools in general practice psychiatry is not without challenges.

The appropriate use and comprehension of such tools rely upon clinicians building a deep understanding of the psychological concepts they embody. Although stimulating progress in the field, e.g., more precise ASD diagnoses from fewer behavioral features gleaned by machine learning, practitioners will continue to experience challenges stemming from a deficiency in training or facilities. Furthermore, the dynamic nature of requirements for diagnosis is set to impact the consistency of practice.

The resolution of these dilemmas through ongoing education and interdisciplinarity lies at the heart of maximum effectiveness for diagnostic tools. Ultimately, the use of these methods adds to patient treatment and broadens the understanding of complex psychiatric diseases in the overall context of general practice psychiatry (Küpper et al., 2020).

3.4.1. Clinical Interviews and Assessments

Clinical interviews and assessments are central to psychiatric practice, particularly in the general practice setting, where PCPs are often also the first point of contact for those afflicted with mental illnesses. Clinical interviews allow clinicians to gain comprehensive information about a patient's mental status, history, and social context, which is priceless for informing diagnosis and treatment. The epidemiology of mental health disorders necessitates that the clinician is skilled in conducting various interviewing styles that provide effective and meaningful information. Building rapport through the interview has a direct effect on information quality, which has an impact on clinical decision-making and patient outcomes. Effective clinical interviews not only build confidence but also facilitate the examination of the patient's symptoms, thoughts, and feelings, which can lead to a better identification of their mental illness issues. Moreover, applying structured clinical assessments acts as an addition to the subjective information gathered from interviews. These assessments often utilize standardized scales that measure and categorize symptoms, providing a blueprint for clinicians to systematically evaluate mental illness. These tools are able to make diagnoses more accurate and guide treatment interventions by identifying particular areas of concern. The use of risk assessment tools, for instance, is able to identify those at risk of harming themselves or others so that practitioners can implement appropriate safeguards. Evidence shows that experienced clinicians use a combination of cues and psychological representations in making well-informed risk determinations involving suicide and neglect, illustrating the complex relationship between clinical judgment and the use of standardized assessments (Buckingham et al., 2008). This combination is crucial, particularly within a primary care setting, where the absence of the availability of vast resources requires effective risk assessment to guarantee PS. Finally, the intricacies of capacity assessments in treating patients highlight the need to employ legal and ethical measures by clinicians during clinical interviews and tests. The Mental Capacity Act 2005 provides a framework for determining a patient's ability to make informed decisions, but, as recent studies have found, legal measures under such an act are typically not carried out adequately in hospital settings (Emmett et al., 2012). This gap can be attributed to the need for greater awareness and adherence to already established guidelines among health professionals. By promoting a deeper understanding of capacity assessments, professionals can ensure that patients are not only treated with dignity but also assisted in making individual health decisions. This double-check approach of combining clinical interviewing rigor with technical observance of legal standards elevates overall general practice psychiatry, eventually leading to better care provision and results in mental health settings that incorporate it (Figure 3.12).

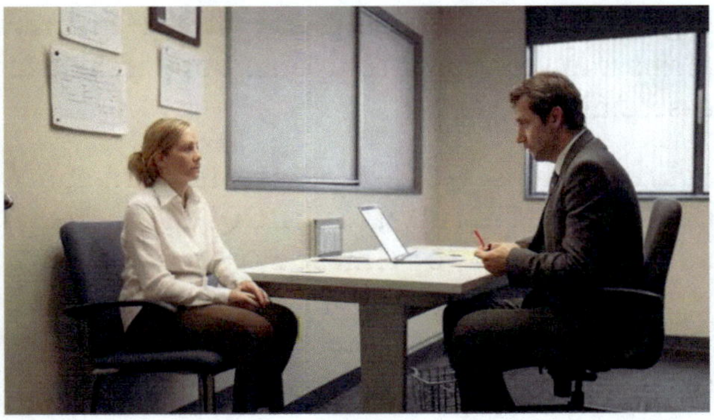

Figure 3.12. Presentation of clinical interview.

Source: https://psychiatristinlahore.com/wp-content/uploads/2024/10/History-Taking.jpg.

3.4.2. Standardized Screening Tools

Use of standardized screening tools in primary care is important in the early identification of psychiatric illnesses, which would otherwise remain undetected until they become full-fledged mental illnesses. The tools allow systematic measurement by PCPs to quantify symptoms of mental illness systematically in diverse patient populations. Specifically, they provide clinicians with empirically supported measures that can effectively detect psychological disorders, such as depression and anxiety, prior to their significantly impairing patients' everyday function. In addition, research indicates that the use of these measures in routine clinical practice directly affects the quality of care provided to patients, eventually leading to timely interventions and improved health outcomes. Use of structured protocols guarantees that practitioners conduct comprehensive health evaluations that form the basis of their effectiveness in handling serious mental health conditions in various environments. Standard screening tool incorporation into the clinical process not only necessitates proper training of healthcare providers but also consistency in monitoring and measuring effectiveness. Successful implementation requires thought for patient populations since various groups may have varying amounts of psychological distress; individualized approaches may enhance the specificity of screenings. New evidence suggests that developmental delays and psychiatric symptoms are widespread but often underdetected, particularly in primary care. Screening tools that are designed to screen for developmental issues, as mentioned in existing literature, point to the development of such tools for the sake of improving the detection and identification of possible mental health issues among clients, particularly children and older people (Sices, 2007). Screening tools need to be adapted and tested regularly for their sensitivity and specificity in identifying the subtlest expressions of mental disorders. Further, the application of standardized screen devices can impede the long-term consequences of untreated psychiatric disorders, such as the exacerbation of depressive symptoms and increased utilization of health care services. A proof is seen in a study among older individuals at home where a nearly 56% prevalence of clinically significant depressive symptoms was recorded among them, emphasizing the importance of effective screening procedures among this vulnerable population (Markle-Reid et al., 2014). With the help of standardized assessments, health professionals can apply evidence-based interventions that reduce depressive symptoms and improve health-related quality of life. Such assessments are particularly vital in enhancing patient outcomes, averting unnecessary hospitalization, and, in the long term, reducing the overall cost of healthcare. As general practice continues to change, so too must the incorporation of such tools remain a central part of encouraging mental health and ensuring that patients are treated in a timely and effective manner across the range of psychiatric services.

3.4.3. Importance of Patient History

Taking patient history forms a central component of much psychiatric evaluation in primary care. A comprehensive understanding of an individual's medical, psychological, and psychosocial history allows practitioners to formulate effective treatment plans on an individualized basis. This comprehensive process includes culturally as well as clinically appropriate factors dictating mental health, such that any concealed issues are investigated and subsequently actively addressed. For instance, knowledge of a patient's history of past experiences with psychiatric interventions, family psychosis, or traumatic life histories can yield useful patterns that assist in the diagnosis of present states and formulation of appropriate therapeutic strategies. Thus, an extensive effort to acquire comprehensive patient histories enables enhanced clinical results and the overall quality of care delivered in psychiatric hospitals. Furthermore, the importance of patient history permeates past single assessments; it plays an important role in suicide risk assessments frequently encountered in EDs. The facilitators and barriers when assessing suicide risk are most commonly identified by health professionals, with the importance of adequate knowledge regarding a patient's history. Multifactorial and coordinated approaches that involve patient history enable providers to address significant issues surrounding suicide risk, such as establishing rapport with the patient and communication strategy (Petrik et al., 2015). Frequent open communication about past trauma and mental illness can lead to more accurate risk assessment and decision-making.

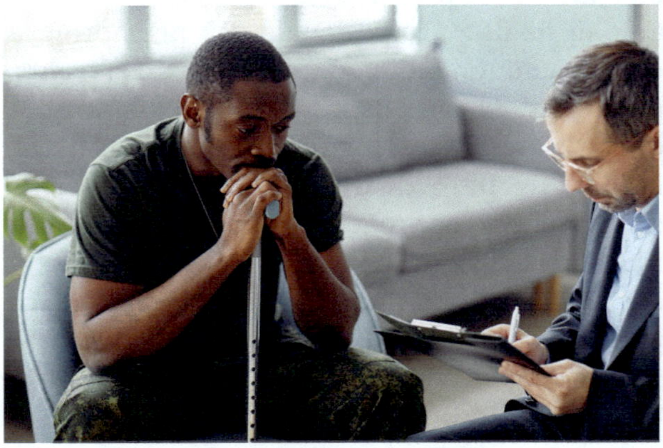

Figure 3.13. Gathering of patient history forms a foundational component of psychiatric assessment.

Source: https://cdn-ikpihob.nitrocdn.com/GJAklxHQfMKMvlVnrUvgDGQlJMJYRDNE/assets/images/optimized/rev-ee31753/therosemarycentre.com.au/wp-content/uploads/2024/11/shutterstock_2150083279-scaled.jpg.

Hence, recalling in-depth patient histories is necessary not only to understand the patient's present context but also to strategically maneuver in intractable clinical dilemmas where risk management is paramount. Finally, aggregating contributions from multiple practitioners indicates that a nuanced appreciation for the factors that bear down upon clinicians' decision-making regarding risk judgment is necessary. Research has discovered that clinical experience mostly dictates patient history interpretation, revealing solid cues that determine risk judgments, such as context and underlying motives (Buckingham et al., 2008). Through the incorporation of these results, healthcare professionals can establish a more nuanced method of evaluating suicide and self-harm risks. This enhances clinical expertise and aids in the construction of evidence-based policies that consider both actuarial data and patient experience. Thus, incorporating patient history not only guides risk judgments but also calls for a holistic approach to mental health in primary care, so that psychiatrists can deliver care that is not only effective but also empathetic and informed (Figure 3.13).

Test Your Knowledge

1. What is the role of clinical interviews in the psychiatric assessment conducted by general practitioners?
2. Which standardized screening tools are commonly used in general practice to identify mental health disorders such as depression and anxiety?
3. How does obtaining a comprehensive patient history contribute to accurate diagnosis in psychiatric cases within general practice?

3.5. Treatment Approaches in General Practice

Learning Outcome

1. Explain the concept of psychopharmacology;
2. Discuss psychotherapy and counseling;
3. Focus on lifestyle modifications and support.

Treatment strategies in family practice, especially in the field of psychiatry, require a combination of evidence-based practices and cooperative dynamics among healthcare professionals. The implementation of research results within clinical practices is essential in improving the quality of psychiatric treatment. A model that has been put forward to address this is the RPI model, which prioritizes collaboration among the principal stakeholders such as the clinicians, patients, and researchers. This model has been highly effective in alcohol and other drug (AOD) dependence treatment, demonstrating how research findings can be translated into practical interventions. Joint initiatives such as this not only improve outcomes from treatment but also create ongoing debate that can lead to the generation of new research questions and generate an ongoing feedback loop that continues to improve clinical practice in psychiatry (Sterling & Weisner, 2006). Another important treatment domain in general practice is sensory processing attention. Sensory information processing has a significant impact on one's mental health, with a tendency to exhibit challenges related to conditions such as anxiety, depression, and post-traumatic stress. Sensory modulation techniques can be extremely effective in offering interventions for individuals who are withdrawn, distressed, or agitated. These strategies offer an alternative to more traditional interventions such as seclusion and restraint, which may result in further psychological harm. Studies have supported that sensory-modulated techniques improve patient engagement and behavior stabilization, reflecting their diverse use across a range of psychiatric conditions. As a result, education of healthcare professionals on these techniques can lead to enhanced models for mental health care within general practice environments (Hoque, 2016). Also, effective intervention within primary care is not solely contingent upon clinical technique but also upon demand for comprehensive staff training and resource allocation. In-service courses regarding sensory modulation strategies have proven to be effective. When staff are properly educated about these strategies, they are better positioned to foster therapeutic environments conducive to patient empowerment and reducing dependency upon more intrusive methods. Assessment of training sessions has revealed that trainees and staff alike favored educational materials to facilitate their practice overall. This points towards a clear pathway for the introduction of new treatment modalities into everyday practice, which would eventually lead to improved patient outcomes as well as overall psychiatric care within general practice environments (Sterling & Weisner, 2006; Hoque, 2016).

3.5.1. Psychopharmacology

In psychiatry, psychopharmacology takes a prominent role in the treatment and disease management of mental illness. The integration of pharmacologic care into primary care has broadened the scope of care to physicians. With the development of medication therapy, professionals need to maintain awareness about new psychotropic medications and their efficacy for treating diseases of vast differences. The subtleties of such treatments highlight the significance of collaboration between the medical profession.

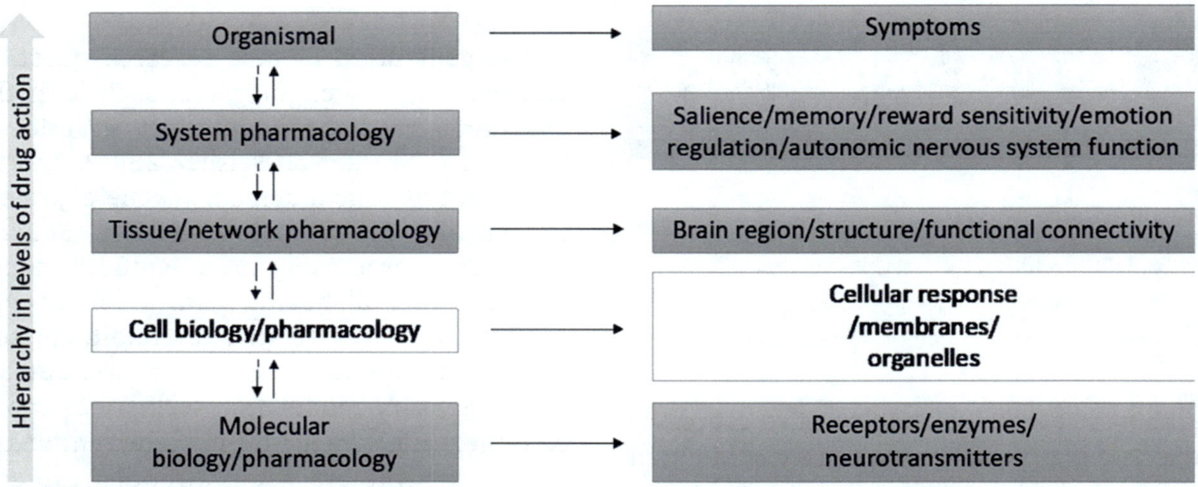

Figure 3.14. Dimensional aspects of drug action in psychopharmacology with special attention to the role of cell-level mechanisms in the understanding of this complex phenomenon.

Source: https://www.researchgate.net/publication/343252120/figure/fig1/AS:918075851419650@1595897748772/Dimensional-aspects-of-drug-action-in-psychopharmacology-with-special-attention-for-the.ppm.

A multidisciplinary approach allows for effective patient care through ensuring therapeutic interventions are of the best practices and patient-specific. In addition, as more GPs are dealing with mentally impaired patients, the ability to manage psychiatric medication becomes important in improving the effectiveness of treatment in an integrated manner. Despite the benefits of psychopharmacological treatments, their inclusion into mainstream medicine remains fraught with challenges. Prescription privileges for psychologists are an issue that underscores the debate regarding the adequacy of training as well as safety concerns. Emphasis has been on interprofessional practice, which highlighted the importance of teamwork to enhance patient care. The American Psychological Association's Ad Hoc Task Force Collaboration Level proposal endorses current healthcare reforms by its favoring of integrated care models over the problematic prescription privileges proposal. Among the criticisms presented is that the variances in educational preparation for psychologists and prescribing professionals raise some very pertinent questions concerning efficacy and PS. Consequently, a shift toward collaborative practice can increase access to treatment and decrease the risk of psychopharmacological intervention while ultimately prioritizing patient welfare over professional grounds. More recent interventions, such as the comprehensive behavioral intervention for tics (CBIT), also shed light upon the effectiveness of non-pharmacologic intervention possibilities, welcoming an open-minded view of mental healthcare. Research on CBIT demonstrates significant reductions in the severity of tics and impairment in children with Tourette disorder, suggesting that behavioral therapies can supplement or, in some cases, complement pharmacologic management. As neurology and pediatric clinics are generally the first contact points for individuals with tics, integrating such therapies into psychiatry is crucial. Positive feedback regarding satisfaction and therapeutic alliance also highlights the significance of an integrated treatment model where various modalities, including psychopharmacology, are utilized in harmony. The establishment of the specialty of psychiatry through a combination of pharmacological and behavioral methods of care enhances the quality of patient care and complies with shifting patterns in healthcare (Figure 3.14).

3.5.2. Psychotherapy and Counseling

The integration of psychotherapy and counseling in general practice is essential in providing holistic mental health care. In contemporary clinical settings, GPs are likely to encounter patients presenting with psychological distress, making mental health a key component of primary care. As practitioners are situated centrally at the interface of physical and mental health, they must have a fundamental conceptual understanding of the various therapeutic modalities, such as psychotherapy. It enables the practitioner to recognize when the patient can be assisted by psychotherapeutic interventions so as to provide more integrated patient care. In addition, the emphasis on mental health enhances overall therapeutic outcomes, ultimately resulting in enhanced management of psychological and somatic symptoms. The development of psychotherapy is increasingly utilizing mindfulness-based interventions, which have become commonplace due to their effectiveness for enhancing therapeutic outcomes. Evidence has opened up the benefits of mindfulness in counseling, proving that not only does it minimize stress but also reinforces clients' control over their emotions and awareness about themselves. As practitioners in general practice are usually the first point of contact for individuals requiring mental health care, it becomes imperative that they are educated about such novel methods. The incorporation of mindfulness in the treatment options can give strength to the practitioner to be able to help their patients with their mental illness more effectively. Mindfulness interventions can also act as a prevention, which will improve mental well-being and hardness, ultimately reducing the burden on the healthcare system. Additionally, the construction of an integrative model, incorporating psychotherapy, together with informal support systems, is necessary for the evolution of mental health care in general practice in the future. Formal psychotherapy and informal social support may overlap, as both avenues play significant parts in the path to emotional health. It has been proven that using these two avenues of psychological assistance could optimize the overall gains of mental health interventions. By accepting the significance of social support in addition to psychotherapeutic treatment, GPs can create a more advanced image of their patients' mental health. This paradigmatic shift triggers the development of collaborative care models, where practitioners of health work together in providing holistic care and fostering a more resilient community through enriched therapeutics (Figure 3.15).

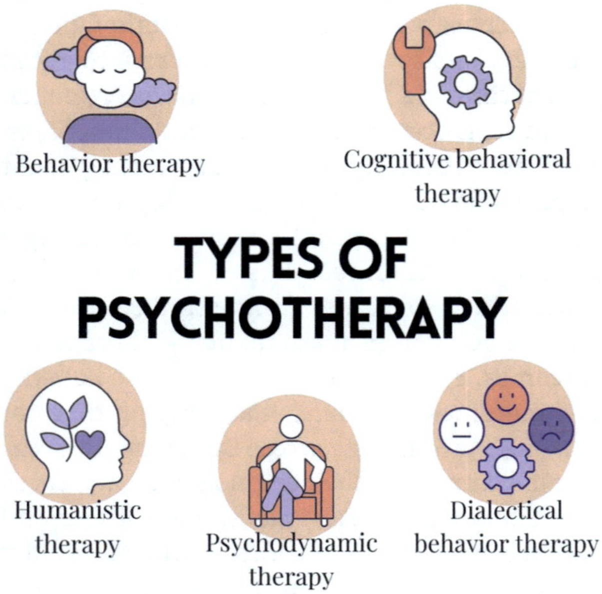

Figure 3.15. Types of psychotherapy.

Source: https://www.simplypsychology.org/wp-content/uploads/Types-of-psychotherapy.jpg.

3.5.3. Lifestyle Modifications and Support

Lifestyle modification is crucial in the management of mental disorders in primary care and puts in the foreground the interconnectedness of body and mind. These may vary from dietary changes, physical activity, sleeping patterns, and social contact, all of which have the capacity to exert a significant influence on emotional states and intellectual processes. For instance, regular exercise has been linked to reductions in symptoms of depression and anxiety, while a healthy diet can enhance mood as well as overall mental health. Both of these lifestyle modifications are especially pertinent in the context of the high prevalence of patients who present with co-occurring medical and mental illness, raising issues regarding mortality rates as well as quality of care. As has been seen, the use of self-management support strategies can facilitate patients to take an active role in their process of care, build resilience, and improve treatment outcomes (The Stern Center for Evidence-Based Policy, 2015). Formal and informal support systems are also very important in facilitating successful lifestyle change. General practice mental health practitioners can guide the patient in creating systematic plans for achieving such change and provide sustained encouragement and motivation. Peer support groups and community resources also enhance the effectiveness of lifestyle interventions by fostering a feeling of membership and accountability among patients with similar issues.

Multidisciplinary collaboration can also enhance care by providing a range of insights into behavioral approaches. The recognition of the social determinants of health underlines the importance of addressing barriers to lifestyle change, e.g., socioeconomic status, which impede an individual's ability to make and sustain changes in favor of mental health (The Stern Center for Evidence-Based Policy, 2015). Tailored healthcare strategies, with applications of tailored medicine, provide promising avenues for integrating lifestyle change into psychiatric care.

The evolving face of technology and genomic profiling offers the promise of personalized interventions, aligning lifestyle change with the individual's own health profile. This strategy can optimize the treatment plan by considering genetic predispositions, lifestyle choices, and psychosocial factors that influence patient engagement and adherence to prescribed change. Since medicine is increasingly shifting towards a systems medicine and biology paradigm, understanding how unique patient attributes impact mental health interventions is increasingly important. These advancements allow clinicians to offer individualized support, thereby maximizing the efficacy of lifestyle modification and overall patient experience of care for patients struggling with mental health issues.

Test Your Knowledge

1. What are the common psychopharmacological treatments initiated by general practitioners for conditions like depression and anxiety?
2. How can general practitioners decide when to refer patients for specialized psychotherapy or counseling services?
3. What role do lifestyle modifications play in the management of mental health disorders in general practice?

3.6. Challenges in Integrating Psychiatry into General Practice

Learning Outcome

1. Discuss about stigma surrounding mental health;
2. Describe time constraints in general practice;
3. Focus on limited resources and training challenges.

The integration of psychiatry into general practice faces enormous challenges, particularly in terms of the readiness of the health system and the allocation of resources. In the majority of the low- and middle-income countries (LMICs), insufficient infrastructure prevents mental health care services from becoming accessible on a large scale. For instance, the PRIME study reports severe shortages in mental health professionals trained and essential medicines within health systems in Ethiopia, India, Nepal, South Africa, and Uganda. These shortcomings pose a considerable hindrance to the delivery of good mental health care in primary care, as GPs may find themselves lacking in the support needed to work on psychiatric disorders. Furthermore, the lack of data for updated coverage of treatment exacerbates problems in implementing scalable mental health integration strategies for which there has been an urgent need for meticulous district plans to harmonize mental health resources with overall health services (Hanlon et al., 2014). The gap in treatment among mental health services also transcends LMICs to other parts of the world that are more developed. A European study cites significant impediments to the delivery of mental health services arising from structural shortcomings and chaotic care provision. Health care practitioners like GPs report ease of access to and availability of mental health services as a problem that constrains their ability to build an integrated chain of care. The complexity in bridging gaps between treatment options and being able to successfully refer only contributes to the layering in the integration process, rendering it challenging for GPs to provide integrated care to psychiatric patients. This systemic disconnection underscores the importance of collaborative models that enhance seamless transition between levels of care and solidify mental health as a core component of the general practice model (Triliva et al., 2020). Furthermore, the development of mental health care in the practice environment must struggle with the prevailing attitudes and stigma surrounding psychiatric illness. Patients, particularly in more ignorant populations, may themselves be resistant to the utilization of mental health care because of societal attitudes that equate failure or weakness with mental illness. Such stigma has the consequence of leading individuals to shun treatment, fueling the widespread mhcGAP reported in studies from different countries. In order to balance this, GPs must not only be clinically competent but also equipped with resources in a bid to increase mental health literacy among patients and their families. By leveraging the use of resources, including e-mental health technologies and community programs, practitioners can make entry easier for patients into mental health care, hence optimizing the integration of psychiatry into general practice and an integrated approach to health care (Triliva et al., 2020).

3.6.1. Stigma Surrounding Mental Health

The mental health stigma is a pervasive barrier that has a very broad impact on individuals who seek help under the backdrop of general practice psychiatry. The stigma manifests in the form of negative stereotyping and societal discrimination in the majority of instances, leading to mountainous issues for the victims of mental health. Fear of stigma and condemnation and also being excluded from a number of patients, can discourage them from seeking suitable treatment or talking openly regarding their conditions.

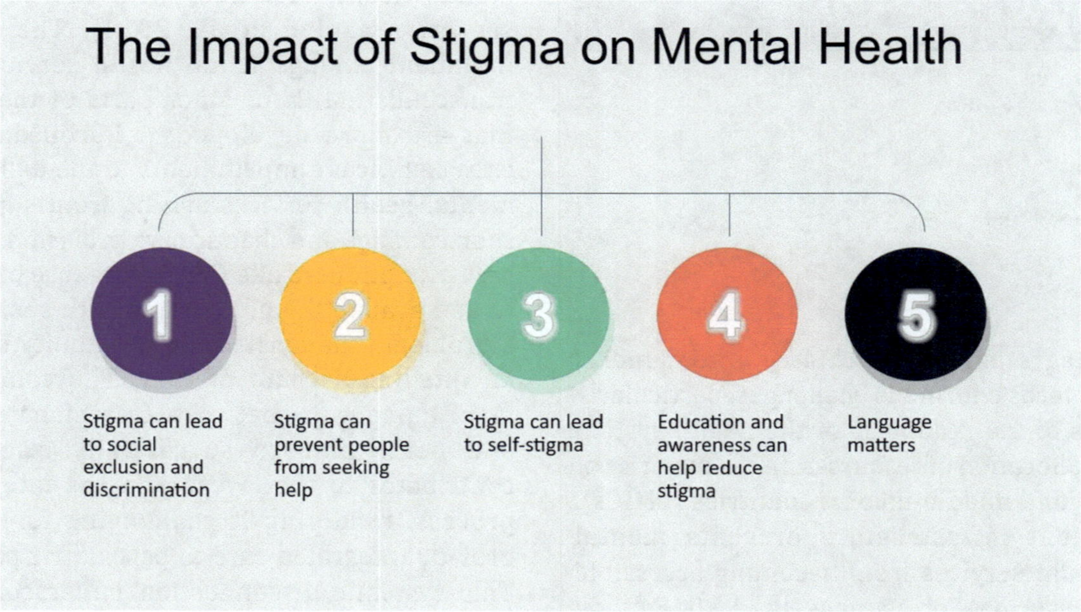

Figure 3.16. The impact of stigma on mental health.

Source: https://fastercapital.co/i/Mental-health--Shattering-Stigmas--Embracing-Mental-Health-and-Distressale--The-Impact-of-Stigma-on-Mental-Health.webp.

Thus, this reluctance not only aggravates their mental illness but also limits channels towards recovery and help. Unless these deep-seated stigmas are properly addressed, the role of psychiatry in general practice can be significantly undermined because a lack of trust in the patient prevents practitioners from effectively providing good mental health services. In addition, studies indicate that the effects of stigma extend beyond personal issues; they also have a strong influence on public health effects. Stigma, according to studies, keeps individuals from accessing basic needs such as housing, job opportunities, and even health centers, creating a cycle of disadvantage and exclusion. The paper points out that stigma is a main barrier to recovery, and eliminating such stigmas is necessary to accept individuals with mental illness as full members of society. Both local and international efforts in stigma reduction are essential in establishing an environment where people get empowered to access mental health care without fear or shame (Hocking B). Consequently, GPs have to be equipped with resources and knowledge in order to combat stigma proactively as part of ordinary practice. In addition, the relationship between physical and mental health stigma further obscures treatment in general practice. Anorexia nervosa, for example, showing a startling prevalence among some patient groups, signifies the integration of mental and physical health (Chelvanayagam et al., 2012). Comprehension of the psychological factors affecting such disorders as anorexia, particularly societal pressure and stigma, is most crucial to GPs. It involves an appreciation beyond the physical extent of a disorder to the psychological reasons underlying which patients may be suffering as a result of stigma. By emphasizing a stigma-free, empathetic treatment of mental health disorders, practitioners can enhance patient participation and a better health care environment that is supportive and open to overall recovery (Figure 3.16).

3.6.2. Time Constraints in General Practice

With today's health care setting, time pressures within general practice have been one of the biggest issues where psychiatric illness is involved. GPs may be pressured to have high volumes of patients for brief periods of consultation. This will dissuade their ability to conduct complete assessments necessary in the detection and diagnosis of mental illness. The problem is compounded even further when it comes to complex conditions like ADHD, which can be more extensively studied to ensure accurate identification and subsequent intervention. GPs as gatekeepers to specialist services can be hesitant to refer patients due to time pressures and self-doubt about their ability to diagnose symptoms of ADHD, leading to underdiagnosis and ineffective delivery of treatment (Tatlow-Golden et al., 2016). Besides, the reluctance of GPs to engage in shared care, particularly psychiatric care, is evidence of yet another feature of the time constraint issue. Some GPs are confused about ADHD because they lack proper training and guidance in managing psychiatric conditions (Tatlow-Golden et al., 2016), according to a systematic review. This vagueness is particularly problematic in general practice's tight agendas, where GPs may prefer to focus on somatic health issues that are seen as more straightforward or urgent. Thus, the critical activity of screening for mental health becomes secondary, and a culture of under-serving for mental health disorders may be fostered and a stigma maintained. Fixing these constraints requires reorientation of the paradigm in training and resource allocation for general practice to maximize the provision of psychiatric care (Tatlow-Golden et al., 2016). A tried approach to the execution of screening and brief interventions (SBI) in general practice can promote better outcomes in mental health despite time limitations. Training general health professionals in SBI strategies has revealed positive effects on healthcare professionals' willingness to address mental health with patients. Whereas the establishment of such programs will likely seem time-consuming at first, the eventual payback could easily be far greater than the initial time cost. By equipping GPs with the tools and protocols necessary to effectively treat mental health issues within their practices, healthcare systems can create an atmosphere wherein psychiatric disorders are addressed more regularly and with less difficulty. In the end, focusing on training and establishing supportive systems that augment a GP's ability will most likely result in better patient outcomes in psychiatric care, avoiding the negative implications of time limits in general practice.

3.6.3. Limited Resources and Training

Good practice in psychiatry is severely handicapped by training and resource shortages. GPs are not typically offered specialist psychiatric training, a barrier to diagnosing and treating mental disorders. There are evidence-based guidelines for the detection and management of psychiatric disorders, and their application is frequently impaired by poor psychiatric training and a deficiency in supportive clinical infrastructures. General practitioners may encounter mixed psychiatric presentations among their patients; however, their ability to intervene may be hindered by inadequate mental health training during the course of their general medical education. This deficit underscores the urgent need for strengthened educational courses that emphasize robust mental health content within primary care training. Furthermore, the integration of psychiatric genetics into general practice represents another area of restricted resources and training. The International Society of Psychiatric Genetics has emphasized the necessity of incorporating genetic information into psychiatric training curricula. While improvements in the identification of the genetic causes of psychiatric disorders are imminent, their clinical application is sporadic. Limitations of genetic testing, such as its limited application in the identification of disorders like autism and intellectual disability, are an essential gap in the skills of GPs. There is a clear need for systematic educational systems that equip practitioners with the skills to interpret and apply genetic information in clinical decision-making (Nurnberger et al., 2018). Also, the overall shortage of general mental health workers worsens the issue of limited resources and training in psychiatry. Congressional initiatives have highlighted the interdependencies of quality, access, and cost of mental health treatment and emphasized the impact that capable providers can have on these measures. Properly trained mental health professionals have a direct influence on how much care is feasible in primary care practice. Further, given the rising need for mental care, the mismatch between the supply of trained professionals and broadened patient demand indicates a key challenge to be addressed by policymakers (Heisler & Bagalman, 2013). Hence, building an adequate mental health workforce through increased training and resource facilitation is essential in fortifying psychiatric care within general practice.

Test Your Knowledge

1. How does stigma surrounding mental health affect patients' willingness to discuss psychiatric symptoms with their general practitioners?
2. In what ways do time constraints during general practice consultations impact the quality of mental health assessments and care?

SUMMARY

The journey into psychiatry within general practice, and it is evident that integration of mental health into primary care is of the highest priority. This convergence of practices not only expands the scope of treatment for patients but also enhances the overall efficiency of the treatment options. GPs educated in the capacity for detection and treatment of psychiatric disorders can reasonably significantly reduce the expense to society of mental illness. A systematic approach that encourages collaboration between mental health professionals and PCPs sustains an environment that is receptive to early intervention and ongoing therapeutic relationships. This collaborative model aligns with emerging evidence that highlights the importance of accessible and comprehensive mental health care as a fundamental pillar of general health. Further, the increasing use of self-monitoring technology by those with illnesses such as bipolar disorder raises the promise of new technology in redefining the management of mental health. Findings suggested in accounts of studies demonstrate that self-measurement strategies enable patients to be active in their own health, with enhanced self-reflection and informative feedback to treatment groups. As testified to by trends in reported experience with digital surveillance, the integration of technology in everyday practice has the potential to deliver personalized support and intervention from real-time data. Thus, such innovation not only simplifies psychiatric treatment in an everyday practice setting but also challenges practitioners to embrace new methods that promote patient empowerment and evidence-based practice (Murnane et al., 2016). Lastly, the variations in mental health treatment noted in other populations like asylum seekers and refugees necessitate understanding of the broader context under which psychiatry must operate. The legal and practical conditions that govern these patients, as in pertinent literature, show an overwhelming need for psychiatric care that is culturally appropriate. Findings of focus groups and quantitative surveys on these groups demonstrate deficits in the knowledge base of their particular psychological needs within general practice, which signals a robust area calling for subsequent research and intervention. Closing these gaps is important because it highlights the demand for advocacy and evidence-based practice within psychiatry, ultimately seeking a more robust and efficient approach to mental health care (Begley et al., 1999).

The integration of psychiatry in general practice has emerged as an essential component of the healthcare landscape of today. The transition is mostly driven by the increasing recognition of the role of mental health in overall health outcomes. GPs are now at the forefront of the identification and management of mental health illnesses, for which they need to be appropriately trained and supported. The texts suggest that an integrated strategy, whereby mental health care is incorporated into primary care, not only improves access to care but also makes for earlier detection and intervention, ultimately decreasing the onset of mental illnesses. Such integration bears witness to usual services, which force a reexamination of how mental health is conceived in the medical community and among patients themselves, establishing a culture wherein mental health is viewed on a par with physical health (Holmwood et al., 2008). Mental health training for GPs is essential in facilitating them to manage psychiatric disorders appropriately. There is evidence that intensive educational programs can enhance GPs' confidence and skill in managing mental health issues significantly. This is required since most patients normally approach with a mix of physical and mental illnesses and require care from a holistic point of view. Besides, the emphasis on models of shared care has greatly contributed to facilitating cooperation between GPs and mental health professionals through a seamless sharing of information and resources.

By creating a more integrated healthcare system, the silos that exist between physical and mental health can be dismantled to create better patient outcomes and satisfaction. Reforms of primary care training for GPs in effect align with the broader objective of making primary practice mental health care more effective (Thornton, 2011). Moreover, the impact that policy will have on reining in mental health care should never be underestimated. The recent years have witnessed radical transformations in national policy efforts towards enhancing the coordination of mental health care in general practice. These changes have been propelling the shift from isolated care models to integrative, community-oriented models with a focus on partnerships among various healthcare providers. The policy milestones have been instrumental in shaping the landscape as they prioritize the key areas of workforce planning, provision of services, and patient activation. The evolving mental health policy environment not only reflects the social change in the idea of mental well-being but also encompasses the requirement of continuous change within the healthcare industry to deal with patients' diverse needs in a unified approach (Holmwood et al., 2008).

KEY TERMS FROM THIS CHAPTER

- Anxiety Disorders
- Attention deficit hyperactivity disorder (ADHD)
- Biomarker identification
- General practice psychiatry
- Hospitalization
- Integrated treatment model
- Mental health assessments
- Mental health stigma
- Mental illness
- Mindfulness-based treatments
- ASD diagnoses
- Behavior stabilization
- Dietary changes
- General practitioners (GPs)
- Human psychological health
- Low- and middle-income countries (LMICs)
- Mental health issues
- Mental health treatment
- Mental sanity
- Patient outcomes

CRITICAL THINKING QUESTIONS

1. **What is the primary role of general practitioners (GPs) in managing mental health?**
   a. Prescribing complex psychiatric medications without specialist input
   b. Identifying, diagnosing, and managing common mental health disorders in the community
   c. Referring all psychiatric cases directly to psychiatrists
   d. Providing psychotherapy exclusively
2. **Which of the following is the most common mental health disorder seen in general practice?**
   a. Schizophrenia
   b. Bipolar disorder
   c. Depression and anxiety disorders
   d. Obsessive-compulsive disorder (OCD)
3. **What is a common first-line treatment approach for mild to moderate depression in general practice?**
   a. Electroconvulsive therapy (ECT)
   b. Immediate referral to inpatient psychiatric care
   c. Psychoeducation, lifestyle modification, and antidepressant medication if needed
   d. Surgery
4. **Which of the following is a major challenge faced by GPs in integrating psychiatric care into general practice?**
   a. Excessive availability of psychiatric resources
   b. Lack of training and confidence in managing mental health issues
   c. Overdiagnosis of mental health disorders in primary care
   d. Too many psychotherapies options
5. **Which diagnostic technique is most important for GPs in identifying mental health issues?**
   a. Brain imaging
   b. Blood tests
   c. Genetic testing
   d. Detailed psychiatric interview and history taking

Short Answer Questions

1. What is the significance of general practitioners as the first point of contact in the identification and management of mental health disorders?
2. Which mental health disorders are most commonly encountered by general practitioners, and how do these impact patient care in primary settings?
3. What diagnostic tools and clinical assessment techniques do general practitioners typically use to evaluate mental health conditions?
4. How important is taking a detailed patient history in the psychiatric evaluation process within general practice?
5. What are the primary treatment approaches used by general practitioners for managing common mental health disorders such as depression and anxiety?

Answers to Critical Thinking Questions

1. (b); 2. (d); 3. (c); 4. (b); 5. (d)

REFERENCES

1. Buckingham, C. D., Adams, A., & Mace, C. (2008). Cues and knowledge structures used by mental-health professionals when making risk assessments. *Journal of Mental Health, 17*(3), 299–314. https://doi.org/10.1080/09638230701498374(accessed on 27th June 2025).
2. Hanlon, C., Luitel, N. P., Kathree, T., Murhar, V., Shrivasta, S., Medhin, G., Ssebunnya, J., Fekadu, A., Shidhaye, R., Petersen, I., Jordans, M., Kigozi, F., Thornicroft, G., Patel, V., Tomlinson, M., Lund, C., Breuer, E., De Silva, M., & Prince, M. (2014). Challenges and opportunities for implementing integrated mental health care: a district level situation analysis from five low- and middle-income countries. *PloS one, 9*(2), e88437. https://doi.org/10.1371/journal.pone.0088437 (accessed on 27th June 2025).
3. Muddiman E, Bullock A, Allery L, MacDonald J, Webb KL, Pugsley L. 'Black sheep in the herd'? The role, status and identity of generalist doctors in secondary care. *Health Services Management Research*. 2016;29(4):124-131. doi:10.1177/0951484816670416
4. (accessed on 27th June 2025).
5. Emmett, C., Poole, M., Bond, J., & Hughes, J. C. (2013). Homeward bound or bound for a home? Assessing the capacity of dementia patients to make decisions about hospital discharge: comparing practice with legal standards. *International journal of law and psychiatry, 36*(1), 73–82. https://doi.org/10.1016/j.ijlp.2012.11.009 (accessed on 27th June 2025).
6. Anderson, J., Bennett, A. J. W., Clayton, P., McKeown, M., et al. (2003). Gender politics and secure services for women: Reflections on a study of staff understandings of challenging behavior. https://core.ac.uk/download/338689.pdf (accessed on 27th June 2025).
7. Mommerency, G., Van den Heede, K., Verhaeghe, N., Swartenbroekx, N., Annemans, L., Schoentjes, E., & Eyssen, M. (2011). Organisatie van geestelijke gezondheidszorg voor kinderen en jongeren : literatuurstudie en internationaal overzicht. Brussel: Federaal Kenniscentrum voor de Gezondheidszorg (KCE).(accessed on 27th June 2025).
8. Whyatt CP and Torres EB (2018) Autism Research: An Objective Quantitative Review of Progress and Focus Between 1994 and 2015. Front. Psychol. 9:1526. doi: 10.3389/fpsyg.2018.01526(accessed on 27th June 2025).
9. Verdejo-Garcia, A., Lorenzetti, V., Manning, V., Piercy, H., Bruno, R., Hester, R., Pennington, D., Tolomeo, S., Arunogiri, S., Bates, M. E., Bowden-Jones, H., Campanella, S., Daughters, S. B., Kouimtsidis, C., Lubman, D. I., Meyerhoff, D. J., Ralph, A., Rezapour, T., Tavakoli, H., Zare-Bidoky, M., ... Ekhtiari, H. (2019). A Roadmap for Integrating Neuroscience Into Addiction Treatment: A Consensus of the Neuroscience Interest Group of the International Society of Addiction Medicine. *Frontiers in psychiatry, 10*, 877. https://doi.org/10.3389/fpsyt.2019.00877(accessed on 27th June 2025).
10. Nurnberger, J. I., Jr, Austin, J., Berrettini, W. H., Besterman, A. D., DeLisi, L. E., Grice, D. E., Kennedy, J. L., Moreno-De-Luca, D., Potash, J. B., Ross, D. A., Schulze, T. G., & Zai, G. (2018). What Should a Psychiatrist Know About Genetics? Review and Recommendations From the Residency Education Committee of the International Society of Psychiatric Genetics. *The Journal of clinical psychiatry, 80*(1), 17nr12046. https://doi.org/10.4088/JCP.17nr12046(accessed on 27th June 2025).

11. Triliva, S., Ntani, S., Giovazolias, T., Kafetsios, K., Axelsson, M., Bockting, C., Buysse, A., Desmet, M., Dewaele, A., Hannon, D., Haukenes, I., Hensing, G., Meganck, R., Rutten, K., Schønning, V., Van Beveren, L., Vandamme, J., & Øverland, S. (2020). Healthcare professionals' perspectives on mental health service provision: a pilot focus group study in six European countries. *International journal of mental health systems, 14*, 16. https://doi.org/10.1186/s13033-020-00350-1(accessed on 27th June 2025).
12. Heisler, E. J. & Bagalman, E. (2013). *The Mental Health Workforce: A Primer*. https://core.ac.uk/download/18615793.pdf (accessed on 27th June 2025).
13. Furnivall, J. and Connelly, G. and Barbour, R. and Bryce, G. and Lockhart, E. and Phin, L. and Stallard, A. and van Beinum, M. and Wilson, Philip (2006) *Only connect : addressing the emotional needs of Scotland›s children and young people.* NHS Health Scotland, Edinburgh, UK.(accessed on 27th June 2025).
14. Bentley, K. H., Boettcher, H., Bullis, J. R., Carl, J. R., Conklin, L. R., Sauer-Zavala, S., Pierre-Louis, C., Farchione, T. J., & Barlow, D. H. (2018). Development of a Single-Session, Transdiagnostic Preventive Intervention for Young Adults at Risk for Emotional Disorders. *Behavior modification, 42*(5), 781–805. https://doi.org/10.1177/0145445517734354 (accessed on 27th June 2025).
15. Sauer-Zavala, S., Wilner, J. G., & Barlow, D. H. (2017). Addressing neuroticism in psychological treatment. *Personality disorders, 8*(3), 191–198. https://doi.org/10.1037/per0000224(accessed on 27th June 2025).
16. Bartram, A. (2012). The performance of pain: The consequences for the performing body and its portrayal of mental health. https://core.ac.uk/download/17352854.pdf (accessed on 27th June 2025).
17. Begley, M., Condon, M., Garavan, K. C., Holland, S., et al. (1999). Asylum in Ireland–A public health perspective. https://core.ac.uk/download/11309246.pdf (accessed on 27th June 2025).
18. Petrik, M. L., Gutierrez, P. M., Berlin, J. S., & Saunders, S. M. (2015). Barriers and facilitators of suicide risk assessment in emergency departments: a qualitative study of provider perspectives. *General hospital psychiatry, 37*(6), 581–586. https://doi.org/10.1016/j.genhosppsych.2015.06.018(accessed on 27th June 2025).
19. Bevan Jones, R., Thapar, A., Stone, Z., Thapar, A., Jones, I., Smith, D., & Simpson, S. (2018). Psychoeducational interventions in adolescent depression: A systematic review. *Patient education and counseling, 101*(5), 804–816. https://doi.org/10.1016/j.pec.2017.10.015(accessed on 27th June 2025).
20. Brabeck, K. M., Holtzman, E. G., Kene, P., et al. (2018). Integrating mindfulness into the training of helping professionals. https://core.ac.uk/download/215489761.pdf (accessed on 27th June 2025).
21. Markle-Reid, M., McAiney, C., Forbes, D., Thabane, L., Gibson, M., Browne, G., Hoch, J. S., Peirce, T., & Busing, B. (2014). An interprofessional nurse-led mental health promotion intervention for older home care clients with depressive symptoms. *BMC geriatrics, 14*, 62. https://doi.org/10.1186/1471-2318-14-62(accessed on 27th June 2025).
22. Bucci, F. (2014). Cultural representations of mental illness in contemporary Japan. https://core.ac.uk/download/74711749.pdf (accessed on 27th June 2025).

23. Camilleri, N., Cassar Parnis, A., & Cassar, J. R. (2009). Problems associated with the diagnosis and the prescribing of anti-psychotic medication in children and adolescents for psychiatric conditions, by non-psychiatric specialists. https://core.ac.uk/download/46602212.pdf (accessed on 27th June 2025).

24. Murnane, E. L., Cosley, D., Chang, P., Guha, S., Frank, E., Gay, G., & Matthews, M. (2016). Self-monitoring practices, attitudes, and needs of individuals with bipolar disorder: implications for the design of technologies to manage mental health. *Journal of the American Medical Informatics Association : JAMIA*, *23*(3), 477–484. https://doi.org/10.1093/jamia/ocv165 (accessed on 27th June 2025).

25. Chelvanayagam, S., Collins, B., Duncan, J., O'Brien, J., et al. (2012). Uncovering anorexia nervosa in a biofeedback clinic for bowel dysfunction. https://core.ac.uk/download/20321227.pdf (accessed on 27th June 2025).

26. Vancampfort, D., Rosenbaum, S., Probst, M., Connaughton, J., du Plessis, C., Yamamoto, T., & Stubbs, B. (2016). What are the top 10 physical activity research questions in schizophrenia?. *Disability and rehabilitation*, *38*(22), 2235–2243. https://doi.org/10.3109/09638288.2015.1116622(accessed on 27th June 2025).

27. Park, M. H., Falconer, C. L., Saxena, S., Kessel, A. S., Croker, H., Skow, A., Viner, R. M., & Kinra, S. (2013). Perceptions of health risk among parents of overweight children: a cross-sectional study within a cohort. *Preventive medicine*, *57*(1), 55–59. https://doi.org/10.1016/j.ypmed.2013.04.002(accessed on 27th June 2025).

28. Ely, L. J., Gilbert, D. L., Lipps, T. D., Mink, J. W., et al. (2015). Pilot testing behavior therapy for chronic tic disorders in neurology and developmental pediatrics clinics. https://core.ac.uk/download/213085584.pdf (accessed on 27th June 2025).

29. Yager, J., Kunkle, R., Fochtmann, L. J., Reid, S. M., Plovnick, R., Nininger, J. E., Silverman, J. J., & Vergare, M. J. (2014). Who's your expert? Use of an expert opinion survey to inform development of American Psychiatric Association practice guidelines. *Academic psychiatry : the journal of the American Association of Directors of Psychiatric Residency Training and the Association for Academic Psychiatry*, *38*(3), 376–382. https://doi.org/10.1007/s40596-014-0046-6(accessed on 27th June 2025).

30. Tatlow-Golden, M., Prihodova, L., Gavin, B., Cullen, W., & McNicholas, F. (2016). What do general practitioners know about ADHD? Attitudes and knowledge among first-contact gatekeepers: systematic narrative review. *BMC family practice*, *17*(1), 129. https://doi.org/10.1186/s12875-016-0516-x (accessed on 27th June 2025).

31. Grey, B. J. (2015). The future of emotional harm. https://core.ac.uk/download/144230394.pdf (accessed on 27th June 2025).

32. Van Gordon W, Shonin E, Griffiths MD (2015) Mindfulness in Mental Health: A Critical Reflection. J Psy Neuro Dis (accessed on 27th June 2025).

33. Holmwood, C., Groom, G., & Nicholson, S.A. (2008). Mental Health Shared Care in Australia 2001: Report for the Commonwealth Department of Health and Aged Care.https://core.ac.uk/download/14931392.pdf (accessed on 27th June 2025).

34. Küpper, C., Stroth, S., Wolff, N., Hauck, F., Kliewer, N., Schad-Hansjosten, T., Kamp-Becker, I., Poustka, L., Roessner, V., Schultebraucks, K., & Roepke, S. (2020). Identifying predictive features of autism spectrum disorders in a clinical sample of adolescents and adults using

machine learning. *Scientific reports, 10*(1), 4805. https://doi.org/10.1038/s41598-020-61607-w(accessed on 27th June 2025).

35. Hocking, B. (2025). A life without stigma. https://core.ac.uk/download/pdf/30676353.pdf (accessed on 27th June 2025).

36. Hoque, S. (2016). *Care team Education on The Use of Sensory Resources in Inpatient Psychiatry.* https://core.ac.uk/download/79664899.pdf (accessed on 27th June 2025).

37. Kallert, T. W., Howardova, A., Kiejna, A., Nawka, P., et al. (2013). To what extent could acute general psychiatric day care reduce inpatient admissions? https://core.ac.uk/download/30698054.pdf (accessed on 27th June 2025).

38. Lucock, M., Leach, C., & Iveson, S. (2005). Using evidence to improve psychological therapies services. https://core.ac.uk/download/57835.pdf (accessed on 27th June 2025).

39. Long, V. (2016). 'Heading up a blind alley'? Scottish psychiatric hospitals in the era of deinstitutionalization. https://core.ac.uk/download/293881690.pdf (accessed on 27th June 2025).

40. Meyer, L., & Melchert, T. P. (2011). Examining the content of mental health intake assessments from a biopsychosocial perspective. *Journal of Psychotherapy Integration, 21*(1), 70–89. https://doi.org/10.1037/a0022907c(accessed on 27th June 2025).

41. Leavey, G., Mallon, S., Rondon-Sulbaran, J., Galway, K., Rosato, M., & Hughes, L. (2017). The failure of suicide prevention in primary care: family and GP perspectives - a qualitative study. *BMC psychiatry, 17*(1), 369. https://doi.org/10.1186/s12888-017-1508-7(accessed on 27th June 2025).

42. Sices, L. (2007). *Developmental Screening in Primary Care: The Effectiveness of Current Practice and Recommendations for Improvement.* https://core.ac.uk/download/71350769.pdf (accessed on 27th June 2025).

43. Sterling, S., & Weisner, C. (2006). Translating research findings into practice: example of treatment services for adolescents in managed care. *Alcohol research & health : the journal of the National Institute on Alcohol Abuse and Alcoholism, 29*(1), 11–18.(accessed on 27th June 2025).

44. Romeo, R., Knapp, M., Hellier, J., Dewey, M., Ballard, C., Baldwin, R., Bentham, P., Burns, A., Fox, C., Holmes, C., Katona, C., Lawton, C., Lindesay, J., Livingston, G., McCrae, N., Moniz-Cook, E., Murray, J., Nurock, S., O'Brien, J., Poppe, M., ... Banerjee, S. (2013). Cost-effectiveness analyses for mirtazapine and sertraline in dementia: randomised controlled trial. *The British journal of psychiatry : the journal of mental science, 202*, 121–128. https://doi.org/10.1192/bjp.bp.112.115212(accessed on 27th June 2025).

45. Thornton, T. (2011). Recent developments for naturalizing the mind. https://core.ac.uk/download/341071.pdf (accessed on 27th June 2025).

46. Zawiła-Niedźwiecki, J. (2016). Antoni Kępiński's philosophy of medicine–An alternative reading. https://core.ac.uk/download/83117222.pdf (accessed on 27th June 2025).

DERMATOLOGY FOR PHYSICIANS

4

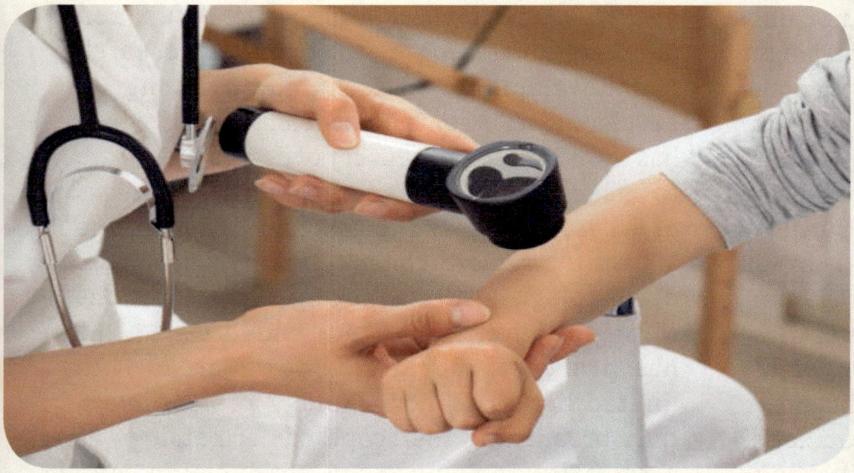

LEARNING OBJECTIVES

After studying this chapter, you will be able to:

1. Understand the anatomy and physiology of the skin;
2. Describe common dermatological conditions;
3. Explain diagnostic techniques in dermatology;
4. Focus on treatment modalities in dermatology;
5. Deal with dermatological emergencies;
6. Discuss the role of dermatology in preventive care.

Introduction

Dermatology is a field that one doctor should be familiar with since it deals with the study of the skin, hair, and nails, which are all aspects of one's well-being. Skin is the body's biggest organ and serves as a protective covering and plays a role in thermoregulation, sensation, and immunity. The essence of dermatology is an exploration of the typical skin anatomy and histology, and pathophysiological mechanisms of common dermatological diseases. Exploration of these conditions by doctors helps in creating a solid foundation for the identification and diagnosis of usual dermatological diseases, which is essential to effective practice. Dermatological knowledge is gaining importance, considering the mounting prevalence of diseases such as melanoma and other skin cancers. Understanding these principles allows physicians to provide holistic patient care in a dynamic medical setting. Even dermatology, with advancements in technology, is also changing, and hence, the use of data mining algorithms and artificial intelligence (AI) is gaining significance. Data mining gives the potential to extract valuable insights out of large collections of medical information, particularly in skin disease cases. Methods like classification, clustering, and association mining play a central role in improving diagnostic methods and patient outcomes (Barati et al., 2011). For example, classification techniques enable dermatologists to diagnose erythematosquamous diseases via solid algorithms that make the diagnosis easier. Likewise, clustering methods sort medical image data, which facilitates better knowledge of disease patterns. These technologies not only allow clinicians to have more accurate diagnostic tools, but also point to the importance of keeping abreast of new technologies in dermatology practice. Coordination between technical experts and dermatologists will be critical to ensuring optimal utilization of AI in clinical settings. As medical professionals embrace AI-driven innovations, they must exercise caution regarding the ethical implications and boundaries of these technologies. Implications of AI are highly promising in melanocytic neoplasms' diagnosis, a refractory area of dermatology that keeps growing despite extensive study (Ghorbani, 2023). Dermatologists may collaborate by making use of AI to support decision-making processes and enhance health care services accessibility. Ongoing training on AI principles and practices will equip doctors with the necessary knowledge in this ever-changing arena. Lastly, the collaboration of medical and technical professionals will promote constant improvement of the practice of dermatology, leading to improved patient health and care.

Definition and Scope of Dermatology

Dermatology, as a branch of medicine, deals with the diagnosis and treatment of skin diseases, encompassing an enormous range of diseases that affect not just the integumentary system, but also related structures such as hair and nails. The field is both medical and surgical in approach to treating conditions ranging from simple diseases such as acne and eczema to severe conditions such as melanoma and psoriasis. In addition, dermatology is not only about general skin health; it is also about understanding the complex relationship between the skin and systemic diseases, hence gaining precious insight into a person's overall well-being. As society struggles with new environmental and lifestyle problems, dermatologists are at the forefront of preventative medicine and the early diagnosis of skin cancers, bearing testament to the essential role of their profession in ensuring public health. Besides clinical practice, the occupation is also flourishing with ongoing research and development in technology. Among its developments is some of the telemedicine, which has transformed the delivery of dermatology care to make it convenient for patients regardless of where they are. Dermatology telemedicine allows for remote consultation, which assists dermatologists in diagnosing skin conditions through digital images and video calls. This has proved to be invaluable in areas with limited access to dermatology professionals, thus broadening the scope of dermatology as a specialty and improving patient outcomes. Recent estimations indicate that adaptation of telemedicine is critical to addressing the growing demand for dermatological care, highlighting the potential as well as the challenges faced in the line of duty (The Stern Center for Evidence-Based Policy, 2015). Besides, the clinical practice of dermatology is increasingly involved with technology advancements, accommodating patient care and interventions. The comprehensive definition of telemedicine includes transmission of electronic medical data via distance to provide effective communication between patients and healthcare professionals (Oliai, 2005). The importance of these technology tools is that they not only increase access to dermatological experts but also enhance the process of diagnosis by enabling real-time collaboration and analysis. The technologies are being applied by dermatologists to incorporate data-driven approaches into practice, which allows for more customized and effective treatment protocols. With the progress of dermatology, the integration of new approaches will undoubtedly shape its future, making it more relevant in the big scheme of healthcare.

Importance of Dermatology in Overall Health

Dermatology is a core area of the health of an individual, playing a significant role in the early diagnosis and management of systemic disorders. The skin is an important barrier as well as a marker of the internal condition of a person, often reflecting underlying diseases such as diabetes, autoimmune conditions, and even certain cancers. As dermatologists assess skin presentations, they are able to identify early warning signs that may prompt timely intervention, thereby enhancing patient outcomes.

For example, skin diseases such as psoriasis have been known to indicate an increased risk for cardiovascular disorders, thus requiring comprehensive care that extends beyond the treatment of the skin and considers systemic implications of health. Therefore, the inclusion of dermatological checks in routine patient analysis is essential to enhance the overall healthcare model, linking dermatology to greater health awareness and preventive care. Furthermore, the psychosocial implications of skin illnesses cannot be overlooked in the greater context of health. Skin illnesses such as acne, eczema, and psoriasis typically lead to long-term emotional distress along with a loss of quality of life for the patients. The visible physical manifestations of such skin conditions frequently result in social discrimination with anxiety, depression, and social isolation. Thus, dermatological management is not merely an issue of physical health but also a significant part of mental well-being. Clinicians need to consider these psychosocial issues while making treatment plans, ensuring that their plans incorporate dermatologic treatment modalities that provide complete well-being. By doing this, not only can dermatologists cure skin illnesses, but they can also facilitate the emotional strength of their patients, which results in a more integrated model of health care. Dermatology is also an entrance into genetic information in medicine with implications for many specialties and patient outcomes. The rapid growth in genetic testing has illuminated the interface between genetic predispositions and dermatologic illness, emphasizing the imperative of interdisciplinary care among medical specialties. As evidence indicates, physicians indicate feeling unprepared to manage genetic services, illustrating an important referral and knowledge gap (Jenevein, 2015). Training physicians in genetic dermatology will allow the medical community to enhance interdisciplinary referrals and improve patient outcomes. Also, subspecialty clinics, such as pediatric dermatology, showcase the value of specialized care in the management of different conditions, as seen in patient demographics and referral patterns studies (Sciberras & Boffa, 2013). This expands the utility of dermatology to be more than its vital contribution to skin health, but also to include comprehensive management of genetic and systemic diseases.

Overview of Common Skin Conditions

One of the most frequent skin illnesses encountered in routine practice, eczema as atopic dermatitis (AD), is vastly significant. It is a chronic illness that not only affects patients' skin but may significantly influence their quality of life, similar to other chronic diseases such as diabetes or asthma. Its presentation is usually with severe itching and redness, which can develop secondary infection if left untreated. The economic burden of eczema is also notable; a systematic review is currently underway to establish the cost-effectiveness of all interventions for prevention and treatment. This is a critical study to enhance the economic case for best use of resources in eczema control so that strategies employed yield maximum outcomes to affected individuals and the overall healthcare system (Sach et al., 2016). In addition to eczema, skin cancer is another serious dermatological condition, accounting as most frequently diagnosed type of cancer in the United States. The disease itself is quite alarming since it is related to sun exposure, which has been associated with all three main types of skin cancer: basal cell carcinoma, squamous cell carcinoma, and melanoma. With melanoma's rate of occurrence being highest among Caucasian populations, it becomes necessary to know the intricacies of skin cancer prevention. In such populations as in Brookfield, CT, increased awareness regarding skin cancer detection and preventive measures is vital. Educational programs that use visual aids, such as informative posters within the hospital or clinic settings, assist in conveying vital information on sun protection and early detection techniques, thereby allowing patients to act proactively against skin cancer (Kolli, 2017).

Psoriasis is also a common skin ailment that needs attention in dermatology. Characterized by red, scaly breaks that typically appear on elbows, knees, and the scalp, psoriasis is an autoimmune condition that possesses the ability to influence psychological well-being significantly. The chronic or recurring nature of psoriasis, sometimes compounded by environmental factors as well as stress, mandates a comprehensive treatment modality that ranges from topical to phototherapy to systemic medication. Moreover, supportive comorbidities of diseases such as cardiovascular disease and psoriatic arthritis demand a holistic approach to the treatment of the disorder rather than the treatment of superficial symptoms. Bridging the gap between dermatological health and general well-being demonstrates how healthcare professionals must adopt a holistic policy in the treatment of psoriasis patients and other chronic cutaneous disorders.

4.1. Anatomy and Physiology of the Skin

Learning Outcome

1. Explain the structure of the skin layers;
2. Discuss the functions of the skin;
3. Describe skin appendages and their roles.

The skin, the largest organ of the body, is a highly evolved barrier as well as a member of the integumentary system. The three main layers—the epidermis, the dermis, and the hypodermis—each contribute to many physiological functions required for homeostasis to be achieved. The epidermis, the most superficial of the three, is made up primarily of keratinocytes, which protect against potentially damaging external substances and create a waterproof barrier. This layer is continuously replaced, as cells emigrate from the basal layer to the surface by a process known as keratinization, which plays a crucial role in the health and integrity of the skin. Knowing these layers is significant for dermatologists as any disruption in their functioning can lead to a number of disorders and diseases of the skin, and highlights the importance of thorough knowledge of the anatomy of skin in clinical practice. Below the epidermis lies the dermis, a thick layer of connective tissue that provides structural support and elasticity to the skin. The dermis harbors essential components such as collagen and elastin fibers, which provide skin resilience and firmness. It also has blood vessels, nerve endings, and appendages such as hair follicles and sweat glands, which all aid in sensory perception and thermoregulation. For instance, sweat glands allow for cooling upon exposure to heat, while the vascular network facilitates the delivery of nutrients and waste removal. Coordination of these structures enables the skin to respond suitably to environmental stimulation. Hence, dermatologists must be familiar with how alterations in dermal structure or function can cause a variety of dermatopathologies, some of which require specific therapeutic maneuvers. Lastly, the hypodermis, or subcutaneous tissue, links the skin to deeper tissues and organs. Made up predominantly of fat tissue, this tissue has a variety of functions, such as insulation, storage of energy, and protection from outer trauma. In addition, the hypodermis provides a pathway for larger vessels and nerves into the skin. It is particularly relevant when applied to skin surgery and other cutaneous procedures, as accurate awareness of this layer can guide effective surgical technique and provide optimal healing of the wound. The distribution of hypodermal fat varies significantly, with relevant implications for the look of the skin and susceptibility to conditions such as cellulite, in practice. Thus, a thorough comprehension of skin anatomy and physiology enables dermatologists to possess the necessary information to treat and diagnose various skin disorders effectively by foregrounding the central role of this basic knowledge in dermatology.

4.1.1. Structure of the Skin Layers

Skin, the largest organ of the body, is structured into three principal layers: epidermis, dermis, and subcutaneous tissue with different but related functions. The epidermis is the outermost layer composed primarily of keratinocytes—cells that produce keratin. The layer is crucial for the formation of a barrier against external irritants, infecting organisms, and water loss, which demonstrates the role of skin in homeostasis.

The thickness of the epidermis is not equal throughout body regions, and the palms and soles are thicker due to the additional stratum corneum, once again emphasizing the adaptive function of the skins. An understanding of the structure of the epidermis is important for dermatologists when making a decision regarding treatment for skin diseases because any disruption of this covering can lead to a plethora of dermatological issues. Dermis exists beneath the epidermis and provides form and elasticity because it is packed with collagen and elastin fibers. It also contains blood vessels, lymphatics, hair follicles, and sensory nerve endings, and therefore plays an essential role in sensation and temperature regulation. Notably, the dermis also possesses immune cells that are extremely significant in the skin's response to injury and infection.

As an illustration, that immune cells are found in this layer underlines the importance of healthy skin for overall immune function. From observation in research into dermatological treatments, for instance, the effectiveness of particular formulations against skin conditions, understanding the dermal architecture can help to tell us what types of products will pass through this layer and be able to impact general skin health (Charruyer et al., 2019). Finally, the hypodermis or subcutaneous tissue serves as an interposed padding between the skin and the deeper elements like bones and muscles while providing insulation and energy storage. It consists primarily of adipose tissue that aids in heat regulation and padding against external trauma.

The structural variations of the subcutaneous tissue in different sites in the body could possibly be the cause for influencing aesthetic and medical outcomes, and hence, its participation in dermatologic operations should be critically assessed. In recent years, advances in imaging technologies, e.g., optical coherence tomography, have enhanced our understanding of skin layer microanatomy, including the hypodermis. With the identification of these differences, physicians can make better diagnoses and treatment recommendations for skin diseases (Adabi et al., 2017). Understanding all three layers' interrelated functions is essential for dermatologists to establish effective treatment plans and improve patient outcomes (Figure 4.1).

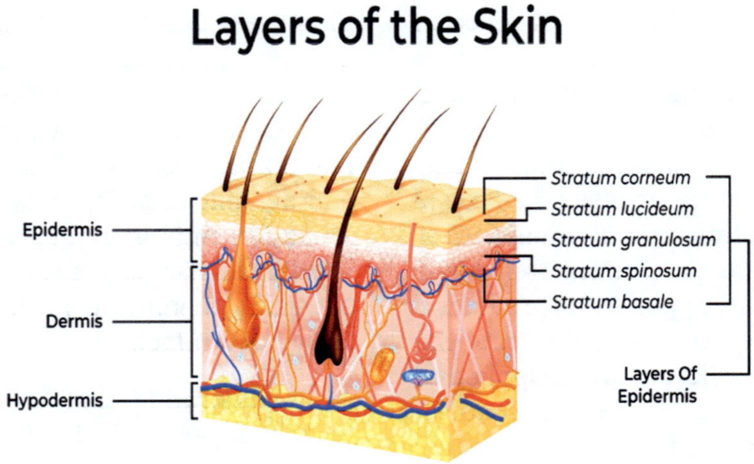

Figure 4.1. Layers of skin.

Source: https://media.geeksforgeeks.org/wp-content/uploads/20230316174511/Layers-of-Skin.png.

4.1.2. Functions of the Skin

The skin serves a variety of key functions that are crucial to health and well-being overall. An important one is its role as a barrier, shielding underlying tissue from mechanical injury, infectious agents, and harmful environmental substances. This barrier function is facilitated by the outer stratum corneum layer of the skin, which prevents transepidermal water loss and maintains moisture. Permeability of the skin also regulates the admission of various substances, highlighting its doubly protective and selective role of acting as an interface between the interior and exterior of the body. In addition, melanocytes in the skin produce melanin that protects the body from ultraviolet (UV) radiation, highlighting the protective role of the skin in the prevention of sun damage and associated dermatological diseases. The skin is not just an external barrier but is also involved in thermoregulation. The skin regulates body temperature through the mechanisms of vasodilation and sweating. If the body is overheated, the sweat glands release perspiration that cools the skin surface via evaporation. In cold conditions, blood vessels reduce in size in order to conserve body heat, illustrating the skin's ability to dynamically react to ambient changes in temperature. This thermoregulatory function is critical in the management of homeostasis and in maintaining that metabolic activities may take place at their best within the body. The skin hence, plays a vital function in the complex interaction of physiological processes controlling stable internal states. Sensory perception is also a significant function played by the skin. The skin possesses several nerve endings sensitive to touch, temperature, and pain, allowing the body to respond to the environment. Such sensory information is critical for protection against damage since it allows individuals to react promptly to injurious stimuli. The skin also plays a role in the general immune response. The presence of immune cells within the dermis, such as Langerhans cells, provides detection and response to infectious agents. The interaction between sensory and immune function identifies the multimodal nature of skin function in dermatology, especially in conditions where these functions may be compromised, making the understanding of skin functions crucial for clinicians in the management of many dermatological conditions (Mercieca & Scerri, 2016; Patton, 2016) (Figure 4.2).

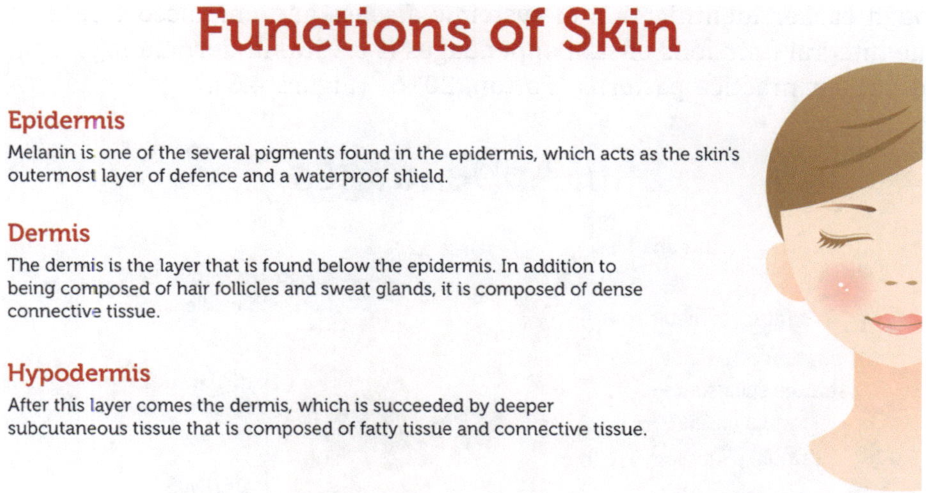

Figure 4.2. Function of skin.

Source: https://assets.lybrate.com/imgs/tic/enadp/function-of-skin.jpg.

4.1.3. Skin Appendages and Their Roles

Skin appendages like hair follicles, sebaceous glands, sweat glands, and nails also play important parts in the integrity of the skin and overall body function. Hair follicles are more than just protective sheaths; they contribute to thermoregulation and perception as well. Sebaceous glands, which are connected to the hair follicles, produce sebum, an oily substance that moisturizes and waterproofs the skin, preventing it from drying out and possibly allowing infectious pathogen penetration. This interaction among sebaceous glands and hair follicles is just one example of how skin appendages cooperate to enhance skin integrity. Secondly, knowledge of the biology of these appendages helps dermatologists to diagnose and manage several types of skin disorders, thus highlighting their significant functions in dermatology practice and patient management. Sweat glands, usually divided into eccrine and apocrine glands, are crucial in thermoregulation and excretion. Eccrine glands are distributed throughout the body, primarily involved in secreting sweat in response to heat increase and physical activity to regulate body temperature. The apocrine glands, which are localized in specific regions such as the armpits, are involved in causing the odor of the body and also become functional at puberty. The glands are influenced by various factors such as hormonal imbalance and external influences. The clinical significance of sweat glands is evident in hyperhidrosis, where excessive sweating can greatly impair patients' quality of life, thus the necessity of specific measures of management. This indicates the necessity of researching these appendages to provide effective dermatological treatment and better patient welfare. Nails, under-estimated, are among skin appendages that serve various functions, including protection, manipulation, and diagnostic information. Composed of keratinized cells, nails protect the distal phalanx and enhance the sense of touch and so play an essential part in everyday functioning. Furthermore, nails can be employed as indicators of systemic health; changes in nail color or texture can signal underlying medical issues such as nutritional deficiency or systemic disease. Dermatologists utilize such information when making diagnoses and devising treatment plans. Here, knowledge about nail health and its significance is critical for dermatology professionals since it can have a profound impact on patient outcomes through earlier identification of systemic disease and enhanced treatment approaches. Highlighting the integral functions of skin appendages is critical in dermatology, upgrading clinical awareness and patient practice patterns (Patton, 2016) (Figure 4.3).

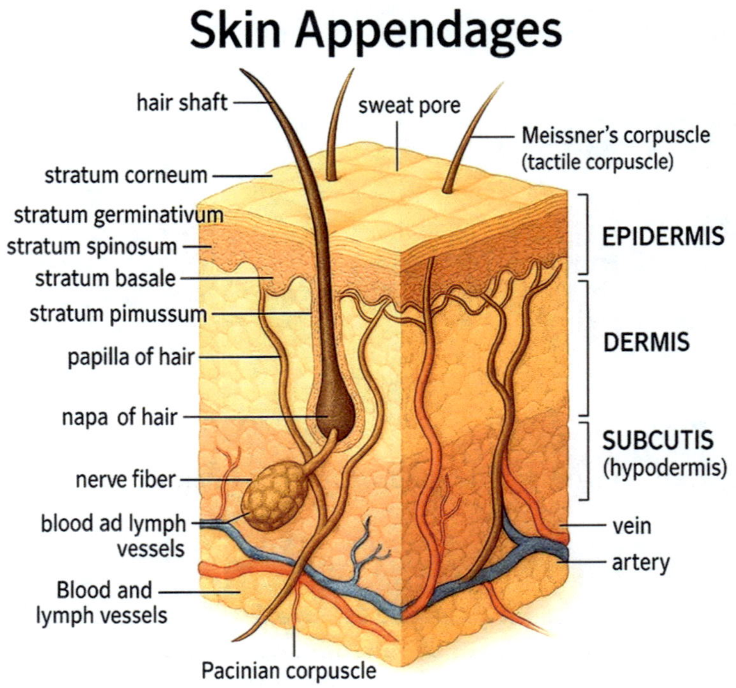

Figure 4.3. Skin appendages.

Source: https://blogger.googleusercontent.com/img/b/R29vZ2xl/AVvXsEg63RDq5OEyRU-0jNp8SpZEQfQEhHm4xeVq2ZH5kax_Q_-t5fMuH_6cAJudfV4wawGIfxJRgthzp0YsII2v0l5mMbDimR590YrL3t3JUz9DsKE-UtzwB35-VbMWvIjj2cDlt24qWaNzB2DGCVdmE4nG0848Yujv9lXtjHEE-zxlIY4y7xX7IybdzI20pUM/s1200/Skin-Appendages.webp.

Test Your Knowledge

1. What are the three main layers of the skin, and what are the primary characteristics and functions of each layer?
2. What roles do skin appendages play in maintaining skin health and homeostasis?
3. How does the skin function as a barrier to protect the body from environmental damage and pathogens?

4.2. Common Dermatological Conditions

Learning Outcome

1. Describe acne and its treatment options;
2. Explain eczema: types and management;
3. Discuss about psoriasis: Causes and therapies.

Among the medical conditions of the many skin diseases, actinic keratosis (AK) is a common and clinically significant condition for physicians. Characterized by rough scaly lesions on sun-exposed skin areas, AK often precedes skin cancer, the most prevalent of which is squamous cell carcinoma. Varying greatly in severity among patients, it is necessary to appropriately evaluate in order to direct therapy. Research in recent years has introduced the creation of the Actinic Keratosis Area and Severity Index (AKASI), a numeric measure to determine AK severity more effectively. The device divides the head into separate regions, enabling complete measurement of the affected surface area degree and severity of significant clinical observations of distribution, erythema, and thickness. Early trials of AKASI were found to be highly correlated with traditional physician global assessment and therefore have the potential to be applied in clinical practice as well as research on novel treatment strategies (Dirschka et al., 2017). One of the usual dermatological diseases is acne vulgaris, which predominantly affects teenagers and young adults but may extend into adult life. Characterized by comedonal, inflammatory, and cystic lesions, acne is the result of a set of factors involving excess sebum production, hormonal changes, and overgrowth of bacteria. While most individuals associate the condition with youth, it may persist much longer, with severe psychosocial effects like low self-esteem and isolation. Treatment involves a combination of topical and systemic therapies, with options varying from benzoyl peroxide and retinoids to oral antibiotics. New advances in treatment methods, including the use of hormonal therapy and isotretinoin, have the potential to significantly impact patient outcomes if used cautiously. Thus, multifactorial causation of acne is crucial to understand for physicians who wish to treat affected patients on a holistic basis. Psoriasis is also very common among dermatological conditions that present certain challenges for both patients and physicians. It is an inflammatory, chronic cutaneous disease characterized by erythematous plaques covered with silvery scales, involving the elbows, knees, and scalp predominantly. It is not merely a cosmetic condition but has associations with systemic conditions like cardiovascular disease and metabolic syndrome, which implies the necessity of integrated care systems. As the incidence of moderate to severe forms increases, a range of treatments has been established, from topical treatment and light treatment to systemic therapy with medications, including biologics. Evidence for psychosocial effects of psoriasis indicates that not only should the physical symptoms be treated, but also mental health to improve the overall quality of life. Thus, an in-depth understanding of psoriasis and its implications is essential for physicians to treat this intricate disease in their patients successfully (Eddy & Duffy, 2019).

4.2.1. Acne and Its Treatment Options

Acne is a multifactorial dermatologic condition that often entails significant physical and psychosocial morbidity in patients. Pathophysiology of acne relies primarily on the inflammatory process of sebaceous follicles, which leads to the formation of comedones, papules, and pustules. Various factors, including hormonal fluctuations, heredity, and environmental influences, contribute to the severity of acne. Treatment of acne is highly diversified and encompasses topical medications, systemic medications, and lifestyle modifications. For instance, benzoyl peroxide and topical retinoids are regular first-line medications due to the fact that they are effective in promoting cellular turnover and countering bacterial colonization. Moderate to severe acne may, however, necessitate oral antibiotics or isotretinoin, particularly in patients who present complicating factors such as scarring, emphasizing the necessity of individualized treatment approaches to counter specific patient needs. Moreover, acne treatment at specific phases of life, i.e., pregnancy, also has to be strictly considered due to the threat to both maternal and fetal well-being.

The professional has to tread the thin line between acne control and safe treatment while pregnant. Kaptanoglu & Mullaaziz (2017) observe that most of the traditional therapies for acne are limited due to the absence of sufficient safety data in pregnant women, thus limiting their application. Accordingly, therapeutic approaches would focus on less invasive options, such as topical products deemed safe but not teratogenic. The issue is not only control of the acne but also control of the emotional and psychological distress it may cause from pregnant women.

Accordingly, holistic evaluation and multidisciplinary management are essential in maximizing treatment regimens while maintaining patient safety. In addition to pharmacological management, patient education and compliance also play important roles in effective acne management. Dermatologists and nurses play a crucial role in encouraging the empowerment of patients through knowledge. Chukwu & Mankila (2018) consider the dermatology nurse's contribution to extend beyond treatment administration; it encompasses systemic patient education about how to care for the skin properly, adherence to recommended regimens, and knowledge of potential side effects. Informed patients with supportive literature are more likely to be actively engaged with their treatment regimen, leading to better outcomes. And, eliminating potential obstacles to compliance, such as cultural differences or insufficient information on the disease, can have a widespread effect on the success of treatment. Here, the integration of individualized patient education efforts into acne care is essential because, in addition to enhancing compliance, it reinforces the patient-provider relationship (Figure 4.4).

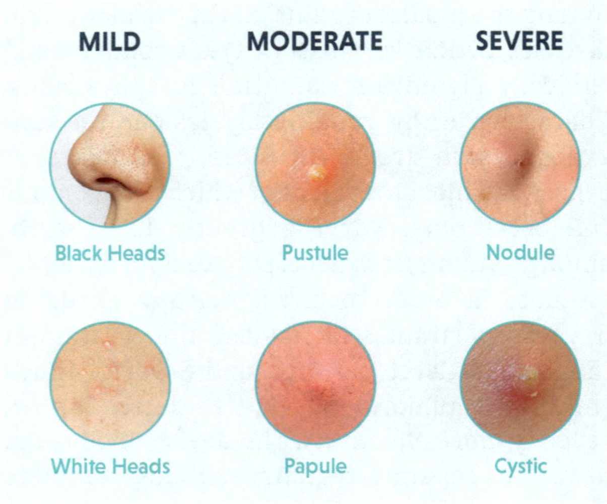

Figure 4.4. Types of acne.

Source: https://www.olivaclinic.com/wp-content/uploads/2024/06/Types-of-Acne.jpg.

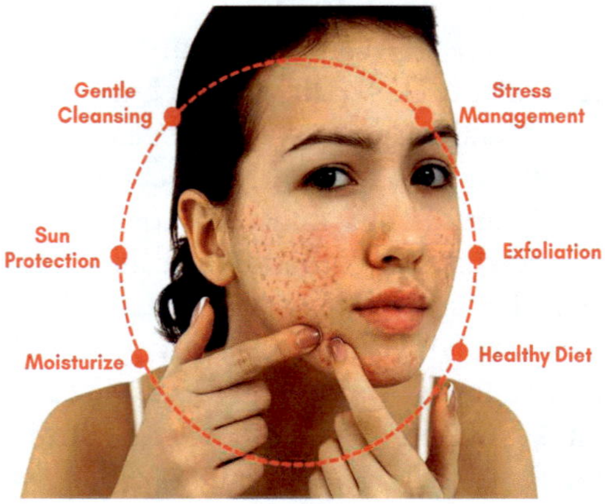

Figure 4.5. Acne treatment.

Source: https://stellaclinics.com/wp-content/uploads/2024/11/Blue-Minimalist-Hair-Treatment-Instagram-Post-2.jpg.

4.2.2. Eczema: Types and Management

Eczema, the common dermatological condition, encompasses varied forms, with most frequent being atopic dermatitis (AD). It is an inflammatory and chronic condition that could be present since birth and persist till adulthood, characterized by heightened pruritus, erythema, and compromised skin barrier. The pathogenesis of AD is multi-factorial, including genetic predisposition and environmental triggers that contribute to its exacerbation. It is crucial to recognize the subtleties of AD, since it can significantly influence the quality of life, cause distress and disrupted everyday functioning. The treatment plans must then consider such multifaceted elements of the disease, echoing the demand for a comprehensive and individualized treatment plan. Accurate diagnosis and determination of the manifestation of the disease are significant, as they serve as a foundation for appropriate therapeutic interventions (Lopes et al., 2020). Eczema control entails a variety of approaches depending on the type and severity of the condition. For AD, the initial treatment regimens would typically be the application of emollients to restore moisture and minimize barrier dysfunction and topical corticosteroids to suppress inflammation. When these initial treatments fail, clinicians may opt for immunomodulators such as calcineurin inhibitors or for systemic therapy, including immunosuppressors and biologics. New treatment options, such as dupilumab, blocking interleukin pathways that play a crucial role in the inflammatory process, hold a new avenue for the management of moderate-to-severe AD (Lopes et al., 2020). Additionally, addressing environmental triggers, such as allergens, through adequate patient education and allergen-specific immunotherapy may bring considerable relief. This multifaceted management approach not only targets physical symptoms but also enhances the psychosocial well-being of eczema patients. The deployment of EHRs is increasingly being viewed as a rich source for maximizing knowledge and management of eczema, such as atopic eczema (AE). Research utilizing these data can elucidate patterns of treatment success and patient outcomes across different populations. One investigation developed a diagnostic algorithm to properly identify AE cases based on a combination of diagnosis and treatment codes, with a high positive predictive value. This validation is required in order to give the precise epidemiologic assessments as well as to appropriately customize management strategies. As clinicians deal with such advanced data platforms, they can improve diagnostic performance and communication within healthcare networks and develop a more efficient process for follow-up of disease course and treatment status. Consequently, integrating EHRs into clinical practice can facilitate not only individual patient management but also broader epidemiological research, ultimately advancing dermatology's understanding of eczema (Figure 4.6).

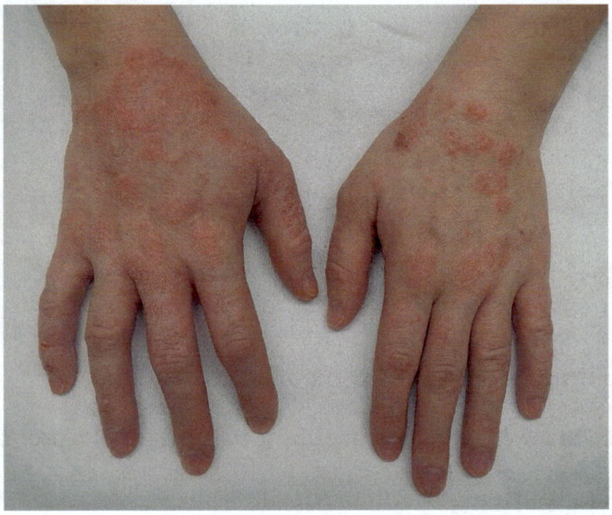

Figure 4.6. A moderate case of dermatitis of the hands.

Source: https://upload.wikimedia.org/wikipedia/commons/thumb/d/de/Dermatitis2015.jpg/800px-Dermatitis2015.jpg.

4.2.3. Psoriasis: Causes and Therapies

Psoriasis is a chronic inflammatory skin condition caused by the multifactorial interaction of environmental and genetic factors. Genetic susceptibility plays a crucial role, with some alleles predisposing to the condition more so than others. Environmental triggers such as infection, stress, and skin trauma further complicate this and can precipitate the formation of skin lesions characteristic of psoriasis. The pathophysiology involves a hyper-proliferation of keratinocytes and a great immune response wherein T cells and other inflammatory mediators are involved in inflammation of the skin. Understanding such causal pathways is essential for dermatologists as it directs preventive and therapeutic measures and, therefore, enhances patient management. Effective management of psoriasis necessitates a multifaceted approach involving topical and systemic therapy. Topical corticosteroids remain the workhorse for localized psoriasis, reduction of inflammation and control of flare.

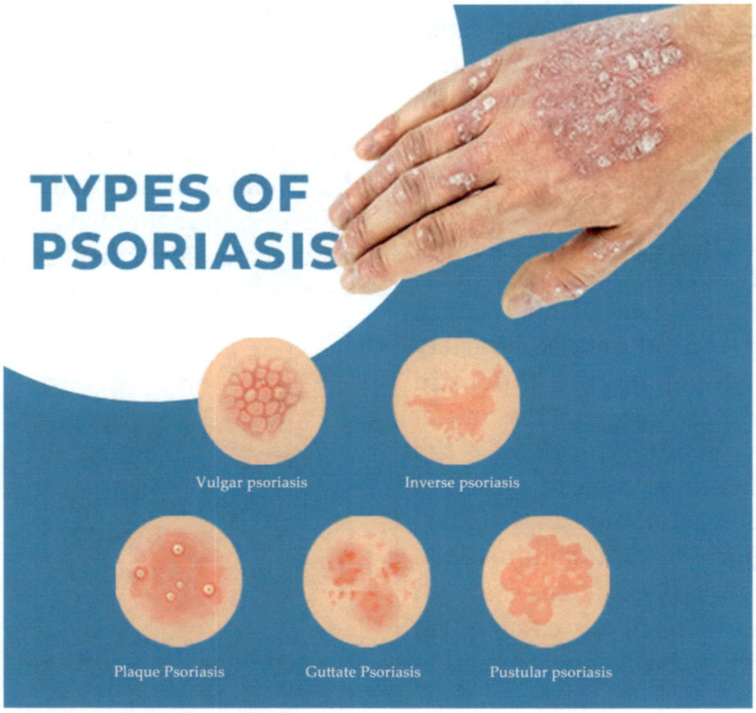

Figure 4.7. Types of psoriasis.

Source: https://drcarehomeopathy.com/wp-content/uploads/2024/02/typesofpsoriasis.jpg.

For patients with moderate to severe disease, however, systemic treatment by biologics and conventional medication cannot be avoided. Biologics, which target distinct mechanisms in the immune response, have transformed psoriasis therapy with sterling potency in patients resistant to traditional treatments. Of interest is that adherence to the therapies is significant, considering that medication non-adherence has been identified as a significant discouragement against effective treatment. Indeed, determinants of adherence include psychological, patient education, and beliefs about drugs, thus suggesting an individualized need for adherence interventions to improve outcomes (Thorneloe et al., 2017). Recent research considers it important to have psychological and habit-driven factors in adherence to medication in psoriasis patients since they can be motivated to enhance treatment effectiveness. For instance, research indicates that people who describe themselves as having more medication problems have higher levels of intentional non-adherence that shape overall health management (Thorneloe et al., 2017). Knowledge of such dynamics enables healthcare professionals to adopt a more personalized approach in treatment programs, engaging patients' underlying assumptions and concerns they have regarding therapy. In addition, patient education and building empathetic therapeutic rapport can significantly enhance patients' rate of adherence, eventually leading to better control of disease and quality of life. While dermatologists are challenged to understand the intricacies of psoriasis care, managing both its clinical and psychosocial aspects is essential to the best possible patient outcomes (Figure 4.7).

Test Your Knowledge

1. What are the main causes of acne, and what treatment options are available for mild, moderate, and severe cases?
2. What are the different types of eczema, and how are they commonly managed in general practice?
3. What are the underlying causes of psoriasis?

4.3. Diagnostic Techniques in Dermatology

Learning Outcome

1. Discuss the role of visual examination and patient history in the practice of dermatology;
2. Describe skin biopsy procedures;
3. Explain the use of dermatoscopy in diagnosis.

Diagnostic method application in dermatology is a multifaceted task that carries great patient outcome implications. With the advancement in technology, clinicians are relying more on clinical evidence technologies (CETs) to enhance diagnostic accuracy. However, in a study of the use of VisualDx, a prominent CET, several barriers and facilitators were found to influence its effectiveness. While PCPs reported that the CET was easy to use, they reported infrequent use of it in practice because of a lack of confidence in dermatology and a preference for traditional sources of information. The findings showed that, although the promise of easier diagnostics and improved patient communication is clear, interface issues and off-target outcomes detracted from the positive effect of CETs on the control of skin disorders, suggesting the need for optimization of these instruments to enhance usability and relevance for practitioners (Burke et al., 2020). Complementing traditional clinical assessments, data mining techniques are emerging as a crucial component in dermatological diagnosis. These methods leverage extensive amounts of medical data for the purpose of recognizing informative patterns that guide clinical decision-making. Among the various data mining methods, classification is particularly critical, particularly for erythemato-squamous disease diagnosis. Such methods as Neural Networks and Genetic Algorithms offer robust foundations for identifying disease characteristics, hence offering early and precise diagnosis. The practical application of these classification techniques, especially in the diagnosis of cancer, lies in their ability to transform dermatological practice. While experts work towards the adoption of these advanced methodologies in clinical practice, overcoming challenges related to data quality and interpretation remains a must in order to maximize the effectiveness of these diagnostic tools (Barati et al., 2011). In dermatology, CET usage in combination with advanced data mining approaches is a more integrative diagnostic approach. While traditional techniques are still the cornerstone of diagnosis, their integration with such advanced methods encourages improved accuracy and outcomes for patients. The knowledge gained through data mining not only improves clinical judgment but also allows medical professionals to individualize treatment based on intricate patterns of information. This combination of technology implies a paradigm shift in dermatology, in which evidence-based expertise and machine systems coexist with traditional clinical experience. However, to best realize their potential, continuous evaluation and refinement of both CETs and data mining methodologies should be prioritized so that they would adapt to evolving needs in dermatologic practice (Barati et al., 2011; Burke et al., 2020).

4.3.1. Visual Examination and Patient History

Thorough visual examination with a rigorous patient history is the foundation of dermatology practice. It is the rudimentary diagnostic tool used by dermatologists to identify and characterize myriad skin diseases. During the visual examination, the doctors assess major features of skin lesions such as morphology, distribution, and color. The variables are extremely useful in distinguishing benign from malignant lesions. With the inclusion of a full patient history, including previous skin conditions, family history, and associated symptoms such as itching or pain, it becomes possible for dermatologists to make a more accurate diagnosis. A good visual examination augmented by patient-derived data has been shown to increase the accuracy of diagnosis and inform future management plans, with an evident key role for these practices in effective dermatology practice. Moreover, correlation of visual findings with patient history also assists in the detection of underlying systemic diseases that present cutaneous symptoms. Diseases like AE, which indeed have salient cutaneous presentations, must be examined and documented carefully regarding the patient's previous therapies, precipitants, and reactions to various therapies. As emphasized in recent studies, standardized measurement tools are crucial in providing consistency in the measurement of dermatological disease across different populations (Vermeulen et al., 2019).

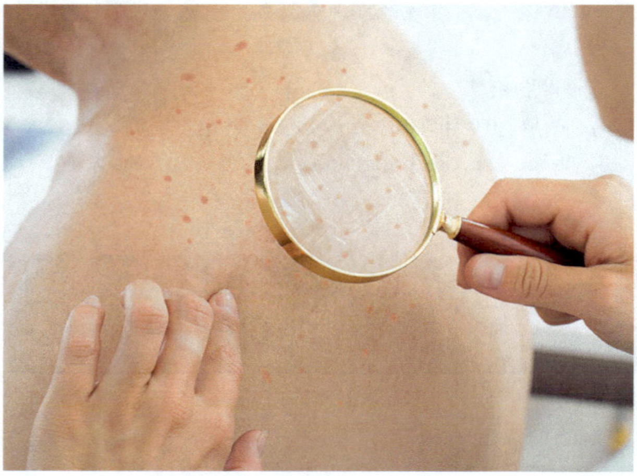

Figure 4.8. Visual examination.

Source: https://walkindermatology.com/wp-content/uploads/2022/10/FBSE-Graphic.jpg.

The consistency not only results in better clinical outcomes but also provides appropriate communication between healthcare providers. Dermatologists, being blessed with hindsight and visual data, can spot trends and patterns that may not be immediately evident and have a full view of chronic as well as acute cutaneous diseases. In addition, visual examination and history are essential in the treatment and forecasting of side effects of therapy, particularly in interventions such as systemic therapy or immunotherapy. The disparate side effects of the interventions manifest themselves first as cutaneous reactions requiring immediate intervention. For instance, immune checkpoint inhibitors have been reported to cause a range of immune-related adverse events presenting dermatologically, thereby highlighting the significance of vigilance and early detection in clinical practice (Puzanov et al., 2017). Through extensive documentation of patient history in conjunction with continuous visual examination, dermatologists are better able to implement timelier interventions and necessary adjustments to treatment plans. By taking a preventive approach, not only does the risk of adverse effects to complicated therapies decrease, but the overall patient experience is optimized, with a more holistic and patient-focused treatment strategy for dermatology (Figure 4.8).

4.3.2. Skin Biopsy Procedures

Skin biopsy surgeries are central to dermatology, playing a vital role in the clinical technique of acquiring tissue samples from the skin to make diagnoses for a range of conditions, such as skin cancers, inflammatory disorders, and infections. The technique is executed in a variety of manners, such as punch biopsies, shave biopsies, and excisional biopsies, each suited to particular clinical contexts. Punch biopsies are indicated for assessing lesions of suspected malignancy since they take a cylindrical sample of epidermis and a bit of dermis. Shave biopsies, however, are typically taken for superficial lesions to heal fast with little scarring. Familiarity with these procedures is essential for dermatologists since the kind of biopsy taken can influence diagnostic accuracy and subsequent treatment plans. In addition, the applicability of skin biopsy tests extends beyond diagnosis; they are essential in monitoring responses to treatments and determining the direction of therapy. In the instance of cutaneous infections or inflammation, the results of biopsies can guide the prescription of drugs, as well as enable clinicians to assess whether ongoing treatments are effective or not.

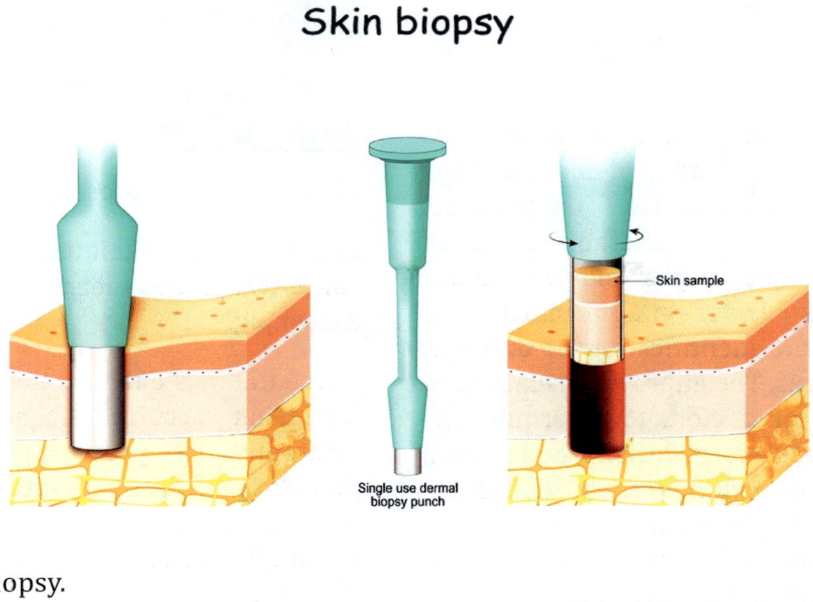

Figure 4.9. Skin biopsy.

Source: https://skinandhairacademy.in/wp-content/uploads/2023/10/Skin-Biopsy.jpg.

The employment of advanced imaging instruments, such as reflectance confocal microscopy (RCM), supplements the traditional biopsy methods by providing real-time, noninvasive evaluations that image and track superficial skin lesions. These invasive and noninvasive instruments together augment the dermatologic arsenal, allowing for an in-depth approach to patient care and management of complex skin diseases (Pimenta et al., 2020). Skin biopsies play a key role in the staging and prognosis of skin cancers, including melanomas. With the rising incidence of melanoma among various populations, particularly those with light skin, the effect of early and accurate diagnosis cannot be exaggerated (Wouters et al., 2018). Multidisciplinary teams have to collaborate to offer the integral treatment from diagnosis through care and follow-up due to the complexity of melanomas. This integrative care model allows for the integration of evidence-based practices and quality measures into the biopsy process, which eventually results in improved patient outcomes. With technology and methods constantly modifying skin biopsy procedures themselves, physicians need to adapt their practice patterns to enhance efficiency, precision, and patient satisfaction in dermatology practice (Figure 4.9).

4.3.3. Use of Dermatoscopy in Diagnosis

The era of dermatology has seen tremendous growth with the incorporation of dermatoscopy in day-to-day diagnostic procedures. Dermatoscopy, an imaging method devoid of invasion, which makes it possible to visualize skin structures under magnification, is responsible for the identification of different types of skin lesions. The improved visualization makes it easier for doctors to determine the morphological features of lesions better than usual examination techniques. By identifying specific dermatoscopic features, professionals can further distinguish between benign and malignant lesions, ultimately improving the accuracy of the diagnosis. The ability to observe structures such as vascular patterns and pigmentation comes in particularly handy during the examination of diseases like melanoma and basal cell carcinoma, where the earliest detection is paramount. Recent studies highlight the benefits of dermatoscopy in the diagnosis of ailments apart from melanoma, including vulvar high-grade squamous intraepithelial lesions (vHSIL) and lichen sclerosus (LS). A clinical trial illustrated the tolerance and practicality of the application of dermatoscopy in combination with dynamic optical coherence tomography (D-OCT) in identifying differentiating features in affected versus unaffected vulvar skin. The dermoscopic studies proved characteristic features such as warty patterns corresponding to vHSIL and sclerotic areas in association with arborizing vessels in patients with LS.

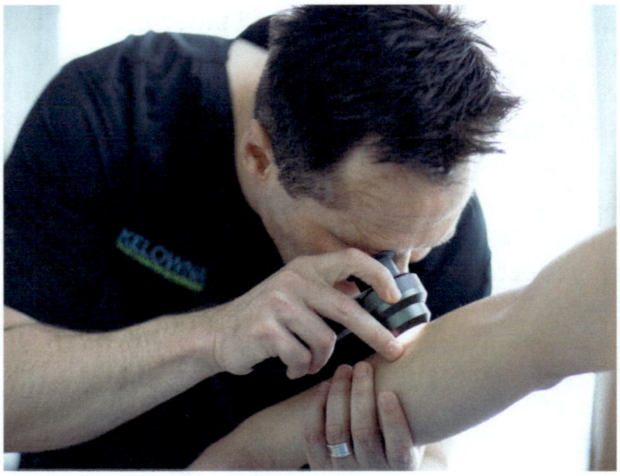

Figure 4.10. Dermoscopy for skin screening.

Source: https://kelownaskincancer.com/wp-content/uploads/dermoscopy-kelowna-skin-cancer.jpg.

These findings enhance the clinicians' capacity for making accurate diagnoses and treatment strategies by providing insight into the pathology of these diseases, which otherwise would be challenging to assess without invasive techniques (Huisman et al., 2023). The uses of dermatoscopy extend beyond diagnosis to include the potential for long-term follow-up and assessment of treatment. As clinicians use dermatoscopy to follow up the development of skin lesions over time, they are able to make therapeutic interventions based on more knowledgeable decisions. For instance, changes in the dermatoscopic presentation of a lesion can reflect treatment response or the need for biopsy. Second, the use of dermatoscopy in clinical practice encourages greater patient interaction in the sense that patients can view their skin condition with their medical care providers. Third, incorporation of dermatoscopy into dermatology is not only a diagnostic tool but also a bridge to improved patient care and education (Burdick et al., 2017) (Figure 4.10).

Test Your Knowledge

1 How does a detailed patient history aid in the accurate diagnosis of dermatological conditions during a visual skin examination?
2. What are the different types of skin biopsy procedures?
3. How is dermatoscopy (dermoscopy) used to assess skin lesions?

4.4. Treatment Modalities in Dermatology

Learning Outcome

1. Discuss topical treatments and their applications;
2. Understand the fundamentals of systemic therapies for severe conditions;
3. Focus on emerging treatments and technologies.

Evolution of treatment modalities in dermatology has immensely enhanced management of a broad spectrum of skin diseases, in line with overall medical innovation trends. Traditional therapies, such as topical corticosteroids and systemic retinoids, have proven to be basic approaches for treating conditions like psoriasis and acne vulgaris. With the evolution of biologic therapies, dermatology has evolved towards targeted therapy, directed at specific pathways involved in inflammatory conditions. These immunosuppressive biologics have been found to be of remarkable efficacy in such diseases as AD and chronic plaque psoriasis, offering hope for patients previously refractory to treatment. Furthermore, the synergistic use of phototherapy with laser treatments has broadened the therapeutic arsenal, tackling conditions ranging from vitiligo to vascular lesions. The evidence does indicate that the integration of these modalities can increase treatment effectiveness and enhance patient outcomes, thus highlighting the dynamic functioning of dermatological care. Advances in dermatological pharmacology have also provided a plethora of topical therapeutic agents formulated to address specific disease entities with minimal systemic impact. For instance, newer forms of calcineurin inhibitors offer corticosteroid alternatives in the management of eczema and minimize the risk of atrophy of the skin that is usually associated with long-term use of corticosteroids. The recent FDA approval of topical Janus kinase (JAK) inhibitors also marks a drastic change in the therapeutic management of alopecia areata and AD, where both oral and topical formulations target intracellular signaling processes. These innovations reflect the recent research and movement toward developing effective, safer dermatologic treatment. But in order to guarantee optimal use of these new drugs, there must be adequate physician education on potential side effects and contraindications, as well as patient compliance with drug regimens to achieve maximum long-term control. The multimodal treatment in dermatology is not without its limitations. A large gap exists between established clinical practice guidelines and their implementation on the ground. As a case in point, recent appraisals of anaphylaxis therapy revealed disturbing discrepancies in guidelines compliance for treatment, with many patients not receiving timely intramuscular adrenaline or adequate follow-up (Grabenhenrich et al., 2012).

These discrepancies point toward the need to strengthen physician training and education on the latest skin therapies. Also, individuals with concomitant conditions, for example, renal disease, present particular challenges in terms of the implementation of certain treatments; there is evidence of an increased risk of nephrogenic systemic fibrosis associated with gadolinium-based imaging contrast agents in vulnerable individuals (Hanna et al., 2014). Overcoming such challenges is central to optimizing treatment methods and, ultimately, patient outcomes in dermatology. Enhanced collaboration and continuing education will be key to bridging the gap between knowledge and practice, leading to increased effective management of dermatological conditions.

4.4.1. Topical Treatments and Their Applications

Topical therapy plays an important role in dermatology, as it offers localized treatment of some skin diseases. Topical medication can treat numerous dermatological disorders, including inflammatory conditions like eczema and psoriasis and infectious conditions like scabies.

The vehicle used in formulating topical preparations usually determines their effectiveness and appropriateness for use in a range of conditions. For instance, vehicles such as creams, ointments, and lotions are able to influence drug penetration and absorption. It is required that the skin type of the patient, the location of skin lesion, and the desired duration of action be considered by dermatologists when giving topical treatment. Effective management of skin diseases relies on knowledge of these nuances, which enhance the effectiveness of treatment as well as minimize potential side effects of inappropriate use. A frequent application of topical treatment is in the case of crusted scabies, which is one of the more severe manifestations with high potential for generating public health issues. Its management involves a complex approach that often includes both topical and systemic medication. For example, one documented case in the context of a nursing home setting illustrated effective management with the use of oral ivermectin and topical scabicidal medication to treat an outbreak of crusted scabies, emphasizing the importance of prompt diagnosis and treatment (Apap et al., 2013).

This figure highlights the way in which topical therapy can make a large contribution to the relief of not only individual patient misery but also broader epidemiological problems in communal living conditions, illustrating their pivotal role in dermatologic therapeutic protocols. Topical treatments are also essential in chronic inflammatory diseases like psoriasis, in which they can provide instant relief of the symptoms. The Goeckerman regimen, where crude coal tar is used in addition to UVB light therapy, is an example of the synergistic effect of topical products in managing this condition. Though not commonly available, a modification of the regimen in the home setting was extremely effective in a patient who was seeking alternatives to systemic treatment, demonstrating patient autonomy and customized care (Reddy et al., 2020). These examples remind us of the versatility and variety of topical treatment in dermatology, in supporting the contention that practitioners must remain vigilant to adapt treatment to meet the diverse needs of their patients (Figure 4.11).

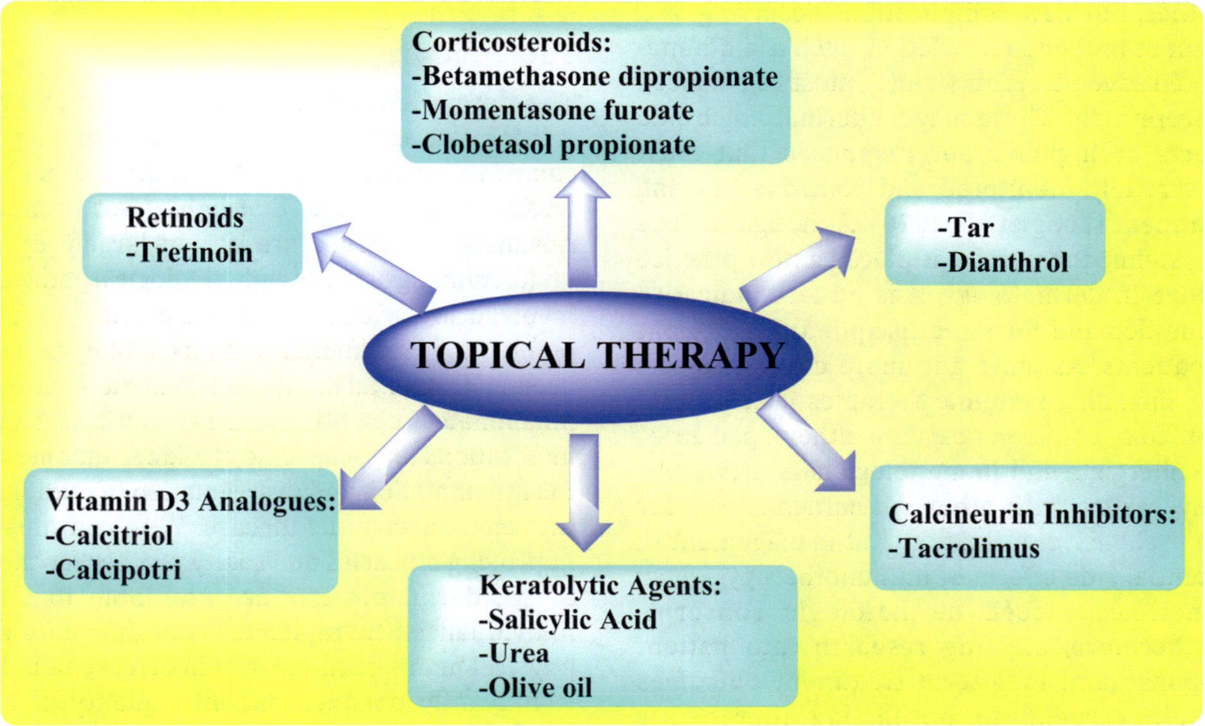

Figure 4.11. Topical therapies in psoriasis treatment.

Source: https://www.researchgate.net/profile/Manjinder-Singh-20/publication/338882307/figure/fig1/AS:936020858109954@1600176171832/Fig-1-Topical-therapies-in-psoriasis-treatment-A-higher-resolution-colour-version.png.

4.4.2. Systemic Therapies for Severe Conditions

In dermatology, the introduction of systemic treatments has greatly transformed the management of severe skin conditions, particularly in those cases where standard topical treatment has not worked. Systemic treatments strive to treat the underlying pathophysiology of diseases such as severe AE, psoriasis, and hidradenitis suppurativa by either modulating immunity or disrupting inflammatory mechanisms. These therapies, such as biologics and immunosuppressants, allow for better patient outcomes by reducing the severity of the disease and improving quality of life. Later consensus efforts have led to the creation of standardized protocols for measuring outcomes in AE patients to allow for greater comparability and merging of data from clinical research registries. This project, based on the TREatment of ATopic eczema (TREAT) Registry Taskforce work, aims to draw evidence-based data from real life regarding the effectiveness and safety of systemic therapies and phototherapy for individuals with severe diseases (Vermeulen et al., 2019). Biologics represent a key advance in systemic therapies, particularly in skin conditions with chronic inflammation. By specifically acting on molecular pathways involved in disease pathophysiology, biologics reduce the risk of systemic toxicities associated with conventional immunosuppressive agents. For instance, monoclonal antibodies targeted against cytokines such as interleukin-17 or interleukin-23 have shown promising results from clinical trials, such as long-term responses for skin clearance and patient satisfaction. These therapies offer hope not just in terms of efficacy but also in their improved safety profiles. But new complications occurring as a result of immune modulation, such as immune-related adverse events (irAEs), must be balanced appropriately. These may be dermatologic side effects or higher-order responses that must be carefully monitored and controlled during treatment (Long et al., 2020). Although the use of systemic therapies has placed a new practice change in dermatology, it is no less indicative of the demand for multidisciplinary treatment of patients. As more and more dermatologists are , including systemic therapies in treatment protocols, convergence with other specialties like allergists and immunologists is inevitable. Convergence with other specialties allows for comprehensive evaluation and management of potential side effects of immunotherapy, which sometimes exceed dermatologic concerns. Furthermore, ongoing research into patient response and long-term treatment outcomes remains crucial to optimizing therapeutic intervention. With data standardization efforts and increasing international cooperation, clinicians are now in a position to obtain significant information regarding systemic treatment long-term effectiveness and improve the overall quality of treatment for patients with severe skin diseases (Vermeulen et al., 2019) (Figure 4.12).

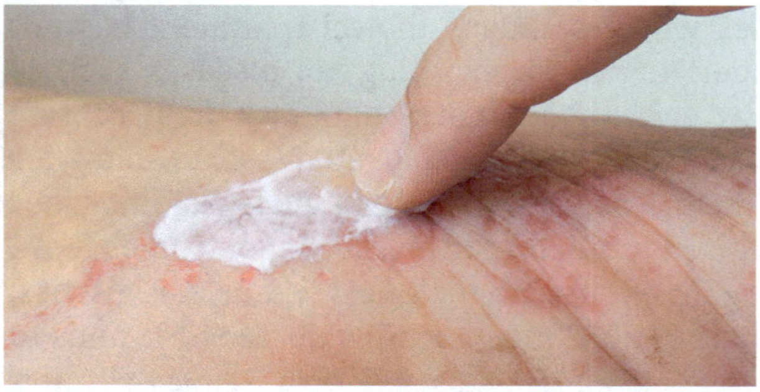

Figure 4.12. Immunosuppressants applied on the skin.

Source: https://amperna.com/cdn/shop/articles/AMPERNA-immunosuppressants_49cd80c6-a1c3-4f68-8a14-201b1f9f15f4.jpg?v=1738196111.

4.4.3. Emerging Treatments and Technologies

The dermal environment is changing at ever greater pace as new treatments and technologies come into prominence, with new avenues for the treatment of patients that hold great promise. Advances in science are driven largely by an understanding of the complex biological pathways involved in various skin diseases. As a case in point, new treatments such as biologics have been instrumental in the management of chronic inflammatory conditions such as psoriasis. These medications target specific cytokines that induce the inflammation and dysregulation of immunity that characterize the disease. With continually improving efficacies and safety profiles for these drugs, dermatologists are now able to offer individualized therapies that not only cure the physical manifestations of skin disease but also significantly enhance patients' quality of life. With the application of these new therapies in clinical practice, dermatologists can control once difficult dermatopathologies more effectively, illustrating the changing nature of dermatologic practice. In addition, continued genetic research further illuminates us regarding the intricate relationship between genetics and dermatologic disease. Recent findings have identified more than sixty psoriasis-related genetic loci and illustrated a strong genetic factor underlying disease susceptibility and severity. This genetic insight informs clinical strategies and opens the door to personalized medicine, wherein treatment can be tightly individualized to a person's genotype. New technologies, such as RNA interference and CRISPR-Cas9 technology, further illustrate the potential for new therapeutic options. These emerging modalities enable the targeted manipulation of disease-related genes, giving new hope to patients with difficult-to-treat skin diseases. With the use of these cutting-edge technologies, physicians can develop more precise and effective therapeutic interventions, in the end, leading to improved patient outcomes and enhanced comprehension of the pathophysiology of skin diseases (Bousquet et al., 2016). Another significant development is in the field of bioprinting of the skin and could potentially transform treatment approaches in dermatology. This new technology allows for the creation of three-dimensional skin tissue based on biocompatible materials and progenitor cells, providing a good solution for most of the challenges, such as graft rejection and donor site morbidity. With readily available bioprinted skin tissues, practitioners can readily tailor the treatment to the unique needs of each patient, thereby ensuring higher efficacy and a reduction in complications. Additionally, the application of bioprinting is not limited to reconstructive therapy and wound healing; it is also able to potentially upgrade the development of experimental models for disease research and drug screening. With dermatology increasingly embracing such technologies, the integration of bioprinting into therapeutic interventions could potentially redefine protocols of standard treatment, thus opening the door to better management of dermatological disorders and patient satisfaction (Bousquet et al., 2016).

Test Your Knowledge

1. What are the most commonly used topical treatments in dermatology?
2. When are systemic therapies indicated in the treatment of dermatological conditions?

4.5. Dermatological Emergencies

Learning Outcome

1. Identify urgent skin conditions;
2. Understand the management of allergic reactions;
3. Focus on effective treatment of infections and infestations of the skin.

Dermatologic emergencies also present a unique challenge for physicians, particularly within the practice of primary care, when family physicians often represent the first contact for patients. They can present themselves in numerous different forms, from life-threatening infections such as necrotizing fasciitis, autoimmune responses like Stevens-Johnson syndrome, or even systemic illness with cutaneous manifestations like Rocky Mountain spotted fever. These conditions need to be recognized early on, as delayed diagnosis may lead to severe morbidity and even death. Family physicians see most patients with skin conditions, and therefore, it is important that they are well-versed with the knowledge of recognizing the signs of these emergencies appropriately. Such abilities not only maximize patient outcomes but further emphasize the need for ongoing education on dermal procedures among PCPs (Alsudairy et al., 2023). During dermal emergencies, differential diagnosis cannot be overstressed. Various skin appearances can mimic one another, and upon close examination, may result in misdiagnosis. For instance, distinguishing between a serious drug reaction characterized by widespread exfoliation of the skin and a minor dermatological condition is vital for proper management. Family physicians must incorporate practices that assist in recognizing specific signs indicating emergencies so that they can make their diagnoses more accurate. Knowledge about referral guidelines is also essential; direct referral to specialists might be the difference in the management outcomes of serious dermatological emergencies. Development of such skills in PCPs bridges several gaps in knowledge and can have a direct impact on patient care (Alsudairy et al., 2023). Training and education in dermato-emergencies must be stressed in the specialty of family medicine. Review of practices indicates that primary care physicians were unable to get proper training in recognition and management of these conditions and hence require a structured curriculum on these topics. Continuing medical education (CME) courses need to include comprehensive modules on dermatological emergencies comprised of clinical case presentations, symptom recognition techniques, and practical workshops that are specifically devoted to emergency care situations. Encouraging family doctors to refer to dermatological literature and participate in special training workshops will significantly improve their proficiency in addressing such emergencies. This does much to establish a more streamlined healthcare system where family physicians can handle complex dermatology issues, which ultimately has the effect of advancing patient care in multiple ways (Alsudairy et al., 2023).

4.5.1. Identification of Urgent Skin Conditions

Identification of emergencies in the skin is critical to physicians since early identification can significantly improve patient outcomes. Cutaneous expression often precedes underlying systemic diseases or emergent life-threatening conditions like infections, autoimmune disease, or malignancy. For instance, necrotizing fasciitis is typified by rapid spread of erythema and edema, for which immediate surgical debridement is necessary. Similarly, toxic drug reactions, such as Stevens-Johnson syndrome, require the immediate identification and cessation of the offending agent—most often a drug. There must be heightened suspicion among clinicians, particularly in those patients who come with atypical rashes along with systemic complaints of fever or respiratory compromise. This presentation can predict an urgent need for care to prevent catastrophic outcomes or death. Besides, the growing application of immunotherapy has introduced diverse immune-related adverse events (irAEs), which can complicate skin assessments. Dermatologists and other healthcare professionals should be familiar with such irAEs because most patients on immune checkpoint inhibitors develop skin reactions that are generally mild to moderate but sometimes life-threatening or severe. Dermatitis, pruritus, and vitiligo are conditions that require supervision and treatment with extreme care to reverse the harmful effects. Because of the inherent difficulty in managing irAEs, guidelines and recommendations have been formulated to provide medical experts with the standards required for effective intervention and treatment at the appropriate time.

The doctors must prioritize the timely detection of such incidents to optimize patient care and prevent advancement, with the paramount role of dermatological evaluation amidst systemic therapies (Puzanov et al., 2017). Besides immunotherapy-related reactions, conditions such as mast cell activation syndrome (MCAS) present unique challenges in the identification of skin disorders in emergencies. MCAS patients may experience allergic-like presentations in which they present with widespread urticaria, flushing, or even anaphylactic responses that can be imitated by other dermatoses. The difficulty in differentiating these presentations is a pointer to the need for cautious clinical criteria in arriving at correct diagnoses. Sensitization to mast cell disorders is critical, especially because the latter may not always follow mastocytosis. Understanding the mast cell activation pathways and their impact on the skin can help practitioners identify patterns that need further investigation and intervention. Finally, understanding these emergent cutaneous conditions ensures that doctors are better equipped to manage potential complications effectively and in a timely fashion, which enhances PS and quality of care (Valent et al., 2011) (Figure 4.13).

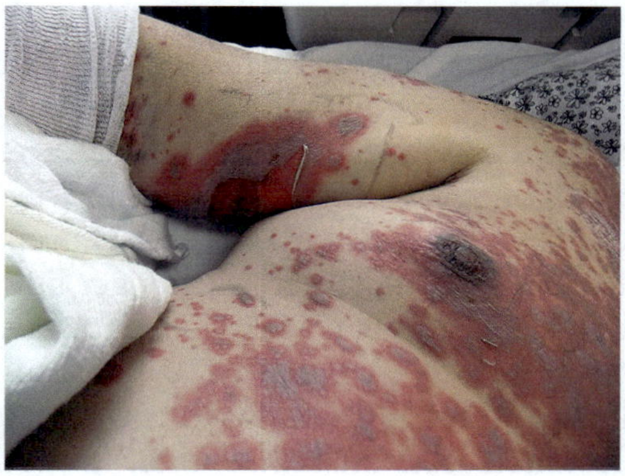

Figure 4.13. Illustration of Stevens-Johnson syndrome.

Source: https://my.clevelandclinic.org/-/scassets/images/org/health/articles/17656-stevens-johnson-syndrome.

4.5.2. Management of Allergic Reactions

Allergic reaction management is an extremely significant part of dermatologic practice, given the skin's key position as a barrier and as an organ of representation of systemic immune events. Allergic reactions may manifest in various ways, including urticaria, eczema, and anaphylaxis, and mandate prompt recognition and management. Optimal management begins with a thorough clinical assessment to establish the precipitating allergen and reaction severity. For mild reactions, the symptoms can be relieved by antihistamines, and in severe reactions, corticosteroids may be indicated to reduce inflammation. Education of the patient as to the necessity of avoidance of recognized allergens is also necessary to avoid subsequent reactions and consequently optimize the long-term prognosis of allergic patients. In more severe situations, particularly anaphylaxis, immediate action is necessary. The recommendations now favor intramuscular delivery of adrenaline, which represents first-line treatment of life-threatening allergic reactions. Though compliance with such recommendations may differ across contexts, evidence indicates a worrisome disparity between practice as recommended and practice as enacted. In a comprehensive study of severe anaphylaxis cases in Germany, Austria, and Switzerland, it was reported that only a fraction of patients received adrenaline as per the guidelines, highlighting significant gaps in the management of anaphylaxis. Such findings underscore the urgent need for enhanced medical education and training, ensuring that healthcare providers are equipped to manage these emergencies effectively and improve PS in clinical practices (Grabenhenrich et al., 2012). To supplement pharmacologic management, dermatologists will also have to deal with ADR-related side effects, particularly if idiopathic pulmonary fibrosis patients are being treated. Administration of pirfenidone, for example, is associated with several gastrointestinal and dermatologic adverse events that make management difficult. Physicians should adopt measures like patient education on drug administration with food and sun protection guidelines to effectively address these side effects (Costabel et al., 2014). The double focus on handling allergic reactions and preventing side effects enables medical doctors to maximize treatment guidelines so that patients can be compliant and achieve maximum clinical results. In conclusion, an interdisciplinary approach with the immediate treatment, education of the patient, and ongoing surveillance is indicated for the effective management of allergic reactions in dermatological clinics.

4.5.3. Treatment of Infections and Infestations

Effective management of skin infections and infestations is a multifaceted process that requires accurate diagnosis and effective therapies. Family doctors and dermatologists come across an array of skin disorders caused by infectious pathogens like bacteria, fungi, and parasites. Recent studies have shown that RCM has been an invaluable diagnostic tool with exceptional sensitivity to identify skin infections. This non-invasive imaging technique allows for real-time visualization of epidermal and superficial dermal alterations observed in infections, thereby making it possible to provide appropriate and timely interventions. Using RCM, dermatologists can rapidly differentiate among various types of infections, thereby providing improved treatment and preventing the application of ineffective therapies. This integration of modern diagnostic technology into common practice signifies ongoing progression in dermatologic care, paving the way for more effective infection control (Pimenta et al., 2020). The role of primary care physicians in skin infection management cannot be overemphasized since they tend to be the first point of contact for patients presenting with dermatologic issues. The majority of the prevalent infections, such as impetigo, cellulitis, and tinea corporis, fall under family medicine. A study examined the identification, management, and referral patterns of family physicians in terms of dermatology and highlighted the vast possibilities of streamlining the modes of treatment. Through targeted education and training measures, PCPs can be trained more effectively to diagnose and treat such diseases. Furthermore, family physicians can establish a robust referral mechanism to specialists in the event of complex conditions to enable integration of holistic care for patients. Enhancing weaknesses in managing dermatological infections will enhance the quality of care and better attend to the needs of patients (Alsudairy et al., 2023). With the progressive development of dermatology, ongoing education regarding the management of infestations and infections is still crucial for both dermatologists and primary care providers. Recent diagnosis technologies, such as RCM, in conjunction with evidence-based training of the family physician, can substantially improve patient outcomes. Increasing awareness of common skin infections and creating successful management plans not only prepares practitioners for immediate challenges but also positions them for long-term advancement in the field. Through collaborative practice and continuing professional development, healthcare professionals can maximize their treatment approaches to infections and infestations, thereby resulting in improved levels of care in dermatology. This emphasis on ongoing learning and adaptation will ultimately lead to better health outcomes and greater patient satisfaction in the treatment of these frequent dermatoses (Pimenta et al., 2020; Alsudairy et al., 2023) (Figure 4.14).

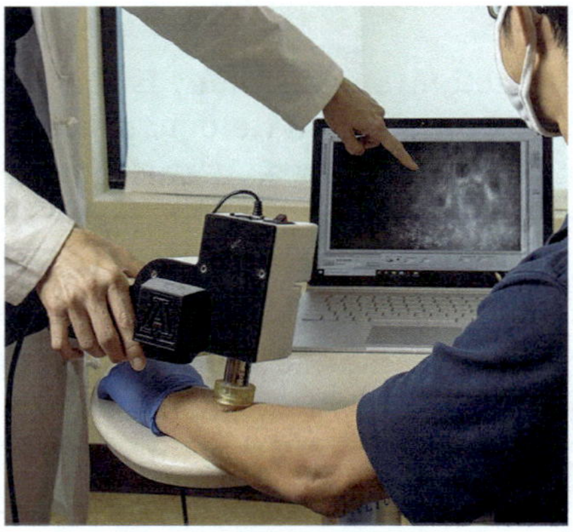

Figure 4.14. Portable reflectance confocal microscopy (RCM) for the identification of skin infections with high precision.

Source: https://www.photonics.com/images/Web/Articles/2022/8/30/thumbnail_68331.jpg.

Test Your Knowledge

1 What are some key clinical signs that help identify dermatological emergencies?
2. How should general practitioners manage acute allergic skin reactions like anaphylaxis or severe urticaria?
3. What are the initial steps in diagnosing and treating rapidly spreading skin infections such as cellulitis?

4.6. The Role of Dermatology in Preventive Care

Learning Outcome

1. Understand skin cancer screening and education for early detection and intervention in dermatologic care;
2. Explain the importance of sun protection;
3. Discuss lifestyle factors affecting skin health.

Placing dermatology within the realm of preventive care is increasingly being viewed as core to overall health care management. Dermatologists are uniquely qualified to detect and treat skin diseases that can be an indicator of more malignant systemic issues, thereby playing a key role in preventive care. Dermatologists are able to detect early warning signs of skin cancers, including melanoma, one of the most lethal cancers, through thorough examinations of the skin. From evidence as evidenced in dermatology literature, an early intervention is highly advantageous to patient results through the establishment of timely management and avoidance of employing even more drastic and costly treatments in the future. The active participation is indicative of the comprehensiveness of dermatology's contribution not only in the treatment of skin disease but also in the prevention of early detection of serious health problems that otherwise would go undetected (Publication Services at Boston University Medical Center, 1989). Besides, dermatologists have a crucial role in executing and spreading public health interventions to inform populations about the skin. This includes advice concerning protection against the sun to avoid developing skin cancers, as well as counseling on the necessity of recognizing and reporting changes in the skin. The effectiveness of these preventive measures manifests itself in various community health programs that have successfully reduced instances of skin ailments through sensitization campaigns. Dermatologists are also prone to collaborate with other medical practitioners to offer comprehensive care, leading to an informed patient population capable of contributing to their care proactively. The multifaceted contribution of dermatologists to promoting education and awareness affirms how prevention is greater than clinical care but encompasses measures in community health (Grabenhenrich et al., 2012). Lastly, continuous research in dermatology continues to support the importance of continued education and patient participation in prevention. Findings of studies comparing anaphylaxis treatment in dermatology, for instance, show that adherence to treatment guidelines is often variable. The data provided indicates stark discrepancies between best practices and practice in the clinic environment. The differences create a call for more training in preventive measures, further showcasing the value of having dermatologists in their current role of being at the forefront of embracing the current standards in a bid to improve patient outcomes. Continuing professional development and excellent patient education are key in the development of dermatology practice to ensure it remains a cornerstone of effective prevention of care (Publication Services at Boston University Medical Center, 1989; Grabenhenrich et al., 2012).

4.6.1. Skin Cancer Screening and Education

Education on skin cancer and screening is critical in promoting early detection and treatment, ultimately leading to improved patient outcomes in dermatological care. Increasing prevalence of skin cancer requires healthcare providers to place a high value on screening procedures that allow the detection of high-risk individuals. Risk factor education, such as UV radiation exposure and genetic predisposition, must be imparted to both patients and physicians. Through educating patients regarding the importance of regular skin check-ups and monitoring moles and lesions for themselves, health workers may empower people to take preventive measures in their own skin. Further, incorporating learning materials and education programs into clinics may promote a culture of awareness, leading to more screening uptake among different populations (Publication Services at Boston University Medical Center, 1989). The technological contribution to education and screening of skin cancer is also imperative since it makes the expansion of accessibility and effectiveness of dermatologic care possible. Improved innovation in clinical evidence technology (CET) has been forthcoming in assisting PCPs with the management and diagnosis of skin disorders. As an illustration, even though the efficacy of certain CET tools, e.g., VisualDx, revealed no discernible effect on patient outcomes in previous studies, they have established both enablers and hinderers that PCPs face daily (Burke et al., 2020). Achieving these nuances enables practitioners to customize their use of technology along with learning content in order to support accurate diagnosis and treatment of skin cancer. To further encourage skin cancer screening programs, collaboration between public health institutions, primary care physicians, and dermatologists is vital. The development of standardized screening guidelines can facilitate greater uniformity in treatment and reduce access differences to dermatologic services. Education-based community programs that target awareness of risks of skin cancer and the importance of early detection among populations that are underserved can also be helpful. Involvement in such collaborative endeavors not only enhances the efficiency of skin cancer screening but also reinforces a broader trend in dermatologic education that can be manifested as improved patient health outcomes (Publication Services at Boston University Medical Center, 1989). Through these concerted measures, providers have an important capacity to impact the well-being of their community while reminding all people of the significance of sustained concern for skin health (Figure 4.15).

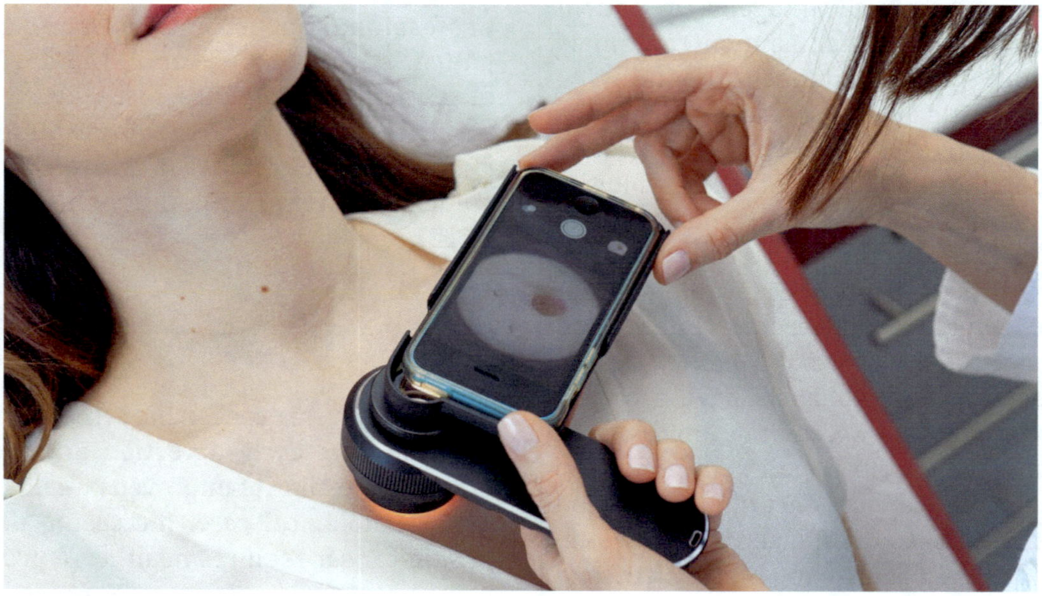

Figure 4.15. Skin cancer screening.

Source: Vhttps://post.healthline.com/wp-content/uploads/2020/04/Skin-Cancer-Screening-1296x728-header.jpg.

4.6.2. Importance of Sun Protection

Protective role of the sun in the foundation of dermatological care cannot be overstressed. One of the main risk factors for skin cancers, namely malignant melanoma and non-melanomatous basal cell carcinoma and squamous cell carcinoma, is exposure to UV radiation. As there have been rising incidences of these around the globe, especially in sun-exposure-prone regions, healthcare professionals must stress effective sun protection methods. These measures include the use of broad-spectrum sunscreens, protective clothing, and staying out of the sun during peak hours. These measures not only reverse the acute erythema of solar exposure but are also important in reducing long-term risk for skin malignancies, and therefore highlight the role of the dermatologist in educating patients on the importance of protective actions against UV exposure. Among the outdoor activities, surfing has a unique challenge for sun protection since it entails prolonged exposure to the sun and the water's reflection capabilities, which have a chance to magnify UV radiation. In research, recreational surfers were found to be at higher risk of developing skin cancers, with findings indicating the incidence of basal cell carcinoma among them (Climstein et al., 2016). This risk underlines the need for certain sun protection practices within recreational and competitive sport groups. For instance, surfers must be reminded to avoid the sun during the highest-risk times (10 AM to 3 PM), to wear protective equipment such as rash vests, and to apply broad-spectrum sunscreen regularly. By emphasizing such precise steps, physicians can better safeguard this group's skin health and cultivate a preventive care culture. Management of skin adverse effects of UV exposure is also extended to clinical practice, where therapies like pirfenidone are being used. Research shows that patients undergoing such therapies need to emphasize sun protection as a measure to avoid skin adverse effects (Costabel et al., 2014). Such patients need to wear protective clothes and high SPF sunscreens for defense against solar damage. Dermatologists play a crucial role in educating patients regarding these preventive measures and thereby enhancing treatment adherence and overall outcome. Clear comprehension of sun protection not only protects susceptible populations against skin cancer but also allows optimization of continued dermatologic treatment, making sun protection an integral part of dermatologic patient care.

4.6.3. Lifestyle Factors Affecting Skin Health

The relationship between lifestyle factors and skin health is significant since the habits influence the condition of the skin. Specifically, diet has a significant influence; a diet rich in antioxidants, vitamins, and essential fatty acids helps maintain healthy skin. For example, vegetables and fruits have nutrients that improve skin elasticity and moisture, while omega-3 fatty acids in fish and flaxseed can reduce inflammation and provide a healthy-looking skin. Conversely, the consumption of processed food and sugars has been linked with the acceleration of skin aging and exacerbation of acne and other skin conditions. Encouraging healthy food habits not only fuels the skin but can also promote a healthy self-perception, which is directly linked to overall mental health and well-being. In addition, the importance of adequate hydration cannot be overlooked if one is considering skin well-being. Adequate water intake is needed to maintain the moisturizing and pliability of the skin, to facilitate the elimination of toxins, and to support the healing of skin damage. Dehydration also leads to dry, flaky skin and exacerbates eczema and psoriasis. Lifestyle factors such as smoking and heavy alcohol consumption are also detrimental to skin health. Smoking will impair blood flow, resulting in the skin appearing sallow, and alcohol dehydrates the skin and can impair its natural barrier function. Patient education regarding the significance of proper hydration and reduction of harmful substances can be a core component of dermatological care that emphasizes the role of lifestyle in healthier skin. Finally, stress management is an often-overlooked but highly significant component of skin health. Higher stress levels can aggravate a number of skin conditions, such as acne, rosacea, and psoriasis, by the release of stress hormones like cortisol that induce inflammation and other negative impacts. Adding stress-reducing measures—like mindfulness training, regular physical exercise, or a hobby—can significantly improve the state of the skin. In nursing patients, the contribution of the dermatology nurse is also paramount in educating patients not only on the correct skin care procedures, but also on the need for a holistic approach, which includes lifestyle modifications to be able to manage stress effectively. A high level of knowledge and guidance pertaining to lifestyle choices can empower the patient since the nurse-patient relationship will be critical in ensuring follow-up in such life-changing practices towards optimal overall skin health (Publication Services at Boston University Medical Center, 1989; Chukwu & Mankila, 2018).

Test Your Knowledge

1. Why is regular skin cancer screening important?
2. What is the role of sun protection in preventing skin cancers and premature aging?
3. How do lifestyle factors affect overall skin health and contribute to dermatological conditions?

SUMMARY

It is important to value the evolving environment in clinical practice and the significant role that technology can play in enhancing diagnostic accuracy and outcomes from treatment. The integration of CETs, like VisualDx, is a significant development in dermatological practice. While the initial expectation had been improved patient outcomes, later studies indicate that implementing CETs cannot always be relied upon to lead to better time of resolution for skin diseases or a reduction in follow-up appointments. As shown in the pragmatic trial results, there were no statistically significant outcome differences where doctors utilized VisualDx, noting that even though technology could be utilized for decision-making support, dermatological diseases may require greater than technological assistance for improved patient outcomes and care (Burke & Littenberg, 2018). Furthermore, this dermatology review highlights physician characteristics as being crucial in the context of industry involvement and influences. The variations observed in industry payments along the lines of sex, years of practice, and medical institution reputation raise serious ethical questions regarding prejudices and their effects on treatment modalities. Since the data indicates, concentricity of industry payments—i.e., that the lion's share goes to a minority of physicians—is potentially influential on clinical choices and can generate unequal access to resources for patients. Such economic forces are worthy of particular attention and discussion, as they can inadvertently influence the broader context within which dermatology is practiced (Inoue et al., 2019). Last but not least, the conclusion must emphasize the immediate need for continuous education and professional training among dermatologists. With the profession facing the rapid development of treatment techniques and the intricacy of skin diseases, continuous training is necessary. They should not only be taught the newest diagnostic technologies and therapeutic interventions but must also learn a sensitivity to the ethical aspects of their practice, particularly as they interface with industry. In doing so, developing a culture of patient-centered care, ethics, and critical thinking will make dermatology progress mean something in terms of real improvements for patients, and thus legitimize physicians' guiding role in shaping such evolving times (Inoue et al., 2019).

In dermatology, data mining has been an essential development in enhancing diagnostic precision and the effectiveness of treatment. With the emergence of advanced technologies, vast amounts of medical data have come within reach, thus presenting an opportunity to identify interesting patterns in skin conditions. It encompasses numerous different methods, including association mining, particularly valuable in rule-building to comprehend multifactorial conditions such as cancer. Furthermore, classification methods, paramount to diagnosing erythemato-squamous disease, play a key role in maximizing patient care. As the literature has emphasized, these data mining approaches not only optimize clinical decision-making but also emphasize the importance of efficient utilization of data in dermatology, thus enabling clinicians to possess robust information to guide their practice effectively (Barati et al., 2011). An additional crucial aspect in dermatology is that new treatment protocols personalized to address individual patient needs are to be followed. Goeckerman therapy, for instance, is an extremely effective method of treatment of moderate to severe psoriasis, involving radiation with UVB plus application of coal tar. However, access is limited because the therapy is only offered by a few centers in the USA. In this manner, patients in regions where centers of this kind do not have facilities might resort to other options, as was evidenced by a case study on a patient who adapted Goeckerman therapy at home. This patient's achievement in achieving full clearance of prescription medications illustrates the worth of modified treatments that are customized to particular circumstances, and the necessity for dermatologists to be flexible and innovative in their treatment modalities (Reddy et al., 2020). Lastly, the integration of data mining with patient-specific treatment modalities is a step in the right direction for dermatology, enhancing the physician's capability to deliver patient-specific care. The integration of advanced AI-based data analytics encourages a closer understanding of skin diseases and sets the stage for accurate, patient-specific treatment regimens. In the same vein, case studies on real-life usage of established therapies highlight the necessity of refining clinical practices to accommodate patient needs optimally. By embracing both data-informed intelligence and patient-specific modifications, dermatologists can maximize their approach to curing various skin conditions, ultimately leading to increased patient outcomes and satisfaction in the practice of dermatologic health. This marriage of technology and individualized medicine is a promising venue for dermatology, solidifying the specialty's intent to enhance medical therapy (Barati et al., 2011; Reddy et al., 2020).

KEY TERMS FROM THIS CHAPTER

- Actinic Keratosis Area and Severity Index (AKASI)
- Allergic reaction management
- Allergic reactions
- Atopic dermatitis (AD)
- Biological pathways
- Chronic condition
- Chronic inflammatory conditions
- Clinical observations
- Community health programs
- Complex skin diseases
- Cystic lesions
- Dermal environment
- Dermatological diseases
- Dermatological health
- Dermatological knowledge
- Dermatological treatments
- Dermatology
- Disease patterns
- Dynamic optical coherence tomography (D-OCT)
- Eczema control

CRITICAL THINKING QUESTIONS

1. **Which of the following layers of the skin is primarily responsible for thermoregulation and insulation?**
   a. Stratum corneum
   b. Dermis
   c. Hypodermis (subcutaneous tissue)
   d. Stratum basale
2. **Which of the following features is most characteristic of psoriasis?**
   a. Target lesions
   b. Silvery scales on erythematous plaques
   c. Vesicles on palms and soles
   d. Hyperpigmented macules in sun-exposed areas
3. **Which of the following is the first-line treatment for mild to moderate acne vulgaris?**
   a. Oral isotretinoin
   b. Systemic corticosteroids
   c. Oral doxycycline
   d. Topical retinoids
4. **Which treatment modality is most appropriate for a superficial basal cell carcinoma?**
   a. Systemic chemotherapy
   b. Surgical excision or Mohs micrographic surgery
   c. Oral antifungals
   d. Phototherapy
5. **Which dermatological condition is considered a medical emergency requiring immediate intervention?**
   a. Stevens-Johnson syndrome
   b. Vitiligo
   c. Atopic dermatitis
   d. Pityriasis rosea

Short Answer Questions

1. What are the primary layers of the skin, and what specific functions does each layer serve in maintaining skin integrity and overall health?
2. Which dermatological conditions are most frequently encountered in general practice, and how can they be clinically differentiated?
3. What diagnostic techniques—, including patient history, visual examination, and dermatoscopy—are essential in accurately identifying skin disorders?
4. When should a skin biopsy be performed, and how do different biopsy methods (e.g., punch, shave, excision) support diagnosis and treatment planning?
5. What are the main topical and systemic treatment options for dermatological conditions, and how is treatment typically tailored based on severity and diagnosis?
6. How should physicians recognize and respond to dermatological emergencies such as Stevens-Johnson Syndrome, anaphylaxis, or severe cellulitis?

Answers to Critical Thinking Questions

1. (c); 2. (b); 3. (d); 4. (b); 5. (a)

REFERENCES

1. Puzanov, I., Diab, A., Abdallah, K., Bingham, C. O., 3rd, Brogdon, C., Dadu, R., Hamad, L., Kim, S., Lacouture, M. E., LeBoeuf, N. R., Lenihan, D., Onofrei, C., Shannon, V., Sharma, R., Silk, A. W., Skondra, D., Suarez-Almazor, M. E., Wang, Y., Wiley, K., Kaufman, H. L., ... Society for Immunotherapy of Cancer Toxicity Management Working Group (2017). Managing toxicities associated with immune checkpoint inhibitors: consensus recommendations from the Society for Immunotherapy of Cancer (SITC) Toxicity Management Working Group. *Journal for immunotherapy of cancer*, *5*(1), 95. https://doi.org/10.1186/s40425-017-0300-z(accessed on 27th June 2025).
2. Abe, R., Akiyama, M., Long, H., McMillan, J., et al. (2007). BMB activity defines refractory and competent hair follicle populations during the propagation of regenerative waves. https://core.ac.uk/download/pdf/97129.pdf (accessed on 27th June 2025).
3. Lopes, A., Sokolova, A., Abreu, C., & Lopes, C. (2020). Atopic Dermatitis Host and Environment Model: Revisiting Therapeutic Options. *European annals of allergy and clinical immunology*, *52*(1), 4–14. https://doi.org/10.23822/EurAnnACI.1764-1489.125(accessed on 27th June 2025).
4. Adabi, S., Clayton, A., Conforto, S., Daveluy, S., et al. (2017). Universal *in vivo* textural model for human skin based on optical coherence tomograms. http://arxiv.org/abs/1706.02758 (accessed on 27th June 2025).
5. Barati, E; Saraee, MH; Mohammadi, A; Adibi, N; Ahmadzadeh, MR (2011). A survey on utilization of data mining approaches for dermatological (skin) diseases prediction. https://core.ac.uk/download/1667194.pdf (accessed on 27th June 2025).
6. Bousquet, J., Hellings, P. W., Agache, I., Bedbrook, A., Bachert, C., Bergmann, K. C., Bewick, M., Bindslev-Jensen, C., Bosnic-Anticevitch, S., Bucca, C., Caimmi, D. P., Camargos, P. A., Canonica, G. W., Casale, T., Chavannes, N. H., Cruz, A. A., De Carlo, G., Dahl, R., Demoly, P., Devillier, P., ... Zidarn, M. (2016). ARIA 2016: Care pathways implementing emerging technologies for predictive medicine in rhinitis and asthma across the life cycle. *Clinical and translational allergy*, *6*, 47. https://doi.org/10.1186/s13601-016-0137-4(accessed on 27th June 2025).
7. Valent, P., Akin, C., Arock, M., Brockow, K., Butterfield, J. H., Carter, M. C., Castells, M., Escribano, L., Hartmann, K., Lieberman, P., Nedoszytko, B., Orfao, A., Schwartz, L. B., Sotlar, K., Sperr, W. R., Triggiani, M., Valenta, R., Horny, H. P., & Metcalfe, D. D. (2012). Definitions, criteria and global classification of mast cell disorders with special reference to mast cell activation syndromes: a consensus proposal. *International archives of allergy and immunology*, *157*(3), 215–225. https://doi.org/10.1159/000328760(accessed on 27th June 2025).
8. Mohammad Alsudairy , Razan Ahmed F Aljuhani , Zahraa Ahmed J Alhassan , Abdulmajeed Saleh A Alharbi, Hamdan Sulaiman Ayed Alshammari , Hamoud Meshal Farhan Alshammari , Abdullah Saad Omar Almalki , Saeed Abdullah Alasmari , Yousef Ahmed Alduhailan , Mohmed Farj Alshmri , Afnan Mohammad Alneami , Sahar Abdullah Mansur , Abdulaziz Khalid A Alhuthayli , Hajar Muhayl Alsahli (2023). Dermatological emergencies in family medicine: Recognition, management, and referral considerations. https://core.ac.uk/download/603897626.pdf (accessed on 27th June 2025).
9. Al-Shabbani, N. H. S., Al-Subaihawi, A. J. K., & Almohammedi, T. G. (2024). Advances in psoriasis treatment: Emerging therapeutic strategies underlying histopathological changes

in psoriasis. https://core.ac.uk/download/639213712.pdf (accessed on 27th June 2025).

10. Apap, C., Boffa, M. J., & Piscopo, T. V. (2013). Crusted (Norwegian) scabies treated with oral ivermectin: A case report and overview. https://core.ac.uk/download/46602448.pdf (accessed on 27th June 2025).

11. Vermeulen, F. M., Gerbens, L. A. A., Bosma, A. L., Apfelbacher, C. J., Irvine, A. D., Arents, B. W. M., Barbarot, S., Deleuran, M., Eichenfield, L. F., Manca, A., Schmitt, J., Vestergaard, C., Wall, D., Weidinger, S., Middelkamp-Hup, M. A., Spuls, P. I., Flohr, C., & International TREAT Registry Taskforce (2019). TREatment of ATopic eczema (TREAT) Registry Taskforce: consensus on how and when to measure the core dataset for atopic eczema treatment research registries. *The British journal of dermatology*, *181*(3), 492–504. https://doi.org/10.1111/bjd.17715(accessed on 27th June 2025).

12. Dirschka, T., Pellacani, G., Micali, G., Malvehy, J., Stratigos, A. J., Casari, A., Schmitz, L., Gupta, G., & Athens AK Study Group (2017). A proposed scoring system for assessing the severity of actinic keratosis on the head: actinic keratosis area and severity index. *Journal of the European Academy of Dermatology and Venereology : JEADV*, *31*(8), 1295–1302. https://doi.org/10.1111/jdv.14267accessed on 27th June 2025).

13. Pimenta, R., Soares-de-Almeida, L., Arzberger, E., Ferreira, J., Leal-Filipe, P., Bastos, P. M., & Oliveira, A. L. (2020). Reflectance confocal microscopy for the diagnosis of skin infections and infestations. *Dermatology online journal*, *26*(3), 13030/qt9qz046f1.(accessed on 27th June 2025).

14. Costabel, U., Bendstrup, E., Cottin, V., Dewint, P., Egan, J. J., Ferguson, J., Groves, R., Hellström, P. M., Kreuter, M., Maher, T. M., Molina-Molina, M., Nordlind, K., Sarafidis, A., & Vancheri, C. (2014). Pirfenidone in idiopathic pulmonary fibrosis: expert panel discussion on the management of drug-related adverse events. *Advances in therapy*, *31*(4), 375–391. https://doi.org/10.1007/s12325-014-0112-1(accessed on 27th June 2025).

15. Wouters, M. W., Michielin, O., Bastiaannet, E., Beishon, M., Catalano, O., Del Marmol, V., Delgado-Bolton, R., Dendale, R., Trill, M. D., Ferrari, A., Forsea, A. M., Kreckel, H., Lövey, J., Luyten, G., Massi, D., Mohr, P., Oberst, S., Pereira, P., Prata, J. P. P., Rutkowski, P., ... Naredi, P. (2018). ECCO essential requirements for quality cancer care: Melanoma. *Critical reviews in oncology/hematology*, *122*, 164–178. https://doi.org/10.1016/j.critrevonc.2017.12.020(accessed on 27th June 2025).

16. Reddy, V., Thomas, S., Thibodeaux, Q., Myers, B., Bhutani, T., & Liao, W. (2020). Psoriasis Vulgaris Successfully Treated with Goeckerman Treatment at Home: A Patient and Physician's Experience. *Dermatology and therapy*, *10*(3), 329–338. https://doi.org/10.1007/s13555-020-00364-0(accessed on 27th June 2025).

17. Inoue, K., Blumenthal, D. M., Elashoff, D., & Tsugawa, Y. (2019). Association between physician characteristics and payments from industry in 2015-2017: observational study. *BMJ open*, *9*(9), e031010. https://doi.org/10.1136/bmjopen-2019-031010(accessed on 27th June 2025).

18. Sciberras, C. & Boffa, M. J. (2013). A review of a pediatric dermatology clinic in Malta. https://core.ac.uk/download/46602353.pdf (accessed on 27th June 2025).

19. Long B, Brém E, Koyfman A. Oncologic Emergencies: Immune-Based Cancer Therapies and Complications. *West J Emerg Med*. 2020;21(3):566-580. Published 2020 Apr 13. doi:10.5811/westjem.2020.1.45898(accessed on 27th June 2025).

20. Burdick, J., Giró Nieto, X., Marques, O., Romero-Lopez, M., et al. (2017). The impact of segmentation on the accuracy and sensitivity of a melanoma classifier based on skin lesion images. https://core.ac.uk/download/87655837.pdf (accessed on 27th June 2025).
21. Burke, M. D., Littenberg, B., Rubin, A., et al. (2020). Barriers and facilitators to use of a clinical evidence technology in the management of skin problems in primary care: Insights from mixed methods. https://core.ac.uk/download/289036096.pdf (accessed on 27th June 2025).
22. Burke, M., & Littenberg, B. (2018). Effect of a clinical evidence technology on patient skin disease outcomes in primary care: A cluster-randomized controlled trial. https://core.ac.uk/download/215154033.pdf (accessed on 27th June 2025).
23. Charruyer, A., Silvander, M., Caputo-Janhager, M., Raymond, I., & Ghadially, R. (2019). Proderm technology: a water- based lipid delivery system for dermatitis that penetrates viable epidermis and has antibacterial effects. *BMC dermatology*, *19*(1), 2. https://doi.org/10.1186/s12895-019-0082-8(accessed on 27th June 2025).
24. Hanna, R. F., Finkelstone, L. A., Chow, D. S., Miloushev, V. Z., Escudero, M. R., Lagana, S. M., & Prince, M. R. (2014). Nephrogenic systemic fibrosis risk and liver disease. *International journal of nephrology*, *2014*, 679605. https://doi.org/10.1155/2014/679605(accessed on 27th June 2025).
25. Chukwu, R., & Mankila, J. (2018). Dermatology nurses' job description: Literature review. https://core.ac.uk/download/161432240.pdf (accessed on 27th June 2025).
26. Climstein, M., Furness, J., Hing, W., Walsh, J., et al. (2016). Lifetime prevalence of non-melanoma and melanoma skin cancer in Australian recreational and competitive surfers. https://core.ac.uk/download/196601611.pdf (accessed on 27th June 2025).
27. Huisman, B. W., Pagan, L., Naafs, R. G. C., Ten Voorde, W., Rissmann, R., Piek, J. M. J., Damman, J., Juachon, M. J., Osse, M., Niemeyer-van der Kolk, T., van Hees, C. L. M., & van Poelgeest, M. I. E. (2023). Dermatoscopy and Optical Coherence Tomography in Vulvar High-Grade Squamous Intraepithelial Lesions and Lichen Sclerosus: A Prospective Observational Trial. *Journal of lower genital tract disease*, *27*(3), 255–261. https://doi.org/10.1097/LGT.0000000000000731(accessed on 27th June 2025).
28. Eddy, L., & Duffy, R. (2019). A study of the skills, education and qualifications of nurses performing dermatological surgery in the United Kingdom. *Dermatological Nursing: The journal of the British Dermatological Nursing Group*, *18*(4), 10-15. https://bdng.org.uk/dn/ (accessed on 27th June 2025).
29. El-Omar, E., Keenan, R. A., Ormerod, A. D., Rice, S., et al. (2013). Topical tacrolimus 0.1% ointment for treatment of cutaneous Crohn's disease. https://core.ac.uk/download/25497467.pdf (accessed on 27th June 2025).
30. Ghorbani, A. (2023). Artificial intelligence in skin cancer: A literature review from diagnosis to prevention and beyond. https://core.ac.uk/download/595875570.pdf (accessed on 27th June 2025).
31. Grabenhenrich, L., Hompes, S., Gough, H., Ruëff, F., Scherer, K., Pföhler, C., Treudler, R., Mahler, V., Hawranek, T., Nemat, K., Koehli, A., Keil, T., & Worm, M. (2012). Implementation of anaphylaxis management guidelines: a register-based study. *PloS one*, *7*(5), e35778. https://doi.org/10.1371/journal.pone.0035778(accessed on 27th June 2025).

32. Jenevein, C. L. (2015). Texas physicians' awareness and utilization of genetic services. https://core.ac.uk/download/46720101.pdf (accessed on 27th June 2025).
33. Kaptanoglu, A. F., & Mullaaziz, D. (2017). Acneiform eruptions and pregnancy. https://core.ac.uk/download/322429544.pdf (accessed on 27th June 2025).
34. Kolli, S. S. (2017). Promoting skin cancer awareness. https://core.ac.uk/download/84397761.pdf (accessed on 27th June 2025).
35. Mercieca, L., & Scerri, L. (2016). 'Food allergy / intolerance testing' in dermatology: Science or hype? https://core.ac.uk/download/83020041.pdf (accessed on 27th June 2025).
36. The Stern Center for Evidence-Based Policy (2015). Addressing the health needs of an aging America: New opportunities for evidence-based policy solutions. University of Pittsburgh. https://core.ac.uk/download/75783019.pdf
37. (accessed on 27th June 2025).
38. Publication Services at Boston University Medical Center, Boston University Medical Center. (1989). *Progress*. https://core.ac.uk/download/142070614.pdf (accessed on 27th June 2025).
39. Oliai, S. (2005). Economic environment and applications of telemedicine. https://core.ac.uk/download/10685681.pdf (accessed on 27th June 2025).
40. Thorneloe, R. J., Griffiths, C. E. M., Emsley, R., Ashcroft, D. M., Cordingley, L., British Association of Dermatologists Biologic Interventions Register, & Psoriasis Stratification to Optimise Relevant Therapy Study Groups (2018). Intentional and Unintentional Medication Non-Adherence in Psoriasis: The Role of Patients' Medication Beliefs and Habit Strength. *The Journal of investigative dermatology*, *138*(4), 785–794. https://doi.org/10.1016/j.jid.2017.11.015(accessed on 27th June 2025).
41. Sach, T. H., McManus, E., Mcmonagle, C., & Levell, N. (2016). Economic evidence for the prevention and treatment of atopic eczema: a protocol for a systematic review. *Systematic reviews*, *5*, 90. https://doi.org/10.1186/s13643-016-0262-0(accessed on 27th June 2025).
42. Patton, E. E. (2016). Nutritional factors associated with acne vulgaris. https://open.bu.edu/bitstream/2144/19444/1/Patton_bu_0017N_12304.pdf (accessed on 27th June 2025).
43. Valparaiso University. (1909). *Old School Catalog 1909–10, Chicago College of Medicine and Surgery*. https://core.ac.uk/download/216810609.pdf (accessed on 27th June 2025).
44. Valparaiso University. (1911). *Old School Catalog 1911–12, Chicago College of Medicine and Surgery*. https://core.ac.uk/download/216810581.pdf (accessed on 27th June 2025).

ALLERGY AND IMMUNOLOGY

5

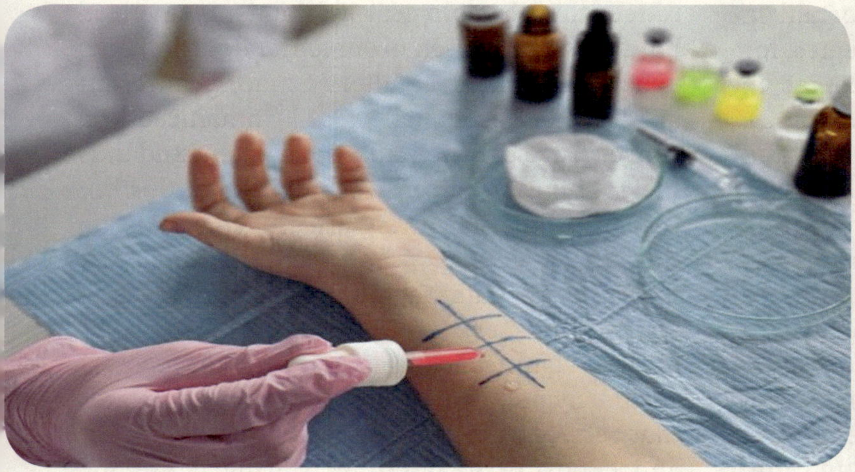

Introduction

Allergy and immunology is a sophisticated specialty that involves the immune system's adverse responses to previously harmless antigens, allergens. Becoming part of the understanding of allergies implies becoming part of the body's immune responses that, while intended to protect against pathogens, in some cases may end up playing harmful roles. Its reaction is not only a physiological process but also subject to an incredibly large number of environmental, genetic, and dietary factors. Scientific research indicates that the duration of exposure to foods with potential allergenicity in early infancy could be a decisive factor in food allergy induction. For instance, some studies have shown that the introduction of delayed solid and allergenic foods in infancy does not always equate to a reduced risk of allergic disorders. Instead, introduction at the right time between 4 and 6 months may be crucial for avoiding future allergy (Larson et al., 2016). Asthma is also a central component in immunology research, such as a stark contrast in control between population groups. In African Americans compared to

LEARNING OBJECTIVES

After studying this chapter, you will be able to:

1. Explain the types of allergies;
2. Understand the mechanisms of allergic reactions;
3. Discuss about diagnosis of allergies;
4. Describe the treatment options for allergies;
5. Define the role of the immune system;
6. Focus on current research in allergy and immunology.

Whites, there are stark contrasts in managing asthma, and there are determinants , including not just contrasts in biology but also contrasts in social determinants of health that accentuate those disparities. Models of research imply a multifaceted approach, classifying determinants into individual, healthcare, community, and sociocultural levels. These guidelines aim to define and transcend the particular challenges of different populations and highlight the need for intervention that is targeted. A grasp of asthma care disparities becomes important in developing effective healthcare strategies for delivering universal access and outcomes in allergy and immunology (Evans-Agnew, 2012). Last but not least, the practice of allergy and immunology necessitates an interdisciplinary strategy that integrates clinical research, public health programs, and education. As our knowledge of allergic diseases continues to develop, it is increasingly important to promote a greater sense of awareness regarding environmental factors, eating habits, and socio-economic variables that affect patients and healthcare systems. Further investigation into the timing of introduction of allergenic foods and determinants of asthma control reinforces the need for multifaceted and participatory approaches that address the needs of both the individual and broader community. By working together, healthcare professionals can better empower families to educate themselves on allergies and asthma, leading ultimately to an avenue toward greater healthcare and quality of life for those affected, no matter their backgrounds.

Definition of Allergies

Allergies represent a significant public health problem, characterized by an excessive reaction of the immune system to otherwise harmless substances termed allergens. These may be anything ranging from environmental exposures like pollen and dust mites to foods like nuts or shellfish. When an individual with a predisposition to an allergy is exposed to an allergen, his or her body recognizes it as dangerous and initiates the secretion of special antibodies called immunoglobulin E (IgE). This immune reaction leads to a variety of symptoms such as breathing difficulties, skin breakouts, and stomach problems, which can impair an individual's lifestyle significantly. While research continues to unfold the complexities of allergic reactions, there remains an urgent need to construct holistic definitions that not only reflect the physiological mechanisms involved but also the socio-environmental determinants driving the rates of allergy among different groups. The onset of allergies is influenced by a convergence of genes and environment and thus their definition becomes complicated. Current research has placed significant emphasis on the role of genetic predisposition, which can increase the vulnerability of an individual to allergic diseases. The environment, however, is no less significant, particularly in the context of the hygiene hypothesis, which postulates that reduced exposure to infectious pathogens and exposure to microbes during childhood can be to blame for the increased prevalence of allergic diseases. Under these circumstances, the concept of allergies extends beyond basic immunological responses to include a greater comprehension of lifestyle determinants and early exposure to modify the immune system. This overlap underscores the importance of interdisciplinarity in the resolution of challenges to the development of allergy, as evidenced in studies of maternal allergy and implications for maternal and infant health outcomes and with the evidence that the prevalence of food allergies is rising in the United States (Seita, 2013). Further, the signs of allergy tend to be varied, which creates various types of allergies and immunology. For example, atopic diseases such as asthma, rhinitis, and AD illustrate the way that allergic reactions can manifest themselves as discrete yet interrelated respiratory and cutaneous illnesses. Such diversity necessitates a complex knowledge of what an allergy is, both in terms of immediate and delayed hypersensitivity reactions. Advances in research technologies, including predictive modeling and omics technologies, can have the potential to enhance our understanding of these diseases and thereby aid the discovery of new therapeutic targets and personalized medicine. Since the proper control of allergies relies very much on accurate diagnosis and understanding of the underlying pathophysiological mechanisms, additional exploration of the pathophysiological mechanisms is going to play a very important role in meaningful design of therapeutic interventions within the discipline of allergy and immunology (Eyerich et al., 2019) (Figure 5.1).

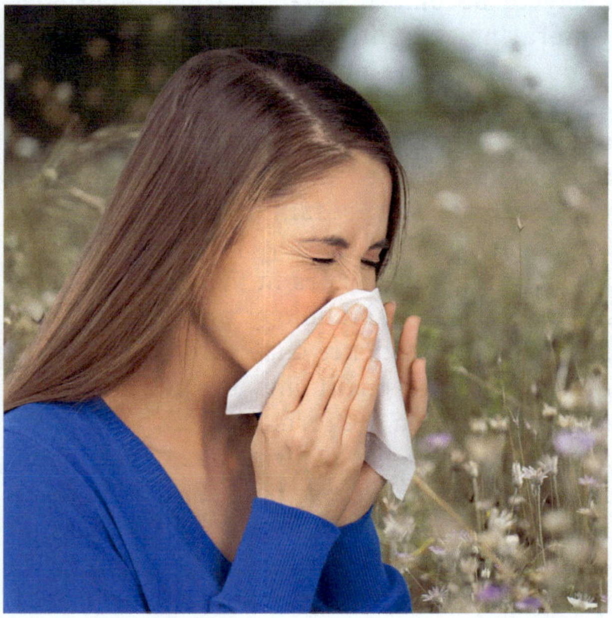

Figure 5.1. Illustration of seasonal allergy.

Source: https://ysm-res.cloudinary.com/image/upload/ar_1:1,c_fill,dpr_3.0,f_auto,g_faces:auto,q_auto:eco,w_500/v1/yms/prod/674942b4-3304-443e-8ddf-73926bd411a2.

Overview of the Immune System

The immune system plays a crucial role in maintaining the homeostasis of the body by defending it against pathogens and contributing to tissue repair. The immune system has two general components: the innate and the adaptive immune system. The first defense mechanism is in the form of the innate immune response, which employs physical barriers such as the skin and mucous membranes, as well as immune cells such as macrophages and neutrophils, which respond immediately to infection. This mechanism responds quickly but is not specific, responding to all pathogens in the same manner. The adaptive immune system, by contrast, provides a specific response to specific pathogens by the stimulation of B and T lymphocytes. Its dual nature is required for effective protection against a number of diseases, such as allergies, in which the immune system may incorrectly perceive innocuous substances as threatening and initiate inappropriate immune activation. The mechanisms involved in immune responses are intricate, typically involving a cascade of signaling pathways and cell interactions. Immune cells communicate by cytokines and chemokines, which regulate the recruitment and activation of immune elements. T helper cells, for instance, coordinate the immune response through the production of cytokines that regulate other immune cell activity, increasing either the humoral or cellular immune response. This aberrantly adapted response, while crucial in actual infections, can sometimes lead to allergic disease. The allergens can initiate undesired immune responses, causing inflammation and damage to the tissues and leading to symptoms such as asthma and rhinitis. Understanding such mechanisms is critical to treating allergic disease successfully. Studies have recently investigated the position of external factors, such as parasitic infection, and their regulation of the immune system. The Hygiene Hypothesis suggests that reduced exposure to infectious agents of diseases, particularly in affluent countries, may be accountable for increased incidence of allergic and autoimmune disease. There is evidence of association with reduced incidence of autoimmune disease after helminthic infection, most likely due to the immunomodulatory impact of such parasites. These worms synthesize various compounds that can modulate immunity, increase anti-inflammatory activity, and uphold general defense against pathogens. This is an intriguing finding, confirming the interdependence and complexity of immune reactions and offering promising leads toward therapeutic interventions against allergic diseases. Understanding these interactions is crucial for advancing the frontiers of allergy and immunology, thereby leading to new therapeutic approaches that can effectively address immune dysregulation, such as in allergic disorders (Seita, 2013; Pineda et al., 2014) (Figure 5.2).

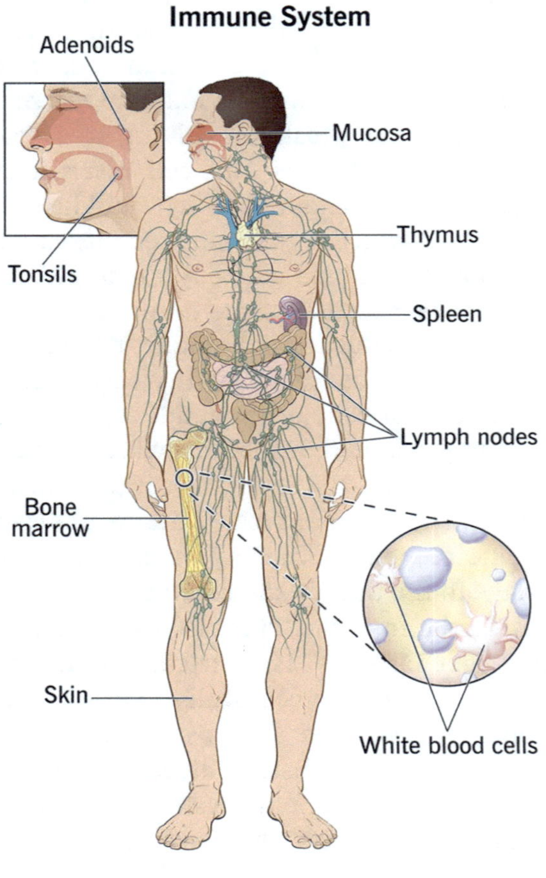

Figure 5.2. Immune system.

Source: https://my.clevelandclinic.org/-/scassets/images/org/health/articles/immune-system.jpg.

Importance of Studying Allergies and Immunology

The significance of the field of allergy and immunology cannot be overstated in the context of the rising burden of allergic disorders worldwide. Present estimates suggest that a substantial proportion of the population, particularly of industrialized nations, carries many allergic diseases like asthma, allergic rhinitis, and food allergy. Understanding the immunological mechanisms underlying these allergies is essential to the development of effective therapeutic strategies. With increasing levels of hygiene and sanitation, changes in lifestyle and diet, the immune system is more likely to become hyper-reactive to allergens, generating amplified allergenic reactions. Understanding the intricate interactions between allergens and the immune system will not only advance our knowledge of these diseases but also pave the way for targeted immunotherapies capable of suppressing symptoms and improving quality of life. Moreover, the role of environmental factors in molding immunity is essential in immunology and allergy. It is suggested by evidence that early exposure to diverse microbial environments could have long-lasting effects on the formation of the immune system and, in the majority of instances, the behavior towards allergens in adulthood. As an example, epidemiologic research indicates that children who grow up in rural settings with greater exposure to animals and environmental pathogens have lower allergy rates. The immunomodulatory effects of various infections, particularly parasitic helminths, account for the potential benefits of maintaining partial microorganism exposure during childhood. This concept is corroborated by evidence for increased rates of autoimmune and allergic disorders in developed countries following the elimination of certain helminth infections and therefore identifying these associations is crucial to plan preventive measures and interventions. Finally, understanding the complex host-helminth interactions presents promising avenues for therapeutic intervention in autoimmune as well as allergic disease. Recent findings on how helminths are able to influence immune responses have opened up their potential use as a therapeutic agent for the treatment of inflammation and hyper-reactivity of allergy. To be more specific, an understanding of adaptive immune mechanisms allowing expulsion of helminths or sustainable chronic infections may guide new directions in vaccine development and immunotherapy. The double role of helminths as immunomodulators and pathogens indicates their therapeutic potential, which means that they can help restore balance to hyperactive immune responses in allergic diseases. Therefore, a comprehensive study of immunology and allergies is not just called for in order to advance medicine but also in order to develop innovative solutions to combat the increasing number of allergic disorders in contemporary society (Pineda et al., 2014).

5.1. Types of Allergies

Learning Outcome

1. Understand food allergies;
2. Define environmental allergies;
3. Describe the prevalence of drug allergies.

The classification of allergies is significant in their occurrence and control in the field of immunology. Allergies are typically classified into two groups: IgE-mediated and non-IgE-mediated responses. IgE-mediated allergies, typically expressed as immediate hypersensitivity reactions, are primarily induced by allergens such as food particles, pollen, and insect stings. These reactions are characterized by the abrupt release of histamines and other mediators from mast cells in response to secondary exposure to a recognized allergen. These reactions can cause symptoms ranging from mild rhinitis to lethal anaphylaxis, necessitating prompt medical attention. Non-IgE-mediated allergies, like contact dermatitis and food protein-induced enterocolitis syndrome, typically comprise delayed reactions. The distinction between the categories is critical to appropriate diagnosis and therapeutic management since they are founded on different immunological principles and treatment approaches. Of the spectrum of IgE-mediated allergies, food allergy constitutes a major public health problem. The rising prevalence of food allergy, particularly in developed countries, has been stressed by recent studies, and calls for a critical evaluation of allergens and their sensitizing potential. Through the application of the adverse outcome pathway (AOP) framework, researchers have begun to systematize the molecular and cellular pathways of IgE-dependent food allergy, expanding our understanding of food proteins' ability to provoke allergic responses (Lozano-Ojalvo et al., 2019). The methodology not only helps scientists consolidate existing test practices but also helps in identifying new assays for allergen sensitivity testing. In addition, increasing awareness regarding food allergy demands rigorous risk assessments before new sources of food are introduced to the market, especially in terms of their potential for causing allergic sensitization in vulnerable populations. The management of allergies also includes specific antigen removal as well as preventive therapies. Environmental allergies, typically caused by pollen, dust mites, mold, and animal dander, may cause chronic diseases such as allergic rhinitis and asthma. In such cases, allergen immunotherapy (AIT) has been a promising therapy. Desensitizing the patients to recognized allergens by controlled exposure, which gradually weakens the allergic response over time, is how this therapy functions. Furthermore, treating doctors have come to appreciate the worth of individualized treatment protocols based on an allergy patient's profile. This is particularly so given that research shows a broad range of effects stemming from different funding approaches in asthma studies, which justifies the ongoing efforts at addressing such complex health disorders effectively (Hanney et al., 2013). Knowledge of different allergy types is hence critical to clinical practice and ongoing research in allergy and immunology.

5.1.1. Food Allergies

The rising prevalence of food allergies has created considerable interest among researchers and doctors, particularly as to what their mechanisms are. Food allergies arise when the immune system inaccurately identifies some of the proteins in food as harmful and, as a result, launches an inappropriate allergic reaction. This immunologic hypersensitivity may provoke an array of symptoms from minor illnesses, such as hives and belly pain, to life-threatening anaphylactic responses that must be treated instantly (Figure 5.3).

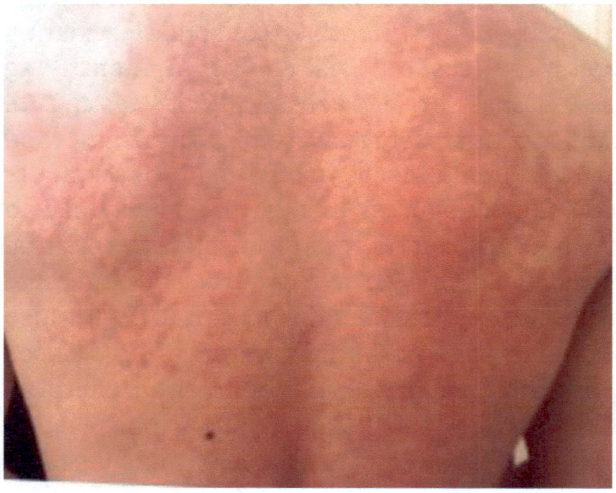

Figure 5.3. Hives on the back are a common allergy symptom.

Source: https://upload.wikimedia.org/wikipedia/commons/b/bb/Hives_on_back.jpg.

Recent studies have determined that food allergy experience persists beyond childhood, with an increase in incidents occurring in adults that is still under-explored. According to insufficiently addressed data, 5.6% of pregnant women suffer from food allergies, paralleling FDA-reported incidence within the general adult population, suggesting that increased investigation into food allergy among adults is warranted (Seita, 2013). Understanding the risk factors that produce food allergies is relevant to effective prevention and treatment approaches. Various factors come into play, including genetic predispositions, environmental factors, and dietary habits, which all work synergistically to produce these hypersensitivities. For instance, infants with allergic parents tend to develop similar sensitivities, and this indicates there is a genetic component. Moreover, recent controversies have brought to attention the important roles of the microbiome and early allergen exposure in regulating immune response. Immune system intolerance failures at an early stage may find their equivalents in aberrant responses during adulthood. Studies exploring such relationships would contribute significantly to our knowledge of food allergies, facilitating the development of targeted interventions capable of preventing their occurrence (Burns, 2019). The impact of food allergies extends beyond individual health conditions to broader public health and safety issues. Since food allergies are more prevalent, their impact on quality of life becomes an issue for healthcare providers and sufferers alike. For pregnant women with food allergies, there is an important need for studies investigating maternal health outcomes in conjunction with infant development. Prior research has not detected a robust correlation between food allergy in the mother and unfavorable outcomes, but the complex problems of pregnancy, diet, and infancy need to be re-explored. Furthermore, strategies for controlling food allergy must evolve to address not only temporary allergic reactions but also the psychosocial aspects of possessing a food allergy. Education and awareness are key to reforming food allergy and management perceptions, thus making the environment more inclusive for individuals with this new health condition (Seita, 2013) (Figure 5.4).

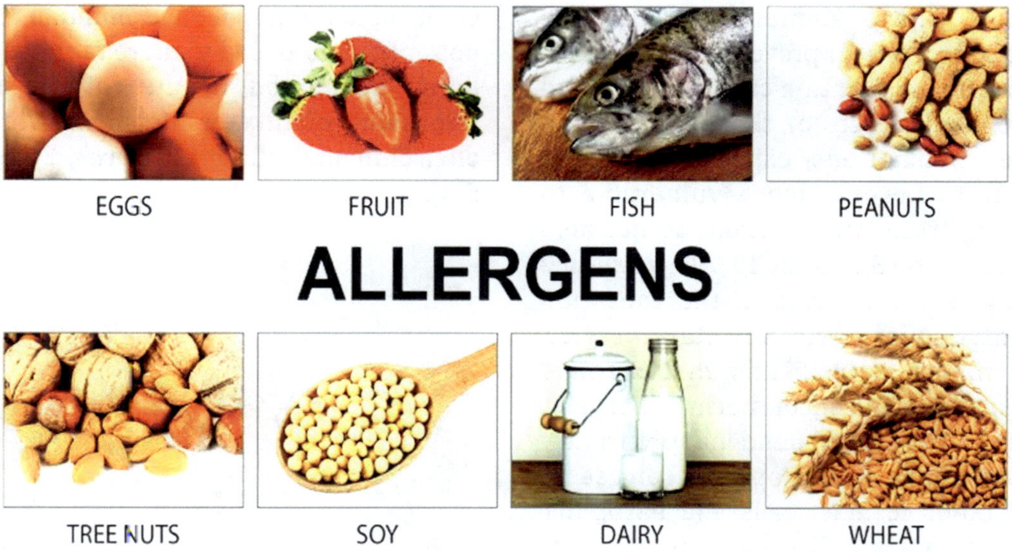

Figure 5.4. Food allergens.

Source: https://www.drbatras.com/sites/default/files/styles/blog/public/2024-04/food-allergies_Header_1.webp?itok=18HBBC8L.

5.1.2. Environmental Allergies

Environmental allergies, or what are commonly referred to as allergic reactions due to varying factors in our environment, are an important aspect of allergy and immunology. They can typically be brought about by contact with pollen, mold spores, dust mites, and pet dander, with symptoms from mild nasal congestion to life-threatening anaphylactic reactions. Environmental allergies have grown increasingly on the increase over the recent decades, a trend that has been attributed to both genetic and environmental factors.

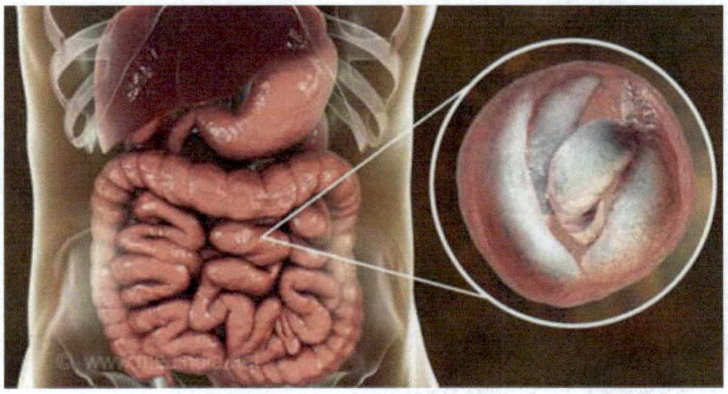

Figure 5.5. Illustration of soil-transmitted helminth infection.

Source: https://www.advancedresearchpublications.com/blog/wp-content/uploads/2024/05/intestinal-parasite-infections.jpg.

Several studies have shown that an individual's susceptibility to environmental allergens may be determined through hereditary inheritance, genetic mutation, and the degree of environmental sensitization. These elements need to be understood so that proper preventative programs and therapeutic intervention can be established to mitigate the impacts of these allergies in the afflicted populations, especially children who appear to become more vulnerable to developing hypersensitive reactions as indicated in recent research (Burns, 2019). The immune system plays a central role in the causation and presentation of environmental allergies, through complex mechanisms that mediate allergic responses. On encountering allergens, the immune system can respond inappropriately and leading to the inappropriate release of IgE, which binds to mast cells and basophils, releasing histamines and other inflammatory mediators. This hyper-reactivity is not only due to contact with allergens but can also be augmented by exposure to other environmental factors, such as pollutants. Recent research has explored the interesting hypothesis of associations between helminth infections and reduced rates of allergic sensitization. Studies have indicated that antigens of helminths have the capacity to induce regulatory immune responses that inhibit allergy, indicating the complex interaction between the multifactorial environmental determinants and the immune response (Rujeni et al., 2012) (Figure 5.5). Management of environmental allergic diseases involves in-depth knowledge of epidemiology and treatment strategies based on patient-specific sensitivities. Public health interventions to minimize exposure to common environmental allergens can reduce the incidence and severity of allergic responses significantly. Perhaps most importantly, improving indoor air quality and adopting hygienic practices that minimize dust and mold accumulation can reduce the burden of allergic disease. Also, increased awareness and knowledge on the part of medical providers and patients about these ubiquitous allergens can result in earlier detection and effective management plans. Continuing research, particularly on how pediatric hypersensitivity operates and whether synergism between environmental impact and immune response is possible, should lead to more targeted therapies being developed in the future, ultimately improving quality of life in individuals with environmental allergies (Burns, 2019) (Figure 5.6).

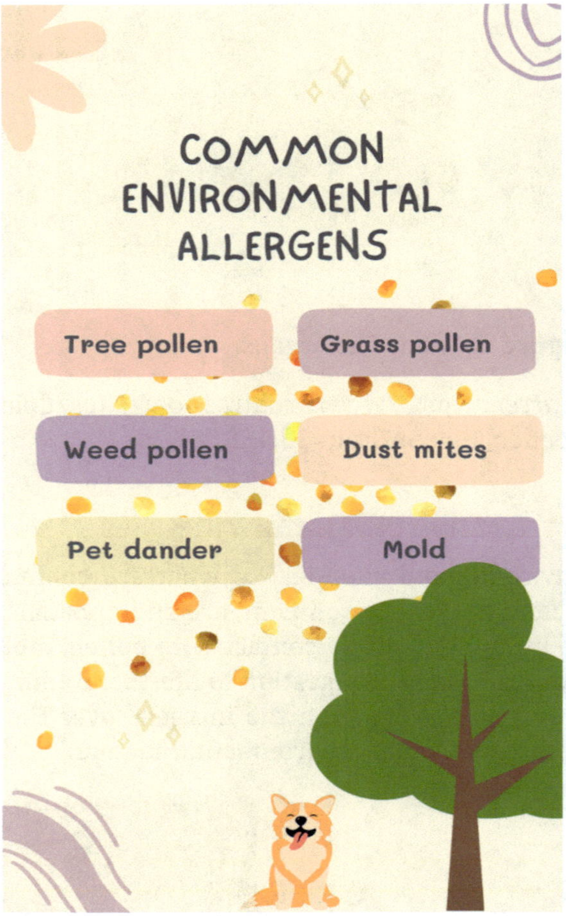

Figure 5.6. Common environmental allergens.

Source: https://foodswithgrace.com/wp-content/uploads/2023/05/Common-environmental-allergens-1-576x1024.png.

5.1.3. Drug Allergies

Drug allergy occurrence is a significant public health problem whose influence is felt on treatment protocols and patient outcomes. Among the drug allergy subgroups, penicillin allergy is in a league of its own, in terms of both prevalence and myths surrounding it. Surprisingly, even as penicillin allergy cases are commonly seen, a study indicates that only approximately 10% of such patients are indeed allergic, resulting in potential deleterious effects on treatment decisions. This inconsistency leads to increased reliance on other antibiotics, which might be less potent or more likely to cause side effects. Therefore, understanding the complexities involved in drug allergies, such as penicillin, is essential for clinicians to maximize patient benefit and minimize risks associated with incorrect allergy diagnosis, ensuring that correct allergy tests are of importance in practice. Drug allergy in pregnant women, even to common therapeutic drugs, holds not only maternal but also fetal health importance. Research, as in the case of a review of the prevalence of food allergy in pregnancy, underscores the need for a clear knowledge base of the impact of allergies on both maternal and infant health status. Though the study revealed that pregnant women's food allergy had no relation to adverse maternal and infant health, it underscores the necessity of studying allergies with varying conditions, such as medications. As they are faced with the complexities of drug allergy during pregnancy, clinicians must balance the risks of allergy therapy against the needs for optimal therapy for mother and fetus alike, ensuring allergies are accurately interpreted and drugs given are safe for this vulnerable population. Drug allergy evaluation and therapy have become increasingly important in outpatient practice. Pharmacists have subsequently begun playing a lead role in conducting penicillin skin testing (PST), by which patients who have a demonstrated penicillin allergy can be re-evaluated. It not only helps de-label the patient but also makes them aware of their actual risk for allergy so that they can be managed appropriately with beta-lactam antibiotics when necessary. The incorporation of allergy evaluation strategies, such as PST, emphasizes changing roles on healthcare teams, depicting how global allergy control can improve therapeutic effectiveness. With continuous education and advocacy striving to build tighter relationships between allergists, pharmacists, and clinicians, the aim is to deliver effective and safe treatments while reducing the burdens caused by inappropriately identified drug allergies, thus making contributions to further developments in allergy and immunology practice (Figure 5.7).

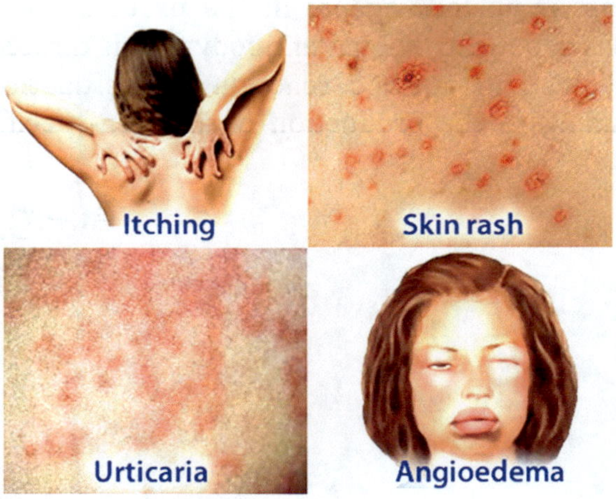

Figure 5.7. Drug allergy.

Source: https://asthmaallergyclinic.in/wp-content/uploads/2023/03/Drug_Allergy_2.png.

Test Your Knowledge

1. What is the primary difference between a food allergy and a food intolerance?
2. Which common environmental allergens are responsible for seasonal allergic rhinitis (hay fever)?
3. What are the typical symptoms of a drug allergy, and how do they differ from common drug side effects?

5.2. Mechanisms of Allergic Reactions

Learning Outcome

1. Explain the role of IgE antibodies;
2. Focus on Histamine release and its effects;
3. Describe anaphylaxis and severe allergic reactions.

Understanding the mechanisms of the allergic reaction is at the heart of allergy and immunology practice. Such a reaction is typically a result of an overactive immune response to otherwise harmless substances, referred to as allergens. Upon exposure to an allergen, the immune system mistakenly views the allergen as foreign and initiates a cascade of events. The most important agents in the process are B cells producing IgE, an antibody that is directly involved in allergic reactions. Sensitization leading to the production of allergen-specific IgE follows a first exposure to an allergen. This IgE binds to the mast cells and basophils and remains latent until the same allergen is again encountered by the individual, at which point degranulation occurs very rapidly and results in the release of inflammatory mediators such as histamine. This process accounts for the fundamental characteristics of allergic reactions and illustrates the central role of IgE as reported in the findings for its clinical relevance (Amarasekera, 2011). The prevalence of allergic reactions has experienced significant growth, particularly in environmental and dietary sensitivities. Of all these, food allergies have emerged as one of the most common presentations of allergic disorders, supplemented by a significant rise in numbers among children. The underlying mechanisms for the increased rate of food allergies remain obscure, prompting significant research interest in environmental causes, genetic predisposition, and microbiome influence.

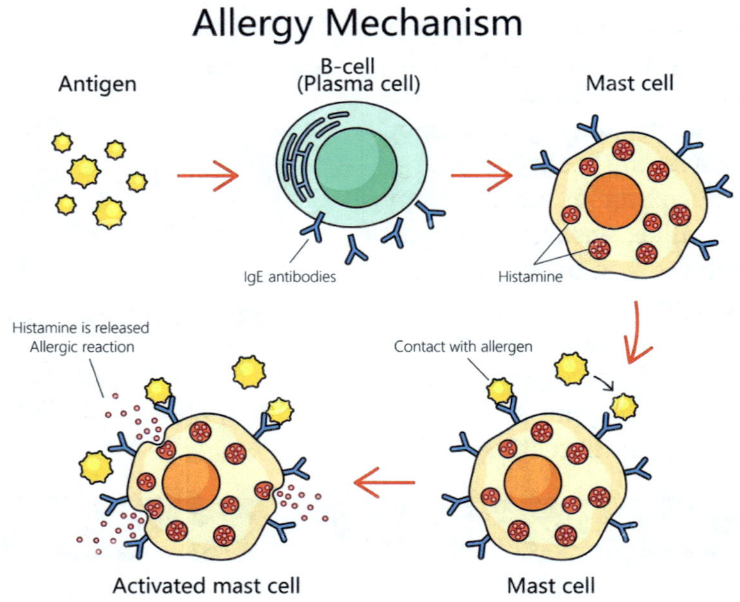

Figure 5.8. Allergy mechanism.

Source: https://thumbs.dreamstime.com/b/mechanism-allergy-action-diagram-medical-science-hand-drawn-schematic-raster-illustration-educational-306245119.jpg.

More recent investigations have also highlighted the social aspects of allergies, with trends in adult populations that were previously not well considered. It has been shown through evidence that maternal food allergies may affect not only their health but also the health of infants, which can potentially influence pregnancy outcomes. These associations are significant to comprehend for clinicians and researchers alike, highlighting the importance of higher awareness and future research in this ever-evolving branch of allergy and immunology (Seita, 2013). To explore further these mechanisms is to appreciate the significant implications in treatment and management regimens in allergic diseases. The central position of IgE in allowing allergic reactions to take place has led to the identification of specific treatments, such as monoclonal antibodies, to block the interaction between IgE and its receptor on mast cells and basophils. New desensitization protocols also attempt to switch the immune response to become tolerant of specific allergens, thereby reducing sensitivity and reaction severity. These advances in allergy therapy enhance not only the patients' quality of life but also the understanding of immunological tolerance and its complexities in the broader Allergy and Immunology community. With research evolving, a framework that is multidisciplinary must be picked up, where clinical findings are being mixed with fundamental immunological phenomena to deal with the growing issue of allergies in current society (Amarasekera, 2011) (Figure 5.8).

5.2.1. Role of IgE Antibodies

The role of IgE antibodies plays a key part in understanding allergy and immunology, particularly when considering hypersensitivity reactions. IgE is arguably best known for its role within the immune response to allergens, triggering the release of histamines and other mediators from basophils and mast cells. This chain reaction leads to the typical symptoms present in allergic reactions, including itching, swelling, and anaphylaxis in extreme cases. The activation of IgE antibodies is also influenced by several factors, including genetic and environmental exposures. The interaction of these factors gives rise to some difficult questions of why some people become allergic and others do not. Investigating these underlying mechanisms remains crucial to the discovery of preventative treatments and therapeutics that can reduce IgE-mediated hypersensitivity. Recent research has underscored the complexity of IgE responses, particularly in comparison with other immune mechanisms, such as helminth infection. Research has demonstrated a negative relationship between sensitization to allergens and the occurrence of helminth infections, suggesting that immune responses to such parasites can modulate IgE production. It has been proposed that helminth antigens can induce regulatory immune responses that may inhibit IgE-mediated pathways that are typically associated with allergies. Such an association raises interesting mechanistic and evolutionary issues about immune adaptation in humans. The ongoing debate on the clinical significance of these findings highlights the intricate nature of protective immune responses and the development of allergic disease, where more effort is needed to gain a comprehensive understanding of the roles of IgE in each case, including its relative dynamics with different immune responses (Rujeni et al., 2012). Moreover, the increasing prevalence of childhood allergies has increased research into the IgE antibodies, further emphasizing the understanding of the specific risk factors behind their production in this vulnerable age group. Genetic inheritance, environmental sensitization, and even nutritional effects have all been attributed as causes within the emerging prevalence of childhood allergies. Studies investigating these elements indicate that exposures in early life can play a powerful role in shaping immune responses, including the tendency to produce IgE antibodies. By studying hypersensitivity pathways, researchers look for potential interventions to reduce allergic responses in pediatric patients. Having a full picture of the factors of risk in children's hypersensitivity strengthens our knowledge about IgE antibodies and guides clinical practice in treating children's alarming rates of allergy (Burns, 2019) (Figure 5.9).

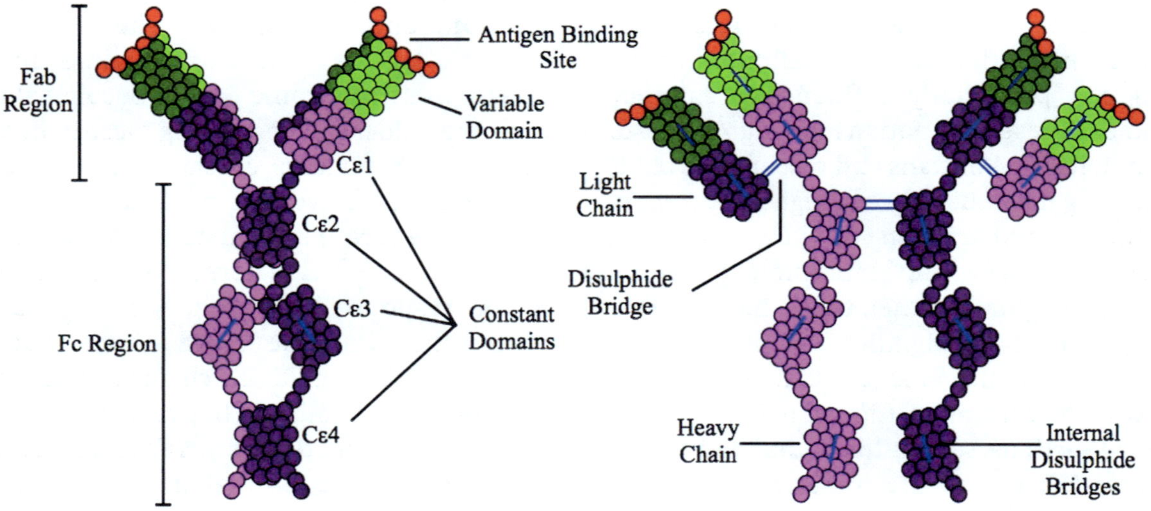

Figure 5.9. The structure of the IgE antibody.

Source: https://upload.wikimedia.org/wikipedia/commons/9/9d/IgE.jpg.

5.2.2. Histamine Release and Its Effects

Histamine release is a basic component of the immune system and plays a central role in allergic responses. The allergens in the body react with specific IgE antibodies on mast cells and basophils and induce degranulation of mast cells and basophils. This is followed by the discharge of several mediators, of which histamine is most critical. Histamine binds to H1 receptors, causing vasodilation, vascular permeability, and smooth muscle contraction, all of which result in the typical allergy symptoms of congestion, swelling, and itching. The complexity of this response explains immune system and environmental stimulus interaction and shows the need for further research into the underlying processes to design effective interventions for individuals afflicted with hypersensitivity reactions (Burns, 2019). It is important to comprehend the effects of histamine when dealing with allergic conditions, particularly in light of the continued rise in childhood allergies. Current studies have focused on determining risk factors in the development of allergic diseases among children and have emphasized both genetic susceptibility and environmental susceptibility. Pediatric hypersensitivities have serious health implications, and it is important to investigate the mechanisms of histamine release and its biological consequences. The connection between environmental sensitization and allergic responses highlights the need for multi-faceted approaches to predict and possibly prevent the rising incidence of such diseases among children (Seita, 2013). Furthermore, the role of histamine is not restricted to acute allergic responses; it plays a part in chronic disorders such as asthma and AD. These diseases illustrate how prolonged histamine release and receptor activation can produce more generalized pathological consequences, elicit a chronic inflammatory process and contribute to tissue remodeling. The intersection of histamine activity with chronic inflammatory disease calls for more understanding of modes of therapy that impact histamine pathways, such that the conditions are alleviated and patient quality of life improved. Investigation into the pharmacological regulation of histamine release and its receptor holds the potential for the development of new therapies for allergic and immunological disorders (Burns, 2019).

5.2.3. Anaphylaxis and Severe Allergic Reactions

Anaphylaxis is the most severe form of allergic reaction, characterized by the capacity to occur rapidly and possibly be life-threatening unless properly managed. It is a systemic response that can be triggered by various allergens, including foods, drugs, insect stings, and latex. The body's immune system reacts excessively to these substances, leading to the secretion of mediators such as histamines, which cause diffuse vasodilation, bronchoconstriction, and increased vascular permeability. As this chain of events goes on, the victim is able to develop potentially fatal conditions such as dyspnea, hypotension, and syncope.

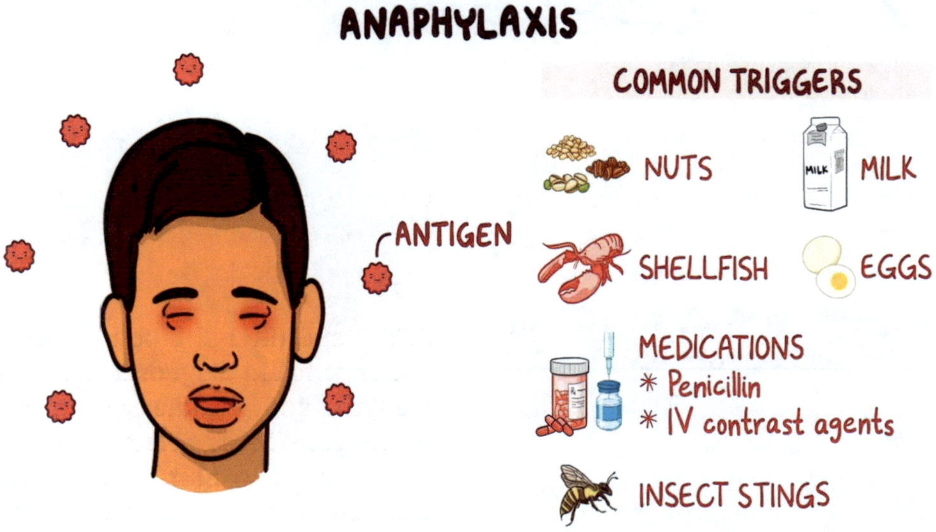

Figure 5.10. Anaphylaxis.

Source: https://www.osmosis.org/_next/image?url=https%3A%2F%2Fd16qt3wv6xm098.cloudfront.net%2F8f5BveRWShieZwwPrO8LAhKnSvy0TNy5%2F_.jpg&w=3840&q=75.

Although anaphylaxis has been noted in multiple age groups, its prevalence appears to be on the rise, particularly food allergy among children, a factor that serves to call for continued research and community education (Seita, 2013). The treatment of anaphylaxis is described through set guidelines with a focus on immediate action. Intramuscular adrenaline administration is the mainstay of treatment, and its adjunct therapies are antihistamines and corticosteroids designed to mitigate symptoms and diminish inflammation. In spite of extensive recommendations, there is a large gap between guidelines and their effective implementation within clinical practice. A study on the management of anaphylaxis in allergy referral centers in Austria, Germany, and Switzerland reported a high level of underreporting of adrenaline injections and related therapy during acute episodes. Specifically, less than a quarter of cases received intramuscular adrenaline, but many did not receive adequate information regarding avoidance of allergen or self-management with epinephrine auto-injectors (Grabenhenrich et al., 2012). Such discrepancies make it necessary to provide improved training and education on anaphylaxis management among healthcare professionals. It is also important to understand the epidemiology of anaphylaxis to address the issue at a larger level. It has been found through research that food allergy is one of the primary reasons for anaphylaxis, particularly in children and young people. However, as the prevalence of such allergies has increased, much epidemiological information regarding adult populations experiencing anaphylaxis still lacks. Research with diverse demographic factors and comprehensive data collection can provide insights into the overall importance of food allergies in public health. Moreover, ongoing investigations on the relationship between maternal food allergies and complications in the perinatal period can provide vital information. As understanding of these complex interactions advances, one can create targeted prevention mechanisms, which show potential to improve control and reduced incidence of life-threatening allergic responses in the population (Seita, 2013) (Figure 5.10).

Test Your Knowledge

1. What role do IgE antibodies play in allergic reactions, and how are they involved in the immune system's response to allergens?
2. Which cells release histamine during an allergic reaction, and what are the typical effects of histamine on the body?
3. How does epinephrine (adrenaline) counteract the effects of anaphylaxis, and why is it the first-line treatment?

5.3. Diagnosis of Allergies

Learning Outcome

1. Discuss skin prick tests;
2. Explain blood tests for allergens;
3. Explain the role of patient history and symptom assessment in the realm of allergy and immunology.

Allergy diagnosis is a critical intersection of clinical experience and patient history in the medical practice of allergy and immunology. Diagnosis requires vigilant review of symptoms, patient history, and typically a series of diagnostic tests. Practitioners begin the assessment by gathering detailed information regarding the patient's medical history, including previous allergic episodes and histories of atopy within their families. This foundation of knowledge helps in identifying potential allergens and tailoring the diagnostic approach. Depending on presentation, clinicians utilize skin prick tests (SPTs), specific IgE blood testing, or oral food challenge to aid diagnoses. Each has its relative strengths and weaknesses, which mandates a careful considered selection according to each case of patient. Skin prick testing is an old cornerstone of the diagnosis of allergies because it is quick and effective in diagnostics. Provided that they are well-performed, SPTs can identify sensitivity to a variety of allergens, including pet hair, pollen, and food substances. Skin prick testing entails applying a minute quantity of an allergen to the skin and observing localized reactions that would be indicative of sensitivity. While this method is typically safe and not likely to be disrupted by a variety of conditions, such as drug use or cutaneous pathology, outcomes can be influenced under such conditions, generating false negative or positive reactions. As a result, to generate an accurate diagnosis of allergy, it becomes important for professionals to compare results to physical exams and clinical histories. Complete diagnostic procedures, then enable more specific use of therapy protocols.

Along with conventional methods, advances in allergy diagnosis are also refining less obvious and patient-tailored approaches. Techniques such as molecular allergology allow for in-depth testing of individual proteins that produce allergic reactions, providing more definitive diagnostic data. By determining the exact molecules triggering a reaction, physicians can provide patients with personalized advice on limiting exposure and symptom management. In addition, national efforts toward promoting standardized practice measurement, as discussed in the process of establishing tracking mechanisms, highlight increasing focus on providing quality care in diagnosing and treating allergy. Efficiency-enhancing strategies that promote patient empowerment in taking health-related decision-making are in line with current shifts toward patient-oriented medical homes in allergy and immunology (The Stern Center for Evidence-Based Policy, 2015; Amaducci et al., 2018).

5.3.1. Skin Prick Tests (SPTs)

The skin prick test (SPT) is a pillar diagnostic tool within the practice of allergy and immunology, primarily employed to identify which specific allergens induce hypersensitivity reactions in patients. During the process, a small amount of suspected allergens is placed into the skin surface, typically the forearm or back. When exposed, if the patient is allergic to a particular substance, then the immune system will respond, resulting in localized inflammation in terms of swelling and redness. The size of the wheal which forms is taken after 15–20 minutes and provides a very good indication of sensitivity to the allergen. Also, skin prick testing is not that complex. It is a low-cost method whose results are known immediately, and it allows doctors to make the most informed judgments regarding other treatments for allergic conditions. One of SPTs' advantages is that it is versatile, as it can be performed against a wide variety of allergens, ranging from pollen and pet dander to dust mites and mold. This multiparametric application allows clinicians to tailor treatment regimens more effectively, based on the appropriate allergens to which an individual is sensitized. SPTs may prove useful in the diagnosis of allergic rhinitis, asthma, and AD through enabling a greater understanding of the related immunological mechanisms at play.

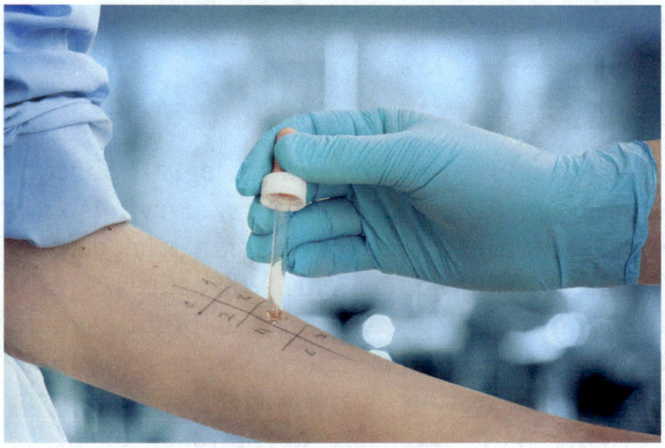

Figure 5.11. A person receiving a skin prick test (SPT).

Source: https://foodallergiesatlanta.com/wp-content/uploads/2022/08/food-allergy-testing.jpeg.

Significantly, the interrelationship of allergen characteristics and patient response has been widely explored. For instance, plant allergens have been of interest based on their complex protein structures, such that features like N-glycosylation affect allergenicity (Blanca et al., 2013). In practice, SPT implementation has been documented to have pragmatic repercussions for diverse populations, including hard-to-reach groups. A pilot cross-sectional study in the Sololá department of Guatemala illustrates this, with data on the prevalence and trends of allergic diseases among an indigenous group. The results of the subsample provided SPTs showed low rates of positivity for several common allergens, and it was assumed that allergic symptoms are relatively rare within this population (Makvandi-Nejad, 2023). Through showing the feasibility of such testing in varied environments, these findings identify the benefit of adapting allergy diagnostic methods in order to better understand and manage allergic diseases in varied populations. Additional information stemming from research like this can ultimately serve as the basis for public health initiatives aimed at improving allergy control and education in underserved communities (Figure 5.11).

5.3.2. Blood Tests for Allergens

Blood tests are now an integral part of diagnosing allergic disorders, serving as a supplementary tool to routine skin prick testing. This test technique primarily measures certain IgE antibodies present in the blood, which are produced against allergens. In situations where skin testing is not advisable, such as in patients with extensive dermatoses or those taking specific antihistamines, blood testing is an acceptable option. Blood tests are also able to provide information about more than one allergen simultaneously, something that could assist clinicians in ascertaining patterns of sensitization. As more knowledge about allergies becomes available, research continues to examine the association between levels of specific IgE and clinical symptoms, refining possibly the precision of allergy diagnosis and treatment protocols in allergy and immunology (Seita, 2013). The worth of blood testing is also discovered in the evaluation of food allergy, which has been increasing, particularly in children. Recent studies have demonstrated that maternal food allergies can similarly affect infant health outcomes, and therefore, there is a complex interaction between gene predisposition and environmental exposure (Seita, 2013). When blood tests are used to identify food allergens, they can help initiate appropriate dietary changes to minimize exposure. Though blood tests are not absolute, they are of immense assistance in minimizing uncertainty and help patients manage their diet and lifestyle based on food sensitivities. Moreover, the relationship between identified food allergies and actual allergic reactions remains a topic of continuous research, such that the need for continuous research in this field is evident. Despite their advantages, blood tests against allergens are not perfect. The interpretative challenges of the IgE levels may lead to false positives or negatives, complicating diagnosis. Also, the cost of such tests may pose accessibility issues for some patients. It is crucial that clinicians place the results of blood tests in the patient's clinical setting and symptomatology to avoid misdiagnosis. The demand for effective diagnostic tools in allergy and immunology has urged constant upgrading of testing methods, suggesting the future promises even more vigorous and accurate assays. Pursuing a comprehensive understanding of allergy mechanisms through such tests will play an essential role in enhancing patient care and management strategies, as the field continues to evolve (Figure 5.12).

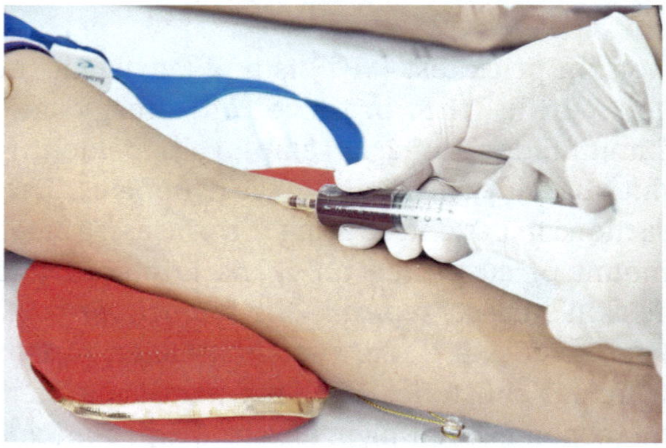

Figure 5.12. Blood tests for allergies.

Source: https://www.allergiesandhealth.com/wp-content/uploads/allergy-blood-testing.jpg.

5.3.3. Patient History and Symptom Assessment

In immunology and allergy, an accurate and comprehensive patient history and symptom assessment are the foundation for successful therapy and diagnosis. The dialogue between the patient and physician generally illuminates the nature of allergic reactions, including causes, frequency, and severity. A thorough patient history should encompass not just information regarding previous allergic reactions but also whether there is an inherited tendency towards allergy or autoimmune disorders. In addition, the background of symptom onset, whether this is seasonal or from contact with certain foods or environments, is valuable information. Adding this type of information allows one to have more individualized management, like the utilization of immunotherapy that has been found to be effective for avoiding symptoms of uncontrollable severe allergic rhinitis, as indicated in the literature (Meadows et al., 2013). Moreover, symptom assessment is critical to the evaluation of the severity and potential complications of allergies. Symptoms such as respiratory distress, skin lesions, or gastrointestinal upset need to be evaluated in detail by doctors to determine the course of action. For instance, anaphylaxis is a life-threatening and serious allergic reaction that needs immediate intervention and intensive initial management. The World Allergy Organization's hypothesized standards underscore the importance of sound clinical diagnosis and timely action, with attention given to patient risk factors as well as establishing a good thought-out emergency plan. This nuanced understanding enables practitioners to determine which symptoms have the potential to be precursors for life-threatening allergic reactions and to adopt practical prevention measures against recurrent instances, thereby facilitating PS and wellness. Finally, patient education in an inclusive manner is an essential part of effective allergy control with a heavy reliance on history and symptom assessment. Increasing sensitization to specific triggers, symptom identification, and the mechanisms required for immediate action can enable patients to manage their conditions proactively. It also establishes lines of dialogue for immunomodulation strategies, such as allergy immunotherapy, designed to optimize long-term outcomes through modification of reactions to an individual allergen. Engaging patients as partners in treatment encourages not only a sense of autonomy but also optimizes the effectiveness of treatment regimens based on their individualized histories and symptomatology. By focusing on the combination of thorough tests with patient education, medical providers can significantly enhance the well-being of patients with allergic diseases.

Test Your Knowledge

1. How does a skin prick test work, and what does a positive result indicate?
2. What information can a blood test provide, and how does it compare to skin testing?
3. Why is a detailed patient history important in diagnosing allergies, even before performing any tests?

5.4. Treatment Options for Allergies

Learning Outcome

1. Understand the role of antihistamines and decongestants for allergies;
2. Discuss the concept of Immunotherapy and allergy shots;
3. Focus on lifestyle modifications and avoidance strategies.

Management of allergies is heterogeneous based on the differential nature and severity of allergic reactions. Avoidance of the responsible allergen is the optimal management in the first place; this is, however, rarely possible in everyday life. Symptomatic control can be achieved through the employment of over-the-counter antihistamines, which are effective very quickly in mild allergic states such as hay fever and cutaneous dermatitis. For more severe cases, like anaphylaxis, urgent medical treatment is indicated. Intramuscular adrenaline is currently recommended by guidelines for severe reactions, backed by antihistamines and corticosteroids to alleviate symptoms after exposure. There has been reported evidence of a substantial gap between guidelines and practice by studies, with suggested education and training of medical staff to optimize patient outcomes (Grabenhenrich et al., 2012). For individuals who suffer from chronic allergic illness, immunotherapy provides an alternative longer-term management. The treatment consists of gradual desensitization of the immune system to specific allergens and works to significantly reduce the severity of an allergic response. Subcutaneous immunotherapy (SCIT) is the most traditional form, which consists of repeated injections over long periods. Sublingual immunotherapy (SLIT) is a newer delivery mechanism that has gained wider usage because it is simple to administer and has a favorable safety record. Research indicates a greater emphasis on home management of acute episodes, particularly in hereditary angioedema due to C1 inhibitor deficiency patients, with high emphasis on availability of emergency therapy and patient education (Longhurst et al., 2015).

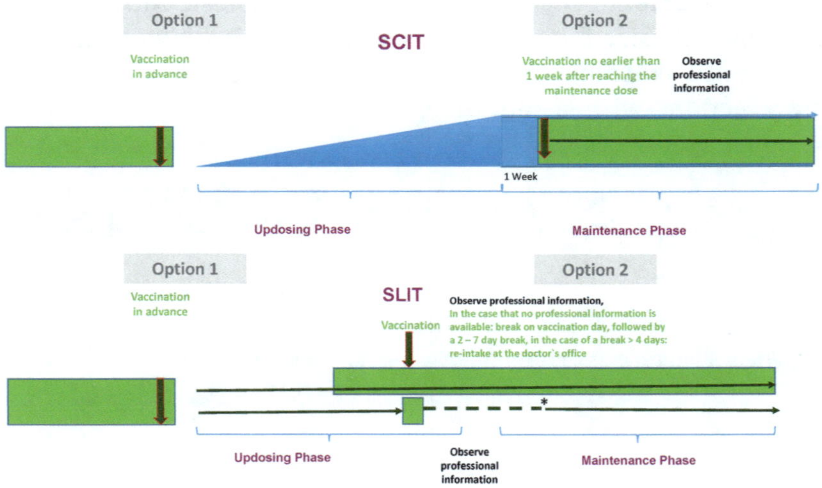

Figure 5.13. Recommendations for subcutaneous immunotherapy (SCIT) and sublingual immunotherapy (SLIT).

Source: https://www.researchgate.net/publication/354185896/figure/fig1/AS:1070957208797184@1632347504928/Recommendations-for-subcutaneous-immunotherapy-SCIT-and-sublingual-immunotherapy-SLIT.png.

This advancement in treatment offers greater individualized management strategies based on individual patient requirements. Moreover, new treatments keep advancing the armada of strategies for allergy management. Biologic drugs targeting distinct immune pathways have shown efficacy for chronic rhinosinusitis with nasal polyps and severe asthma, providing relief to patients previously unresponsive to standard pharmacotherapy. These new therapies could require careful patient selection and ongoing follow-up since they represent a paradigm shift in allergy management. With the immune system coming to be understood, so too does the future for new interventions increase, with the potential to improve the clinical outcome and quality of life for millions with allergies. Research and multidisciplinary collaboration between healthcare staff, patients, and researchers will be at the forefront of developing care and ensuring that treatment practice is updated with the latest evidence (Figure 5.13).

5.4.1. Antihistamines and Decongestants

Antihistamines and decongestants play a very crucial role in the management of allergic rhinitis and other associated conditions. Antihistamines exert their action by blocking the histamine receptors; therefore, the action of the allergic reaction, such as sneezing, itching, and a runny nose.

Antihistamines are divided into first-generation antihistamines and second-generation antihistamines. First-generation antihistamines have efficacy but also produce sedation since they penetrate the blood-brain barrier. However, second-generation antihistamines are less apt to induce somnolence, thus they would be more appropriate for patients who need awareness during the progression of daily activity. Application of antihistamines with other treatments, such as SNIs, can also optimize patient responses in terms of managing allergic symptoms, hence improving the overall quality of life, as in the articles on the treatment of allergic rhinitis (Tran et al., 2011). Decongestants, on the other hand, provide symptomatic relief by making the blood vessels of the nasal passages smaller, thus reducing swelling and congestion. They are applied in both allergic and non-allergic rhinitis conditions. Decongestants can be administered orally or topically, with the latter tending to provide slower relief. Frequent application of topical decongestants, however, leads to rebound congestion, a disease known as rhinitis medicamentosa. This phenomenon reaffirms the need for caution and responsible usage of decongestants as excessive consumption may result in prolonged nasal obstruction and other diseases, such as sinusitis and the development of nasal polyps (Kalinowska et al., 2025). Thus, physicians suggest a rational approach to the utilization of decongestants that yields relief from symptoms effectively and minimizes the side effects of prolonged therapy. While antihistamines and decongestants are effective therapies, these therapies should be included within an overall strategy for treating allergic rhinitis. These treatments might include allergen avoidance maneuvers and other therapies, such as intranasal corticosteroids, which are the key to treatment in the control of inflammation. By using these approaches together, it is possible to have simultaneous action on many inflammatory processes caused by allergens and gain improved control over symptoms. In addition, individualized treatment regimens, which can include immunotherapy for long-term relief, are important to deal with each patient's unique allergic profile. As our knowledge in allergy and immunology progresses, ongoing research endeavors seek to further optimize these pharmacological treatments and their applications, leading to improved patient outcomes and a reduction in allergy-related disease burden (Tran et al., 2011) (Figure 5.14).

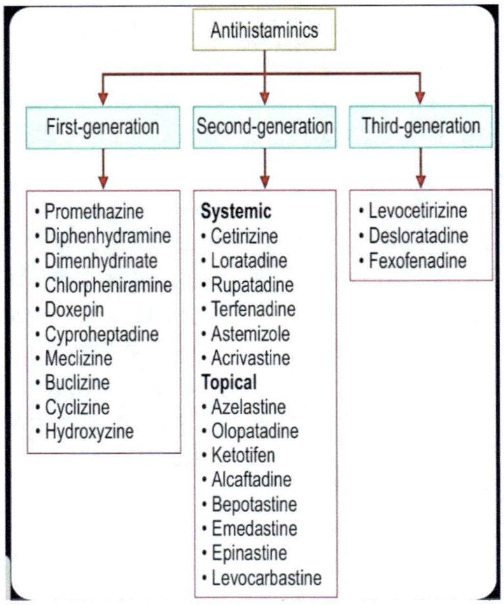

Figure 5.14. Antihistamines.

Source: https://encrypted-tbn0.gstatic.com/images?q=tbn:ANd9GcSB82zGnaJbV17Mr7gWuhYmVAoFBrcpAPXRdQ&s.

5.4.2. Immunotherapy and Allergy Shots

Immunotherapy is one of the primary forms of treatment in addressing a variety of allergies, particularly through the allergy shots and oral immunotherapy (OIT) practices. SCIT, or allergy shots, refers to the method of incrementally introducing higher doses of allergens to produce immunity in the immune system.

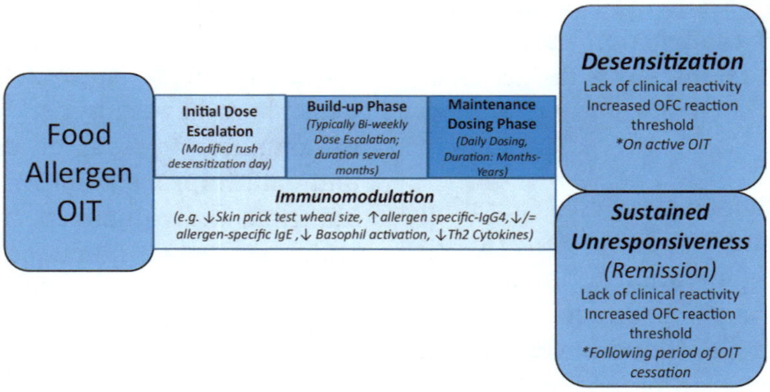

Figure 5.15. Overview of food allergen oral immunotherapy (OIT), including phases of treatment and clinical outcome.

Source: https://www.researchgate.net/publication/344033391/figure/fig1/AS:11431281261054562@1721320597233/Overview-of-food-allergen-oral-immunotherapy-OIT-, including-phases-of-treatment-and.png.

The method has been extensively researched, and it has been proven to effectively reduce symptoms of seasonal and perennial allergies. By immunizing the immune system to react less violently to familiar allergens, patients often experience a significant reduction in the symptomatology of allergies. Extensive use of this treatment has rendered it a norm of allergy treatment, providing long-term improvement in millions of individuals suffering from chronic allergic disease. In recent years, the evolution of OIT has introduced a new approach to immunotherapy, and most notably, for food allergy. As highlighted by current studies, OIT allows patients to slowly consume food allergens in the clinic to create a desensitized immune response. The treatment is best for those with a life-threatening food allergy, such as peanuts, which is a huge risk if eaten, such as anaphylaxis (Rauscher, 2015).

While OIT is not a food allergy cure, the imposition of this therapy represents a significant milestone in the management of allergies, releasing patients and families from the constant anxiety and quality-of-life issues of food allergy. Research into OIT has stimulated the development of specialty programs in private and academic settings to better understand the general impact and safety of this therapy. With ongoing advancements within the field of allergology, the function of mixing immunotherapy in both forms of allergy injections as well as OIT necessitates extreme care with respect to efficacy and safety. Ongoing studies continue to be pivotal towards maximizing these therapies, particularly with increased utilization. For instance, knowledge of variability in response to therapy among patients and potential dangers of desensitization (Olson, 2019) is necessary. As more and more clinical trials with outcomes become available, focus will be directed at refining these treatments so that they are both available and effective across broad populations of patients. The ultimate hope is to enhance the quality of life in those afflicted with allergies by reducing the effect of these diseases and the pervasive fear of a reaction (Figure 5.15).

5.4.3. Lifestyle Modifications and Avoidance Strategies

Lifestyle modification and avoidance strategies take center stage in the management of allergic disease in the field of allergy and immunology. Allergy-prone individuals must adopt strategic interventions to minimize exposure to allergens in the environment. These include vigilant label reading to identify potential allergens in food, as traces of these allergens produce adverse reactions. In addition, inhabitants can also benefit from the reduction of dust mites and mold by applying air purifiers, humid control, and standard cleaning methods. These modifications lead to opportunities towards a better living environment and reduce exposure to allergens, emphasizing preventive features in health care. Social factors are also relevant while planning lifestyle modifications because allergic reactions significantly impact everyday life and social engagement. People with food allergies, for instance, experience restrictions when eating out or engaging in shared meals. To cope with such challenges adequately, it is vital for people to express their allergies freely to friends and relatives to establish a network of understanding individuals who know what they can or cannot eat. On top of this, the utilization of resources such as allergy action plans is able to guide individuals and their caregivers to respond appropriately to allergic attacks, emphasizing awareness and readiness in social situations. As social methods are modified, they enhance the quality of life as well as security among individuals with allergies. Higher rates of allergy diseases call for an integral approach towards lifestyle choices, particularly for the elderly portion of the population. When a person ages, the vulnerability to developing and exacerbating allergies is higher, and there is a requirement for lifestyle modifications to accommodate physiological changes and heightened sensitivity. The encouragement of regular physical exercise becomes a key point not just for overall well-being but also for the maintenance of asthmatic respiratory allergies. Besides, the addition of AIT to the treatment protocol can provide extended benefits for the elderly by markedly improving the quality of life and decreasing the burden of allergic diseases. Healthy lifestyle changes encourage comprehensive knowledge of allergy management and stress the need to learn about the effects of aging on the immune system and allergic responses more profoundly (Ventura et al., 2017; Olson, 2019).

Test Your Knowledge

1. Explain the role of forensic pathologists.
2. Write a short note on post-mortem computed tomographic angiography (PMCTA).
3. What is exhumation?

5.5. The Role of the Immune System

Learning Outcome

1. Differentiate between Innate and adaptive immunity;
2. Discuss about Immune response to allergens;
3. Understand tolerance and sensitization.

The immune system is crucial to the maintenance of homeostasis and defense of the body against pathogenic invasion. It is composed of a highly complex network of cells, tissues, and organs that function in concert to identify and eliminate foreign pathogens, such as bacteria, viruses, and allergens. Central to this defense mechanism are two essential responses: the innate and adaptive immune responses. Innate immunity is the primary defense and employs barriers like skin and mucous membranes, and cellular elements like macrophages and neutrophils. The immune system of adaptation is characterized by its ability to remember a given pathogen through immunological memory, and this is facilitated by T and B lymphocytes. This is an important distinction, particularly with allergies, where the immune system misidentifies harmless material as harmful and mounts inappropriate hyperactive responses that require further examination and study. The behavior of the immune system in allergic responses shows the delicate balance it must maintain. Allergies are mostly mediated by IgE, a type of antibody produced in response to specific allergens. This aberrant activation of the immune system stimulates mast cells and basophils to degranulate and secrete inflammatory mediators such as histamines, which cause the symptoms of allergic responses. Recent developments in allergy research have placed firm emphasis on the necessity of rigorous risk assessments prior to new dietary proteins being introduced into the market. In particular, the AOP framework has been proposed to elucidate mechanistic pathways that function in IgE-mediated food allergies. The framework provides a structure for combining in vitro methods and establishing gaps that are likely to hamper successful testing for the sensitizing capacity of food proteins, thus enhancing understanding of immune system interaction with allergens (Lozano-Ojalvo et al., 2019). Furthermore, the immune response is regulated by many external factors , including exposures to the environment and infections.

Epidemiological data suggest that individuals in low-infection environments can develop hyperreactive immune responses that can lead to allergies and autoimmune disease. Immune modulation by parasitic infection is an interesting topic; helminths, in particular, have been found to suppress inflammation and thereby can be investigated for their therapeutic potential for regulating inflammatory conditions. This exchange challenges the timing and character of immune conditioning—how early exposures sculpt immunity versus those influences that come later in life. With continued discovery of the regulatory mechanisms at play, the duality of immune function as protective apparatus and potential origin of dysregulation becomes more evident, emphasizing its central position in the field of allergy and immunology (Maizels et al., 2014).

5.5.1. Innate versus Adaptive Immunity

Innate immunity is the body's immediate defense against pathogens, comprising physical barriers and instant non-specific immune responses. Innate immunity has a number of components, such as epithelial cells, phagocytic cells, and natural killer (NK) cells, which react rapidly to intruders. Activation of innate immunity occurs within a few hours following exposure to pathogens, and its components cannot adapt or remember the pathogens with which they are involved. Of particular interest, innate immune reactions are capable of activating adaptive immunity, thereby forming a vital link between the two. Allergically, innate immune cells like type II innate lymphoid cells (ILC2) have a key role to play because they release Th2 cytokines that promote allergic inflammation and further add to the complexity of the immune response repertoire. It is vital to appreciate the role played by innate immunity to formulate therapeutic interventions against allergic disorders (Lund et al., 2013). Adaptive immunity works with a delay, typically days, to gain maximum efficiency. It is characterized by its antigen-specific responses and ability to recall antigens of those pathogens one has been exposed to before, grâce to the work of specialized cells such as T and B lymphocytes. Adaptive immunity itself is also divided into humoral and cell-mediated responses; both are named for the production of antibodies by B cells and the activation of T cells that can directly kill infected host cells or help other immune cells. This memory and specificity are the foundation of vaccine effectiveness and a permanent defense against reinfection. However, when dysregulated, adaptive immunity can be the cause of non-normal responses such as allergies, in which sensitized B cells produce IgE antibodies in a non-normal fashion. This connection between the innate and adaptive pathways illustrates the intricacies of the immune response as well as its role in allergic disease. The intricate interaction between innate and adaptive immunity is observed in a very distinct manner in the case of the hygiene hypothesis, where lesser exposure to microbes may lead to a different immune response and make the individual susceptible to allergic disease. With the new lifestyle changes lowering exposure to complex microbial settings, the development of the immune system is left with a devastating impact. Scientific evidence suggests that low exposure to microbes may restrict the production of regulatory immune cells, thus predisposing individuals towards hypersensitivity and the development of allergy. The effect is not limited to early childhood but extends even into fetal life, where maternal microbial interactions shape the immune environment of the developing fetus. These data underscore the multifactorial nature of allergic disease and the impact of early microbial exposure on the establishment of disparate immune trajectories (Apostol et al., 2020) (Figure 5.16).

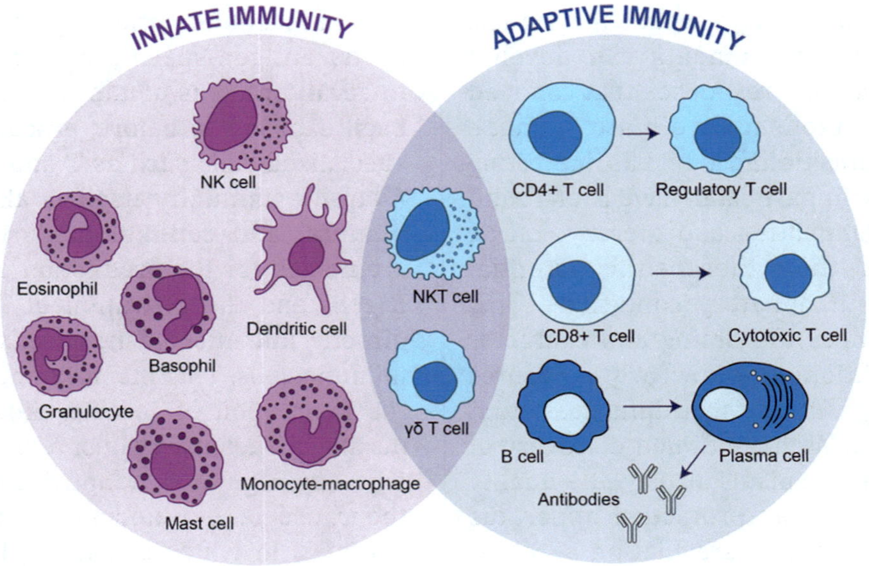

Figure 5.16. Innate immunity vs adaptive immunity.

Source: https://www.researchgate.net/publication/383092819/figure/fig1/AS:11431281271426097@1723615474820/Innate-immunity-vs-adaptive-immunity-The-innate-immunity-is-the-first-line-of-defense.tif.

5.5.2. Immune Response to Allergens

The allergic immune reaction is a complex interaction of the varied components of the immune system, characterized by hypersensitivity reactions mediated by IgE. In first-time exposure to an allergen, the immune system identifies the allergen as a foreign substance and activates T and B cells specific to the allergen. This results in the production of IgE antibodies that activate mast cells and basophils. During repeated exposure to the same allergen, these sensitized cells secrete histamines and other mediators, resulting in the classic features of allergic reactions, such as sneezing, itching, and, in very severe cases, anaphylaxis. Awareness of this original sensitization is significant for the construction of effective interventions, as it forms a foundation for a general strategy of allergy control, allowing for clinical as well as therapeutic treatment in immunology. In recent years, researchers have been examining mechanisms of immune-mediated hypersensitivity reactions with increased focus on pediatric populations. Much evidence is now appearing that the timing of exposure to the environment, genetic predisposition, and the introduction timing of allergens have a large contribution to allergy development. Allergies in children in the form of hypertonic response to harmless substances create a need for detailed investigation of causative factors and mechanisms. By illuminating the factors, scientists seek to delineate intervention critical windows that would prevent or at least decrease the incidence of allergies in children. The understanding obtained from such studies not only broadens knowledge about pediatric hypersensitivity but also points towards the importance of individualized prevention plans and potential new treatments in this susceptible group (Burns, 2019). Aside from environmental and genetic influences, the innate immune system has a crucial role in establishing the allergenic response. The more recent enhancement of utilizing the AOP framework provides an organizational means of understanding cellular and molecular mechanisms behind IgE-mediated food allergies. The method is useful in the identification of recognized in vitro methods employed to characterize the sensitizing capability of diverse food proteins and other allergens. Measuring the natural immune response generally produces fewer complex assays compared to those applied in measuring the adaptive immune response due to the lack of allergen-specific T and B cells. Incorporation of new ex vivo culture methods is likely to improve our understanding of the mechanisms of sensitization and, in the long term, contribute to reduced dependency on animal models and stimulate the initiation of specific countermeasures against allergic reactions (Lozano-Ojalvo et al., 2019) (Figure 5.17).

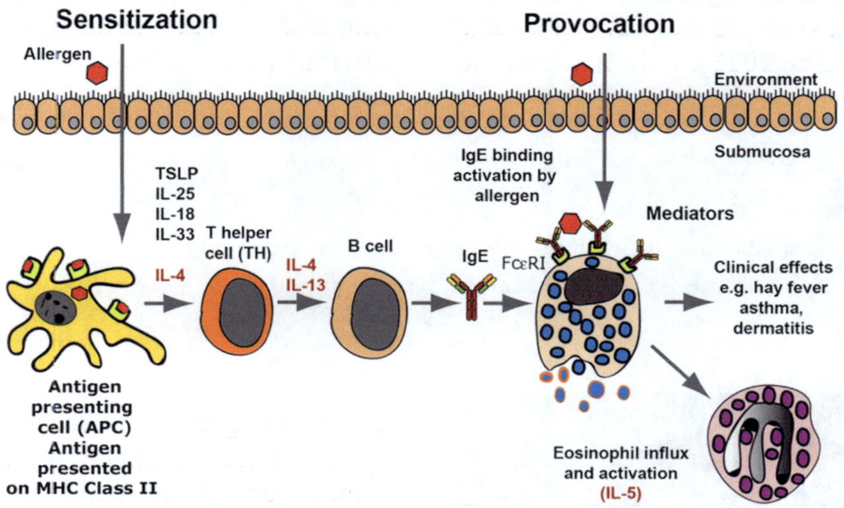

Figure 5.17. An allergic immune response.

Source: https://www.researchgate.net/publication/321914428/figure/fig1/AS:11431281250087553@1717756813163/An-allergic-immune-response-The-figure-presents-a-schematic-overview-of-an-allergic.tif.

5.5.3. Tolerance and Sensitization

The concepts of sensitization and tolerance are core to understanding the dynamics of allergic reactions when considering immunology. Tolerance refers to the capacity of the immune system to recognize and tolerate the presence of some allergens without invoking a reaction. The mechanism is necessary in preventing excessive responses to harmless substances within the environment and homeostasis. Conversely, sensitization occurs when the immune system is presented with an allergen and develops a hyperimmune response, which is usually in the form of the liberation of IgE antibodies. With time, repeated exposure to the allergen with insufficient tolerance can lead to the development of most allergic diseases, each affecting the individuals differently based on the genetic aspects and environmental factors. Recent research has established the exposure timing of allergens in infants and the effects on tolerance or sensitization development. A systematic review showed that late introduction of food that is possibly allergenic did not significantly reduce the risk for allergic disease; it was instead associated with increased risk for food allergies in high-risk and low-risk infants (Larson et al., 2016). This finding points to the significance of early diet exposure to the creation of immune tolerance. Clinicians now have the recommendation to suggest introducing food allergens at four or six months, which might be utilized for creating immune tolerance rather than causing sensitization. With such associations, clinicians can organize more effective allergy prevention strategies during the developmentally important periods. The incidence of food allergies and sensitization processes is not limited to children; indicators show towards an alarming trend in adult populations as well. Research that has examined pregnant women has determined that maternal food allergies affect neonatal health outcomes but found no significant correlation between maternal allergies and adverse effects on child health (Seita, 2013). This points to the complexity of immune responses and allergy-inducing factors across different stages of life. As exposures in the environment and genetics converge, ongoing efforts in research strive to dissect the intricate mechanisms of tolerance and sensitization. An understanding of these events is imperative for the development of targeted interventions and policy measures that reduce the burden of allergic disorders across different populations.

Test Your Knowledge

1. What is the primary difference between the innate and adaptive immune systems?
2. Define immunological tolerance and explain how its failure can lead to allergic reactions.

5.6. Current Research in Allergy and Immunology

Learning Outcome

1. Understand the advances in allergy treatments;
2. Discuss genetic factors in allergies;
3. The impact of climate change on allergy prevalence.

Present developments in allergy and immunology research show a fast-growing understanding of the genetic and environmental determinants of asthma, particularly in nations like Pakistan, where the illness is rapidly developing. The prevalence is estimated at around 20% of the children's population, this percentage boosted by urbanization, air pollutants, and heredity. Earlier, the emphasis had been placed on environmental influences, but recent research points to the role of several genes in disease manifestation. Over 100 such genes for asthma have been identified worldwide, but irrefutably, further work in the Pakistani context is required. Scientists have initiated research on the genetics of asthma, recognizing that environmental factors and genes collaborate with each other to have profound effects on disease outcomes in local populations, which necessitates having targeted studies that address unique genetic and demographic subtleties in asthma prevention and control measures (Sabar et al., 2018). At the same time, research into natural product therapeutic agents is a hopeful avenue in allergy and immunology research. Natural products, including those of medicinal plants, have been employed for centuries in traditional medicine, and recent scientific studies are beginning to demonstrate their efficacy. Carnosol, a Rosmarinus officinalis diterpenoid, has been the subject of interest due to its potential therapeutic benefits against autoimmune conditions such as multiple sclerosis. Research has established that carnosol not only represses symptomology in animal models of autoimmune encephalomyelitis but also interferes with the underlying inflammatory mechanisms by inhibiting important pathways for disease progression. By inhibiting differentiation of Th17 cells and reducing inflammatory infiltration, carnosol is dual effective against autoimmune responses. These findings suggest the integration of traditional medicinal knowledge with the techniques of contemporary research to develop new therapeutic strategies in allergy and immunology (Li et al., 2018). Overall, the convergence of genetics, environment, and natural curative drugs represents the frontline of research in allergy and immunology. As the science of complex interactions causing allergic diseases unfolds, there is a crucial need for new strategies encompassing both genetic studies and natural pharmacological progress. There can be greater collaboration between researchers, practitioners, doctors, and traditional practitioners to offer integrative perceptions towards enhancing prevention, diagnosis, and treatment of allergic diseases. By taking a multidimensional perspective, researchers can demystify the intricacies of allergic and immunologic diseases and open doors for individualized therapies to reflect individualized genetic signatures, environmental exposures, and health practices for arriving at an improved response to these pervasive health challenges in diverse populations (Li et al., 2018; Sabar et al., 2018).

5.6.1. Advances in Allergy Treatments

New advances in allergy treatment have significantly altered the management of allergic disorders, enhancing patients' quality of life. One of the promising directions of therapeutic progress is the application of biologic agents, and monoclonal antibodies that selectively bind to IgE and other allergen-activating mediators are of special interest. These biologics, such as omalizumab, have been discovered to be very effective in reducing the severity and frequency of allergic attacks, particularly in patients who experience moderate to severe allergen-induced asthma. This molecular therapy allows for a more personalized treatment regimen, with interventions being adapted according to individualized patient profiles and thereby increasing treatment compliance and efficacy. Furthermore, the invention of SLIT has expanded the treatment scope for allergies, particularly environmental allergens such as pollen and dust mites. Compared with traditional SCIT, SLIT offers improved convenience and a more favorable safety profile to become an option for a greater population of patients. Recent studies indicated that SLIT could safely immunize patients against specific allergens and establish long-term tolerance even after discontinuing the treatment (Figure 5.18).

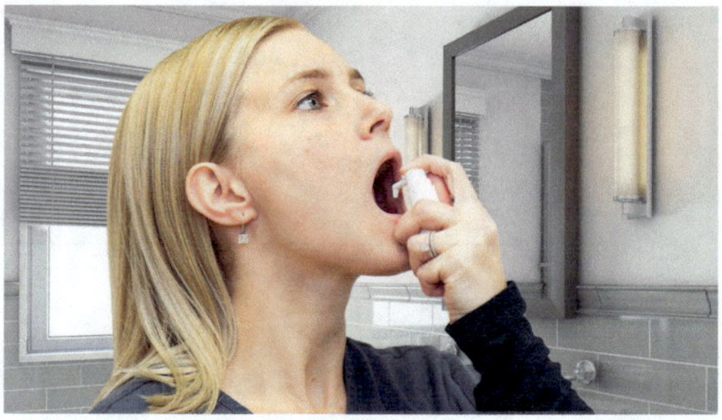

Figure 5.18. Sublingual immunotherapy (SLIT)–allergy relief without injections.

Source: https://www.phillymag.com/wp-content/uploads/sites/3/2016/10/AASpost4.jpg.

By means of controlled allergen exposure, SLIT not only decreases symptoms but also alters the underlying pathophysiologic mechanisms of allergic disease and therefore represents a potential disease-modifying treatment capable of transforming long-term management practices in allergy and immunology. One such area of interest garnering attention in allergy therapies is the use of digital health solutions and personalized medicine. This convergence allows healthcare practitioners to utilize mobile apps and online platforms to monitor symptoms and compliance with medication, and to adjust treatment plans in accordance with real-time data. Digital solutions can also support patient education regarding triggers and avoidance strategies, which are central to allergy management. These innovative approaches mesh with broader movement in healthcare toward more interconnected and patient-centered care. With research developing, it is vital to examine these technologies further and how they are integrated into existing treatment options so that patients can be given balanced and holistic care that meets their immediate symptoms and long-term health status, as such endeavors as those referenced in Bousquet et al. (2016) and Van Cleemput et al. (2019) continue to prove (Figure 5.19).

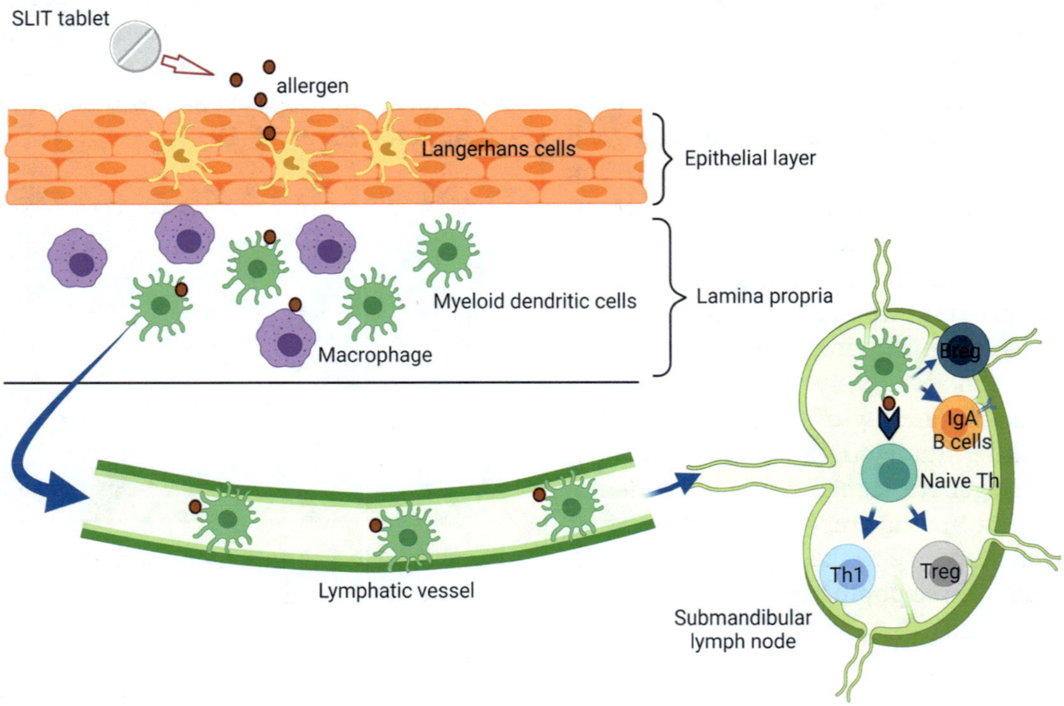

Figure 5.19. Immunologic mechanism of sublingual immunotherapy (SLIT). Substantial amounts of allergens from the SLIT tablet are captured by Langerhans cells in the epithelial layer. Next, the allergen is processed and migrates transmucosally by myeloid dendritic cells (mDCs) to draining lymph nodes. In the lymph node, these cells interact with T and B cells, priming them to regulate immune tolerance.

Source: https://www.researchgate.net/publication/355702578/figure/fig1/AS:1083867603705857@1635425582881/Immunologic-mechanism-of-sublingual-immunotherapy-SLIT-Substantial-amounts-of.png.

5.6.2. Genetic Factors in Allergies

The role of genetic factors in susceptibility to allergies has been a focus of research in the area of immunology. It has been established that susceptibility to allergic disease is inherited through large-scale studies, and genetic polymorphisms affecting various components of the immune system have been identified. Such variations can affect cytokine production, IgE responsiveness, and the integrity of the skin. Particularly, the etiology of diseases like AD has been related to genetic elements that influence the skin's barrier function and immune system. Although the specific genotype associations with AD development remain underresearched, more research is increasingly identifying some of the predominant genetic markers. A deeper understanding of such genetic determinants is required for the creation of personalized therapeutic regimens and prophylactic strategies in treating allergy, representing a critical juncture between genetics and allergy research (Martyna, 2013). Moreover, environmental interactions with genes also have a prime role in inducing an individual's allergic response. For instance, the hygiene hypothesis proposes that decreased levels of exposure to pathogens in early life can result in greater allergy prevalence. This influence can be quantified within the context of genetic immune function as well. Genetic predispositions would interact with environmental stimuli such as allergens and helminths in an effort to alter pathways within the immune system, potentially explaining why some individuals become allergic and others do not. Notably, evidence has revealed an inverse relationship between allergic sensitization and helminth infection, suggesting that genetic influence modulations of immune processes may be multifactorial and complex. Exploration of such interactions is further building the understanding of the mechanism of allergy underlying and could potentially play a pivotal part in formulating intervention (Rujeni et al., 2012). Generally, allergy research incorporating genetics calls for a deeper understanding of both environmental issues and genetic predisposition. As investigators probe deeper into the intricate genetic underpinnings of diseases like AD, it becomes increasingly clear that genetics determines not just susceptibility but also the overall immune status of affected individuals. In addition, an understanding of how genetic risk factors interact with environmental exposures, and specifically exposures to infectious agents like helminths, can create new avenues in the prevention and treatment of allergies. Against such a background, ongoing research activity continues to be critical to elucidating the entire picture of genetic contributions to allergic disease, and laying the foundation for more specific and effective immunological treatments in allergy and immunology (Rujeni et al., 2012; Martyna, 2013).

5.6.3. The Impact of Climate Change on Allergy Prevalence

The intricate interplay of global change and the prevalence of allergies is increasingly understood as a significant public health concern. With the warming of the globe, the rising concentration of allergens in the air, particularly pollen from grasses, trees, and weeds, poses an increasing risk to populations prone to allergic reactions. An increase in temperature prolongs the plant life cycle and promotes enhanced pollen emission, and exposure times are prolonged among susceptible populations. In addition, elevated levels of carbon dioxide enhance plant growth and allergen production, further exacerbating symptoms for those with respiratory allergy. Comprehension of these climate-influenced dynamics thus provides valuable insights into allergy epidemiology and the induction of asthma-like disease strongly linked with environmental change evolving with advancing climate change. Besides the basic effect of increased temperatures on allergen levels, climate change is a critical factor in modifying weather patterns, which will indirectly impact the occurrence of allergies. Increased precipitation and humidity create an ecosystem where molds will grow as a major indoor allergen. Therefore, people who might not have previously had allergies to molds are most likely to become susceptible to them as these fungi propagate as a result of modified climatic conditions. Re-emergence and re-emergence of the allergens in new regions can also cause an increase in the prevalence of allergic diseases in urban populations that are not normally exposed to such risks. According to recent studies, the broader public health implications of climate change demand a re-examination of current management strategies for allergens and emphasize the necessity for anticipatory measures in allergy prevention. Besides, public health interventions should also be altered to address the developing threat of climate change to allergy control and prevention. Coordination between global and national health agencies is important, according to current research, in order to determine more complete strategies of fighting climate change-allergic disease interface with shared research objectives. This involves not only monitoring variations in the level of allergens but also performing public sensitization campaigns about the potential health impacts tied to increasing allergens in the environment. For instance, actions such as improving indoor air quality and ventilation facilities can minimize the effects of allergens, although studies indicate that interventions may be of different levels of effectiveness when applied in real-life conditions (Wright et al., 2009). Lastly, encouraging well-informed communities with knowledge about how climate change affects the prevalence of allergies is important for enhancing overall public health outcomes (Petruzelli, 2020).

Test Your Knowledge

1. What are some recent advances in immunotherapy for treating allergies?
2. How do genetic predispositions influence an individual's likelihood of developing allergies?
3. In what ways is climate change believed to affect the prevalence and severity of allergic diseases?

SUMMARY

The abstract of an essay on Allergy and Immunology not only provides a synopsis of the major findings but also an interpretation of the implications of these findings for clinical practice and future research. Bringing together the different strands of the argument, important steps forward in our understanding and control of allergy highlight the importance of a multi-faceted response. For instance, the recent anaphylaxis care review has revealed intimidating inconsistencies between published guidelines and actual practice within clinical settings. Not only are the inconsistencies difficult for PS, but they also highlight a pressing need for increased medical education and training for severe allergy treatment, as the analysis of data at allergy referral sites (Grabenhenrich et al., 2012) shows. These will necessitate ongoing efforts from healthcare practitioners and policymakers. Being aware of food allergy distribution and severity, especially among high-risk groups such as pregnant women, is important for designing targeted interventions. Recent studies indicate that while food allergy prevalence among pregnant women is similar to that of the entire adult population, additional explorations of their actual influences on maternal and infant health outcomes are still required. The retrospective analysis establishes that while maternal food allergies are in normal ranges, their association with adverse health outcomes needs further exploration (Seita, 2013). Thus, promoting studies in this arena may provide useful points that improve practice management and healthier standards, ultimately leading to healthier infant and maternal care. Ultimately, growth in the field of Allergy and Immunology relies on bridging knowledge gaps dictated by current studies and clinical reports. The evident inequality in the practice of anaphylaxis treatment guidelines necessitates a united effort towards the standardization of practice and more education regarding the management of allergies among the populace. Furthermore, in light of the increasing issue of food allergies in a multicultural society, it is important that future research examines the complex etiology of these conditions. By emphasizing interdisciplinary collaboration and integrating new knowledge into clinical practice, the field can look to improve patient outcomes significantly and establish an environment in which allergic diseases are comprehended and managed more effectively.

The Allergy and Immunology specialty encompasses a broad range of health concerns that accentuate the investment in research and impact assessment. Asthma UK, as one of the key players in this field, has focused on quantifying multi-faceted impacts achieved through its research funding. Using the Payback Framework, researchers were able to measure the paybacks from society and academia generated through various funded studies. This systematic review identified that, although the majority of society's impacts were derived from a minority of projects, tangible advances, such as the development of novel asthma treatments, were evident. This indicates the significant role of targeted funding approaches to creating impactful research that can influence clinical guidelines and make substantial contributions to the benefits of patients' health (Hanney et al., 2013). Another matter of urgency in Allergy and Immunology is the management of anaphylaxis, especially patient self-management. Despite the recommendation of carrying epinephrine auto-injectors by patients who are at risk, numerous individuals do not do so. Research has shown that barriers such as inconsistent advice provided by healthcare professionals, subjective stigma associated with carrying the device, and lack of training significantly hinder successful self-management. In-depth interviewing reveals that patients often forget the need to wear their auto-injectors out of assumptions about emergency response or unfamiliarity with the device's design. Addressing these issues through greater education and enhanced device usability is critical to building patient empowerment for allergy treatment (Money et al., 2013). The coordination of findings from both lines of research, such as asthma research and anaphylaxis therapy, uncovers a broader discourse in Allergy and Immunology. Research impact and attempts to engage patients form an integral whole, together with a compelling push toward integrative practices for balancing clinical practice and advances in research. With patient organizations and health professionals joining forces, being there for the support network is the goal of promoting a culture of improved health outcomes. The emphasis on patient education, self-care adherence to recommendations, and product design creativity is key to their success. Ultimately, the unified system that quantifies both research impact analysis and patient empowerment will solidify Allergy and Immunology as a discipline and improve the health of people with allergic disorders (Money et al., 2013; Hanney et al., 2013).

KEY TERMS FROM THIS CHAPTER

- Adaptive immune system
- Allergic reactions
- Allergy diagnosis
- Asthma
- Chronic inflammatory disease calls
- Diet exposure
- Environmental sensitization
- Food allergy induction
- Healthcare strategies
- Helminths
- Allergen immunotherapy (AIT)
- Allergy and immunology
- Anaphylaxis
- Chronic allergic disease
- Cutaneous illnesses
- Environmental allergies
- Food allergens
- Genetic predisposition
- Helminthic infection
- Histamine release

CRITICAL THINKING QUESTIONS

1. **Which immunoglobulin is primarily involved in immediate allergic reactions?**
   a. IgA
   b. IgG
   c. IgM
   d. IgE
2. **What is the role of mast cells in allergic reactions?**
   a. They produce antibodies
   b. They destroy infected cells
   c. They release histamine and other mediators
   d. They inhibit inflammation
3. **Which of the following is a common cause of food allergies?**
   a. Gluten
   b. Soy
   c. Shellfish
   d. All of the above
4. **What is the gold standard for diagnosing an IgE-mediated allergy?**
   a. Total IgE level
   b. Skin prick testing
   c. Eosinophil count
   d. Chest X-ray
5. **Which medication is commonly used as first-line treatment for anaphylaxis?**
   a. Diphenhydramine
   b. Hydrocortisone
   c. Epinephrine
   d. Loratadine

Short Answer Questions

1. What are the four main types of hypersensitivity reactions, and which ones are typically involved in allergic responses?
2. Describe the process of sensitization and re-exposure in an IgE-mediated allergic reaction.
3. Name two common diagnostic tests for allergies and describe how they work.
4. List and briefly explain three common treatment strategies for allergic conditions.
5. How do food allergies differ from food intolerances in terms of immune involvement?
6. What is anaphylaxis, and what is the first-line treatment?

Answers to Critical Thinking Questions

1. (d); 2. (c); 3. (d); 4. (b); 5. (c)

REFERENCES

1. Amarasekera M. Immunoglobulin E in health and disease. *Asia Pac Allergy*. 2011;1(1):12-15. doi:10.5415/apallergy.2011.1.1.12(accessed on 27th June 2025).
2. Bousquet, J., Hellings, P. W., Agache, I., Bedbrook, A., Bachert, C., Bergmann, K. C., Bewick, M., Bindslev-Jensen, C., Bosnic-Anticevitch, S., Bucca, C., Caimmi, D. P., Camargos, P. A., Canonica, G. W., Casale, T., Chavannes, N. H., Cruz, A. A., De Carlo, G., Dahl, R., Demoly, P., Devillier, P., ... Zidarn, M. (2016). ARIA 2016: Care pathways implementing emerging technologies for predictive medicine in rhinitis and asthma across the life cycle. *Clinical and translational allergy*, *6*, 47. https://doi.org/10.1186/s13601-016-0137-4(accessed on 27th June 2025).
3. Wright, G. R., Howieson, S., McSharry, C., McMahon, A. D., Chaudhuri, R., Thompson, J., Donnelly, I., Brooks, R. G., Lawson, A., Jolly, L., McAlpine, L., King, E. M., Chapman, M. D., Wood, S., & Thomson, N. C. (2009). Effect of improved home ventilation on asthma control and house dust mite allergen levels. *Allergy*, *64*(11), 1671–1680. https://doi.org/10.1111/j.1398-9995.2009.02098.x(accessed on 27th June 2025).
4. Sabar, M.F., Akram, M., Awan, F. I., Ghani, M. U., Idrees, F., et al. (2018). Awareness of asthma genetics in Pakistan: A review with some recommendations. https://core.ac.uk/download/268082381.pdf (accessed on 27th June 2025).
5. Pineda, M. A., Al-Riyami, L., Harnett, W., & Harnett, M. M. (2014). Lessons from helminth infections: ES-62 highlights new interventional approaches in rheumatoid arthritis. *Clinical and experimental immunology*, *177*(1), 13–23. https://doi.org/10.1111/cei.12252(accessed on 27th June 2025).
6. Tran NP, Vickery J, Blaiss MS. Management of rhinitis: allergic and non-allergic. *Allergy Asthma Immunol Res*. 2011;3(3):148-156. doi:10.4168/aair.2011.3.3.148 (accessed on 27th June 2025).
7. Alvarez-Twose, I., Muraro, A., Arga, M., Armstrong, K., Arroabarren, E., Sheikh, A., Barnett, D., et al. (2014). International consensus on (ICON) anaphylaxis. https://core.ac.uk/download/28978204.pdf (accessed on 27th June 2025).
8. Amaducci, S., Bacci, E., Baldacci, S., Bartoli, M., et al. (2018). Inhalation therapy in the next decade: Determinants of adherence to treatment in asthma and COPD. https://core.ac.uk/download/152415584.pdf (accessed on 27th June 2025).
9. Apostol, A. C., Beaudin, A. E., & Jensen, K. D. C. (2020). Training the fetal immune system through maternal inflammation—A layered hygiene hypothesis. https://core.ac.uk/download/288432714.pdf (accessed on 27th June 2025).
10. Longhurst, H. J., Tarzi, M. D., Ashworth, F., Bethune, C., Cale, C., Dempster, J., Gompels, M., Jolles, S., Seneviratne, S., Symons, C., Price, A., & Edgar, D. (2015). C1 inhibitor deficiency: 2014 United Kingdom consensus document. *Clinical and experimental immunology*, *180*(3), 475–483. https://doi.org/10.1111/cei.12584(accessed on 27th June 2025).
11. Avery, L. M., Bookstaver, P. B., Justo, J. A., Kufel, W. D., et al. (2019). Penicillin allergy assessment and skin testing in the outpatient setting. https://core.ac.uk/download/231841951.pdf (accessed on 27th June 2025).
12. Money, A. G., Barnett, J., Kuljis, J., & Lucas, J. (2013). Patient perceptions of epinephrine auto-injectors: exploring barriers to use. *Scandinavian journal of caring sciences*, *27*(2), 335–344. https://doi.org/10.1111/j.1471-6712.2012.01045.x (accessed on 27th June 2025).

13. Meadows, A., Kaambwa, B., Novielli, N., Huissoon, A., Fry-Smith, A., Meads, C., Barton, P., & Dretzke, J. (2013). A systematic review and economic evaluation of subcutaneous and sublingual allergen immunotherapy in adults and children with seasonal allergic rhinitis. *Health technology assessment (Winchester, England)*, *17*(27), vi–322. https://doi.org/10.3310/hta17270 (accessed on 27th June 2025).

14. Daniel Lozano-Ojalvo, Sara Benede, Celia M. Antunes, Simona L. Bavaro, Grégory Bouchaud, et al.. Applying the adverse outcome pathway (AOP) for food sensitization to support in vitro testing strategies. Trends in Food Science and Technology, 2019, 85, pp.307-319. ⟨10.1016/j.tifs.2019.01.014⟩. ⟨hal-02623081⟩(accessed on 27th June 2025).

15. Eyerich, K., Brown, S. J., Perez White, B. E., Tanaka, R. J., Bissonette, R., Dhar, S., Bieber, T., Hijnen, D. J., Guttman-Yassky, E., Irvine, A., Thyssen, J. P., Vestergaard, C., Werfel, T., Wollenberg, A., Paller, A. S., & Reynolds, N. J. (2019). Human and computational models of atopic dermatitis: A review and perspectives by an expert panel of the International Eczema Council. *The Journal of allergy and clinical immunology*, *143*(1), 36–45. https://doi.org/10.1016/j.jaci.2018.10.033(accessed on 27th June 2025).

16. Blanca, M., Blanco, C., Cuesta-Herranz, J., Diaz Perales, A., et al. (2013). Enriched mannose glycosylation contributes to Act d 2 allergenicity. http://oa.upm.es/30046/1/INVE_MEM_2013_164273.pdf (accessed on 27th June 2025).

17. Ventura MT, Scichilone N, Paganelli R, et al. Allergic diseases in the elderly: biological characteristics and main immunological and non-immunological mechanisms. *Clin Mol Allergy*. 2017;15:2. Published 2017 Feb 3. doi:10.1186/s12948-017-0059-2(accessed on 27th June 2025).

18. Burns, H. (2019). The development of hypersensitivity reactions in the pediatric population: A review. https://core.ac.uk/download/213464303.pdf (accessed on 27th June 2025).

19. Lund S, Walford HH, Doherty TA. Type 2 Innate Lymphoid Cells in Allergic Disease. *Curr Immunol Rev*. 2013;9(4):214-221. doi:10.2174/1573395510666140304235916(accessed on 27th June 2025).

20. Else, K. J., Garcia, F. T., McSharry, C., Nakajima, H., Oku, Y., Pawlowski, Z., Petit-Frere, C., et al. (2014). Mucosal immune responses following intestinal nematode infection. https://core.ac.uk/download/29469509.pdf (accessed on 27th June 2025).

21. Evans-Agnew, R. A. (2012). Asthma management: An Eco social framework for disparity research. https://digitalscholarship.unlv.edu/cgi/viewcontent.cgi?article=1011&context=jhdrp (accessed on 27th June 2025).

22. Van Cleemput, J., Poelaert, K. C. K., Laval, K., Impens, F., Van den Broeck, W., Gevaert, K., & Nauwynck, H. J. (2019). Pollens destroy respiratory epithelial cell anchors and drive alphaherpesvirus infection. *Scientific reports*, *9*(1), 4787. https://doi.org/10.1038/s41598-019-41305-y(accessed on 27th June 2025).

23. Grabenhenrich, L., Hompes, S., Gough, H., Ruëff, F., Scherer, K., Pföhler, C., Treudler, R., Mahler, V., Hawranek, T., Nemat, K., Koehli, A., Keil, T., & Worm, M. (2012). Implementation of anaphylaxis management guidelines: a register-based study. *PloS one*, *7*(5), e35778. https://doi.org/10.1371/journal.pone.0035778(accessed on 27th June 2025).

24. Larson, K., McLaughlin, J., Stonehouse, M., Young, B., & Haglund, K. (2017). Introducing Allergenic Food into Infants' Diets: Systematic Review. *MCN. The American journal of maternal*

child nursing, *42*(2), 72–80. https://doi.org/10.1097/NMC.0000000000000313(accessed on 27th June 2025).

25. Kalinowska, Z., Krężel, M., Matera, W., Snoch, M., et al. (2025). Drug-induced rhinitis as a complication of using mucosal decongestants. https://core.ac.uk/download/656518361.pdf (accessed on 27th June 2025).
26. Maizels, R. M., McSorley, H. J., & Smyth, D. J. (2014). Helminths in the hygiene hypothesis: Sooner or later? https://core.ac.uk/download/287602009.pdf (accessed on 27th June 2025).
27. Makvandi-Nejad, S. (2023). Prevalence of allergic diseases in Mayan population of Lake Atitlan, Guatemala: A cross-sectional pilot study. https://core.ac.uk/download/580972364.pdf (accessed on 27th June 2025).
28. Rujeni N, Taylor DW, Mutapi F. Human schistosome infection and allergic sensitisation. *J Parasitol Res.* 2012;2012:154743. doi:10.1155/2012/154743(accessed on 27th June 2025).
29. The Stern Center for Evidence-Based Policy (2015). Addressing the health needs of an aging America: New opportunities for evidence-based policy solutions. University of Pittsburgh. https://core.ac.uk/download/75783019.pdf
30. (accessed on 27th June 2025).
31. Olson, K. (2019). Pilot study: Program evaluation of peanut oral immunotherapy in a private clinic. https://core.ac.uk/download/223074370.pdf (accessed on 27th June 2025).
32. Petruzelli, N. (2020). The influence of climate change on disease and public health. https://core.ac.uk/download/322826252.pdf (accessed on 27th June 2025).
33. Rauscher, B. (2015). Use of immunotherapy in the treatment of peanut allergies in the pediatric population. https://core.ac.uk/download/58826198.pdf (accessed on 27th June 2025).
34. Seita, H. M. (2013). Food allergies in pregnant women: A study of prevalence in expecting mothers and association with neonatal outcomes. https://open.bu.edu/bitstream/2144/12219/6/Seita_Helene_2013.pdf (accessed on 27th June 2025).
35. Hanney SR, Watt A, Jones TH, Metcalf L. Conducting retrospective impact analysis to inform a medical research charity's funding strategies: the case of Asthma UK. *Allergy Asthma Clin Immunol.* 2013;9(1):17. Published 2013 May 7. doi:10.1186/1710-1492-9-17(accessed on 27th June 2025).
36. Li, X., Zhao, L., Han, J. J., Zhang, F., Liu, S., Zhu, L., Wang, Z. Z., Zhang, G. X., & Zhang, Y. (2018). Carnosol Modulates Th17 Cell Differentiation and Microglial Switch in Experimental Autoimmune Encephalomyelitis. *Frontiers in immunology*, *9*, 1807. https://doi.org/10.3389/fimmu.2018.01807(accessed on 27th June 2025).

ENVIRONMENTAL AND OCCUPATIONAL MEDICINE

6

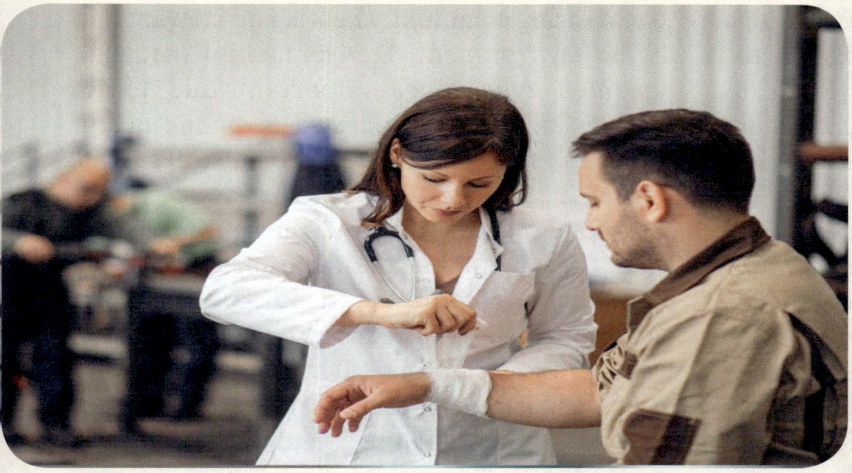

Introduction

Environmental and occupational medicine is a significant cross-disciplinary area of study concerned with the interrelationship between environmental conditions and health status in the workplace. The study addresses how employees' exposure to some environmental elements—such as pollutants, toxic substances, and even psychological stressors—can adversely affect employees' health and productivity levels in the workplace. Such understanding not only improves the health of individuals but also informs policy formulation and adoption to enhance workplace safety. The importance of this field has become increasingly evident as industries change and as global environmental issues continue to worsen, warranting a critical look at occupational and environmental health practice impacting diverse populations in different settings. To further place into perspective the relevance of occupational and environmental medicine, there has been escalating recognition of models such as the International Classification of Functioning, Disability and Health (ICF). The model provides

LEARNING OBJECTIVES

After studying this chapter, you will be able to:

1. Understand the historical background of environmental and occupational medicine;
2. Describe major environmental health hazards;
3. Discuss occupational health risks;
4. Focus on assessment and diagnosis of health issues stemming from exposure to hazardous substances;
5. Deal with preventive strategies in environmental and occupational medicine.

a formal evaluation of the impact of health across various perspectives and facilitates its application across professions , including nursing, occupational therapy, and public health. Although the ICF model is not old, its inclusion in occupational and environmental studies holds the prospect of refining the categorization and conceptualization of health outcomes in such settings. However, the implementation of the ICF in practice has been faced with little empirical research on how it is used in clinical settings, showing the necessity for further investigation into the utilization of systems established to promote workplace health programs (Bruyere et al., 2005). Moreover, the multilevel character of employee mental health outcomes in the workplace also highlights the necessity of multidimensional analysis techniques. The interplay between individual variables, group processes, organizational policy, and social contexts is central to understanding employee well-being. A necessity for studies using multilevel measures that adequately reflect these dynamics is present, and it is in the form of how work-related variables can influence mental health outcomes more generally. Such an approach not only justifies the formulation of more advanced interventions but also reiterates the value of occupational and environmental medicine in enhancing employee health and company performance (Martin et al., 2016). The evolution of this field towards more integrated practices will be instrumental in meeting the challenges of occupational health and safety management in the contemporary world.

Definition of Environmental Medicine

Environmental medicine may be characterized as a clinical discipline that explores the interactions between environmental exposures and health. The specialty is interested in an understanding of how multiple environmental exposures, including air and water pollutants, toxic substances, and particular physical stressors, impact health results. By utilizing principles derived from epidemiology, toxicology, and public health, environmental medicine educates disease avoidance and control of environmentally linked health issues. For instance, the growing incidence of respiratory disease can often be explained as being caused by compromised air quality and exposure to allergens, which means clean air initiatives become important environmental health practices. Professionals in this field assess health risks and develop policies aimed at minimizing exposure, the key to enhancing community health and stewardship of the environment. Environmental medicine becomes even more important due to its function of fighting widespread public health concerns associated with environmental causes. Traffic injury-related problems, as identified in recent studies, are a major public health issue that highlights the need for this branch of medicine. Traffic medicine as a specialty endeavors to investigate the intersection between transportation systems and health, subsequently offering practices and policies capable of reducing rates of injury and, by extension, morbidity and mortality. This highlights how environmental medicine goes beyond standard clinical practice as it entails multi-sector efforts integrating transportation, city planning, and health. The use of environmental medicine research in policymaking can help improve more effective public health interventions, demonstrating its necessity in addressing the evolving health concerns our environment poses (Groneberg-Kloft et al., 2013). Environmental medicine further entails the monitoring of occupational exposures that impact workers' health and safety significantly. As demonstrated by research that looked into carpal tunnel syndrome (CTS), the field is concerned with understanding correlations among work conditions and health outcomes. By applying job exposure matrices (JEMs), researchers are able to correlate job requirements physically with the development of musculoskeletal disorders (MSDs) and therefore, highlight the need for ergonomic measurements in occupational health interventions. By intervening in such health problems, environmental medicine not only makes an input in the training of healthcare policy but also in ensuring safer working conditions and ecologically friendly practices. Results of such investigations go towards maximizing both individual and community health, emphasizing the continued relevance of environmental medicine in addressing contemporary health challenges of occupational environments (Evanoff et al., 2014) (Figure 6.1).

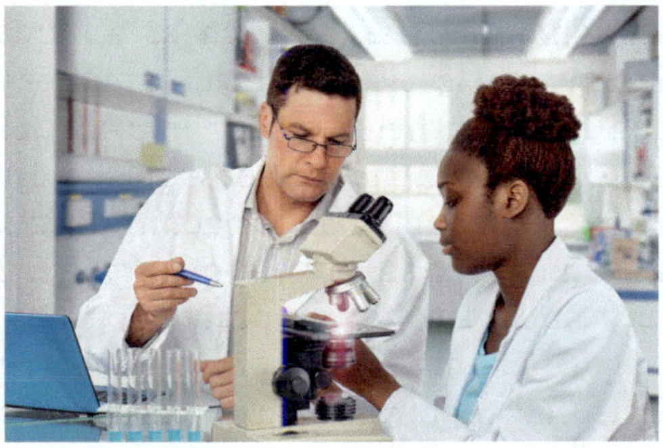

Figure 6.1. Medical research in the field of environmental medicine.

Source: https://www.aamc.org/sites/default/files/Research-laboratory-993475228.jpg.

Definition of Occupational Medicine

Occupational medicine is a vital specialty that encompasses the prevention, treatment, and assessment of occupational injury and illness. It not only concerns the physical health of employees but also entails an overall understanding of the environmental hazards that can impact their well-being. With the progression of industries, particularly with the advent of unconventional modes of employment like the gig economy, occupational medicine will be forced to face new challenges in preserving health and safety. According to existing literature, non-traditional work arrangements between part-time workers and independent contractors have been known to lead to adverse health impacts due to a deficiency in occupational health protection (Tran & Sokas, 2017). The practice of occupational medicine is thus widening to accommodate the multi-faceted demands of a diverse population, making it critical to continue researching and developing intervention plans optimized for this new setting. The professional practice of occupational medicine is not only about treating injury but also about preventive care to enhance the health of the workers. These may be risk assessment, health surveillance, and education on workplace hazards. Because most of the workers are currently in gig jobs without the traditional employer protections, the profession must adjust its model in order to provide health equity. New research highlights the reality that gig workers are subjected to tremendous vulnerabilities due to the lack of access to safety nets such as workers' compensation and health insurance (Tran & Sokas, 2017). Consequently, these healthcare professionals owe it to themselves to treat single instances of cases of health conditions, yet they also have the responsibility to raise their voices in advocating for systemic changes that safeguard the occupational health of all workers, regardless of work status. Furthermore, occupational medicine's integrated view emphasizes the interaction between physical health, mental wellness, and working conditions affecting employees. As awareness of their corporate social responsibility grows, firms are now incorporating mental health assessments into occupational health programs. This acknowledges that psychological disturbance may be a consequence of job insecurity, prevalent among gig and contingent workers. By broadening the definition of occupational medicine to include mental health, the profession can more effectively meet the changing needs of the workforce and address ongoing and rising health inequities. Ultimately, a comprehensive definition of occupational medicine not only acknowledges the need to protect physical health but also addresses the psychological and environmental factors that collectively influence the health of workers in varying contexts (Figure 6.2).

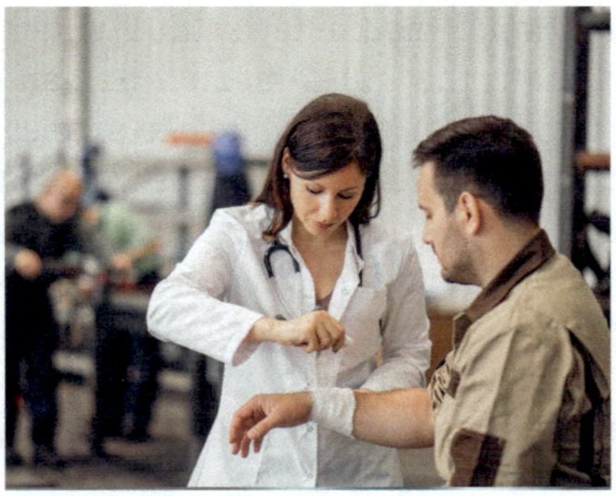

Figure 6.2. An occupational health worker treating a patient.

Source: https://healthmanagement.co.uk/wp-content/uploads/2022/01/occupational-health-worker-treating-patient.jpg.

Importance of the Field in Public Health

Environmental and occupational medicine is highly important in public health as it addresses the health issues associated with environmental exposures and occupational exposures. The field is of high importance because it uses science to identify and mitigate hazards that have the potential to lead to disease and injury. Exposure to toxic chemicals in the air we breathe or in which we are exposed at work can result in chronic diseases that affect quality of life and the health and productivity of the workforce. Therefore, the interface between environment, work, and health must be comprehended for developing strategies meant to improve individual health status and protect community health. The findings that emanate from environmental and occupational medicine support the encouragement of policies that enhance further healthier work and living conditions. Moreover, the research conducted on presenteeism—a condition where employees report to work ill—shows the intersection of health and productivity in this field. Research identifies multiple determinants of presenteeism, including general ill health, workplace stressors, and policies at work that deter absenteeism (Miraglia & Johns, 2015). This criticism demonstrates the extensive effects of workplaces on the health of the public. Minimization of presenteeism advantages not only individual health interests but also organizational efficiency, as healthy employees can work more efficiently. Hence, inclusion of minimization measures in work health programs shows the economic benefits from investing in workers' well-being and creating sympathetic workplaces. Aside from occupational health, public health influences and is influenced by environmental issues such as air quality. Measurement of levels of particulate matter (PM) through research helps gather information on human exposure in mobile settings, the driving conditions being noted as impacting air quality within (Uibel et al., 2012). Air quality dynamics are very important to comprehend, given that prolonged exposure to pollutants greatly accounts for respiratory and cardiovascular disease. By discovering the context of personal exposure to environmental pollutants, public health interventions can be engineered to reduce the risk of the effects of pollution. Ultimately, environmental and occupational medicine is the foundation discipline for improving public health by being the key to disease prevention and healthier communities.

6.1. Historical Background

Learning Outcome

1. Understand the evolution of environmental medicine;
2. Focus on the development of occupational medicine;
3. Deal with key milestones in the integration of both fields.

Environmental and Occupational Medicine is of early 20th-century origin, an outcome of a growing recognition of the link between workplaces and health states. Industrialization brought with it a range of toxic exposures, and along with them, the realization that there was a necessity to look systemically at how some occupations resulted in health risks. Specifically, industry working conditions were underpinned as a location for the assessment of exposures to dangerous chemicals like benzene with increased risk for leukemia. Epidemiological studies initiated during this period formed the background for comprehending occupational disease. As an example, review meta-analyzing several studies has found the relationship between exposure to benzene and leukemia, whereas the effect sizes yielded a definite dose-response trend, hence corroborating the importance of tracking occupational exposure in safeguarding worker health (Khalade et al., 2010). As the discipline improved, procedures for measuring and controlling occupational health risks needed to be formulated. Organizational structures were put in place to oversee the health of employees, thus creating organizational bodies dedicated to occupational health and safety regulation. The interpretation of biomedical data became the cornerstone of these programs, and guidelines were developed for complete medical history and medical examination with regard to specific occupational hazards. The assessment of conditions in the workplace was also improved by the addition of advanced techniques of collecting toxicity data, which assisted in emphasizing early detection and management of occupational health anomalies. These advancements not only improved the health results of the workers but also assisted in greater comprehension of how environmental factors are interconnected with occupational safety (The Stern Center for Evidence-Based Policy, 2015). The field has registered tremendous advancements over the past decades, with the use of research evidence in public health policy and occupational health laws. The critical examination of epidemiological relations between occupational exposures and workplace health hazards has led to the opening of the door for strategically targeted interventions. Policymakers have grown to adopt evidence-based advice to prevent exposure to toxic substances in the workplace. For example, mounting evidence regarding exposure to benzene necessitates strict regulatory limits, reflecting the impact of scientific research on policy legislation. As this field continues to evolve further, the history of this development highlights the necessity of ongoing vigilance in handling occupational risk factors in order to guarantee both employee safety and public health issues at a wider scale (Khalade et al., 2010).

6.1.1. Evolution of Environmental Medicine

Environmental medicine growth heavily relies on grasping the complex interaction between the environment and human health. Historically, the field grew in response to the negative effects of industrialization, urbanization, and lifestyle on health. Established guidelines and research methods have served a central purpose in addressing the challenges of environmental health. For example, the Global Burden of Diseases, Injuries, and Risk Factors Study has given us valuable information on how different occupational and environmental exposures contribute to outcomes for global health. Such a study shows that treatment of risks like pollution and dangerous conditions can drastically change the course of health among populations, highlighting the importance of a multi-faceted approach in environmental medicine (The Stern Center for Evidence-Based Policy, 2015). It is therefore essential to possess a comprehension of these dynamics so that public health policy can be fashioned to minimize the risks associated with environmental exposure. Over the years, since the field of environmental medicine has matured, it has increasingly embraced interdisciplinary approaches. Collaborative efforts among environmental scientists, epidemiologists, and healthcare professionals have improved the degree of sophistication with which ecological dynamics such as climate change and biodiversity loss impact human health. These advancements have highlighted the importance of merging biological and ecological perspectives in assessing health consequences. New research holds that environmental health must not be thought of in terms of a collection of distinct elements but as an integrated system. For example, rising metabolic disease and mental illness among populations is likely to have its genesis in environmental determinants, and therefore necessitates a wide-ranging approach to prevention and treatment (Robert, 2016). It is where interdisciplinary collaboration is essential in coming up with policies and practices that consider the complex nature of modern health issues. Finally, the evolution of environmental medicine has revealed the necessity of health-supporting public policies that emphasize prevention over intervention. This shift is evident in the greater emphasis on health promotion practices that prioritize clean air, pure water, and sustainable levels of living. The public health policies now increasingly depend on comprehensive data to advance legislative reforms as well as community-based interventions targeting environmental health disparities. For instance, restricting exposure to harmful chemicals within workplaces is not only beneficial to the individual workers but to overall community health. It is crucial to comprehend the influence of social determinants in environmental health to develop policies that decrease risk and enhance health equity (The Stern Center for Evidence-Based Policy, 2015). Since environmental medicine continues to expand, its paradigm of holism will be crucial in managing future health challenges as and when they come up and in building a healthy and sustainable future for all populations (Figure 6.3).

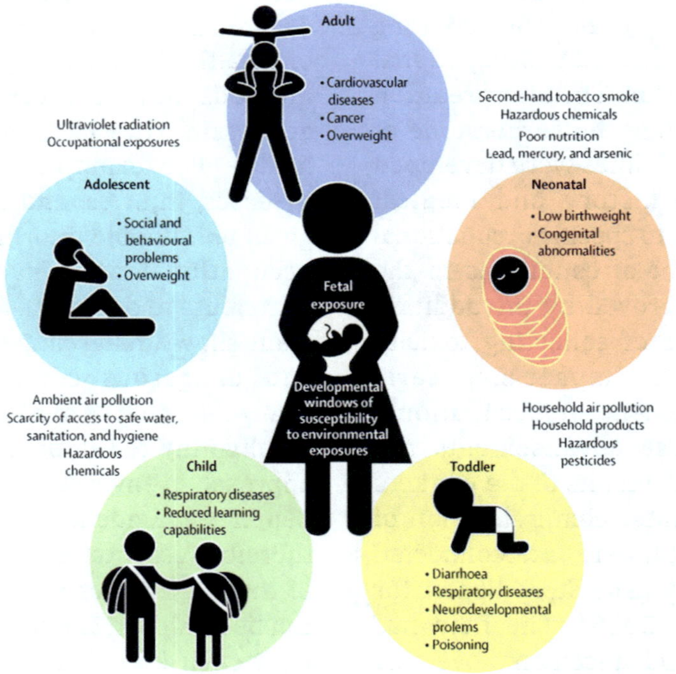

Figure 6.3. The effects of environmental hazards across generations.

Source: https://www.thelancet.com/cms/10.1016/S2542-5196(17)30048-7/asset/fa7f597c-4d25-4759-8f6f-983af21717cd/main.assets/gr1.jpg.

6.1.2. Development of Occupational Medicine

The development of occupational medicine has undergone a significant transformation since its inception, reflecting broader changes in industrial practices and public health priorities. Initially emerging in the late 19th century, occupational medicine primarily focused on the identification and management of diseases caused by hazardous workplace conditions. With growing industries and evolving labor legislation, the field increasingly incorporated a more holistic notion of employee health, one that was concerned not just with the prevention of disease but with promoting all-around well-being.

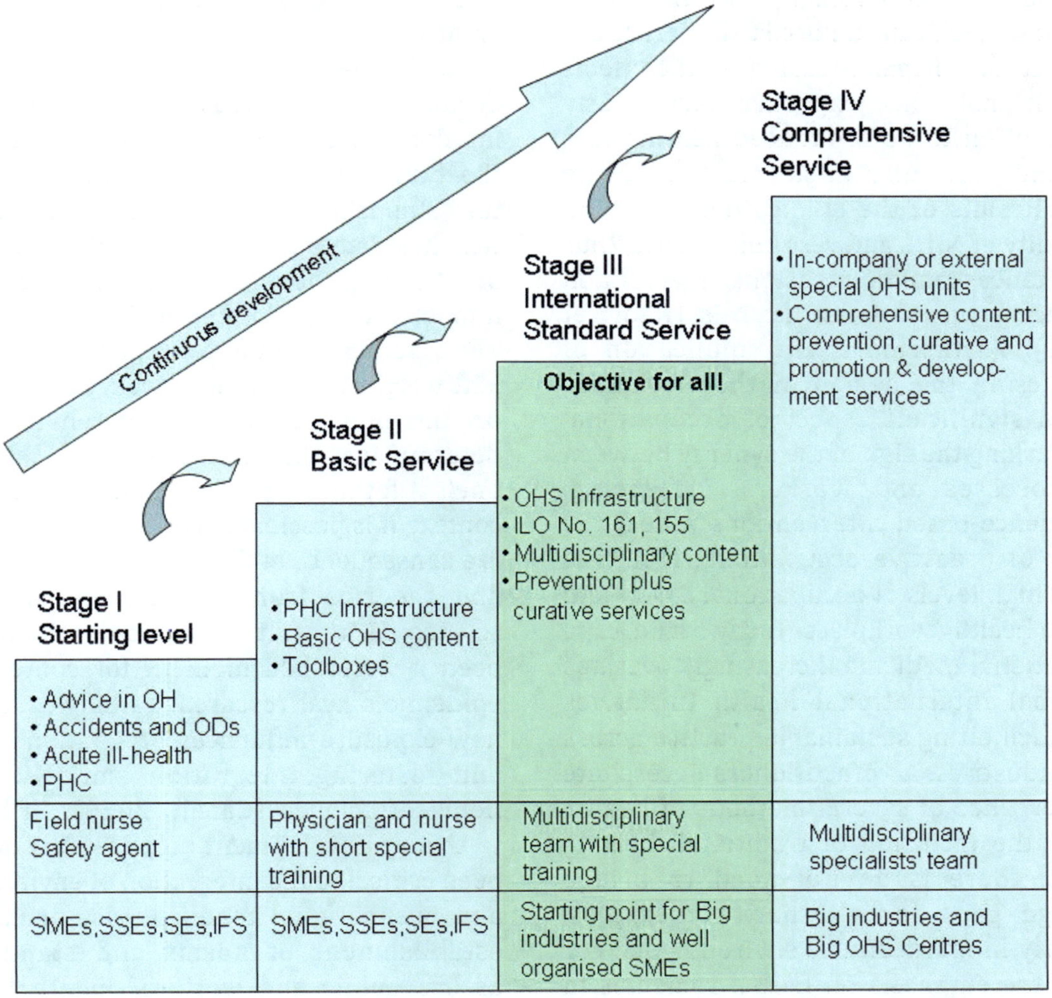

Figure 6.4. Stepwise development of occupational health services.

Source: https://www.researchgate.net/publication/290010291/figure/fig5/AS:669630444105743@1536663747344/Stepwise-development-of-occupational-health-services-Note-From-J-Ranranen-Basic.png.

This shift occurred in tandem with the emerging recognition of the social and psychological aspects of work, as experts grew to understand that occupational health is determined by an extensive variety of factors beyond the physical realm of exposure. A turning point in this evolution was the development of official systems for the surveillance of workers, allowing for the establishment of trends in occupational disease and, consequently, informing preventive interventions and policy interventions. As the specialty of occupational medicine evolved, research on individual occupational risks came to the forefront, emphasizing the function of intervention specifically tailored to limit risk. For instance, studies began focusing on the effects of occupational noise exposure, particularly its contribution to noise-induced hearing loss (NIHL) and vestibular impairment in textile workers. Results of the studies demonstrated co-morbidity of NIHL and vestibular issues, thus the importance of multidimensional intervention in mitigating occupational hazards (Nadri et al., 2024). Furthermore, the application of ergonomics in the design of the workplace became a significant aspect of occupational health, marking the sign of the synergy between work processes and workers' well-being. Such evidence-based interventions reflect the necessity of proactive occupational medicine to expect high levels of occupational safety and promote a healthy workplace. Today's landscape of occupational medicine increasingly overlaps with global international health initiatives towards facilitating sustainable practice across various industries. As practitioners necessitate the convergence of several methods of health, including the inclusion of traditional healing practices, there is a vital need to bridge knowledge gaps for alternative therapies, particularly in multicultural environments. For example, the emphasis on herbal remedies in South Africa illustrates the necessity to integrate indigenous practice in modern healthcare programs so that health practitioners have a better grasp of patient choice (Mashigo et al., 2024). This integrative emphasis not only augments future occupational medicine professionals' knowledge base but also instills a culture of respect for cultural health beliefs and inclusivity. These developments in occupational medicine strengthen a total system that benefits not only environmental sustainability but also worker health, ultimately setting a healthier workforce for the future (Figure 6.4).

6.1.3. Key Milestones in the Integration of Both Fields

The mutual pollination of occupational and environmental medicine has been advanced over the past decades, and that marks the evolution of an increasing appreciation of the interconnectedness of the two fields. One of the building blocks of this intersection was the establishment of multidisciplinary systems, which started to emphasize the importance of studying how environmental exposures impact individuals' health in the workplace. The emergence of the concept of exposome has lent weight to this link as well, as it speculates on the immense number of environmental determinants that influence health throughout one's lifetime. By placing the exposome in context, it is possible to realize how its invention is a consequence of the development of methods and theories from outside life and health science. As a result, exposure development has been a watershed moment for contemporary epidemiological research, guiding inquiry into how exposure influences occupational disease and fostering integration among disparate fields of science (Canali, 2020). In addition to theory development, applications have also been critical to the integration of environmental and occupational medicine. Particularly, the establishment of norms and standards to assure public and workers' health has seen considerable collaboration between experts from both disciplines. For example, health organizations and state agencies have developed occupational safety laws that consider potential environmental hazards to which employees are exposed. The guideline regulations have spurred more research and development in the identification of hazardous work exposures and their relationship with environmental issues. The concurrent development of these guidelines has worked to enhance occupational health protections while giving more emphasis to the necessity of a whole-person approach to health hazards at workplaces and homes. Such convergence is needed in order to generate effective prevention programs and improve overall health outcomes (Constant et al., 2010). The ongoing advancement in technology and methodology of research has been another milestone, playing a significant role in the merging of occupational and environmental medicine. New technologies, such as biomonitoring and epidemiology software, allow more precise establishment of correlations between occupational health and environmental exposures. Through these technologies, scientists are better placed to obtain and analyze data that point towards significant health patterns that are linked with environmental factors among workers. Moreover, the increase in cross-disciplinary initiatives, including scientific collaborations and business alliances, has provided an environment for different skill sets to unite in order to address difficult health issues. Such multidisciplinary collaboration is pivotal in addressing the pressing issues that are being presented by environmental determinants and how they influence occupational health, paving the way for new solutions and overall public health interventions (Canali, 2020).

Test Your Knowledge

1. Name one key historical law or regulation that significantly advanced occupational health and safety.
2. How has the relationship between environmental and occupational medicine evolved over time?

6.2. Major Environmental Health Hazards

Learning Outcome

1. Discuss air pollution and its effects;
2. Focus on water contamination and health risks;
3. Deal with chemical exposures in the environment.

Among the most important environmental health hazards are air pollutants with critical impacts on public as well as occupational health. They encompass a vast array of substances, including PM, nitrogen dioxide, and volatile organic compounds, which can lead to a whole range of acute and chronic effects on health. Workers in industries such as manufacturing, construction, and agriculture are extensively exposed to poisonous emissions that damage their respiratory and cardiovascular systems. Along with direct health effects, long-term exposure to air pollution aggravates chronic conditions, leading to enhanced healthcare costs and reduced productivity. Added to this, certain occupational categories experience synergistic effects due to co-exposure to multiple pollutants, for which improved protective measures need to be enforced to mitigate associated risks. Proper regulatory measures and workplace safety protocols must be established based on an integrated perspective of these environmental risks. Another significant environmental health hazard is contact with harmful chemicals, which is prevalent in most industries like agriculture, construction, and manufacturing. Employees exposed to pesticides, solvents, and other dangerous chemicals have the highest risk of developing immediate injuries and long-term health effects like cancers and reproductive issues. The issue lies with the often-incomplete assessment and regulation of chemical exposure, which can lead to underreporting of disease and a lack of protective action. Adding to this is the difficulty of quantifying exposure levels and distinguishing among agents. For instance, a newer study acknowledged MSDs as a priority health concern among dentists, referring to the need to assess not only chemical but also ergonomic hazards in occupational medicine. One can detect and manage such risks of chemical exposures in workplaces using new technologies such as Digital Twin simulations (Moussa et al., 2024). Night work is a general environmental health hazard that has occupied the minds of occupational medicine due to its effects on circadian rhythm and overall health. Prevention of normal sleep patterns due to night shifts is proven to yield a variety of adverse health effects, such as sleep disorders, cardiovascular disease, and compromised immunity. Other determinants such as light at night exposure and related workplace hazards have been argued to further complicate the intricate relationship between shift work and health. For instance, evidence in maternal night shift work has shown potential urogenital abnormality among children, highlighting the long-term effects of circadian desynchrony (Peters & Hall, 2021). In light of greater awareness of the medical perils of night shifts, there is a genuine need for comprehensive action to mitigate these risks in the shape of education on circadian health, monitoring of work rotation, and active enforcement of policies that place emphasis on staff well-being.

6.2.1. Air Pollution and Its Effects

Air pollution is a significant public health concern, and PM has been a significant cause of respiratory and cardiovascular diseases. The effects of air pollutants such as PM10 and PM2.5 have been well established in the practice of environmental and occupational medicine. Research indicates that exposure to PM, particularly in high-traffic urban areas, has been linked to increased rates of asthma, chronic bronchitis, and even lung cancer. Most importantly, workers who participate in jobs involving exposure to such pollutants as a necessary requirement, such as those in the transportation or manufacturing sector, face increased health risks. The poisonous character of such airborne particles, often from motor emissions and industrial processes, reinforces the need for extensive measurement and innovative methods to avoid or minimize exposure in the general and occupational atmospheres. New methods have only recently been applied to measure air quality in mobile contexts, enabling greater insight into levels of individual exposure. For instance, the mobile air quality study (MAQS) examined why levels of PM vary under different vehicle conditions. It was determined that PM10 levels were greater with the roof open in a vehicle, refuting the assertion that enclosed conditions provide equal protection for occupants from hazardous air quality. Moreover, despite time of day and ventilation having a strong influence on exposure, the study emphasized that local conditions, such as driving practices and neighborhood emissions, could lead to varying levels of pollution. These findings highlight the need for individualized estimates of exposure and related recommendations in reducing aggregate health hazards due to air pollution, particularly for persons frequently exposed to these conditions, in informing more general public health regulations. The association of PM2.5 exposure with harmful health impacts also finds evidence in longitudinal cohort studies. The research specifically conducted in distinct working environments and sectors, such as the aluminum sector, has established PM2.5 to be a better predictor than total particulate matter (TPM) for the risk of ischemic heart disease (IHD). Highly exposed workers showed significantly higher hazard ratios for the formation of IHD, highlighting the importance of monitoring fine particulate emissions on large measurements. These findings highlight the importance of establishing more accurate exposure surveillance programs that target PM2.5 monitoring as a requirement to guarantee worker health and guide risk management practices. Thus, occupational health practice in risk industries for high-air pollution must evolve based on the new causality evidence between some of the pollutants and acute health effects in order to augment preventive intervention and ensure public protection from harm (Figure 6.5).

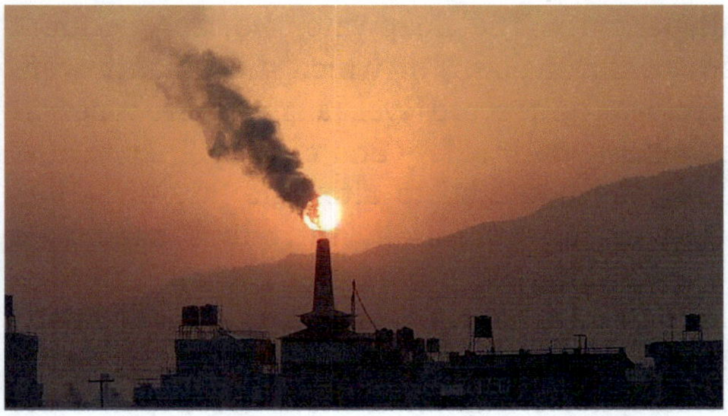

Figure 6.5. Air pollution by brick factories.

Source: https://upload.wikimedia.org/wikipedia/commons/thumb/0/0d/Air_pollution3.jpg/1024px-Air_pollution3.jpg.

6.2.2. Water Contamination and Health Risks

Water contamination poses enormous health hazards that call for close examination in the discipline of Environmental and Occupational Medicine. Contaminated water sources can contain a treasure trove of toxic substances like heavy metals, infectious pathogens, and chemical toxins, all of which pose harmful effects on human health. Consumption of contaminated water has been linked to certain acute and chronic health problems, such as gastrointestinal diseases, neurological disorders, and cancer. In addition, vulnerable populations like children, pregnant women, and the aged are all significantly susceptible to these health impacts, according to their emerging or weakened immune system. Thus, it is crucial to identify the public health impacts of water quality to inform policy change for guaranteeing safe drinking water, since water management breakdowns will increase existing healthcare inequalities and medical costs in the long run. The geographical history of the population is a key consideration in establishing exposure to contaminated water and resulting health effects. Identification of where the individuals have lived throughout their lifetime can cast informative light on potential extended exposure to water-borne toxins, which typically have delayed latency periods from exposure to clinical manifestation. For instance, geographic history is particularly beneficial in the analysis of diseases such as cancer, where time and exposure to the environment overlap strongly. Such a stringent methodology increases the application of medical geology in medical practice, where practitioners are better placed to analyze environmental risk factors for individual patients. In this context, interdisciplinary collaboration becomes imperative in responding to water pollution because the integration of epidemiology, geoscience, and biomedical research gives health professionals tools with which they can predict, forecast, and prevent health hazards involving environmental contaminants, thereby ensuring a successful prevention strategy. Experiments establishing the function of environmental factors, such as temperature stresses, also establish the complex relationship between the environment and health responses. A review of IHD mortality risk with respect to temperature variation is illustrative of the importance of considering local climatic conditions in assessing health hazards. While temperature variability will exacerbate some health conditions, contaminated water will likely do the same by exacerbating existing medical conditions or introducing entirely new health risks. It is therefore important to learn how these synergistic interactions between environmental exposures—climate and water quality, for example—transpire to generate effective public health interventions. Improved monitoring and health policy that accounts for these interactions will ultimately result in a more robust system for protecting public health and lessening the pervasive problems of water pollution and its health consequences in various communities (Figure 6.6).

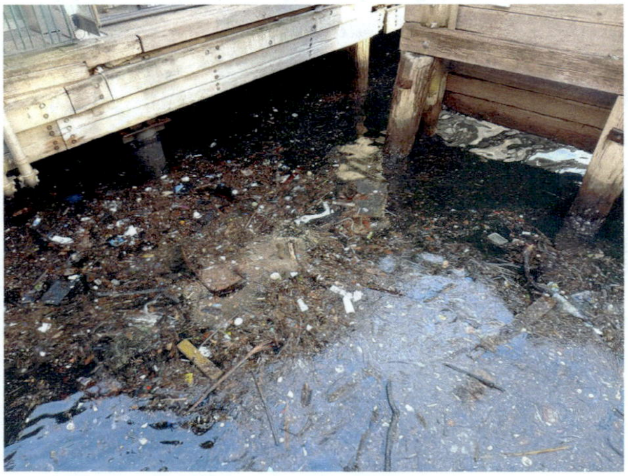

Figure 6.6. Garbage and other junk floating in the water.

Source: https://upload.wikimedia.org/wikipedia/commons/thumb/a/a0/Garbage_floating_around_in_Circular_Quay.jpg/800px-Garbage_floating_around_in_Circular_Quay.jpg.

6.2.3. Chemical Exposures in the Environment

The prevalence of chemical exposures in the environment is a serious public health issue, particularly since industrial activities and agricultural use continue to rise. Chemicals released into the air, water, and soil have the potential to cause widespread pollution, impacting ecosystems as well as human beings. Not only are these exposures linked to a range of adverse health outcomes—ranging from respiratory ailments, neurological conditions, and cancer—but they also create socioeconomic consequences that disproportionately affect the most susceptible members of society. The risks associated with these exposures are often compounded by the inadequacy of effective regulatory frameworks and the synergistic interaction of numerous chemical agents. This intricately terrained situation demands an interdisciplinary approach to occupational and environmental medicine that includes the detection and control of chemical hazards, effective health surveillance, and risk communication programs engaging the community. Environmental disasters such as oil spills further complicate the issue of chemical exposures through the use of chemical dispersants. The Deepwater Horizon accident is a case in point, in which dispersants were deployed on a record level, raising severe concerns regarding their safety and efficacy. Dispersants have the potential to alter the fate of spilled oil and can potentially introduce poisonous chemicals into the marine ecosystem and even into human bodies. Thus, agency evaluations such as those of the National Oceanic and Atmospheric Administration (NOAA) indicate the need for thorough scrutiny of the state-of-the-science on chemical dispersants and their impact. Moreover, debates on the use of chemical dispersants acquire particular importance in ecologically sensitive Arctic regions with abysmal conditions that make responding to spills ineffective and could enhance adverse health and environmental impacts, as quoted by the Coastal Response Research Center (2019). Chemical exposure management demands the formulation of comprehensive health monitoring systems to create protection for worker health and community health. Proper medical surveillance is necessary for the early detection of occupational disease and the prevention of disproportionately exposed employees from being subjected to abuse by toxic chemicals. Collection of medical history and toxicity data, emphasized in health protocol assessments such as those at NASA medical facilities, is very important in occupational settings. These assessments are a move towards optimizing health maintenance practice and make the requirement of adaptive clinical reactions more difficult, which can respond to emerging environmental threats. With investments in robust occupational health programs and prioritizing preventive strategies, stakeholders have the ability to effectively minimize the damage related to chemical exposures and, ultimately, enhance public health and develop resilient populations (Figure 6.7).

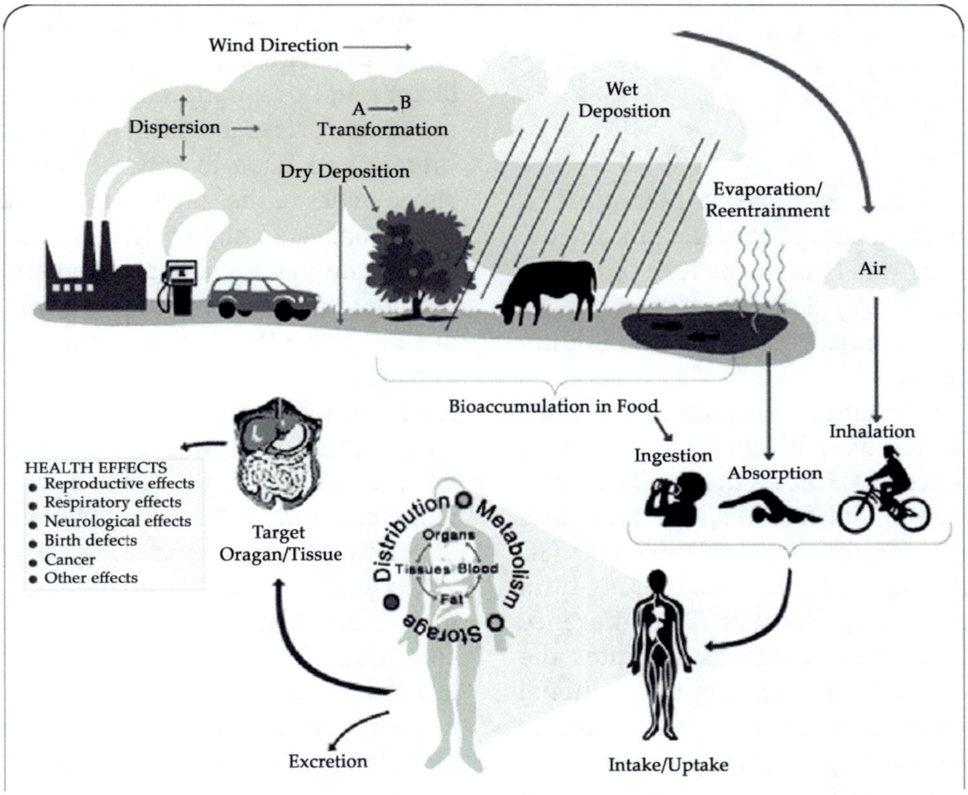

Figure 6.7. Illustration how people are exposed to chemicals in the environment and the effect of such chemicals on human health.

Source: https://www.researchgate.net/publication/297731586/figure/fig4/AS:668874479505410 @1536483511077/llustration-how-people-are-exposed-to-chemicals-in-the-environment-and-the-eff-ect-of.png.

Test Your Knowledge

1. What are the primary health effects associated with exposure to fine particulate matter (PM2.5) in air pollution?
2. Name three major sources of outdoor air pollution and one common indoor air pollutant.

6.3. Occupational Health Risks

Learning Outcome

1. Describe common workplace hazards;
2. Explain the impact of ergonomics on worker health;
3. Understand the role of safety regulations in mitigating risks.

The mining industry is a classic example of a high-risk industry in occupational health, and the major reason for this is the exposure to whole-body vibration (WBV) that operators of heavy earth-moving machinery, i.e., load-haul-dump (LHD) vehicles, are exposed to. The operators get exposed to prolonged periods of vibration and shocks, which have been identified with a greater incidence of MSDs. As the recent studies have uncovered, quantification of health risks with standards like ISO 2631-1:1997 and ISO 2631-5:2018 is required to analyze the long-term consequences of such exposure. The difference in findings from such standards indicates the complexity involved in assessing occupational hazards, requiring a gentle approach in setting up health standards, particularly in countries with growing mining industries. Identification of such risks gives room for improving safety strategies and employees' well-being in this difficult circumstance (Sharma & Mandal, 2024). In addition to structural deficiencies typical of industries such as mining, adverse waste management practices also present health concerns, and are a significant occupational health risk. For instance, improper handling of fecal sludge presents several public health risks, including exposure to harmful gases and PM. Experiments conducted in Dar es Salaam have pointed to new methods, such as the production of carbonized briquettes from fecal sludge and organic binders, as a means to reduce airborne toxins in workplaces and homes. Experiments on the fumes emitted by the briquettes revealed varying amounts of carbon monoxide and PM, which demonstrated the critical role binder choice can have in enhancing air quality. These findings underscore the importance of sustainable waste management practices that, besides mitigating hazards to occupational health, contribute to the accomplishment of more general public health objectives (Puig et al., 2024). The convergence of environmental factors and occupational safety is necessary in minimizing risks to health in various industries. Interactions used to control and manage such risks need to balance safety and operating performance. In high-risk industries like mining and waste management, stringent studies and modifications of operations are imperative. The ongoing research on mining operators' vibration exposure indicates a proactive approach toward the protection of workers' health, while advancements in waste management reflect an innovative path toward environmental enhancement. As industries evolve, a concerted effort to integrate technological advancement with sound health recommendations will play a key role in enhancing better working conditions. Through these channels, industries are in a position both to protect their workers and support the general goals of occupational and environmental medicine (Puig et al., 2024; Sharma & Mandal, 2024).

6.3.1. Common Workplace Hazards

A variety of common work hazards present serious threats to the health and safety of employees, requiring careful notice in the context of occupational and environmental medicine. Perhaps most common among these hazards are chemical agents, including but not limited to, solvents, heavy metals, and harmful chemicals, that employees come in contact with in a variety of work processes. Prolonged exposure to these chemicals may lead to acute or chronic health problems such as respiratory diseases, skin issues, or long-term neurological deficits. Physical hazards like slips, trips, and falls are also hardly ever taken into consideration, despite being the major occupational injury causes. To manage such risks, there are effective safety protocols, regular training, and a definite understanding of the dynamic interaction between workspace layout and staff behavior so that risks are minimized and safety performance maximized in different workplaces (Pouliakas & Theodossiou, 2010). The second most important thing to manage is ergonomics, which defines how employees work with tools and workspace. Poor ergonomics results in MSDs like backache, CTS, and repetitive strain injury. Over recent decades, heightened awareness of the significance of ergonomics in the workplace and the need for organizations to assess workspaces and provide necessary accommodations has emerged. Creation of workspaces with ergonomic accommodations enhances comfort improves productivity and reduces injury-absenteeism. Moreover, the economic benefit of ergonomics improvement is substantial as it can reduce healthcare costs and enhance worker morale, thus leading to a healthier workforce (Pouliakas & Theodossiou, 2010). Last but not least, the influence of psychosocial risk factors presents an increasingly recognized problem in modern workplaces. Workplace violence, bullying, stress, and inadequate support measures are some of the factors that can lead to a toxic culture and low employee well-being. Mental health is becoming a subject of discussion when the issue of occupational safety and health is raised, particularly as it leads to absenteeism and low job satisfaction. It is most likely that vulnerable groups, such as ethnic minorities, will suffer from higher stress and poor health status in the workplace and complicate these issues. Therefore, developing a constructive work culture with supportive frameworks for open communication and good mental health provisions can be a key driving factor to counteract psychosocial risks and enhance workplace health in general (Figure 6.8).

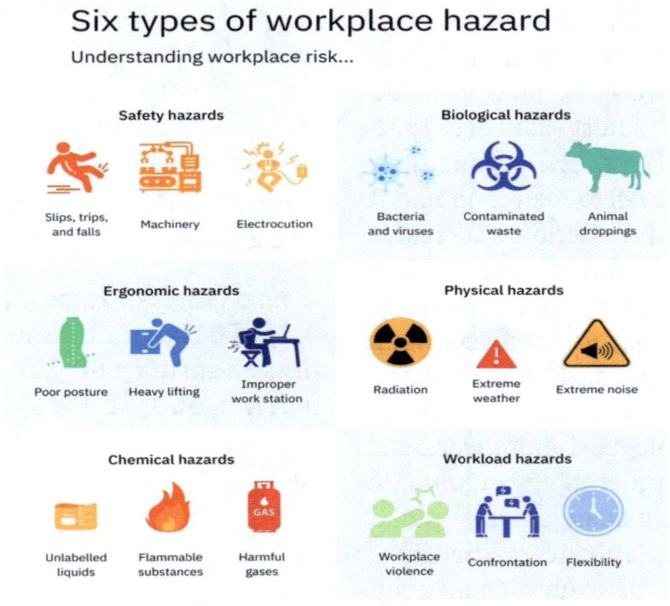

Figure 6.8. Six types of workplace hazards.

Source: https://cdn-ilcjceb.nitrocdn.com/VtFsciNiiemJiXTnmldbhHuQqIuDijYB/assets/images/optimized/rev-e1275c6/www.ecoonline.com/wp-content/uploads/2025/01/Six-types-of-workplace-hazard-724x1024.webp.

6.3.2. Impact of Ergonomics on Worker Health

Workplace ergonomics is essential in the promotion of employee health and in reducing the possibility of MSDs. Poor ergonomic practice leads to work-related musculoskeletal disorders (WMSDs), impacting labor productivity as well as employee well-being. A significant limiting factor in improving ergonomic conditions is the involvement of employers and workers in risk assessment and developing solutions. A recent participatory ergonomics intervention among construction workers illustrated that high worker participation rates and multiple ergonomic solutions existed, yet a lack of contractor support stopped these changes from being successfully implemented. Thus, intervention must not only inform workers about ergonomic methods but also actively involve management to deliver an environment for long-term change (Dale et al., 2016). Moreover, communication mechanisms such as toolbox talks (TBTs) can improve the positive impact of ergonomic interventions on the health and safety of workers. Toolbox talks provide room for the airing of safety concerns and stimulating discussions on work ergonomics. However, traditional TBTs fail to realize potential avenues for meaningful interaction and result in superficial worker engagement. Research has established that participatory TBTs, whereby workers are invited to engage in discussions around ergonomics, significantly enhance the acceptability and appropriateness of safety messages. Through employees' empowerment to become responsible for identifying ergonomic issues and recommending changes, the uptake of healthier practices is enhanced, therefore reducing the incidence of injury caused by improper ergonomics (Kaskutas et al., 2016). Lastly, the management of the impact of ergonomics on worker health must be holistic in its approach, with a combination of education and active participation. Engaging workers in the process of ergonomic evaluation and solution increases their awareness as well as establishes a culture of safety in the workplace. To ensure effective long-term outcomes, it is critical that worker observations and contractor reactions are linked to deliver the necessary support and implementation of the ergonomic interventions. By creating a work environment focusing on ergonomics and engaging workers in all phases, companies can mitigate risk associated with unhealthy work practices and enhance overall worker health and productivity, thus emphasizing the applicability of integrating ergonomic principles into the broader practice of environmental and occupational medicine (Dale et al., 2016; Kaskutas et al., 2016) (Figure 6.9).

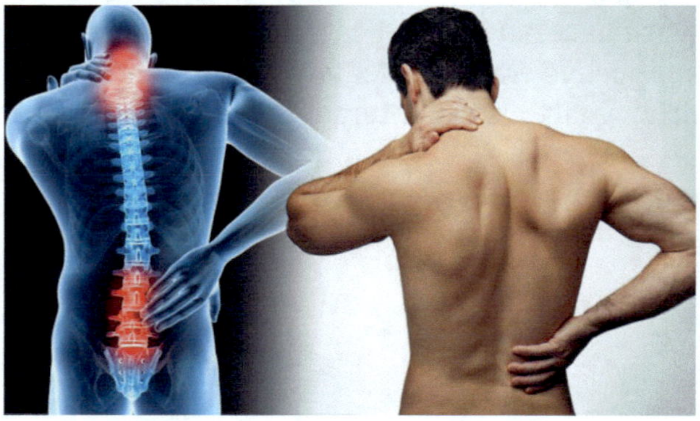

Figure 6.9. Illustration of work-related musculoskeletal disorders (WMSDs).

Source: https://media.licdn.com/dms/image/v2/C5612AQEnBFBmos0gOQ/article-cover_image-shrink_600_2000/article-cover_image-shrink_600_2000/0/1600035051926?e=2147483647&v=beta&t=kyazinVGMho5S2-QlXKl_5oXWNac8d6hpcVBKu-RArY.

6.3.3. Role of Safety Regulations in Mitigating Risks

Enforcement of safety regulations is paramount in the discipline of occupational and environmental medicine as a baseline to mitigate risks posed by various work environments. By establishing rigorous guidelines, safety regulations have a tendency of providing a framework that limits the capability of employees, particularly those in high-risk sectors such as construction, manufacturing, and food processing, from being exposed to hazards. These codes not only require compliance with health and safety procedures but also promote a safety culture within both management and workers. For instance, codification of procedures in ergonomics and chemicals has direct effects on the workers' health outcomes by guarding them from unwanted exposure to harm that can cause long-term health problems or acute trauma. By encouraging such practice, organizations can enhance their operational efficiency while simultaneously guarding their workforce from injury. Second, safety legislation is also important in regulating the multifaceted risks that extend beyond labor to include contiguous communities and the environment. Public health concerns, such as air and water pollution, which are often an industrial byproduct, can have far-reaching impacts on the well-being of people, going full circle to environmental justice. Regulations on emissions and waste disposal not only safeguard workers but also minimize risk to the health of the environment, opening the doors to a sustainable future. The connection between occupational safety and environmental health is most evident in instances that are associated with meat production, whose employees' and the general populace's health is endangered by harmful processes in abattoirs (Holdier, 2016). By implementing strict safety protocols, we can reduce these threats, thus promoting a healthier natural balance and community welfare. By heading in the direction of a holistic occupational health culture, the importance of personalized methods incorporating safety protocols becomes a concrete reality. Literature review shows a shift in paradigm from traditional measures of disease treatment to measures of disease prevention through active reduction (Karanika-Murray & Weyman, 2013). This development emphasizes organizational leadership for health and well-being beyond compliance with safety regulations. By addressing organizational drivers such as leadership and job design, organizations are able to create workplaces that are safer by nature and that place a high value on mental and physical health. In this case, the role of safety rules shifts from mere regulatory necessity to being an approach to creating workplace well-being and resilience. Consequently, this holistic strategy not only enhances worker safety but also contributes to overall organizational performance, illustrating the central role of safety regulations in minimizing occupational and environmental risk.

Test Your Knowledge

1. What are three common categories of workplace hazards, and give one example for each?
2. What are psychosocial risks in the workplace, and how can they impact worker health?

6.4. Assessment and Diagnosis

Learning Outcome

1. Explain the methods for evaluating environmental exposures;
2. Describe the techniques for assessing occupational health;
3. Discuss the importance of interdisciplinary approaches.

In environmental and occupational medicine, the diagnosis and assessment of diseases resulting from exposure to harmful chemicals are paramount to safeguarding public health. It is critical to have precise assessment methods for identifying risk groups and delineating the health impact of environmental poisons. These assessments typically involve taking full occupational histories, including detailed descriptions of the type and duration of exposure. Health practitioners widely employ a blend of clinical structured interviews and subjective symptom questionnaires to assess psychological distress and other illnesses among exposed populations. For instance, research indicates that sheep farmers with previous low-level exposure to organophosphate pesticides present greater self-reported depression and anxiety than unexposed controls, where the requirement for extensive psychological assessment in occupational medicine clinics is highlighted (Harrison & Mackenzie, 2016). Diagnosis in occupational and environmental medicine entails the correct distinction between occupational-related disease and other conditions. Temporal association between agent exposure and the onset of clinical symptoms is the key to a diagnosis. For example, in occupational asthma, a culpable history correlating the start of symptoms with specific work exposures is good evidence for making a diagnosis. Correlation of objective tests, such as pulmonary function tests, with occupational exposures is valuable in the determination of symptom-occupation relationships. Identification of specific agents responsible for conditions such as asthma is difficult and requires a multi-axial approach to consider patient history as well as environmental etiologies. Failure to properly diagnose such conditions may lead to prolonged disability and compromised quality of life, and therefore, care must be taken in clinical assessment (Lombardo & Balmes, 2000). Further, early intervention is then absolutely essential upon confirmation of the diagnosis. Early diagnosis of occupational diseases may permit early withdrawal of the patient from noxious exposure, a step that is capable of halting the progression of conditions such as asthma or chronic obstructive pulmonary disease (COPD). Where prolonged exposure is unavoidable, early initiation of therapeutic interventions, such as inhaled corticosteroids, can mitigate the severity of symptoms and improve patient outcomes. Preventive measures are prioritized, since they reduce the number of new cases due to deleterious exposures in various occupations. With the advanced research undertaken in environmental and occupational medicine, more advanced assessment tools will enhance diagnostic precision and result in better patient management practices, eventually leading to a healthier occupational work environment for workers (Lombardo & Balmes, 2000).

6.4.1. Methods for Evaluating Environmental Exposures

In environmental and occupational medicine, the evaluation of environmental exposures is interdisciplinary in nature. The most prominent approach is through an epidemiological study that quantifies the relationship between health effects and environmental risk factors. These are either descriptive, establishing the distribution of events related to health among populations, or analytical, testing the exposure-disease hypothesis. For instance, cohort studies track individuals over time to observe how diseases unfold in relation to particular environmental exposures, such as air toxics or hazardous waste. This is the strength of the methods since it has the ability to measure temporal associations, thereby illuminating causation. That being said, researchers should be careful about confounding variables that might obscure the real nature of such associations, and most importantly, rigorous study design and execution are essential in order to make sound inferences. Another useful method for the evaluation of environmental exposures is biomonitoring, which quantifies the presence of chemicals or their metabolites in biological fluids, e.g., blood or urine. This scientific approach offers direct proof of exposure and is more representative of the dose-response relationship than is environmental monitoring alone. By measuring the actual human body concentration of toxins, scientists are able to more appropriately link exposure levels to health outcomes, as demonstrated by studies of the effects of organophosphate pesticides on mental health (Harrison & Mackenzie, 2016). Second, biomonitoring provides quantitative data on populations at risk in terms of biological susceptibility, thereby facilitating targeted public health intervention. Notwithstanding, there are limitations such as the need for validated exposure markers and problems related to sample timing that can constrain the usefulness of the findings. Lastly, geospatial analysis has proven to be a valuable tool in environmental exposure evaluation and the integration of geographic information systems (GIS). By geospatial mapping of hazard distributions in the environment against health data, researchers can identify patterns and relationships that may be otherwise concealed. This, in fact, enhances significantly the visualizing and evaluating capacity for how environmental determinants influence health outcomes within different populations (Kyle et al., 2006). For example, GIS can reveal disease clusters that relate to proximity to industrial centers or traffic areas and hence assist in public health policy and allocation of resources. But the technique also has to be applied cautiously as regards data quality and the ecological fallacy, where group data may not reflect individual exposure. Lastly, the unification of the diversified strategies reinforces the broad vision of environmental determinants of health in the context of environmental and occupational medicine.

6.4.2. Techniques for Assessing Occupational Health

Occupational health assessment is a multifaceted process that employs a variety of methods with the aim of identifying hazards, assessing risks, and implementing preventive measures in the workplace. Of these methods, epidemiological studies are especially effective tools to assess occupational exposures and subsequent health effects. Through data collection and analysis from exposed and unexposed groups, scientists are able to determine disease patterns and establish causal relationships that guide public health interventions. In addition to assisting in the understanding of the magnitude and character of occupational health hazards, this process also assists policymakers in creating laws that reduce these hazards. For instance, a systematic review of zoonotic diseases in Bangladesh explains how such epidemiological data can inform interventions and influence future studies on occupational health, specifically where pathogen exposure is significant (Samad, 2025). Biomonitoring is another important way of assessing occupational health by quantifying chemicals, their metabolites, or biological effects in human samples. This method has become a routine component of exposure assessment, providing quantifiable evidence of occupational and environmental exposure. Biomonitoring enables the scientist to quantify the levels of chemicals in the body, thus facilitating the identification of exposure pathways and corresponding health risks. Furthermore, it helps in meeting predetermined exposure guidelines and assisting occupational health research and surveillance. Effective biomonitoring depends on the appropriate selection of biomarkers and the appropriate timing of sample collection, which play major roles in the validity of results. Such strict measurements can serve as a basis for interventions, evaluate the efficiency of such interventions, and ultimately result in better health outcomes among workers (Mourad, 2024). Finally, environmental monitoring is another key approach which functions parallel to biomonitoring to quantify occupational health risks. By the quantification of exposure levels in the environment, this technique provides a model for understanding the occupational hazards to which the workers are submitted. It is interested in assessing the degree of dangerous agents existing in the workplace, like the air, water, and soil, thereby delimiting potential exposure scenarios to workers. This quantification is critical while preparing complex risk management plans aimed at protecting workers' health. Furthermore, integration of environmental monitoring with biomonitoring provides a comprehensive picture of the exposure risks, addressing sources as well as effects of the toxic chemicals. Occupational health professionals can formulate effective interventions through constant surveillance and targeted assessment, promoting safer workplaces and reducing the disease burden of occupational diseases (Figure 6.10).

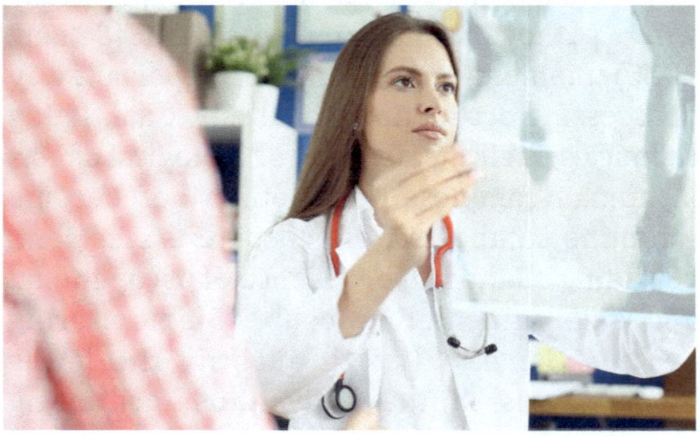

Figure 6.10. Occupational health assessment.

Source: https://www.co-health.co.uk/wp-content/uploads/2023/12/occupational-health-assessment.png.

6.4.3. Importance of Interdisciplinary Approaches

The contribution of interdisciplinary thought to occupational and environmental medicine cannot be overstated, given the fact that these fields often overlap in highly complex and multidisciplinary ways. In addressing health issues arising from exposure to the environment, there is a need for health hazards to be considered from various different aspects, including geology, epidemiology, and biomedical sciences. For instance, environmental health problems often require medical professionals to be aware of patients' histories of exposure to toxins and pollutants, which requires interdisciplinary integration of knowledge. By applying an integrative model, health practitioners will be in a good position to effectively assess the impacts of environmental factors on individuals' and groups' health. As emphasized in contemporary studies, a holistic view that combines epidemiological data and personal health histories is essential to properly diagnose and treat various chronic diseases, particularly those with long latency periods, such as cancer and respiratory illnesses (Boulos & Le Blond, 2016). In the pursuit of effective environmental and occupational medicine, the development of interconnected models that involve multiple actors is essential. Specialists in other professions, including physiotherapy and occupational therapy, can provide fresh experience and ideas to treatment strategies aimed at facilitating improved patient recovery. Team working in the rehabilitation service environment, for example, is reported to enhance communication and interprofessional mutualism among healthcare professionals. This facilitates the integration of many factors influencing patient health, including environmental conditions and social determinants, in addition to clinical choices. The acknowledgement of such variegated dimensions eventually results in facilitating holistic care designed for particular needs and context-specificities, which is exceptionally vital in empowering health and well-being among variegated groups (Suddick & De Souza, 2007). With the growing dominance of interdisciplinary approaches in environmental and occupational medicine, they facilitate various scientific methods being integrated. This is particularly the case in the emerging field of medical geology, where geological conditions are explored in their interaction with human health. Achievement of purposes in prediction, prevention, and tailored treatment involves coordinated effort across disciplines such as toxicology, public health, and environmental science. Findings from every discipline are significant to provide for more effective interventions for diseases governed by environmental controls. In general, encouraging interdisciplinarity not only increases the wealth of knowledge that is available about health risks but also provides innovative ways of handling and mitigating the risks, ultimately leading to improved public health outcomes and informed decision-making (Boulos & Le Blond, 2016).

Test Your Knowledge

1. What are two common methods used to assess an individual's exposure to environmental pollutants?
2. Name three common tools or techniques used to evaluate workplace hazards and worker health.
3. Why is obtaining a detailed occupational and environmental exposure history crucial in diagnosing related health issues?

6.5. Prevention Strategies

Learning Outcome

1. Focus on public health initiatives for environmental protection;
2. Discuss workplace safety programs and training;
3. Explain the role of legislation in promoting health.

Preventive policy in environmental and occupational medicine is most critical for the protection of worker and community health. The policy has a focus on strong proactive action versus reactive action, risk assessment, and the minimization of potential hazards in the workplace. Effective approaches can include minimizing workplace ergonomics, creating comprehensive health education programs, and promoting mental health in workers. Elements such as psychosocial elements play a key role in determining health outcomes, further strengthening the importance of addressing overall work environments to promote improved physical and mental health. Such programs aim to reduce the frequency of work-related injuries and disorders, hence enhancing employees' productivity and health. Multidisciplinary intervention is necessary in terms of designing effective prevention strategies that incorporate elements pertaining to environmental health. The collaboration of health workers, environmental scientists, and policymakers is significant in order to counter the diverse array of determinants of health, particularly in the healthcare service sector. As Davies & Lowe (1999) put it, there exists massive upstream management potential, particularly in reducing the environmental impact of healthcare activities. Transition to green practices, such as minimizing waste generation and the utilization of sustainable materials, can contribute significantly to reducing the environmental footprint of healthcare buildings. Realization of direct and indirect impacts generated by service sector operations underscores the necessity for continuous evaluation and incorporation of sustainable practices into organizational processes. The success of prevention initiatives further relies on increased community involvement and awareness. Public awareness of occupational and environmental health risks can have the power to enable individuals to demand improved working conditions and safer environments. Training sessions that equip employees with knowledge of preventive measures for health, such as waste disposal, ergonomics, and detection of occupational disease signs at an early stage, play a significant role in developing a culture of safety. Through community-based initiatives, the emphasis on holistic employee training and services not only promotes the short-term well-being of workers but also contributes to long-term community sustainability. As such, these prevention efforts ultimately result in a healthier and more productive workforce that benefits global public health initiatives as well.

6.5.1. Public Health Initiatives for Environmental Protection

The integration of public health programs and environmental protection is necessary in lessening risk to health arising from environmental degradation. Such programs are increasingly being accepted as part of environmental and occupational medicine, in which community health is interconnected to the quality of the environment in which it lives. With clean air, safe water, and green waste management, public health interventions reduce exposure to harmful substances that can lead to serious diseases. For instance, since healthcare facilities are great polluters, they can adopt green practices that not only enhance health outcomes but also lower their environmental footprint. The trend towards healthier, greener medical practice encompasses actions aimed at minimizing waste, recycling, and adopting alternative materials, thereby eradicating the adverse effects of medical waste incineration and chemical dumping (Davies & Lowe, 1999). Moreover, health campaigns to create awareness on environmental threats can be instrumental in influencing behavior and policy. These programs have a tendency to focus on educating communities regarding the impacts of pollution and preventive health measures, which can lead to healthier outcomes. One of the main goals of these programs is to engage the public in discussion pertaining to occupational health and safety regulation, particularly in high-risk industries. However, the implementation of these regulations is hindered, primarily by a lack of political commitment and implementation machinery.

The lack of adequate advocacy and policy commitment continues to erode the effectiveness of public health programs in responding to environmental health issues. Therefore, building these programs requires a multifaceted process that includes participation of the community, educational mobilization, and effective policy implementation to ensure that environmental health and public safety are given top priority (Lethbridge, 2008). Finally, the integration of environmental conservation into public health strategies needs multidisciplinary collaboration. Environmental and occupational medicine experts must work in collaboration with community stakeholders, regulators, and healthcare providers to ensure that there are coordinated strategies are created and implemented. This multidisciplinary practice can enable the sharing of resources, knowledge, and best practices that advance public health and environmental responsibility. For instance, initiatives to reduce emissions from health care facilities can not only reduce the industry's impact on the environment but also bring about healthier working environments for staff at risk of disease. Further, engaging upstream suppliers with their environmental practices can bring rich rewards, leading to an integrated approach that incorporates consideration of the health of the population alongside the integrity of the ecosystems. Through supporting these partnerships, we can build a healthier and more sustainable future where health and environmental quality are considered together (Davies & Lowe, 1999) (Figure 6.11).

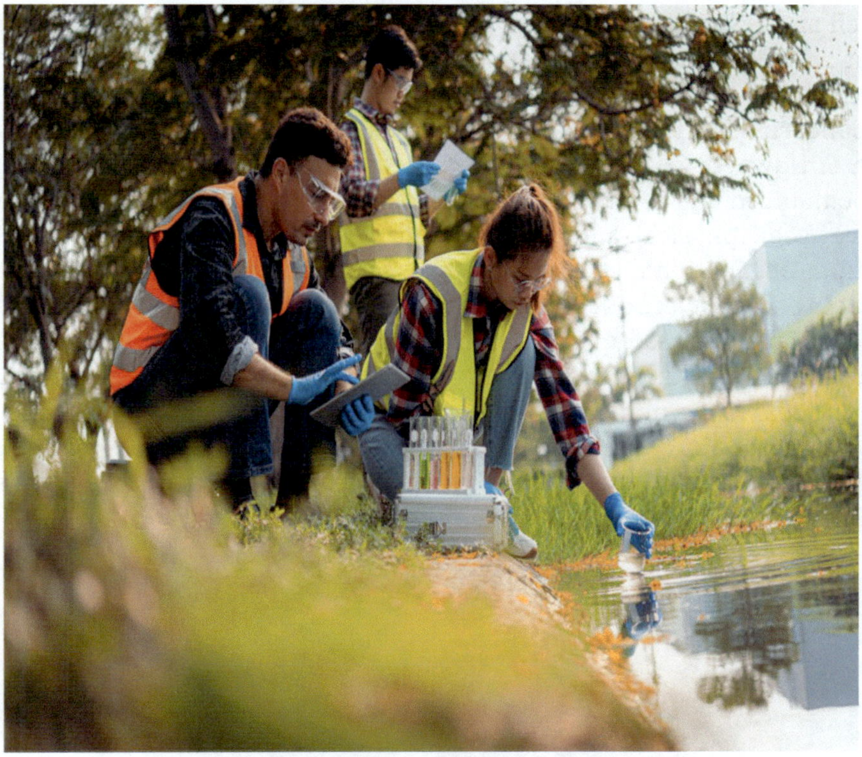

Figure 6.11. Public health initiatives and environmental protection.

Source: https://eu-images.contentstack.com/v3/assets/bltf2605c1a31475f8b/blt87388c460a523c44/65425181139351040a0f63cc/ACC_celebrates_35_years_of_environmental_program.jpg?width=1280&auto=webp&quality=80&format=jpg&disable=upscale.

6.5.2. Workplace Safety Programs and Training

Safety training programs and workplace safety are at the core of the discipline of Environmental and Occupational Medicine since they directly impact worker health and well-being. Not only do the programs emphasize the importance of following safety procedures, but they also promote a culture of awareness in an organization. Successful safety training equips staff members with the ability to recognize and manage hazards, reducing the likelihood of illness and injury in the workplace. In addition, understanding the psychosocial aspects of the workplace can help increase the effectiveness of these programs even further. By incorporating discussion topics related to physical and mental health, companies can foster a better work environment that supports overall wellness and productivity. This integrated model is crucial as it recognizes that worker health is influenced by more than a single factor, including stress, workload, and organizational support (Chapman & Naweed, 2015). Workplace safety programs are most needed in risky industries where the possibility of accident occurrence is significantly heightened, such as transportation and construction. For instance, it has been shown by research that prevention programs for health promotion, in the direction of avoiding issues like obesity, can yield measurable benefits in safety-critical employment. In the Australasian rail and road industries, chronic lifestyle diseases like obesity can decrease cardiac and fatigue-related risks prevalent in these industries. Health interventions such as personalized health profiles and improved food options within the premises, in addition to not only demonstrating enhanced employee well-being but also considerable returns on investment, remind us that safety training must extend beyond immediate hazards to encompass broader health concerns and thereby offer a comprehensive approach to occupational health and safety (Chapman & Naweed, 2015). Moreover, the efficiency of occupational safety programs can be significantly enhanced by adding mental health support and services. The identification of the interaction between physical and mental health is crucial in terms of promoting a healthy working population. Occupational stressors such as high demands and low control can exacerbate health issues, leading to poor productivity and increased absenteeism. Therefore, safety programs that encompass both physical safety policies and mental health interventions offer an integrated approach that centers on health. Second, organizations need to continually assess and adjust their safety training protocols to maintain up-to-date with emerging trends in health and evidence-based practice. In doing so, they not only remain compliant with the law but also create an environment in which employees are valued and locked in, ultimately leading to higher job satisfaction and retention (The Stern Center for Evidence-Based Policy, 2015) (Figure 6.12).

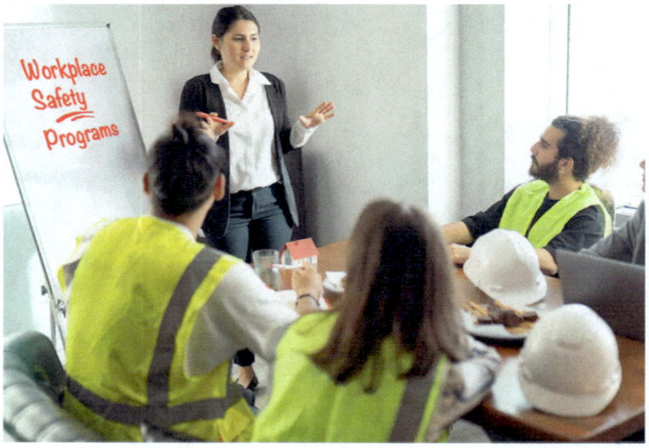

Figure 6.12. Workplace safety programs.

Source: https://www.realtimenetworks.com/hubfs/WPS-PP-top-hero-banner-1200x832-3.jpeg.

6.5.3. Role of Legislation in Promoting Health

The role of law in health promotion is an integral part of environmental and occupational medicine, particularly for the establishment of safe and healthy working environments. Comprehensive legislations have been enacted globally in a bid to address health issues brought about by various occupational exposures. Such laws not only aim to set the standards of workplace safety but also to ensure workers' protection from unsafe conditions that can adversely affect their physical and mental health. By mandating workers to perform frequent inspections and improvement of the workplace, laws are a necessary instrument in building healthier workplaces. As has been argued in literature, the material context and psychosocial factors of work enter into interaction with health outcomes, again emphasizing the necessity of robust legal provisions placing such factors to the forefront of workplace conditions (The Stern Center for Evidence-Based Policy, 2015). In addition to placing the short-term interests of workers' safety in the spotlight, the law plays an important role in promoting more general public health initiatives. Legislation to manage environmental health issues, such as air and water quality, helps minimize occupational exposure-related health risks. In addition to safeguarding individual workers, the law also affects the overall well-being of society by applying extremely rigorous standards to environmental pollutants. In other regions, such as Malawi, research gaps in environmental health have required deliberate legal action to effectively address the issues. Recommendations ensuing from such analyses require action plans involving inclusivity that can be accommodated within legislative agendas for the betterment of health outcomes, evidence of the complementary role that legislative intervention has in enhancing environmental health (Morse et al., 2010). In addition, public education and awareness campaigns can be utilized to enhance the impact of health-promoting legislation. Through engaging the labor force and society in understanding the consequences of law, there is a greater likelihood of compliance and promotion of health-promoting policies. Education can bridge the knowledge gap on rights and obligations in the workplace, forcing employers and workers to see the significance of health. Successful health promotion through legislation relies not only on the passage of law but also on sustained support and obedience to such law. In the long term, as legislation evolves to address emerging issues in environmental and occupational health, an integrated strategy with education, advocacy, and enforcement will be essential in securing effective health protection for all (The Stern Center for Evidence-Based Policy, 2015).

Test Your Knowledge

1. What are two major public health initiatives aimed at reducing environmental pollution and protecting community health?
2. How do workplace safety training programs help prevent occupational injuries and illnesses?

SUMMARY

The science of Environmental and Occupational Medicine has a very crucial role to play in understanding the interrelated complexities of public health with occupational environments. The science not only seeks to avoid the detrimental effects of environmental agents on workers but also stresses the significance of an integrated strategy to health promotion across sectors. An understanding of the multifaceted determinants of health underscores the imperative to embrace a multilevel analysis that accounts for individual, organizational, and population-level influences. Recent research indicates that interventions that only address individual-level measures may overlook significant contextual effects. Thus, including a broader perspective can also solidify evidence-based strategies for improving employee well-being and mental health on the basis of evidence that states multilevel assessment of psychosocial work environments is the gateway to continuing organizational interventions (Martin et al., 2016). Systematic exploration of traffic medicine as a confluence of occupational and environmental health cannot be overemphasized. Traffic trauma is a large public health issue, often complicated by matters of road infrastructure, urban planning, and driving practices. History reveals a highly gigantic disparity in research output in this field, with the United States being a leader in traffic medicine research (Groneberg-Kloft et al., 2013). Improved understanding of such dynamics can be employed to inform policy-making and public health interventions, in turn reducing morbidity and mortality rates arising from road traffic crashes. Such inclusion of traffic medicine within the broader context of Environmental and Occupational Medicine not only justifies more research efforts but also highlights the implications of practical application to community health and safety. Finally, the future of Environmental and Occupational Medicine depends on collaborative action that encourages interdisciplinary study and practice. Involving diverse stakeholders—from policymakers and health professionals to industries and communities—is essential to addressing the intricacies of environmental and occupational health. Also, as emerging threats to health continue to evolve, so must intervention strategies and preventive tactics. By embracing a comprehensive, multi-level research and solution approach, we are more capable of meeting the immediate needs of workers and society. This way, we not only provide improved health but also contribute to a future that is sustainable in the sense that there is occupational health as well as environmental integrity.

The role that Environmental and Occupational Medicine plays will also help explain how factors in the environment and workplace correlate with human health. More importantly, such vital points include determining risks of exposure to environmental toxins, which will have impacts on the results for public health. This includes, for instance, air, soil, and water pollutants that will lead to chronic illness and acute health complications. The exercise accentuates the need for objective assessment in order to understand these environmental threats in appropriate terms. Besides, occupational exposure to harmful substances such as chemicals and biological agents necessitates monitoring and intervention measures in order to protect workers. The utilization of epidemiological data in addition to environmental science provides a foundation on which to base guidelines for risk reduction, implying the need for interdisciplinary collaboration in this context. Moreover, the use of assistive devices and activity of daily living (ADL) training is required in patients with mobility impairments post-surgery, as has been found from the literature review. These interventions not only work in the recovery arena but also are impressive in the quality of life experienced by patients. The review shows that the results of patients' outcomes who may undergo procedures such as hip arthroplasty can be very vulnerable to hip precautions education, environmental interventions, and assistive device use. Such information gives credence to individually based rehabilitation programs that share aspects of both physical and environmental interventions leading to recovery and independence, pointing to a direct relationship between medical intervention and environmental support systems in occupational health interventions (Smith et al., 2013). Lastly, the rigorous scrutiny of work tasks, particularly in highly stressful jobs such as law enforcement, reaffirms the necessity for optimal ergonomic designs in protective gear. A systematic review has enlightened the biomechanical challenges associated with the body armor of officers, which can compromise performance during emergencies. Primary findings demonstrate noteworthy increases in perceived effort and longer task completion times when officers use traditional armor (Tomes et al., 2017). This underscores the need for research on the physical demands made on workers in dangerous occupations and adaptive techniques to enhance their performance and health. The factors finally indicate the complex interplay between environmental conditions, occupational safety, and overall health outcomes, calling for evidence-based policies to ensure safety and efficiency in many occupational contexts.

KEY TERMS FROM THIS CHAPTER

Air pollution
Chemical toxins
Environmental exposures
Environmental medicine
Exposure assessment
Health disparities
Health inequities
Healthcare providers
IHD mortality risk
Mental wellness
Carpal tunnel syndrome (CTS)
Environmental contaminants
Environmental health practice
Environmental threats
Health consequences
Health education programs
Health outcomes
Heavy metals
Job exposure matrices (JEMs)
Multidimensional analysis techniques

CRITICAL THINKING QUESTIONS

1. **Which of the following best describes the historical origin of environmental and occupational medicine?**
   a. It began with the Industrial Revolution due to increased factory-related illnesses.
   b. It started during the 20th century with the rise of chemical industries.
   c. It originated in ancient times with recognition of occupational diseases among miners and craftsmen.
   d. It was established after World War II in response to nuclear hazards.
2. **Which of the following is NOT typically considered an environmental health hazard?**
   a. Air pollution
   b. Noise pollution
   c. Radiation exposure
   d. Ergonomic stress at a workstation
3. **Which occupational health risk is most commonly associated with prolonged exposure to asbestos?**
   a. Hearing loss
   b. Lung cancer and mesothelioma
   c. Skin dermatitis
   d. Lead poisoning
4. **What is the primary purpose of biological monitoring in the assessment of health issues from hazardous exposures?**
   a. To measure the concentration of hazardous chemicals in the environment
   b. To evaluate clinical symptoms in workers exposed to hazards
   c. To detect levels of chemicals or their metabolites in biological samples from exposed individuals
   d. To implement workplace safety protocols
5. **Which preventive strategy is most effective in reducing occupational health risks?**
   a. Providing personal protective equipment (PPE) only after exposure symptoms appear
   b. Implementing engineering controls to eliminate or reduce exposure at the source
   c. Conducting annual health check-ups without modifying workplace conditions
   d. Relying solely on administrative policies without physical interventions

Short Answer Questions

1. What are the main health effects of prolonged exposure to fine particulate matter (PM2.5) in air pollution?
2. Name three common categories of workplace hazards and provide one example for each.
3. What methods are commonly used to assess an individual's exposure to environmental toxins?
4. Why is a detailed occupational exposure history essential in diagnosing work-related illnesses?

Answers to Critical Thinking Questions

1. (c); 2. (d); 3. (b); 4. (c); 5. (b)

REFERENCES

1. Smith, T. O., Jepson, P., Beswick, A., Sands, G., Drummond, A., Davis, E. T., & Sackley, C. M. (2016). Assistive devices, hip precautions, environmental modifications and training to prevent dislocation and improve function after hip arthroplasty. *The Cochrane database of systematic reviews*, *7*(7), CD010815. https://doi.org/10.1002/14651858.CD010815.pub2(accessed on 27th June 2025).

2. Harrison, V., & Mackenzie Ross, S. (2016). Anxiety and depression following cumulative low-level exposure to organophosphate pesticides. *Environmental research*, *151*, 528–536. https://doi.org/10.1016/j.envres.2016.08.020(accessed on 27th June 2025).

3. Dale, A. M., Jaegers, L., Welch, L., Gardner, B. T., Buchholz, B., Weaver, N., & Evanoff, B. A. (2016). Evaluation of a participatory ergonomics intervention in small commercial construction firms. *American journal of industrial medicine*, *59*(6), 465–475. https://doi.org/10.1002/ajim.22586(accessed on 27th June 2025).

4. Holdier, A.G. (2016). Holdier, A. G. (2016). Speciesistic Veganism: An Anthropocentric Argument. In Jodey Castricano & Rasmus Rahbek Simonsen, Critical Perspectives on Veganism. United Kingdom: Palgrave-Macmillan. pp. 41-66.(accessed on 27th June 2025).

5. Martin, A., Karanika-Murray, M., Biron, C., and Sanderson, K. (2016) The Psychosocial Work Environment, Employee Mental Health and Organizational Interventions: Improving Research and Practice by Taking a Multilevel Approach. *Stress Health*, 32: 201–215. doi: 10.1002/smi.2593.(accessed on 27th June 2025).

6. Lombardo, L. J., & Balmes, J. R. (2000). Occupational asthma: a review. *Environmental health perspectives*, *108 Suppl 4*(Suppl 4), 697–704. https://doi.org/10.1289/ehp.00108s4697(accessed on 27th June 2025).

7. Kyle AD, Balmes JR, Buffler PA, Lee PR. Integrating research, surveillance, and practice in environmental public health tracking. *Environ Health Perspect*. 2006;114(7):980-984. doi:10.1289/ehp.8735 (accessed on 27th June 2025).

8. Bruyere, S. M., Peterson, D., & VanLooy, S. (2005). The International Classification of Functioning, Disability and Health: Contemporary literature overview. https://core.ac.uk/download/5124461.pdf (accessed on 27th June 2025).

9. Canali, S. (2020). What is new about the exposome? Exploring scientific change in contemporary epidemiology. https://core.ac.uk/download/323306328.pdf (accessed on 27th June 2025).

10. Coastal Response Research Center. (2019). *2019 State-of-the-Science of Dispersants and Dispersed Oil (DDO) in U.S. Arctic Waters: Public Health and Food Safety*. https://core.ac.uk/download/215540593.pdf (accessed on 27th June 2025).

11. Amelie F. Constant & Bienvenue N. Tien & Klaus F. Zimmermann & Jingzhou Meng, 2010. "**China's Overt Economic Rise and Latent Human Capital Investment: Achieving Milestones and Competing for the Top**," Discussion Papers of DIW Berlin 1062, DIW Berlin, German Institute for Economic Research.(accessed on 27th June 2025).

12. Costello, S., Cullen, M. R., Eisen, E. A., Hammond, S. K., et al. (2016). Ischemic heart disease incidence in relation to fine versus total particulate matter exposure in a U.S. aluminum industry cohort. https://core.ac.uk/download/323081294.pdf (accessed on 27th June 2025).

13. Evanoff, B., Zeringue, A., Franzblau, A., & Dale, A. M. (2014). Using job-title-based physical exposures from O*NET in an epidemiological study of carpal tunnel syndrome. *Human factors, 56*(1), 166–177. https://doi.org/10.1177/0018720813496567(accessed on 27th June 2025).
14. Kaskutas V, Jaegers L, Dale AM, Evanoff BA. Toolbox Talks: Insights for Improvement. *Prof Saf.* 2016;None:33-37. (accessed on 27th June 2025).
15. Davies, Terry & Lowe, Adam I., 1999. "**Environmental Implications of the Health Care Service Sector**," Discussion Papers 10857, Resources for the Future.(accessed on 27th June 2025).
16. Suddick, K. M., & De Souza, L. H. (2007). Therapists' experiences and perceptions of teamwork in neurological rehabilitation: Critical happenings in effective and ineffective teamwork. *Journal of Interprofessional Care, 21*(6), 669–686. https://doi.org/10.1080/13561820701722634(ac cessed on 27th June 2025).
17. Fallon, E., Bopp, M., & Webb, B. L. (2013). Factors associated with faith-based health counselling in the United States: Implications for dissemination of evidence-based behavioral medicine. *Health & Social Care in the Community, 21*(2), 129–139. https://www.semanticscholar.org/paper/4b05ac3f88f7170e02b45e64c906c905cc631380 (accessed on 27th June 2025).
18. Uibel, S., Scutaru, C., Mueller, D., Klingelhoefer, D., Hoang, D. M., Takemura, M., Fischer, A., Spallek, M. F., Unger, V., Quarcoo, D., & Groneberg, D. A. (2012). Mobile air quality studies (MAQS) in inner cities: particulate matter PM10 levels related to different vehicle driving modes and integration of data into a geographical information program. *Journal of occupational medicine and toxicology (London, England), 7*(1), 20. https://doi.org/10.1186/1745-6673-7-20 (accessed on 27th June 2025).
19. Forouzanfar, M. H., Alexander, L., Anderson, H. R., Bachman, V. F., Biryukov, S., Bräuer, M., Burnett, R., et al. (2016). Global, regional, and national comparative risk assessment of 79 behavioral, environmental and occupational, and metabolic risks or clusters of risks, 1990–2015: A systematic analysis for the Global Burden of Disease Study 2015. *The Lancet, 388*, 1659–1724. https://doi.org/10.1016/s0140-6736(16)31679-8 (accessed on 27th June 2025).
20. Groneberg-Kloft, B., Klingelhöfer, D., Scutaru, C., Zitnik, M., et al. (2013). Traffic medicine–related research: A scient metric analysis. https://core.ac.uk/download/16213823.pdf (accessed on 27th June 2025).
21. Guidotti, T. (2018). Environmental health needs a new paradigm, I. Getting back in focus. *Archives of Environmental & Occupational Health, 73*, 267–269. https://www.semanticscholar.org/paper/8c141001cd94a5294073d08bc1e432bd0f573b2e (accessed on 27th June 2025).
22. Miraglia, M., & Johns, G. (2016). Going to work ill: A meta-analysis of the correlates of presenteeism and a dual-path model. *Journal of occupational health psychology, 21*(3), 261–283. https://doi.org/10.1037/ocp0000015(accessed on 27th June 2025).
23. Kamel Boulos MN, Le Blond J. On the road to personalised and precision geomedicine: medical geology and a renewed call for interdisciplinarity. *Int J Health Geogr.* 2016;15:5. Published 2016 Jan 28. doi:10.1186/s12942-016-0033-0(accessed on 27th June 2025).
24. Karanika-Murray, M., & Weyman, A. K. (2013). Optimising workplace interventions for health and well-being: A commentary on the limitations of the public health perspective within the workplace health arena. *International Journal of Workplace Health Management , 6*(2),

104-117. Article 17089837. https://doi.org/10.1108/IJWHM-11-2011-0024(accessed on 27th June 2025).

25. Khalade, A., Jaakkola, M. S., Pukkala, E., & Jaakkola, J. J. (2010). Exposure to benzene at work and the risk of leukemia: a systematic review and meta-analysis. *Environmental health : a global access science source, 9*, 31. https://doi.org/10.1186/1476-069X-9-31(accessed on 27th June 2025).

26. Lethbridge, J. (2008). Occupational health regulations and health workers: Protection or vulnerability? https://core.ac.uk/download/67329.pdf (accessed on 27th June 2025).

27. Morse, Tracy and Lungu, Kingsley and Taulo, Steven (2010) Gap Analysis of Environmental Health Research in Malawi : Report to the National Commission of Science and Technology. National Commission for Science and Technology (Malawi), Malawi.(accessed on 27th June 2025).

28. Mashigo, M., Risenga, I., & Dukhan, S. (2024). First-year health sciences students' perspectives on indigenous knowledge and medical practices. *African Journal of Research in Mathematics, Science and Technology Education, 28*, 422–436. https://www.semanticscholar.org/paper/64b61d8118e4f5810793bf1350c2a56365b51b77 (accessed on 27th June 2025).

29. Mourad, H. (2024). Biomonitoring in occupational medicine (Review article). *Egyptian Journal of Occupational Medicine.* https://www.semanticscholar.org/paper/5cbd162d4be4a7c2af8fd955781258e08eb8e8e3 (accessed on 27th June 2025).

30. Moussa, A., Hayouni, M. M., Rassas, I., Merchaoui, I., & Amri, C. (2024). P-158 5P medicine: A digital twin model for hospital-based occupational medicine. *Occupational Medicine.* https://www.semanticscholar.org/paper/2c03afb2b0596bfce2a27d8fcfba94dd574b7156 (accessed on 27th June 2025).

31. Nadri, H., Khavanin, A., Kim, I. J., Akbari, M., Nadri, F., & Yeganeh, R. (2024). Association between noise-induced hearing loss and vestibular dysfunction in workers chronically exposed to occupational noise. *Indian Journal of Occupational and Environmental Medicine, 28*, 189–193. https://www.semanticscholar.org/paper/73c8da8b7aa68d07b6589177525879178c74f4d4 (accessed on 27th June 2025).

32. Chapman, J. & Naweed, A. (2015). Health initiatives to target obesity in surface transport industries: Review and implications for action. Evidence Base, issue 2, 2015, , ISSN 1838-9422, version 1 https://core.ac.uk/download/pdf/30671333.pdf (accessed on 27th June 2025).

33. Tomes, C., Orr, R.M. & Pope, R. The impact of body armor on physical performance of law enforcement personnel: a systematic review. *Ann of Occup and Environ Med* **29**, 14 (2017). https://doi.org/10.1186/s40557-017-0169-9(accessed on 27th June 2025).

34. Peters, S., & Hall, A. (2021). Is a JEM an informative exposure assessment tool for night shift work? *Occupational and Environmental Medicine, 78*, 780–781. https://www.semanticscholar.org/paper/da1ffbda5786be41cb9e9431de27025f7cc78c11 (accessed on 27th June 2025).

35. Pouliakas, K., & Theodossiou, I. (2010). An inquiry into the theory, causes and consequences of monitoring indicators of health and safety at work. https://core.ac.uk/download/177141.pdf (accessed on 27th June 2025).

36. Rovira Puig, M., Mbonaga, S. S., Seco, J., & Chacha, N. (2024). P-453 Assessing gas emissions from fecal sludge fuel briquettes; good practices for tackling occupational safety and health

concerns in Tanzania. *Occupational Medicine.* https://www.semanticscholar.org/paper/21bdc594b29c1e2a94a9ee8e66b85ff5b2664c35 (accessed on 27th June 2025).

37. Samad, M. A. (2025). A systematic review of bacterial zoonotic diseases in the light of 'One Health' approach with multidrug resistance status in Bangladesh. *Journal of Veterinary Medical and One Health Research.* https://www.semanticscholar.org/paper/e37c68e79b37e2241b29a8b570dec93d34e0ff3a (accessed on 27th June 2025).
38. Sharma, A., & Mandal, B. B. (2024). A critical assessment of boundary limits of health risks associated with WBV exposure based on field studies on LHD vehicles in Indian underground coal mines. *Indian Journal of Occupational and Environmental Medicine, 28*, 198–206. https://www.semanticscholar.org/paper/657517549f9e945622ffa4ecaa926b283860dfea (accessed on 27th June 2025).
39. Sikes, R. S. (2016). 2016 Guidelines of the American Society of Mammalogists for the use of wild mammals in research and education. *Journal of Mammalogy, 97*, 663–688. https://doi.org/10.1093/jmammal/gyw078 (accessed on 27th June 2025).
40. Tran, M., & Sokas, R. K. (2017). The gig economy and contingent work. *Journal of Occupational and Environmental Medicine, 59*, e63–e66. https://doi.org/10.1097/jom.0000000000000977 (accessed on 27th June 2025).

EMERGENCY MEDICINE IN GENERAL PRACTICE

7

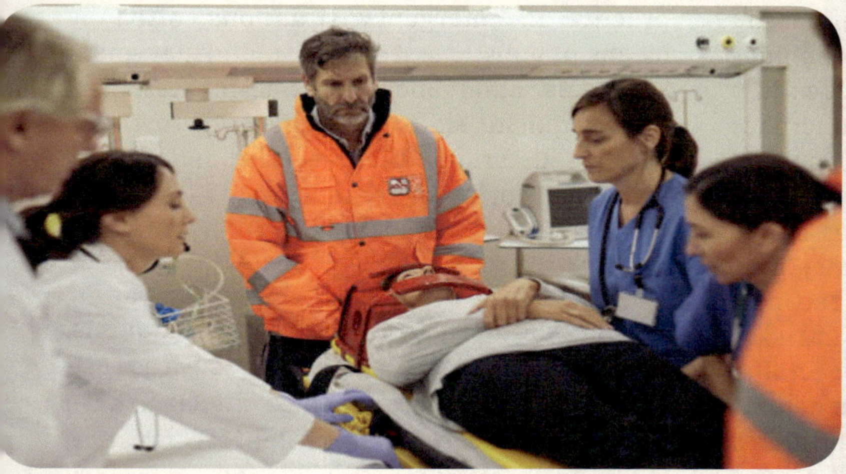

LEARNING OBJECTIVES

After studying this chapter, you will be able to:

1. Explain the role of general practitioners in emergency situations;
2. Describe common emergencies encountered in general practice;
3. Discuss training and skills required for general practitioners;
4. Focus on challenges faced by general practitioners in emergency medicine;
5. Understand the integration of technology in emergency medicine;
6. Deal with case studies and real-life applications.

Introduction

Emergency medicine, a health care necessity, is a vital component in the context of general practice settings, which endeavor to address acute medical conditions requiring immediate treatment. Incorporating emergency medicine into general practice not only enhances the capacity of PCPs but also optimizes patient results through timely interventions. As general practitioners (GPs) are often the first contact point for patients, equipping them with the necessary skills and knowledge to handle emergencies can significantly contribute to reducing morbidity and mortality from acute medical conditions. Furthermore, such inclusion allows for a more comprehensive approach to patient handling, bridging the difference between emergency and routine health handling. Incorporating emergency medicine education into general practice involves various strategies, including the implementation of standardized guidelines and protocols that facilitate effective decision-making within acute environments. Creating these protocols should prioritize evidence-based practice, the most important aspect to ensure maximum delivery of care within emergency environments. For instance, more recent contributions to health care research highlight the importance of having a formal system for the management of conditions that are common in general practice, such as low back pain, which, if left untreated can progress to severe disability. Systematic review has shown that more than 50% of individuals with low back pain present to the doctor, and hence there is a need for efficient emergency care in general practice in order to enable the correct identification and management of such conditions (Buchbinder et al., 2020). Furthermore, the dynamic nature of emergency medicine necessitates adherence to continuous education and training for GPs. Remaining current with contemporary research, treatments, and best practices is necessary to optimize the effectiveness of emergency care provided within general practice settings. For promoting knowledge transfer and skill acquisition, collaboration with specialist emergency medical practitioners is also helpful. Second, in establishing the Medical Research Council's revised framework, there is a need to prioritize research on emergency medicine interventions in primary care so that their effectiveness and efficiency can be maximized (Skivington et al., 2021). Lastly, expanding the role of emergency medicine in general practice not only improves patient outcomes but also builds a more flexible and responsive healthcare system.

Definition of Emergency Medicine

Emergency medicine is a distinct field of medicine that has emerged to deal with the acute, often life-threatening illnesses presented in the clinical setting. It embraces a broad spectrum of cases, from trauma, cardiac arrests, and acute disease, where prompt diagnosis and intervention are needed. Being an action-oriented field, emergency medicine requires specialized training and skills in healthcare providers to rapidly assess and stabilize patients. The extent of emergency medicine further extends beyond intervention during crises alone; it further entails the utilization of protocols and debriefing mechanisms in a bid to boost clinical outcomes, as well as maintain performance standards in cases involving acute care. The specialty is thus a crucial component of the healthcare system, with the vision of having patients get speedy and effective interventions at the moment that they need them most (Nadir et al., 2016). Emergency medicine is characterized by its patient-focused practice in emergency situations, often by means of holistic assessment and management strategies. Emergency medicine professionals with requisite skills have the duty to triage patients, determine their severity, and classify them by priority for treatment.

The ED environment is changing, typically exposed to a variety of factors such as volume and variety of patient presentations. Incorporation of existing practices, such as real-time debriefing, through which clinicians have a clear time to reflect and improve practice, is key to the attainment of a good emergency care environment. Debriefing procedures help ensure teamwork and communication among health care practitioners with the overall goal of shaping the general objective of promoting best patient outcomes in emergency medical facilities (Nadir et al., 2016). Besides, the connection between emergency medicine and general practice is becoming increasingly vital to the broader health environment. Many of those visiting EDs have conditions that can be handled by their regular doctors, hence system inefficiencies.

Consequently, interventions have been established to decongest EDs by opening up more efficient access to primary care services, particularly in non-emergency situations. By redeeming the boundaries between emergency medicine and general practice, the healthcare system can better allocate resources and make sure that EDs are kept available for true emergencies. With such collaboration, a more efficient process of healthcare provision is achieved, addressing the problems of the patients more efficiently (Figure 7.1).

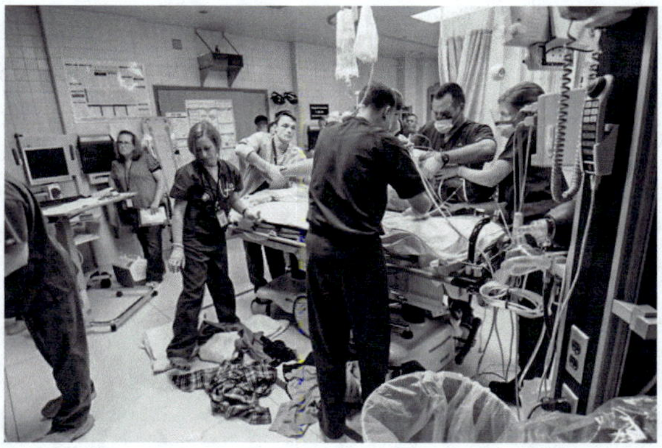

Figure 7.1. Emergency physicians conducting a trauma resuscitation.

Source: https://upload.wikimedia.org/wikipedia/commons/a/a3/10530-banner-Lives625-6-14.jpg.

Importance of Emergency Medicine in General Practice

Integrating emergency medicine in general practice is important on several accounts with the prime being towards enhancing patient outcome. The essence of emergency conditions is that it is high priority to take rapid decisions and act upon them; thus, having a sound foundation in emergency medicine gives GPs the skillset to deal with such exigent situations. For instance, studies prove that early intervention in the form of imaging and procedural handling is directly proportional to better morbidity and mortality outcomes in trauma. It is particularly relevant to pediatric populations, where effective trauma protocol reduced time to necessary imaging and surgical intervention and has led to better outcomes. By understanding and applying emergency procedures, GPs can ensure that the patient is given the right and timely care, which is crucial in avoiding complications as well as maximizing recovery processes (Nti et al., 2019). Further, the coming together of emergency medicine and general practice not only addresses immediate health issues but also maximizes the productivity of healthcare systems as a whole. If GPs are adequately trained in emergency situations, it cuts down on unnecessary referrals to specialists and EDs, thus ultimately leading to reduced overcrowding in these facilities.

Particularly in urban areas where EDs experience patient volumes that are unbearable. For example, it comes out in surveys that the majority of acute complainants, such as those with chest pains, can have the underlying issues—such as substance abuse—that are easily addressed by competent GPs. This dual approach—confronting the emergency cases while stabilizing core chronic conditions—results in an integrated hospital delivery system that is responsive to patient demand and is cost-efficient (Meredith et al., 2004). Lastly, the incorporation of emergency medicine into general practice allows medical practitioners to take preventive steps that are likely to thwart the occurrence of emergencies.

Early detection of risk factors and symptoms allows GPs to deploy preventive measures that minimize the occurrence of acute medical conditions. Education and training in emergency medicine work to not only enhance clinical expertise but also instill a culture of readiness among medical practitioners. This is vital in guaranteeing community health resilience, especially in disaster-risk or public health emergency zones. As such, GPs not only respond first in the event of emergencies but also serve as agents of importance for public health, encouraging preventive care habits that eventually reduce the burden on emergency medical services (EMS) and improve population health (Nti et al., 2019).

7.1. Role of General Practitioners in Emergency Situations

Learning Outcome

1. Understand initial assessment and triage;
2. Focus on stabilization of patients;
3. Deal with referral to specialized care.

In emergency care, GPs have a pivotal role that extends well beyond their routine clinical case load. Being drawn into the immediacy of emergency situations, either acute medical emergencies or life-threatening disasters, allows for more holistic treatment of patients. With their in-depth understanding of patients' medical histories, GPs can quickly assess and establish priorities for treatment, thus being of huge value in processing cases in emergencies. By virtue of their knowledge of local healthcare services and facilities, GPs are well-placed to coordinate additional treatment, e.g., emergency referrals and continuity care. This role is particularly salient in the setting of community health, where GPs often lead public outreach efforts tasked with educating individuals on how to recognize emergency signs, thus enhancing the general level of resilience in the community towards medical emergencies (Bickerton et al., 2010). In addition, GPs' ability to face ethnic and cultural diversity in emergent circumstances speaks volumes regarding their role in ensuring equitable access to healthcare. With the increase in population heterogeneity within communities, GPs play a central role in addressing racially and ethnically heterogeneous patients. Racial and ethnic differences in healthcare delivery have been proven to result in significant health inequalities (Wankhede et al., 2014). With cultural competence and patient-specific information, GPs are able to overcome language barriers and cultural misperceptions that lead to discontinuity in care. By doing so, not only do they facilitate continuity and trust between clinicians and patients, but they also improve clinical judgment and diagnostic acumen. Through active participation and being aware of the unique contexts of their diverse patient populations, GPs can ensure that lifesaving medical interventions are optimally tailored and successfully applied in emergency cases. Additionally, the role of GPs in emergency situations is emphasized through the fact that they can provide immediate and life-saving treatments. Where time is of the essence, GPs are also capable of conducting speedy assessments and starting treatment procedures pending specialist emergency services.

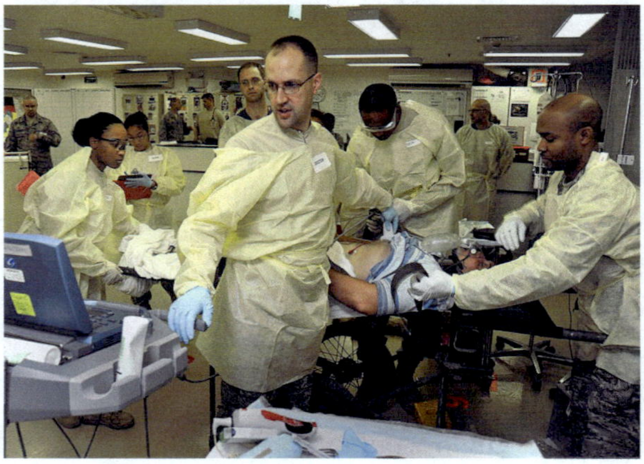

Figure 7.2. Medical personnel simulate emergency treatment.

Source: https://upload.wikimedia.org/wikipedia/commons/thumb/3/3b/Emergency_medicine_simulation_training_exercise_in_Balad%2C_Iraq.jpg/800px-Emergency_medicine_simulation_training_exercise_in_Balad%2C_Iraq.jpg.

Their exposure to emergency identification and management, coupled with their ability to perform core procedures such as airway management or cardiac resuscitation, renders them essential first responders in the health system. In addition to that, GPs frequently participate in emergency readiness training, which allows them to gain skills valuable in efficiently responding to mass casualty incidents or public health crises. This active participation not only improves individual GP abilities but also strengthens the entire emergency response system in communities such that there is organized health crisis management (Bickerton et al., 2010) (Figure 7.2).

7.1.1. Initial Assessment and Triage

In the field of emergency medicine, triage and initial assessment are critical elements in having efficient control over patient care. This is accomplished through the systematic assessment of patients on arrival at EDs, where health practitioners rapidly establish the severity of their conditions. An effectively carried out initial evaluation not only allows for the prioritization of patients based on the urgency of their needs but also streamlines the whole process within healthcare facilities. Additionally, the process of triage should be adaptable enough to accommodate the dynamic health setting in order to allow for a customized response to differing patient profiles. Utilization of structured triage systems ensures that resources are utilized effectively, taking into consideration the added pressures put upon emergency services by contemporary society. Triage practices may vary widely between health systems, and both the strengths and weaknesses of use should be apparent. For example, in Indonesia, the existing triage system does not seem as solid as other nations' because a great number of hospitals utilize a rather primitive sorting process that tends not to integrate re-triage properly. Rochana et al. (2016) state that although some features of Indonesian triage are consistent with the rest of the world, the lack of a systematized re-triage process is of concern regarding efficiency as well as patient outcome. This identifies the necessity of ongoing evaluation and updating of the triage protocols to ensure that they represent evolving healthcare needs and that they support enhanced patient care. An important consideration in the triage is the role played by healthcare professionals in the assessment of potential risk factors that are associated with conditions presented. For instance, the detection of substance abuse, such as cocaine, among patients with chest pain, is significant while providing certain interventions and appropriate management plans. The identification of this issue indicates that a large proportion of patients are bound to come with drug-related undiagnosed complications, which obscure their clinical picture (Meredith et al., 2004). Therefore, inculcating in-depth assessments of incorporating identification of such risk factors in the process of triage is necessary to ensure effective emergency response. By prioritizing comprehensive assessments, healthcare practitioners can improve PS and health outcomes, and ultimately uphold the overall tenets of emergency medicine in daily practice (Figure 7.3).

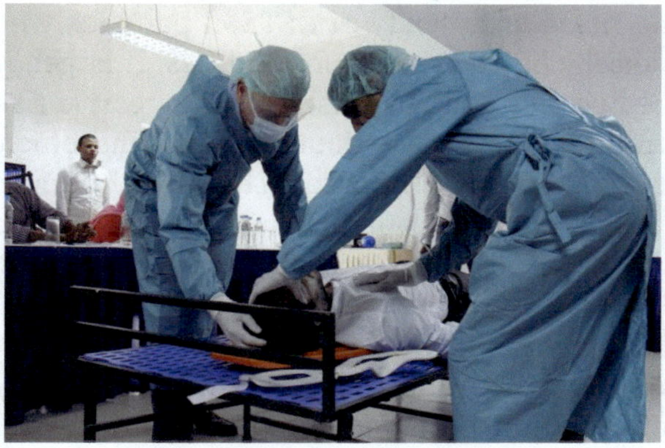

Figure 7.3. Initial assessment.

Source: https://www.icrc.org/sites/default/files/wysiwyg/Bangladesh/_mg_4880low.jpg.

7.1.2. Stabilization of Patients

In emergency medicine, the stabilization of patients is a critical preliminary process in the management of acute medical conditions. Stabilization is the immediate assessment and management of life-threatening conditions, respecting the priority needs of the patient. For instance, adherence to the Emergency

Medical Treatment and Labor Act (EMTALA) focuses on the legal and ethical obligation of health workers to stabilize patients as a precondition for referral to another hospital. The prevalence of EMTALA violations for obstetric emergencies registers egregious disparities in recognizing and meeting pregnant patients' needs. Out of 232 EMTALA settlements, nearly 40% were for obstetric emergencies, wherein the majority alleged failures to conduct appropriate screening examinations and stabilizing treatment, indicating an urgent need for education on the part of EDs to perform stabilization appropriately to avoid negligence and give PS (Terp et al., 2020). The importance of effective patient stabilization is also valid in cardiovascular emergencies, including non-ST-segment elevation myocardial infarction (NSTEMI). The condition necessitates immediate intervention, in which the oxygen supply and demand of the myocardium are optimized. With the rising complexity of NSTEMI patients, who typically have several comorbidities, emergency medicine physicians must apply aggressive risk stratification along with tailored pharmacologic regimens. Guideline-based instructions optimize patient outcome potential and minimize the likelihood of readmission or recurrent events. By being adept at the continuum of NSTEMI management, emergency medical personnel can better coordinate care and institute timely interventions, thus highlighting the pivotal role of stabilization in improved prognoses for patients presenting with acute coronary syndromes (Amin et al., 2019). In comprehending the vital significance of stabilizing patients, it is obvious that ongoing education and training are crucial to health practitioners working in emergency medicine. Investment in more robust training programs that focus on compliance with emergency protocol and assessment scenarios will be capable of providing practitioners with the means to deal with a variety of emergencies efficiently. This proactive approach is especially important in environments where resources that are currently available may be scarce, and timely decision-making can significantly impact patient outcomes. Further, developing a knowledge base of the legal framework surrounding patient stabilization, for example, under circumstances of EMTALA violation, enables medical professionals to successfully navigate the intricacies of emergency care. This pledge ensures patients receive the comprehensive, effective treatment they need in times of need, thereby assisting with the principal guidelines of emergency medicine within general practice (Figure 7.4).

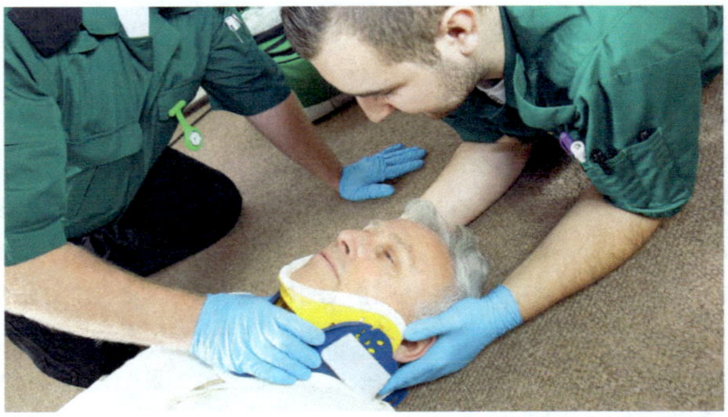

Figure 7.4. Manually stabilize a patient's head.

Source: https://www.c2cfirstaidaquatics.com/wp-content/uploads/2021/04/methods-to-manually-stabilize-a-patient-s-head-Coast2Coast-3-min.jpg.

7.1.3. Referral to Specialized Care

Referral to specialized care is the most important aspect of ensuring that patients receive the optimum care and treatment for their conditions in emergency medicine. GPs are usually faced with complex cases that are more than they can handle in the immediate moment. These types of cases need timely referral to specialists, and this is not only crucial for the patient's outcome, but for the efficiency of the health system as well. By facilitating such referrals, GPs can eliminate delays in diagnosis and treatment and prevent morbidity and mortality from various medical conditions. Such seamless integration of care between the specialists and GPs is crucial, particularly while handling emergent health issues that must be treated urgently and treated as such. Inequities in access to healthcare, however, can contribute significantly to the process of referral for specialist care. Insurance and economic status also typically dictate the extent of care that patients receive, particularly in racial and ethnic minority groups. Literature has suggested that disparities also exist in the diagnosis and treatment of diseases such as heart disease, with factors concerning income and health coverage emerging as barriers to access to specialized care (Mead et al., 2006). Consequently, GPs must possess an acute perception of these difficulties as they navigate through the referral process, so that their patients are not simply informed of their options for specialty treatment but are actually given real paths to those treatments. The tiered model is therefore illustrative of the emphasis on thorough and equitable healthcare provision in the emergency medicine setting. Also, the evolving landscape of specialty healthcare facilities impacts full-service general hospitals and emergency care as much as it impacts general practice. While specialized hospitals and ambulatory surgery centers strive to improve the quality and efficiency of care, literature indicates that their development does not always have a positive impact on full-service general hospitals (De Regge et al., 2013). In fact, the competitive grounds of these specialized centers should be examined critically because their multiplication holds the potential to destabilize healthcare systems as a whole unintentionally. GPs must be attentive to these dynamics so that the referrals to specialist care would not undermine the fundamental premise of an integrated system of healthcare where accessible, patient-centered service at every level of care is the top priority. Recognition of the complex interplay between generic and specific care is crucial in enhancing patient outcomes and maintaining the reputation of emergency medicine (Figure 7.5).

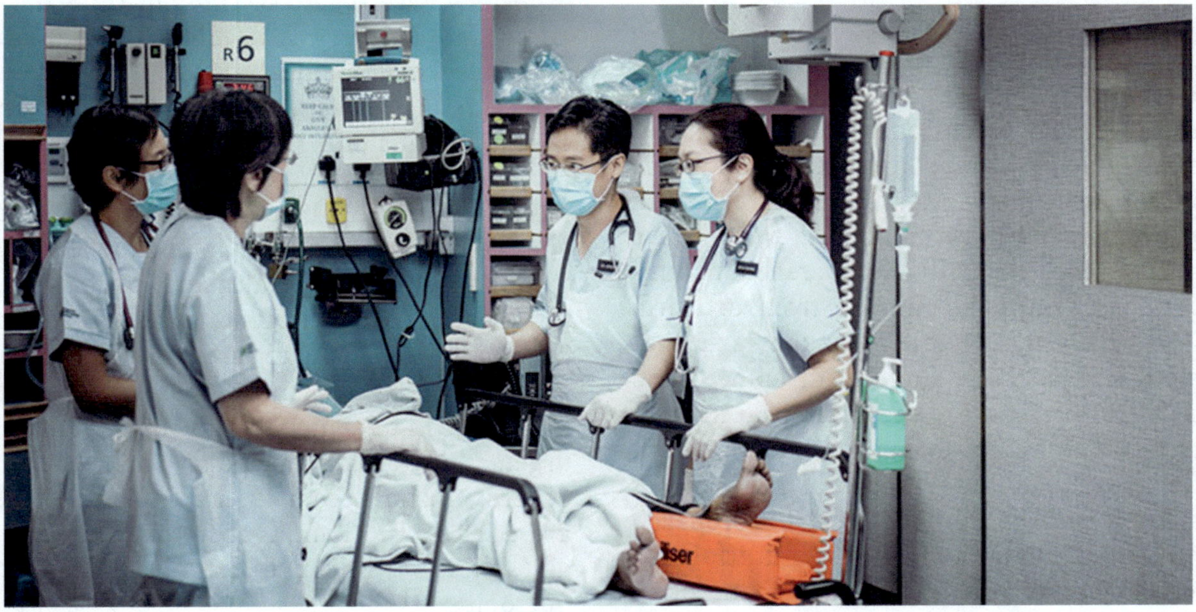

Figure 7.5. Doctors discussing the referral of the patient to specialized care.

Source: https://www.sgh.com.sg/patient-care/specialties-services/PublishingImages/Dept-Banner/EmergencyMedicine.jpg.

Test Your Knowledge

1. How do general practitioners effectively prioritize patients in emergency situations to ensure timely care and appropriate resource allocation?
2. What are the key steps a general practitioner should take to stabilize a critically ill or injured patient?
3. How do general practitioners coordinate referrals to emergency departments or specialists to ensure continuity and effectiveness of care?

7.2. Common Emergencies Encountered in General Practice

Learning Outcome

1. Understand cardiac emergencies;
2. Discuss respiratory distress;
3. Describe trauma and injuries.

In general practice, medical professionals encounter a variety of emergencies that must be addressed quickly and effectively. Acute asthma attacks, allergic reactions, and myocardial infarcts are the common ones to refer to general practitioners as emergencies. Asthma attacks, for instance, tend to get worse very fast, so timely intervention is essential to prevent respiratory failure. Likewise, those patients presenting with allergic reactions may experience symptoms ranging from urticaria that is hardly perceptible to anaphylaxis that is fatal, and so ready supplies of epinephrine and vigorous emergency treatment are required. The ability to quickly stabilize such patients can mean a great deal in terms of outcomes, and hence, GPs must be prepared for various acute conditions. Additionally, emergency gastrointestinal management forms a significant component of general practice consultations. Situations such as appendicitis, bowel obstruction, and gastroenteritis may arise acutely and mandate immediate evaluation and treatment. Appendicitis is typically presented with abdominal pain and might entail potential surgical interventions if not given immediate attention. Bowel obstruction, however, can present in a myriad of ways, and comprehensive evaluation and potentially life-saving interventions might be needed. In order to better manage such situations, GPs are required to have ongoing education and adhere to evidence-based methodologies, thus, optimal care pathways for such emergent states, as observed in the creation of standardized guidelines for handling particular emergencies (Biega, 2024). Obstetrical emergency care is an added set of challenges in general practice, especially with regard to complications during labor and delivery. The EMTALA mandates all emergency medical facilities to provide necessary stabilizing care for emergency conditions, including active labor specifically. However, recently there has been an alarming increase in EMTALA breaches related to obstetric emergencies, reflecting a gap in knowledge and compliance among healthcare professionals (Terp et al., 2020). Incidents such as the lack of conducting an adequate screening examination or not being able to transfer pregnant women in distress in time highlight the importance and urgency of training and policy intervention in general practices to make sure that practitioners are equipped to handle obstetric emergencies and thereby improve fetal and maternal outcomes.

7.2.1. Cardiac Emergencies

Cardiac emergencies are an acute subset of events that occur in daily practice, and they underscore the critical need for practitioners to possess sound knowledge and preparedness. These emergencies, ranging from such events as cardiac arrest, acute myocardial infarction, and unstable angina, require urgent and effective interventions towards the end of enhancing patient outcomes. Proper training in cardiopulmonary resuscitation (CPR) and in the use of automated external defibrillators (AEDs) is important for healthcare workers in general practice. In particular, a review of the literature identifies that school nurses, for instance, say that they are some way prepared to manage sudden cardiac arrest cases, which indicates that the same training model can be used across all healthcare workers dealing with cardiac emergencies, as 44% of participants indicated they had adequate resources and support to efficiently manage such emergencies (Dahlen, 2014). Having an awareness of all forms of cardiac emergencies is crucial in terms of early diagnosis and intervention. GPs must be competent to recognize warning signs of impending cardiac arrest, for example, chest pain, shortness of breath, and arrhythmias, as these are typically premonitory signs of more severe complications. As a result of the aging population, comorbidities make the clinical presentation complicated and require immediate evaluation and intervention. To illustrate, a study on dentists' preparedness to deal with medical emergencies found that recent graduates were more competent in diagnosing and addressing the same than their senior counterparts (de Bedout et al., 2018). This aspect proves the necessity of constant education and training in emergency medicine, not only in dental medicine but for every field of medicine, as it is possible for old techniques to seriously hamper treatment at a critical moment. Combining formal emergency response procedures and regular training sessions is bound to prepare a practitioner for cardiac emergencies to a great extent. A systematic approach, as practiced in hospitals where priority is accorded to emergency response planning, facilitates coordination and reinforces emergency performance. For example, implementing similar procedures utilized in schools to respond to sudden cardiac arrest can transform general practices by ushering in the culture of preparedness. As proposed in existing literature, these response systems need to be tested regularly to allow healthcare practitioners to respond to new challenges in emergency medicine. An effective communication system and regular training prepare practitioners better while providing members of the healthcare team with confidence, ultimately improving patient care (Dahlen, 2014) (Figure 7.6).

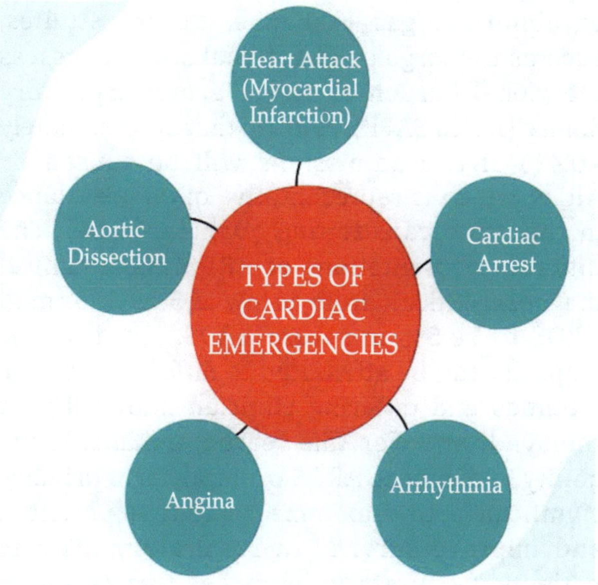

Figure 7.6. Types of cardiac emergencies.

Source: https://linkhospitals.in/blog/cardiac-emergencies:-symptoms-and-types.

7.2.2. Respiratory Distress

Respiratory distress is an acute illness that mandates prompt diagnosis in the field of emergency medicine. It manifests itself as symptoms of shortness of breath, hypoxia, and work of breathing, which can be due to a variety of pathologies, such as infection, allergic disorders, and chronic pulmonary disease. In general practice, particularly, the initial assessment of a patient presenting with respiratory distress is extremely important. Clinicians need to do a comprehensive assessment, such as clinical history, physical examination, and vital sign monitoring, to determine the severity and possible etiology of distress. Early treatment and diagnosis will prevent complications and increase patient outcomes in acute instances significantly, validating the emergent nature of diagnosing this condition in the emergency department. One of the most significant causes of respiratory distress is acute respiratory distress syndrome (ARDS), which is characterized by widespread inflammation in the lungs leading to abnormal gas exchange. Recent studies, such as the large observational study to assess the global burden of severe acute respiratory failure (LUNG SAFE), confirm that approximately 10.4% of ICU admissions will be caused by ARDS, which is representative of its prevalence in the acute care setting (Dahlen, 2014). The different presentations of ARDS make clinical diagnosis difficult, from as low as 51.3% for mild ARDS to 78.5% in severe ARDS. Much of this disparity can be attributed to differing practice methods and differing clinician knowledge of the syndrome. For this reason, enhancing the ability to diagnose ARDS promptly is of primary significance to maximize treatment potential and improve survival in respiratory distress patients. Respiratory distress is treated on an individual case basis, particularly with respect to mechanical ventilation interventions in ARDS patients. Low tidal volume ventilation is required, considering that fewer than two-thirds of ARDS patients are actually receiving sufficient tidal volumes according to recent research (Dahlen, 2014). This underutilization represents a practice deficit that can impact morbidity and mortality quite significantly, as ARDS carries a hospital mortality of only 34.9% for mild cases, increasing to 46.1% for severe cases. Adjunctive therapies such as prone positioning have also been shown to increase oxygenation but remain underused, with the process being implemented in only 16.3% of severely compromised patients. It is important that practitioners of general practice are aware of these guidelines to improve the delivery of care for patients presenting with respiratory distress, with the overall aim of improved clinical outcome (Figure 7.7).

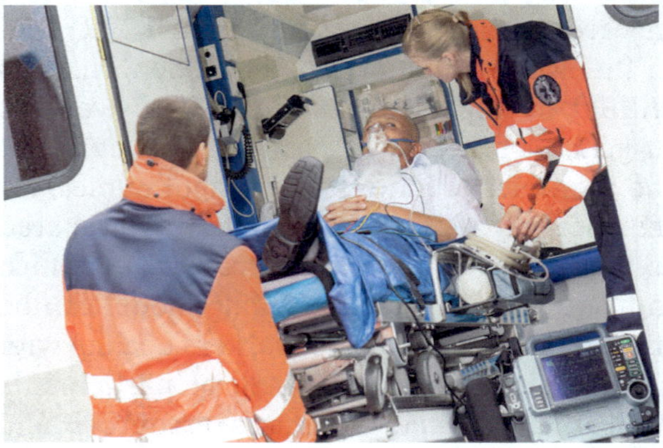

Figure 7.7. An illustration of respiratory emergency.

Source: https://blog.sscor.com/hubfs/Blog/rsz_gettyimages-154972130.png.

7.2.3. Trauma and Injuries

In emergency medicine, the prevalence of injury and trauma makes it a significant task for GPs. In the elderly, the severity of traumatic injury is greater because of existing health conditions that complicate the quality of injuries. For instance, a study at Shinyanga Regional Hospital in Tanzania noted that geriatric trauma was responsible for 22.7% of all admissions for trauma, with the average patient age being 68.5 years. The range of injury prevalence—largely due to assault, falls, and road traffic injury—is a very telling indicator of the imperative need for targeted interventions for this risk group. The findings confirm that elderly trauma not only results in increased hospitalization but is also linked to increased mortality, and this highlights the importance of prevention as well as intervention at an early stage in order to reverse such adverse consequences (Chalya et al., 2012). The causes of trauma and injury are multifactorial, with individual as well as environmental determinants often interacting. In all but a few cases, geriatric patients are at higher risk of suffering injury from falls in their own homes, which accounted for over 81% of the cases in the aforesaid study. This statistic invites interrogation into existing safety and community support measures that are instituted to guard the aged. Furthermore, the prevalence of soft tissue injuries and fractures among this group also creates a critical need for healthcare professionals to act proactively towards injury prevention. With the progress of community education programs and enhancement in the living environments of vulnerable populations, healthcare professionals can play an essential role in preventing such injuries, thereby improving overall health outcomes and lowering healthcare expenditure (Chalya et al., 2012).

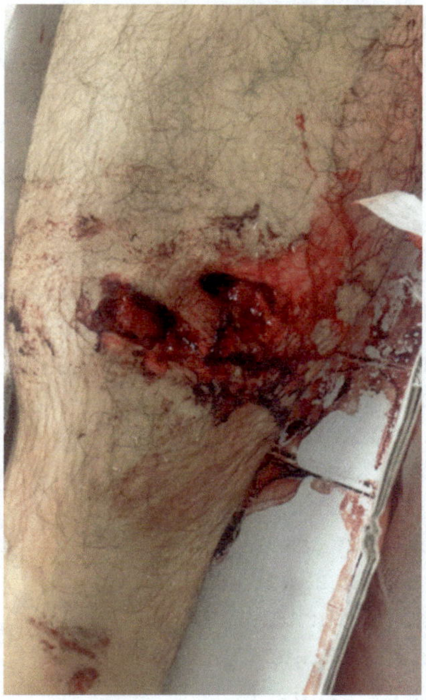

Figure 7.8. The patient, who applied to the emergency department after a gunshot injury, has tibia fracture and severe soft tissue injury in the crural region.

Source: https://www.researchgate.net/publication/378872291/figure/fig1/AS:11431281282472243@1728352202986/The-patient-who-applied-to-the-emergency-department-after-a-gunshot-injury-has-tibia.jpg.

Besides, the integration of research networks in EMS will significantly enhance the level of comprehension of trauma management in general practice. The pediatric emergency care applied research network (PECARN) is a good example of how systematic research culminates into better treatment protocols and improved outcomes for trauma patients. By emphasizing evolving evidence and practice translation, PECARN offers a model which is applicable across all ages, from the elderly. This type of research work is advantageous not only for the development of tailored injury prevention interventions but also for the training of new researchers in the field. This emphasis on education and best evidence practice is important because it guarantees the sustainability and evolution of emergency medicine in a way that assists practitioners in effectively treating trauma and injury in diverse populations (Figure 7.8).

Test Your Knowledge

1. How should a GP assess and manage a patient presenting with acute shortness of breath?
2. What initial steps should a GP follow in managing a patient with suspected head trauma?

7.3. Training and Skills Required for General

Learning Outcome

1. Discuss about medical education and residency;
2. Understand continuing medical education and certifications;
3. Explain practical skills in emergency procedures.

GPs' training is primarily needed to meet the dynamic requirements of emergency medicine in the premises of primary care. The educational system must be robust enough to encompass extensive clinical exposure and organized teaching in fields applicable to emergency cases. Literature thus far has pointed to a critical gap with regard to certain sub-specialties, such as otolaryngology, and this is significant because 25% of the complaints addressed by primary care consist of this specialty. By incorporating certain modules in the emergency management of otolaryngological conditions in the curriculum, GPs can become more competent in managing common conditions, thus improving patient outcomes during emergencies.

Moreover, novel pedagogy in the form of simulation-based education and case-based reasoning must be taken into account as a strategy to address the knowledge gap present within the areas of emergency care and specialist areas, emphasizing the calls for curriculum reform in GP training courses (Thal & Zapanta, 2016). To be able to adequately equip GPs with the diversity of emergencies they may encounter, there is an emphasis on continuous learning and skill acquisition. The more the number of emergency cases, the greater the responsibility of GPs to deal with such cases professionally. Pre-graduation training must be strict with focused attention to emergency medical care (EMC) practice so that practitioners remain competent in resuscitative skills. Critical analyses of professional journals have indicated that the efficiency of emergency care offered by GPs depends directly on the quality of training received. Long-term learning strategies such as workshops, refresher, and joint training programs can enable GPs to maintain pace with evolving practice and emergency care algorithms, in effect preparing them more aptly to tackle emergencies in the community (Dahlen, 2014). Moreover, translation of theoretical knowledge into effective application of skills is critical in GPs' training. In emergency conditions, GPs are normally the first port of call and must be empowered with information and confidence to act quickly. Combining practical sessions of simulation-based learning, where GPs can undergo actual situations with the guidance of experienced mentors, can prove very beneficial. Experiential exposure like this maximizes the practitioner's skill sets in performing assessments and interventions critical in emergency medicine. By stimulating preparedness culture and confirming the theory base of emergency care with practice education, the skill of GPs in emergency situations can be significantly improved in the long term, potentially leading to better patient outcomes in life-threatening medical conditions (Dahlen, 2014).

7.3.1. Medical Education and Residency

The evolution of medical training and residency education, particularly in emergency medicine, has also become increasingly important with the evolving nature of healthcare demands. The practice of emergency medicine has also progressed well, particularly in nations like Oman, where a new national healthcare system is in rapid development. The current progress in local residency training programs and the development of emergency nursing have enhanced the ability of healthcare professionals to provide immediate care. This trend in organizing education in emergency medicine enhances the skill level of professionals and places them at international emergency care standards. The inclusion of formal training pathways assures that emerging clinicians are properly equipped to address the dynamic character of EDs and, by extension, indirectly affect patient outcomes in real-world practice settings (Al-Harthi et al., 2009). Post-simulation debriefings have been emphasized in academic emergency medicine as holding potential for maximizing learning experiences among residents. Studies indicate that early, non-critical incident debriefs have the potential to crystallize educational principles, although much remains unreported on prevalent practices in EDs. The debriefs provide residents with the chance to ponder experience, establishing a culture of constant improvement. Early findings from a New York City multicenter study indicate that clinicians recognize the value of these debriefing processes in educational settings, but a majority report having no formal training in conducting effective debriefings. As more emergency medicine is integrated into primary care, residency programs have to ensure that they prioritize such learning resources so residents are properly equipped for what they will face in practice (Nadir et al., 2016). Cooperation between medical education and the reality of emergency medicine can be a substantial determinant of general practice efficiency as a whole. Since emergency medicine prioritizes the importance of high-stakes, high-pressure decision-making, residency programs need to put a focus on interprofessional collaboration and hands-on training. High-pressure simulation in emergency-type scenarios is necessary to allow residents to concentrate on clinical judgment and communication. In addition, increased focus on building educational infrastructure within emergency medicine allows for networking opportunities and mentorship, key elements for residents whose careers are beginning. By establishing a robust learning environment incorporating hands-on skills in addition to theoretical competence, medical education can ensure that potential practitioners are proficient in emergency settings as well as ready to translate their knowledge to everyday practice, thus enhancing patient care (Al-Azri, 2009; Nadir et al., 2016) (Figure 7.9).

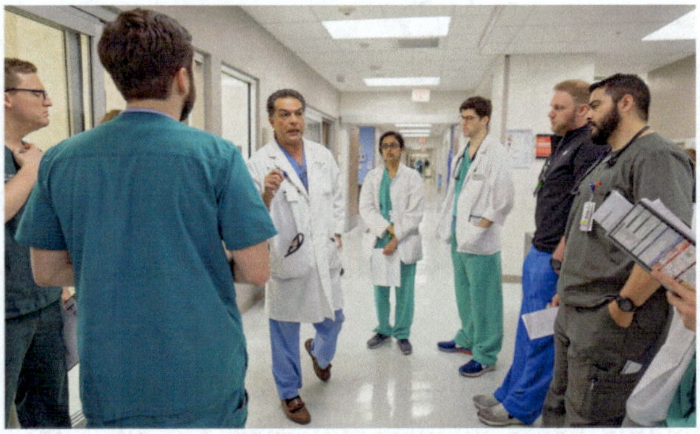

Figure 7.9. Briefing the staffs for emergency situation.

Source: https://lsom.uthscsa.edu/emergency-medicine/wp-content/uploads/sites/144/2020/12/EM-meded-1_2018_EmergencyRoomShots_001_39-800x486.jpg.

7.3.2. Continuing Medical Education (CME) and Certifications

Continuing medical education (CME) is essential in keeping doctors current and proficient, and informed of the evolving trends in emergency medicine. With advancing medical science at a never-before pace, general practice doctors must attend continuous education events to maintain their licensure and certifications. These learning opportunities not only develop clinical skills but also promote the adoption of new procedures and technologies that may assist in improving outcomes for patients. CME is emphasized by the discovery that professionals who pursue such training are more likely to be trusted in making decisions, especially in high-stakes environments like emergency departments. This ongoing education enables them to manage the complexities of emergency cases with ease and some level of preparedness that is a matter of utmost significance in life-or-death cases. Certifications are tangible evidence of a practitioner's dedication to his or her field, particularly in specialties such as emergency care.

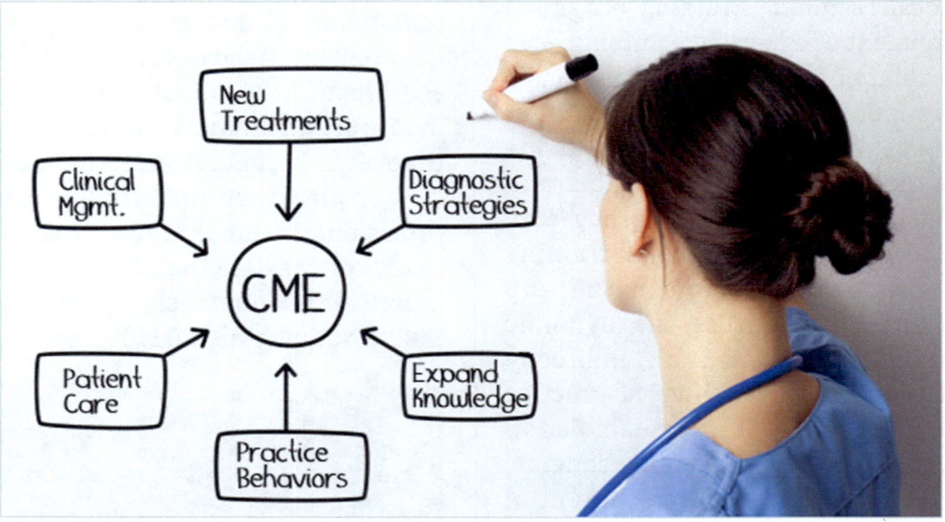

Figure 7.10. Continuing medical education (CME).

Source: https://www.medicalmagazine.in/wp-content/uploads/2020/04/cme-medical-equipment.jpg.

These certifications ensure that the physician has the training and experience necessary to handle acute medical illnesses. For instance, ACLS or trauma life support certifications would positively influence patient survival in emergency situations. These certifications would typically entail participation in intensive training courses as well as adherence to maintenance standards, perhaps in the form of periodic re-certification courses and skills assessment. These organized systems of education equip GPs not only with obedience to the best practice of the moment but also with competency to respond to unforeseen medical events, hence enhancing the overall quality of care during crisis situations. Further, inclusion of simulation-based education (SBE) in CME and certification procedures has been shown to be an innovative method of training healthcare practitioners. This method allows practitioners to rehearse realistic scenarios within a controlled environment, refining their methods without jeopardizing PS. The theory of "deliberate practice," as emphasized in current education policy, reinforces the belief that "practice makes perfect" and plays a vital role in learning complex procedures within emergency medicine. Running low-cost simulation models, as demonstrated in recent studies, can enhance emergency training by means of experiential learning channels. Through the use of these technologies within CME courses, medical instructors can ensure that practitioners are well equipped for everyday as well as emergency events, and thus inculcate a culture of excellence in emergency care (Puentedura et al., 2016; Alinier, 2018) (Figure 7.10).

7.3.3. Practical Skills in Emergency Procedures

Practical skills in emergency care are essential to efficient patient management in general practice settings, where clinicians are usually the initial front line in acute presentations. Competence in skills like airway management, CPR, and wound management is important in stabilizing the patient and improving outcomes. Simulation training courses help practitioners build their skills in simulated environments, so they can tackle the uncertain emergency case environment. For instance, it was discovered through a study that individuals reporting to emergency with chest pain have substance abuse cases and therefore there is a necessity to accelerate the assessment and intervention procedures in emergency units (Meredith et al., 2004). Hence, through rigorous training and genuine field application, medical professionals can achieve the level of competence needed in handling a multitude of emergency situations, ultimately enabling better PS and continuity of care. Of equally paramount importance in the domain of emergency procedures is enforcing procedure protocols for the detection of specific cases, i.e., child abuse in EDs. As frontline professionals, GPs need to know how to recognize and act on signs of abuse, as EDs are likely to be the first point of contact for vulnerable children (Biu et al., 2007). High levels of adherence by EDs in England and Northern Ireland have been reported in relation to written child protection procedures, with 91.3% reporting operational guidelines. These protocols encourage consistency and effective management in instances of suspected abuse. Clinical education courses need not just equip clinicians with the technical skills for immediate action but also emphasize the importance of respecting psychosocial considerations, thereby ensuring that emergency care is balanced. It is this combined focus on practical expertise and sensitivity that is necessary to produce well-rounded practitioners with improved abilities to overcome the pediatric emergency challenges. Lastly, practical skill priority extends beyond individual clinician ability; it incorporates additional priorities on emergency teamwork and communication. Collaborative practice by clinicians is essential in a successful response during emergency scenarios.

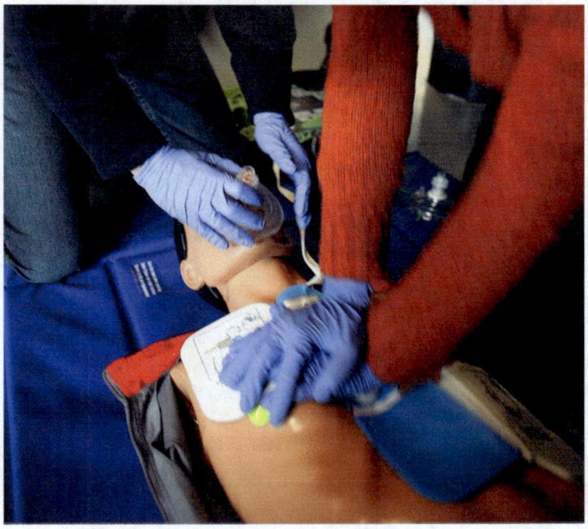

Figure 7.11. Cardiopulmonary resuscitation (CPR) being performed on a medical training.

Source: https://upload.wikimedia.org/wikipedia/commons/thumb/5/58/CPR_training-04.jpg/800px-CPR_training-04.jpg.

For instance, the successful execution of a resuscitation protocol relies on coordination among nurses, physicians, and ancillary staff. Simulating multi-disciplinary team responses can significantly improve the quality of emergency care delivery. Through this team co-operation role-play, health teams are able to counteract the high-speed dynamics of emergencies with more certainty and precision. Strategy and practice in training programs can develop critical thinking and adaptability, enabling emergency medicine specialists to react both with technical expertise and with the ability for leadership and teamwork, thereby enhancing patient outcomes in everyday practice settings (Figure 7.11).

Test Your Knowledge

1. What core emergency medicine competencies are typically included in the medical education and residency training of GPs to prepare them for frontline emergency care?
2. Why is continuing medical education essential for GPs in maintaining proficiency in emergency care?

7.4. Challenges Faced by General Practitioners in Emergency Medicine

Learning Outcome

1. Explain how resource limitations in rural areas impact the delivery of emergency medical services (EMS);
2. Understand time constraints and patient volume;
3. Discuss emotional and psychological stress.

The general practice landscape of emergency medicine has some problems that need to be resolved daily by practitioners. One significant problem here is the unpredictability of emergency cases, which must be met with an immediate, firm response and thereby put GPs under tremendous pressure. These practitioners are handicapped by limited resources at their command, particularly in the management of acute conditions. In rural or deprived environments, the unavailability of specialist medical support can be a compounded version of the issues faced by GPs, forcing them to handle greater variability in medical issues with restricted backup. The need to handle advanced emergencies is one factor that adds to the thinking demands since clinicians have to immediately assess and prioritize interventions, making sure that high levels of patient care are sustained. Communication barriers go a long way in complicating emergency care across various groups of patients. GPs often encounter patients of several racial and ethnic backgrounds, all with their own unique health beliefs and language capacity. Research indicates that differences in the delivery of healthcare result from inadequate cross-cultural communication, leading to potential second-best treatment or misdiagnosis of minority patients (Wankhade et al., 2014). This is particularly critical in emergency care, where the need for speed does not leave time for detailed patient histories or adequate communication plans. The resultant disconnection between patient need and practitioner expectation can destabilize good clinical decision-making, ultimately impairing the quality of care for vulnerable patients. It is thus of paramount importance that communication skills and cultural competence are enhanced in GPs in the emergency setting. Additionally, integration of emergency medicine within general practice tends to emphasize training and preparedness gaps. The majority of GPs may not be equipped with extensive education in relation to emergency procedures since they are trained in preventive care and long-term disease management in primary healthcare. This deficiency creates vagueness in dealing with severe emergencies, thereby affecting patients' outcomes. Ongoing professional development and specialized training sessions aimed at equipping GPs with essential emergency skills are important (Rogers, 2004). Through providing favorable learning and adaptation conditions, healthcare systems can enhance GPs' skills in emergency medicine. In the long term, remedies to such systemic training deficits will enable GPs to effectively meet needs in emergency care and provide quality services to their patients.

7.4.1. Resource Limitations in Rural Areas

The lack of resources in rural areas highly affects the provision of EMS, with particular challenges for general practice. Rural healthcare providers are primarily faced with a lack of both human and technological resources required for effective emergency care. Specialist and advanced medical equipment access is poor, which undermines the ability to handle critical situations when necessary. Moreover, rural areas usually experience logistical challenges in moving patients to larger medical facilities, especially in emergent situations. The effects of such limitations are drastic since they can lead to delayed treatment, poorer patient outcomes, and overall decreased levels of quality care. In light of such challenges, there is a critical need for new innovations that expand resource availability and ensure ready access to EMS in such underserved regions, and thus the necessity of ongoing research and development in this area. The addition of education and training programs designed specifically for rural EMS providers can help to address some of these resource limitations. As examined through various EMS fellowship programs, such as those described by Weston et al. (2020), innovative ways of teaching the curriculum are essential to the formation of medical practitioners capable of practicing effectively within remote communities. These programs adapt their curricula to address the unique needs of rural settings through distance education modules and experiential training to enhance practitioners' ability to respond to emergencies. Furthermore, such education programs can also consolidate healthcare professionals to work together for collaboration and hence improved delivery of emergency services. Providing practitioners with the skills and knowledge needed that are pertinent to the realities of rural healthcare, such programs can fill the EMS gap significantly and end the long-standing hassles created by the scarcity of resources. Apart from training and education, relieving the financial constraints on rural health centers is imperative in order to enhance EMS. The majority of the hospitals and clinics in these areas operate under tight financial constraints that do not allow them to purchase necessary medical equipment or replace critical facilities. The cash flow distress is detailed by a survey represented by Tammy (2011), indicating that the exorbitant cost of labs, equipment, and drugs significantly limits the capacity to perform. Short of resources and financing, rural health facilities cannot sustain providing full services, which may leave individuals within the area vulnerable in times of emergencies. Policymakers need to prioritize financing projects aimed at upgrading rural healthcare facilities so that they are capable of acting in times of emergencies and providing patients with the quality of care that they deserve and need.

7.4.2. Time Constraints and Patient Volume

The intersection of time pressures and patient volumes puts emergency medicine under severe strain. With EDs dealing with increasing patient flow, pressure mounted on emergency physicians (EPs), making patient care and triage decision-making difficult. A recent study points to EPs strongly prioritizing the severity of illness and requirement for ICU interventions over the logistical demands of bed availability in deciding on admissions to intensive care units (ICUs). Approximately 61.3% of EPs mentioned the high volume of patients as a primary concern while dealing with patients on the waiting list for ICU admission, which indicates the intrinsic dilemma between medical necessity and the fact of overcrowded ED settings (Mathews et al., 2020). Thus, understanding time limit dynamics in situations with clinical volumes is crucial for developing strategies to optimize the outcomes of patients and maintain the level of care within the emergency medicine limit. The pandemic of COVID-19 has also added to pre-existing time pressures and patient loads in emergency medicine. The EDs have become flooded with acute infection patients, the majority of whom develop aggravated emotional distress and anxiety due to their health status. This has caused the clinicians to be accountable for not only completing the physical requirements of the patient but also the psychological requirements of the patient. The traditional methods of empathetic communication have been rendered more challenging, predominantly due to increased patient numbers and the constraints imposed by infection control regulations (Sonis et al., 2020). However, despite these challenges, there remains a necessity for prioritizing humanistic care. By implementing strategies to boost empathy and communication, emergency practitioners can establish a friendly environment that listens to patient concerns without disregarding the complex nature of their work. With these challenges in mind, the impact of time pressure and volume of cases in emergency medicine goes beyond immediate clinical decisions to affect the overall experiences of both patients and healthcare providers. The demands of rapid and effective decision-making under pressure may lead to clinician burnout and increased stress levels, ultimately affecting the quality of care delivered. Successful management of these factors requires new solutions that aim at both efficiency and patient-focused care. EDs benefit from embracing system-level reforms such as improved staffing ratios, use of telehealth options for triage of non-emergency patients, and better coordination with outpatient facilities. Such measures may indeed alleviate some of the concomitant burdens with high patient volumes, but ensure EPs remain authorized to provide timely and compassionate care (Mathews et al., 2020; Sonis et al., 2020) (Figure 7.12).

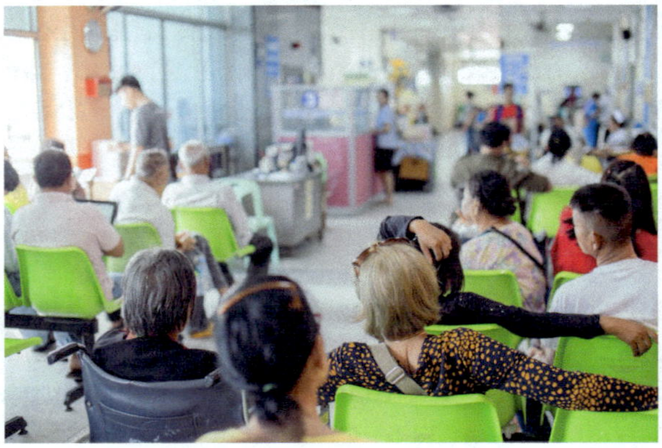

Figure 7.12. High patient volume in emergency care.

Source: https://www.erexpress.com/wp-content/uploads/2023/03/shutterstock_1142067620-scaled.jpg.

7.4.3. Emotional and Psychological Stress

Emotional and psychological stress has a profound impact on healthcare providers, particularly emergency medicine providers. The high-stakes decision-making situation with exposure to traumatic events that accompany emergency care can be a prescription for extreme stress and burnout for providers. Research has shown that medical personnel providing services in emergency departments indicate high levels of emotional distress from long workdays and the severity of patient conditions. This environment can create a cycle of stress that, in addition to affecting the individual doctor, affects the overall quality of patient care. The Accreditation Council for Graduate Medical Education has recognized this as an issue, with initiatives to promote resident wellness and reduce burnout in residency training programs. By utilizing individual-level and system-level interventions, institutions can foster a healthier work environment that can mitigate the destructive consequences of psychological stress among healthcare professionals and enhance care delivery (Parsons et al., 2020). Where emotional stress intersects with patient interaction, particularly in emergency medicine, is of particular interest. Practitioners will, on occasion, be confronted with patients of acute psychological distress from life-threatening situations, which can result in a highly empathetic response. This empathy, though essential to delivering effective patient care, also results in vicarious trauma among health professionals. They are observed grappling with the emotional tolls of their patients' histories, thereby compromising their own psychological well-being. Moreover, the high prevalence of trauma conditions among specific populations—such as Latino and African-American boys—highlighted in more recent research further calls for interventions conducted with trauma-informed care methods to be created. By recognizing and treating the psychological impacts of trauma in patients, emergency medical responders are not only improving patient outcomes but also creating a more effective support clinical environment for themselves and other professionals (Rich et al., 2009). For emergency medicine physicians, managing emotional and psychological stress is not only vital for individual well-being but also for optimal patient care. Effective strategies against these stressors include mindfulness courses, peer support groups, and institutional systems of support for increasing psychological well-being. An urgent requirement for care institutions is addressing mental health programs specifically designed to address the unique stressors that emergency medicine professionals face. With the effective implementation of aggressive well-being programs and open discussion of mental health concerns, one is able to develop clinicians' resilience. Such initiatives can potentially foster a culture of support and compassion, thereby enhancing patient and provider experience in the long run. As the practice adapts with these emerging needs, recognition of emotional and psychological stress as a core component of emergency medicine will drive the development of the resilience and efficacy of healthcare providers (Parsons et al., 2020) (Figure 7.13).

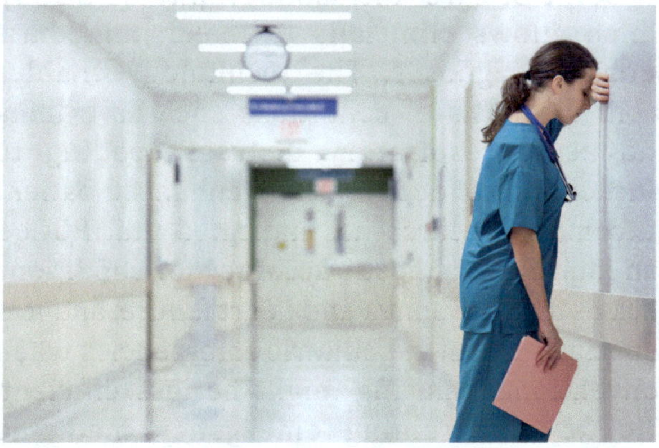

Figure 7.13. A lady doctor with psychological stress.

Source: https://s3-prod.modernhealthcare.com/s3fs-public/022221-feature-iStock-526223747_WEB.jpg.

Test Your Knowledge

1. How do limited medical supplies, equipment, and specialist access in rural or remote areas impact a general practitioner's ability to manage emergency cases effectively?
2. What strategies can general practitioners employ to manage high patient volumes and time-sensitive emergencies?
3. What are the common sources of emotional and psychological stress for GPs in emergency situations?

7.5. Integration of Technology in Emergency Medicine

Learning Outcome

1. Understand telemedicine and remote consultations;
2. Discuss the role of electronic health records and data management;
3. Explain the use of mobile applications for emergency protocols.

The application of technology in emergency care has significantly transformed the patient care environment, enhancing both diagnostic processes and treatment efficacy. Among the significant enhancements is the application of point-of-care ultrasonography (POCUS), which allows clinicians to make immediate bedside diagnoses. The technology enables rapid diagnosis of conditions such as trauma and acute respiratory distress, leading to quicker clinical decisions and enhanced patient outcomes. Research has indicated that POCUS can improve diagnostic accuracy for conditions such as acute dyspnea and heart failure, and it is especially useful in pediatric emergencies when conventional imaging might be less efficient. The key to training emergency medicine residents in POCUS is to guarantee that the full potential of this technology is fulfilled in practice, ultimately making EDs more efficient care settings (Hashim et al., 2023). Secondly, the interoperability of EHRs has reduced the manipulation of patient records, and it has enhanced inter-professional communication. The retrievability of patient history, allergies, and drug interactions is enhanced by EHRs, which is very critical in emergency situations when time is of the essence. Technology not only facilitates immediate access to patient records but also real-time documentation of care, reducing the errors that impact PS. Moreover, integration of EHRs with telemedicine allows for specialist consultations, providing immediate expert assessment to guide treatment plans. Such collaboration is the best manifestation of how technology not only enhances patient care but also broader health care systems by ensuring continuity of care and collaborative practice among professionals (Hashim et al., 2023). Finally, technologies such as machine learning and AI are beginning to have an influence in emergency medicine through predictive analytics that can identify at-risk patients in advance. These technologies can dig through vast databases to recognize patterns or anomalies that might be overlooked under standard reviews and alert practitioners to looming crises before they occur. The analytical power of AI assists in more effective triaging of patients, allowing those in greatest need to receive interventions in a timely manner. With emergency medicine changing, the need for incorporating such sophisticated technologies becomes increasingly clear. Bringing real-time analysis of data and enhanced clinical tools together allows for more informed decision-making and can significantly support PS and satisfaction within emergency environments (Hashim et al., 2023).

7.5.1. Telemedicine and Remote Consultations

The integration of telemedicine and remote consultation into emergency medicine provides a range of opportunities and challenges, including within general practice. Healthcare professionals are able to utilize technology in order to access patients who cannot or will not come to a clinic for their care. This shift is most significant for patients in rural or underserved areas where access to emergency care is typically limited. The inclusion of telemedicine minimizes barriers such as issues with transportation, as well as enables immediate diagnosis and treatment, essential in case of emergencies. However, the development of telemedicine requires robust legislative and regulatory frameworks to drive its widespread integration, as realized through the issues raised in The Stern Center for Evidence-Based Policy, 2015. These issues need to be solved so that distant consultations reach their full potential and do not complicate current healthcare systems, but rather supplement them. Furthermore, access inequalities also impact telemedicine performance deeply, and the industry urgently needs equal solutions. Vulnerable populations, including racial minorities and low-income individuals, are disproportionately disadvantaged by barriers to specialty care and emergency services, as shown by Bhavaraju et al. (2016). Telemedicine can be used to reduce these disparities by enhancing access to specialized consultation without geographic constraints. However, the underlying socio-economic determinants of health inequities—i.e., lack of internet access, gaps in insurance, and discriminatory providers—should be systematically addressed. Remote consultations should therefore be integrated into broader strategies for improving health equity for emergency medicine. Through collaboration between policymakers, healthcare providers, and community groups, telemedicine can help bridge these gaps. Finally, using telemedicine in emergency situations effectively means ensuring that there are protocols and training for healthcare providers. Inasmuch as they have to adapt to the latest technology, comprehensive training enables providers to utilize telemedicine platforms effectively while providing quality care. Additionally, complete guidelines on patient consent, data security, and remote triage processes need to be in place, particularly in emergency cases where speed of decision-making is critical. Telemedicine integration is also made difficult by the variations in insurance schemes and reimbursement systems, which could affect its sustainability and availability to patients across the board, as revealed by The Stern Center for Evidence-Based Policy, 2015. Constructing a culture that facilitates seamless integration of telemedicine into common practice not only enhances patient care but also has a pivotal role to play in overcoming systemic inefficiencies in emergency medicine. Together, the transition to remote consultation is a paradigm shift towards the evolution of healthcare provision, and concerted efforts are needed to address existing setbacks (Figure 7.14).

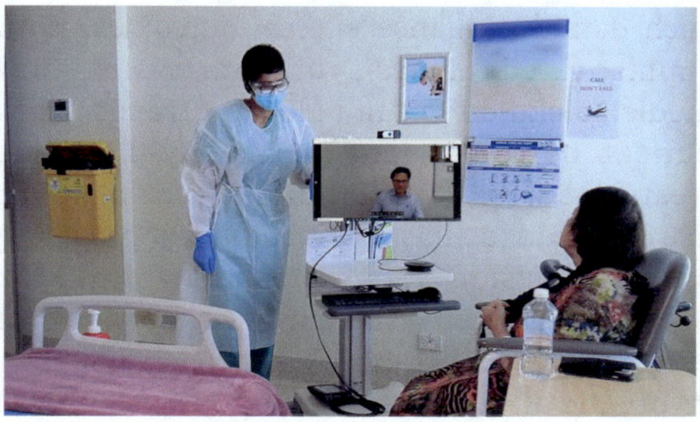

Figure 7.14. Illustration of telemedicine.

Source: https://dtresearch.com/blog/wp-content/uploads/2022/06/HPA_video3-1-1024x607.jpg.

7.5.2. Electronic Health Records (EHRs) and Data Management

In emergency medicine within general practice, the implementation of EHRs significantly enhances patient data availability and management. EHRs provide a centralized place to keep patient information so that health care providers can access and update important medical histories, medications, and allergies instantly. Such immediate accessibility becomes instrumental in emergency care, where timely decision-making can be the difference between life and death. Further, EHRs enhance continuity of care through their support for communication among clinicians more easily and more frequently across care settings and providers, thus reducing the likelihood of errors due to data fragmentation. This is the same with the use of EHRs in emergency medicine, where it emphasizes the requirement of an efficient healthcare delivery system since it enables practitioners to make decisions based on uniform treatment protocols established across various facilities (Bhavaraju et al., 2016). Data management methods associated with EHR systems are part of improving the quality of care in emergency care. Good management does not just involve collecting and warehousing patient information, but also structuring and analyzing such data to enhance clinical outcomes. With sophisticated analysis of data, emergency medicine clinicians can make out trends, track patient outcomes, and ultimately fine-tune treatment algorithms. EHRs also encourage the use of evidence-based practices by providing clinical decision support tools, which walk practitioners along standardized pathways of care. This evidence-based approach not only favors the direct treatment of patients but also general public health programs by allowing for disease surveillance and outcome measurement (Scott et al., 2017).

Effective data management in EHR systems is thus fundamental in the future development of emergency medicine in general practice. Despite the undeniable benefits of EHRs in emergency care, there are some issues that must be resolved for their maximum potential to be realized. The interoperability issues among dissimilar EHR systems can thwart free data exchange and cause gaps in patient information that can adversely affect emergency care processes. Additionally, concerns involving patient confidentiality and data protection are still significant barriers as health organizations struggle to comply with tighter regulations while managing sensitive health data. Strengthening infrastructure, improving regulatory environments, and re-engineering payment models is essential to overcoming such barriers and ensuring maximum coordination of information between providers (Bhavaraju et al., 2016). Overcoming these barriers will allow healthcare systems to realize the full potential of EHRs, in time creating a more efficient and streamlined emergency medicine model of general practice.

7.5.3. Use of Mobile Applications for Emergency Protocols

The integration of mobile apps into emergency response protocols significantly enhances the efficiency and effectiveness of EMS. Mobile apps are vital tools for medical professionals in various roles, ranging from immediate patient assessment to real-time interfacing with caregiving teams incorporated. First responders, for instance, can utilize mobile apps to capture and share crucial patient information such as history and vital signs, which can save lives during emergency situations. By ensuring quick access to life-critical information, such technologies facilitate informed decision-making during emergencies. Patients may be given the appropriate resources in time. Timely information transfer can seal the gaps in communications between emergency responders and hospitals in emergency medicine, leading to improved outcomes for patients. Moreover, the use of mobile applications facilitates greater readiness among the public and healthcare professionals alike. Such apps can have extensive emergency procedures, teaching their users procedures to follow during various emergencies, such as cardiac arrest or trauma. By equipping users with easily accessible instructions and guidelines, mobile apps allow people to act assuredly when every second counts, risking their lives. Democratization of knowledge relating to emergency medicine contributes to community readiness and resilience, enabling more people to participate in emergency response activities. Therefore, the technology trend of smartphones and user-friendly interfaces facilitates broader access and education regarding emergency health processes, and such applications become a standard component of general practice emergency care. Moreover, further development of wireless technology facilitates the development and deployment of mobile healthcare software, simplifying emergency protocols. The shift to mobile and wireless solutions in healthcare delivery in recent times has made it possible to shift from common models that rely on continuous network accessibility. This shift facilitates clinicians to access and share patient information anywhere and at any time, thereby creating a more responsive system in emergency situations (Omogbadegun & Ayo, 2007). This infrastructure facilitates the accurate capture and real-time transmission of vital patient information, leading to prompt intervention and improved patient management. The implementation of these technologies is, however, threatened by issues like data security and the need for standardized protocols, which must be addressed for the maximum potential of mobile applications in emergency medicine to be fully actualized. Thus, with advancements in mobile technology, its integration into emergency procedures offers broad potential for improving the delivery of healthcare in general practice (Eadie et al., 2015) (Figure 7.15).

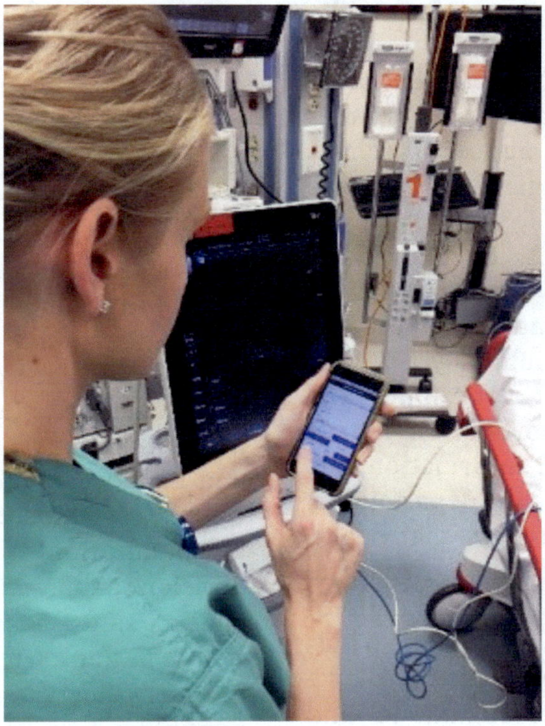

Figure 7.15. A clinical provider uses the massive transfusion protocol mobile app to determine whether a trauma patient just admitted to the emergency room requires a massive blood transfusion.

Source: https://blogger.googleusercontent.com/img/b/R29vZ2xl/AVvXsEgN5myhbrsNd4PK_tO7V1-HSJ9Hy20ECB2uQBRdmNbvdM5qWg-tJ8MNieRDl1OnOr4ClKSe4lFILahuO4o2VumbjNJ34hxC2gvn8A4oapP8-SjUw8RosrNrQ6HMpOMoV1-481PfOEOofYwF/s1600/MTP+fig+02.png.

Test Your Knowledge

1. How can telemedicine support general practitioners in managing emergency cases in remote or underserved areas?
2. In what ways do electronic health records enhance the efficiency and accuracy of emergency care provided by GPs?

7.6. Case Studies and Real-Life Applications

Learning Outcome

1. Discuss successful emergency interventions by general practitioners;
2. Focus on lessons learned from emergency scenarios;
3. Understand the impact of emergency medicine on patient outcomes.

Successful communication of patient handovers in the emergency department has broader implications for general practice outcomes. To illustrate, research into handover practice across three NHS emergency care pathways determined that the majority of failures are caused by the challenges of managing patient flows and organizational agendas. The research concluded that handovers could play a variety of roles, such as offloading responsibility and managing capacity, but more often led to inadequately communicated information due to time constraints and conflicting departmental agendas. The results substantiate that health care workers are faced with inherent conflicts in handovers, where conflicting demands of urgency and completeness are crucial. Thus, innovations in handover protocol need to take into account such dynamics so that PS and care continuity are fostered, substantiating the imperatives of effective communications during emergencies as brought forth by within the conclusions of the study's findings (Sujan et al., 2014). Application of improved handover techniques in practical terms is also seen in hospitals adopting structured models of communication, which lower handover failure significantly. By using models that integrate quantifiable data and qualitative knowledge, more understanding about patient care flows and interdepartmental relationships can be obtained by hospitals. This allows more cohesive consideration of patient management, as evident in ongoing efforts towards hospital department interrelationships. This integrated approach can be used to inform operational workflow improvements with consideration of the specialty-specific needs of emergency medicine. Hence, EDs that implement teamwork-focused and organized handover practices are likely to have fewer patient data errors, ultimately leading to better patient outcomes. These strategies exemplify how clinical pathways can reduce ambiguity in patient flows and optimize departmental cooperation, further entrenching emergency medicine's place in broader general practice (Vanberkel1 et al., 2009). Furthermore, taking a sociotechnical approach to handover practices can also make a significant impact in changing the delivery of emergency care. The emphasis on departmental collaboration and organizational culture, as highlighted in the studies, suggests the importance of a departmental and intra-departmental mindset that would place greater emphasis on intra-high-stakes communication. By recognizing the interaction between patient flow management and handover quality, healthcare systems can create environments that promote teamwork and communication, which are essential for hasty decision-making in emergency situations. This cultural shift is capable of equipping clinicians with the ability to navigate the complexities of emergency care more efficiently, making it possible for critical patient information to be relayed consistently. In this manner, healthcare providers can respond appropriately to patient needs within a due time, thereby improving the general effectiveness of emergency medicine within practice settings.

7.6.1. Successful Emergency Interventions by General Practitioners (GPs)

The GP's function in emergency medicine is crucial, particularly in rural and resource-poor settings where access to specialized facilities may be slimited. In these situations, sound emergency management by GPs may have a direct impact on patient outcomes. Acute respiratory illness, trauma, and cardiovascular emergencies, for instance, are frequently managed by GPs, and these require not only medical expertise but also the ability to make instant decisions. Their training equips them to conduct preliminary assessments, stabilize patients, and determine the need for referral to a specialist where necessary. The ability to promptly recognize life-threatening conditions can minimize complications and enable higher recovery levels. Thus, adding emergency medicine training to the curriculum of GPs can enhance their capacity for providing timely and effective care in situations of emergency by emphasizing their vital position in the healthcare system. Also, by addressing emergencies in their practice, GPs tend to prolong the immediate medical interventions. Successful interventions often involve holistically caring for the social and psychological aspects of a patient's health. GPs need to address patients with complex health needs on the basis of socioeconomic factors, complicating their management for health. GPs need to address these needs through care management that not only handles short-term conditions but also focuses on long-term outcomes. Follow-up processes and continuity of care, for example, are crucial to handle hospital readmission and improving health. The nuanced awareness of the contexts of patients that is gained through regular interaction enables GPs to craft sensitive interventions that are tailored to particular requirements. Thus, this practice underscores the importance of an integrated approach to health in managing emergency conditions with compassion and efficacy. Finally, new technology is a key to enhancing the efficacy of GPs in emergency medicine. The introduction of technology, such as telemedicine and remote monitoring, has revolutionized how GPs can potentially address emergencies. Technologies that support virtual consultations allow GPs to assess and treat patients in real time, significantly enhancing the accessibility of care among people residing in remote areas. However, as demonstrated through existing studies, there are built-in constraints in utilizing these technologies, particularly pertaining to patient engagement and retention in care management. For instance, while virtual interventions have the potential to improve outcomes, technology access and patient literacy barriers may impede their impact. Therefore, it is necessary for GPs to reconcile patient-centered care with the use of technology in a way that ensures interventions in emergencies are not only successful but also equitable, thereby enhancing the overall quality of healthcare provision in everyday practice (Berry-Millett & Bodenheimer, 2009; Tambakis et al., 2017) (Figure 7.16).

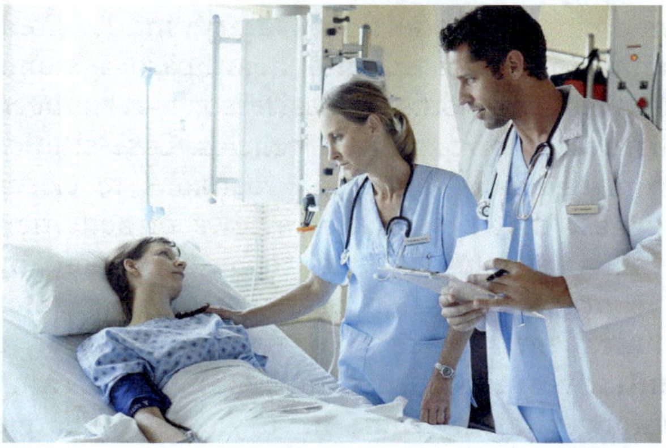

Figure 7.16. General practitioners (GPs) in emergency medicine.

Source: https://www.verywellhealth.com/thmb/wNRSrF2ctZbU3Csyx7_3-gqfSCo=/1500x0/filters:no_upscale():max_bytes(150000):strip_icc()/doctors-talking-to-patient-in-hospital-icu-493216255-583452e15f9b58d5b1b967c7.jpg.

7.6.2. Lessons Learned from Emergency Scenarios

In emergency medicine, front-line experience in previous emergencies is able to significantly enhance the effectiveness of interventions in normal practice. From an examination of the experiences of such organizations as Médecins

Sans Frontières (MSF), some important lessons are gained about responding to urban health emergencies. MSFs transition from being reactive to proactive highlights the necessity of recognizing the specific needs of vulnerable urban populations that are not only affected by natural disasters but also by violence and exclusion. It allows for the critical analysis that makes possible the application of particular medical approaches and operational responses that can appropriately respond to the specific challenges posed in urban settings. These findings are critical for GPs to know, who may themselves be encountering equivalent emergency landscapes, and whose conduct necessitates the application of durable and contextualized research methods in emergency medicine. In addition, safety innovations being incorporated into healthcare systems demonstrate another critical lesson that has been discovered through emergencies. Case studies from health organization reactions to crises suggest that systematic reviews of activities, results, and lessons has to be conducted by the organizations in order to develop safer clinical environments. For example, innovative initiatives that promote collective learning among clinical teams have yielded effective innovations to enhance PS. These partnerships emphasize that insights gained should feed into best practices in the future, allowing healthcare professionals to reduce risks and improve patient outcomes during crisis situations. The ability to learn from and adapt on the basis of past experience during emergencies is a key factor in building a culture of safety in general practice for the ultimate good of patients and practitioners. Furthermore, the essential aspect of being ready for emergency care simply cannot be overstressed. The ability to conduct effective assessments and establish measurable indicators of vulnerability is the foundation of an effective response to health emergencies. The experiences learned from MSF's operational challenges highlight the importance of customized security management and timely closure of operations that were central during crises. Through reviews with such analyses, GPs are able to predict and coordinate the specific needs of their patients during emergencies better. Therefore, these lessons reiterate the necessity of continuous evaluation and adjustment in emergency care practice within general medicine in order for practitioners to continue to be competent to respond effectively and sympathetically to the diverse and changing issues they may face.

7.6.3. Impact of Emergency Medicine on Patient Outcomes

Even the integration of emergency medicine in general practice has also reflected in the patient outcomes, particularly with regard to accurate diagnosis. Emergency conditions usually demand a quick and correct assessment to save life-threatening disorders. In such cases, advances such as POCUS have been most beneficial. By enhancing the diagnostic capability, POCUS enables clinicians to make timely treatment decisions regarding treatment options, particularly acute dyspnea and acute decompensated heart failure (ADHF), where rapid intervention is paramount. The systematic review of pertinent interest detailed in recent studies indicates that not only does POCUS change diagnostic impressions, but most importantly, profoundly impacts management plans and, therefore, patient care and outcomes in general. Therefore, emergency medicine equipment, as well as procedures, are important in improving the management of complex cases within regular practice, highlighting the need to incorporate such technologies into standard healthcare operations (Hashim et al., 2023). Furthermore, leadership and collaboration within EDs also play an important role in determining PS outcomes. Experiencing a positive safety climate can have a significant influence on the effectiveness of medical treatments. As shown in a study that was carried out in Southern Ontario, senior leadership commitment and teamwork climate were always associated with favorable outcomes in overall perceptions of PS. This suggests that when safety is felt to be endorsed by effective leadership, healthcare workers are inclined to work more collaboratively with safety improvement initiatives. Significantly, the research also indicated that positive supervisory leadership could balance lower senior leadership, demonstrating the nuanced dynamics of emergency care settings. Accordingly, enhancing these perceptions through effective leadership training and team-building activities has a key function in reinforcing safety and improving patient outcomes during emergencies, demonstrating the relationship between organizational culture and clinical effectiveness (Zaheer et al., 2018). Lastly, ongoing training and education of emergency medicine practitioners are essential in improving patient outcomes. Incorporation of POCUS in training has been proven to facilitate its use among emergency medicine residents and is consistent with enhanced efficiency in patient management. This area of learning not only prepares practitioners with the skills required but also fosters ongoing improvement and a culture of flexibility within emergency rooms. Besides, hosting workshops in critical soft skills such as conflict management can support interdepartmental cooperation, thereby improving cooperation and communication in high-stress situations. By highlighting technical knowledge as well as interpersonal relationships, healthcare centers can ensure patient needs are still addressed in emergency medicine while enhancing overall quality of care. Finally, the multidimensional educational paradigm, together with emerging technologies, facilitates the positive trend of patient outcomes in emergency medicine (Zaheer et al., 2018; Hashim et al., 2023).

Test Your Knowledge

1. Can you describe a real-life case where a general practitioner successfully stabilized a patient in a life-threatening emergency before referral?
2. How have GPs adapted emergency care delivery during public health crises?

SUMMARY

Inclusion of emergency medicine into general practice is a necessary transformation in health care that addresses the immediate needs of patients and promotes more integrated patterns of care. As the healthcare setting continues to change, the necessity for PCPs to be equipped with emergency medicine becomes imperative. Such training not only hastens the management of acute medical conditions immediately but also improves patient outcomes by enabling timely interventions. The knowledge obtained from ED providers identifies key barriers and facilitators of suicide risk assessment, emphasizing the importance of streamlined processes and multi-agency strategies. These findings underscore the need for interdisciplinary collaboration in addressing complex medical conditions and improving the quality of care delivered within both emergency settings and general practice (Petrik et al., 2015). Furthermore, the emphasis on integrated models of care becomes increasingly significant in addressing medically vulnerable populations' complexities. Severely mentally ill patients, for example, have high comorbid medical illnesses but may present to emergency services for their acute presentation rather than utilize preventive care or primary healthcare services. This misalignment generates inefficiency and poor results, making it unavoidable to have an integrative approach to handling their care. Providing a collaborative method between primary care physicians and mental health professionals can decrease these issues to a very significant level. By facilitating communication and the integration of care environments, healthcare systems can improve access to care, increase patient satisfaction, and eventually decrease pressures on emergency services (Read, 2016). The ultimate model for healthcare provision to diverse populations is the integration of emergency medicine and general practice. As principles of emergency medicine are being increasingly integrated into the framework of general practice, healthcare professionals can make significant leaps towards treating acute and chronic ailments with comparable efficiency, creating a proactive rather than reactive patient care regimen. The evidence provided by current studies and practitioner responses should be the blueprint for making practice and policymaking efforts better in the future. By ongoing improvement and application of effective practices, healthcare systems can improve the delivery of service such that patients are treated quickly and appropriately, easing the burden on EDs (Petrik et al., 2015; Read, 2016).

The integration of emergency medicine as part of general practice is increasingly being viewed as an essential aspect of providing full patient care. One of the central supports of such inclusion is the adequate training of doctors in the treatment of acute medical emergencies, and particularly obstetric emergencies. It needs to be handled with specialized skills and knowledge that would be encountered less often in routine practice, filling a lacuna in readiness among GPs. Active learning methods that optimize learning, such as board games conveying labor and delivery scenarios, have also been successful in facilitating key knowledge and skills transfer to residents. During the process, utilizing interactive learning materials facilitates collaboration and improves retention of essential details. As highlighted in learner feedback, these novel pedagogical tools significantly enhance learning results compared to the traditional lecture, with the students highly valuing the education, showing their effectiveness in prepping practitioners to implement in the real-world context (Chen et al., 2019). Moreover, principles for effective debriefing techniques following simulated clinical practice are core in promoting ongoing enhancement in emergency medicine training. Debriefing gives an opportunity for students to reflect on what has already happened, therefore reinforcing their knowledge and enhancing their ability to manage similar situations during actual clinical practice. Reflective practice, apart from improving performance at the individual level, harmonizes team behavior in health institutions in order to ensure safety and quality of care. Debriefing guidelines, as outlined in professional texts, emphasize the creation of a respectful and supportive environment, with the need to acknowledge the feelings of learners as a part of their action and decision analysis. Facilitating a systematic debriefing process can assist instructors in guaranteeing knowledge reinforcement and the identification of gaps and near misses in the performance of trainees, thereby directly contributing to enhanced PS (Oriot & Alinier, 2017). As the landscape of healthcare evolves, interoperability between emergency medicine and general practice remains pertinent. The implementation of novel pedagogical methods like formal debriefing and game-based learning represents a progressive approach to skill development in managing emergencies in an efficient manner. Its persistent use and refinement are vital to the development of healthcare professionals for a proper response to emergent conditions faced during clinical practice. Interestingly, such training not only facilitates technical proficiency but also critical thinking and teamwork abilities, critical in high-risk settings. Accordingly, the emphasis on emergency medicine in general practice training not only equips practitioners with critical technical expertise but also helps foster responsiveness and safety culture, ultimately leading to better patient care outcomes in various medical settings.

KEY TERMS FROM THIS CHAPTER

- Acute decompensated heart failure (ADHF)
- Adjunctive therapies
- Cardiac emergencies
- Cardiopulmonary resuscitation (CPR)
- Continuing medical education (CME)
- Emergency case environment
- Emergency cases
- Emergency medicine
- Emergency response activities
- EMTALA breaches
- Gain skills
- General practitioners (GPs)
- Healthcare practitioners
- Healthcare team
- Heart disease
- Hospital delivery system
- Life-threatening illnesses
- Management plans
- Medical conditions
- Medical practitioners

CRITICAL THINKING QUESTIONS

1. **What is the primary role of a general practitioner (GP) in emergency situations?**
   a. To provide long-term specialist care for chronic diseases
   b. To refer all emergencies to hospital-based emergency departments
   c. To assess, stabilize, and initiate management of acute conditions
   d. To perform complex surgical procedures in a primary care setting
2. **Which of the following is one of the most common emergencies encountered in general practice?**
   a. Cardiac tamponade
   b. Acute myocardial infarction
   c. Severe trauma with multiple fractures
   d. Stroke requiring neurosurgery
3. **What essential training or skill is most crucial for GPs dealing with emergency situations?**
   a. Advanced neurosurgical training
   b. Specialized radiology certification
   c. Dialysis machine operation
   d. Basic life support (BLS) and advanced cardiac life support (ACLS)
4. **One of the main challenges faced by GPs in emergency medicine is:**
   a. Overstaffing in rural clinics
   b. Inadequate access to emergency diagnostic tools
   c. Too many ambulances in close proximity
   d. Excessive training in emergency procedures
5. **How is technology increasingly integrated into emergency medicine within general practice?**
   a. By replacing GPs with fully autonomous AI systems
   b. Through paper-based records and faxes
   c. Via telemedicine consultations and portable diagnostic tools
   d. Through home visits replacing clinic consultations

Short Answer Questions

1. What are the key responsibilities of general practitioners during emergency situations, and how do they contribute to the initial stabilization and triage of patients?
2. What are the most frequently encountered emergency conditions in general practice (e.g., chest pain, respiratory distress, trauma), and how should GPs prioritize their management?
3. How do general practitioners determine which emergency cases require immediate referral to secondary or tertiary care, and what information should be communicated during the referral?
4. Which practical and theoretical skills should GPs possess to effectively manage emergencies?
5. What are the main challenges faced by general practitioners when providing emergency care, particularly in rural or resource-limited settings?

Answers to Critical Thinking Questions

1. (c); 2. (b); 3. (d); 4. (b); 5. (c)

REFERENCES

1. Sonis, J. D., Kennedy, M., Aaronson, E. L., Baugh, J. J., Raja, A. S., Yun, B. J., & White, B. A. (2020). Humanism in the Age of COVID-19: Renewing Focus on Communication and Compassion. *The western journal of emergency medicine, 21*(3), 499–502. https://doi.org/10.5811/westjem.2020.4.47596(accessed on 27th June 2025).
2. Hashim A, Tahir MJ, Ullah I, Asghar MS, Siddiqi H, Yousaf Z. The utility of point of care ultrasonography (POCUS). *Ann Med Surg (Lond).* 2021;71:102982. Published 2021 Nov 2. doi:10.1016/j.amsu.2021.102982(accessed on 27th June 2025).
3. Al-Azri NH. Emergency medicine in Oman: current status and future challenges. *Int J Emerg Med.* 2009;2(4):199-203. Published 2009 Dec 11. doi:10.1007/s12245-009-0143-6(accessed on 27th June 2025).
4. Alinier, G. (2018). Cost-effective extracorporeal membrane oxygenation simulation. https://core.ac.uk/download/288394195.pdf (accessed on 27th June 2025).
5. Oriot, D. & Alinier, G. (2017). Pocket book for simulation debriefing in healthcare. https://doi.org/10.1007/978-3-319-59882-6 https://core.ac.uk/download/159073196.pdf (accessed on 27th June 2025).
6. Allen, T. J. (2011). Addressing resource gaps in the U.S. health care safety net: An assessment of the free clinic network. https://core.ac.uk/download/71357645.pdf (accessed on 27th June 2025).
7. Amin, A., Cohen, M., Deitelzweig, S., DiLascia, J., et al. (2019). Contemporary NSTEMI management: The role of the hospitalist. https://core.ac.uk/download/322850160.pdf (accessed on 27th June 2025).
8. Melissa De Regge, Jeroen Trybou, Paul Gemmel, Philippe Duyck, and Lieven Annemans, 2013: Physician-Owned Specialized Facilities: Focused Factories or Destructive Competition?. *Proceedings,* 2013, https://doi.org/10.5465/ambpp.2013.13667abstract(acce ssed on 27th June 2025).
9. Terp, S., Wang, B., Burner, E., Arora, S., & Menchine, M. (2020). Penalties for Emergency Medical Treatment and Labor Act Violations Involving Obstetrical Emergencies. *The western journal of emergency medicine, 21*(2), 235–243. https://doi.org/10.5811/westjem.2019.10.40892(accessed on 27th June 2025).
10. Wankhade, P., Cook, I. G., & Halsall, J. P. (2014). Ethnic Minorities and Their Health Needs: Crisis of Perception and Behaviours. *Illness, Crisis & Loss, 22*(2), 145-158. https://doi.org/10.2190/IL.22.2.e (Original work published 2014)
11. (accessed on 27th June 2025).
12. Omogbadegun, Z. O. & Ayo, C. K. (2007). Impact of mobile and wireless technology on healthcare delivery services. https://core.ac.uk/download/19447815.pdf (accessed on 27th June 2025).
13. Parsons M, Bailitz J, Chung AS, et al. Evidence-Based Interventions that Promote Resident Wellness from the Council of Emergency Residency Directors. *West J Emerg Med.* 2020;21(2):412-422. Published 2020 Feb 21. doi:10.5811/westjem.2019.11.42961(accessed on 27th June 2025).

14. Zaheer, S., Ginsburg, L. R., Wong, H. J., Thomson, K., & Bain, L. (2018). Importance of safety climate, teamwork climate and demographics: understanding nurses, allied health professionals and clerical staff perceptions of patient safety. *BMJ open quality*, *7*(4), e000433. https://doi.org/10.1136/bmjoq-2018-000433(accessed on 27th June 2025).

15. Nadir, N. A., Bentley, S., Papanagnou, D., Bajaj, K., Rinnert, S., & Sinert, R. (2017). Characteristics of Real-Time, Non-Critical Incident Debriefing Practices in the Emergency Department. *The western journal of emergency medicine*, *18*(1), 146–151. https://doi.org/10.5811/westjem.2016.10.31467(accessed on 27th June 2025).

16. Meredith, C., Treacy, C., Bandeeri, N. (2004). The prevalence of cocaine-associated chest pain in a London hospital. Emergency Medicine Journal(21:e4), pp. 4-(accessed on 27th June 2025).

17. Petrik, M. L., Gutierrez, P. M., Berlin, J. S., & Saunders, S. M. (2015). Barriers and facilitators of suicide risk assessment in emergency departments: a qualitative study of provider perspectives. *General hospital psychiatry*, *37*(6), 581–586. https://doi.org/10.1016/j.genhosppsych.2015.06.018(accessed on 27th June 2025).

18. Berry-Millett, R., & Bodenheimer, T. (2009). Care management of patients with complex health care needs. https://core.ac.uk/download/71346306.pdf (accessed on 27th June 2025).

19. Biega, B. (2024). SCARES: A clinician guide to spinal cord awareness, response, and emergency support creation and implantation of SCARES protocol among hospitalist advanced practice providers. https://core.ac.uk/download/619611492.pdf (accessed on 27th June 2025).

20. Biu, T., Goldsworthy, L. L., & Sidebotham, P. (2007). Child protection procedures in emergency departments. https://core.ac.uk/download/45517.pdf (accessed on 27th June 2025).

21. de Bedout, T., Kramer, K., Blanchard, S., Hamada, Y., Eckert, G. J., Maupome, G., & John, V. (2018). Assessing the Medical Emergency Preparedness of Dental Faculty, Residents, and Practicing Periodontists: An Exploratory Study. *Journal of dental education*, *82*(5), 492–500. https://doi.org/10.21815/JDE.018.058(accessed on 27th June 2025).

22. c, P.T. , Boucherie, R. J., Hans, E. W., Hurink, J. L., Litvak, N., et al. (2009). A survey of health care models that encompass multiple departments. https://core.ac.uk/download/pdf/11471201.pdf (accessed on 27th June 2025).

23. Buchbinder, R., Underwood, M., Hartvigsen, J., & Maher, C. G. (2020). The *Lancet* Series call to action to reduce low value care for low back pain: An update. *Pain, 161*, S57–S64. https://doi.org/10.1097/j.pain.0000000000001869 (accessed on 27th June 2025).

24. Bhavaraju, N. , Sholk, J., Nanni, J., Peterson, K., Smith, L. A., & Carlson, C., (2016). Breaking the barriers to specialty care: Practical ideas to improve health equity and reduce cost–Increasing specialty care availability. https://core.ac.uk/download/75785770.pdf (accessed on 27th June 2025).

25. Chalya, P. L., Dass, R. M., Gilyoma, J. M., Mabula, M., et al. (2012). Geriatric injuries among patients attending a regional hospital in Shanyang Tanzania. https://core.ac.uk/download/pdf/18410878.pdf (accessed on 27th June 2025).

26. Chen, E. H., & Silverio, L. M. (2019). L&D in the ED: A game-based approach to learning high-risk obstetric emergencies. https://core.ac.uk/download/323074437.pdf (accessed on 27th June 2025).

27. Sujan, M., Spurgeon, P., Inada-Kim, M., Rudd, M., Fitton, L., Horniblow, S., Cross, S., Chessum, P., & W Cooke, M. (2014). *Clinical handover within the emergency care pathway and the potential risks of clinical handover failure (ECHO): primary research.* NIHR Journals Library. https://doi.org/10.3310/hsdr02050(accessed on 27th June 2025).

28. Weston, B. W., Gaither, J., Schulz, K., Srinivasan, S., Smith, J. J., & Colella, M. R. (2020). Innovative Approaches to Emergency Medical Services Fellowship Challenges. *The western journal of emergency medicine, 21*(2), 429–433. https://doi.org/10.5811/westjem.2019.10.43830(accessed on 27th June 2025).

29. Scott PJ, Cornet R, McCowan C, Peek N. Addendum to Informatics for Health 2017: advancing both science and practice. BMJ Health & Care Informatics. 2017;24:. https://doi.org/10.14236/jhi.v24i3.969f (accessed on 27th June 2025).

30. Bickerton, J., Procter, S., Johnson, B. *et al.* A Video Life-world Approach to Consultation Practice: The Relevance of a Socio-Phenomenological Approach. *Hum Stud* **33**, 157–171 (2010). https://doi.org/10.1007/s10746-010-9162-9(accessed on 27th June 2025).

31. Nti, B. K., Laniewicz, M., Skaggs, T., Cross, K., Fallat, M. E., & Rominger, A. (2019). A novel streamlined trauma response team training improves imaging efficiency for pediatric blunt abdominal trauma patients. *Journal of pediatric surgery, 54*(9), 1854–1860. https://doi.org/10.1016/j.jpedsurg.2018.12.013 (accessed on 27th June 2025).

32. Dahlen, P. (2014). School district assessment for sudden cardiac arrest preparation. https://core.ac.uk/download/162576263.pdf (accessed on 27th June 2025).

33. Tambakis, G., Darby, J., & Jiwa, M. (2017). What is the scope to test a smoking cessation intervention aimed at young people admitted to hospital?. The Journal of Health Design, 2 (2), 2-9. (accessed on 27th June 2025).

34. Eadie, L. H., Mort, A. J., & Wilson, P. M. J. (2015). Technology to support rural health and well-being. https://core.ac.uk/download/29465861.pdf (accessed on 27th June 2025).

35. Mead, H., Regenstein, M., & Lara, A. (2007). The heart of the matter: the relationship between communities, cardiovascular services, and racial and ethnic gaps in care. *Managed care interface, 20*(8), 22–28.(accessed on 27th June 2025).

36. Mathews, K. S., Nelson, J. E., Richardson, L. D., Rodriguez, R. M., et al. (2020). Triage and ongoing care for critically ill patients in the emergency department: Results from a national survey of emergency physicians. https://core.ac.uk/download/287622005.pdf (accessed on 27th June 2025).

37. Rochana, N., Morphet, J., & Plummer, V. (2016). Triage process in Emergency Departments: an Indonesian Study. Nurse Media Journal of Nursing, 6(1), 37-46. https://doi.org/10.14710/jil.%v.%i.27-37(accessed on 27th June 2025).

38. The Stern Center for Evidence-Based Policy (2015). Addressing the health needs of an aging America: New opportunities for evidence-based policy solutions. University of Pittsburgh. https://core.ac.uk/download/75783019.pdf

39. (accessed on 27th June 2025).

40. Osborn, L., & Rossi, A. (2020). A case report of angioedema and anaphylactic shock induced by ingestion of polyethylene glycol. https://core.ac.uk/download/305124170.pdf (accessed on 27th June 2025).

41. Read, T. L. (2016). Emerging needs in behavioral health and the integrated care model. https://open.bu.edu/bitstream/2144/17694/1/Read_bu_0017N_11995.pdf (accessed on 27th June 2025).

42. Puentedura, E. J., Slaughter, R., Reilly, S., Ventura, E., & Young, D. (2017). Thrust joint manipulation utilization by U.S. physical therapists. *The Journal of manual & manipulative therapy*, *25*(2), 74–82. https://doi.org/10.1080/10669817.2016.1187902 (accessed on 27th June 2025).

43. Risso, A. V., Alvarez, J., Bellani, G., Bettini, A., et al. (2016). Epidemiology, patterns of care, and mortality for patients with acute respiratory distress syndrome in intensive care units in 50 countries. https://core.ac.uk/download/54529633.pdf (accessed on 27th June 2025).

44. Rogers, W. A. (2004). Reducing health inequalities: Ethical issues in a Scottish child health home visiting program. https://core.ac.uk/download/14935808.pdf (accessed on 27th June 2025).

45. Skivington, K., Matthews, L., Simpson, S. A., Craig, P., Baird, J., Blazeby, J. M., Boyd, K. A., Craig, N., French, D. P., McIntosh, E., Petticrew, M., Rycroft-Malone, J., White, M., & Moore, L. (2021). A new framework for developing and evaluating complex interventions: update of Medical Research Council guidance. *BMJ (Clinical research ed.)*, *374*, n2061. https://doi.org/10.1136/bmj.n2061(accessed on 27th June 2025).

46. Thal, A., & Zapanta, P. (2016). Otolaryngology for internal medicine: Increasing exposure to otolaryngology using computer-assisted instruction. https://core.ac.uk/download/230828860.pdf (accessed on 27th June 2025).

47. Rich, J., Rich, L., Wilson, A., Bloom, S., Evans, S., & Corbin, T. (2009). Healing the hurt: Trauma-informed approaches to the health of boys and young men of color. https://core.ac.uk/download/71360851.pdf (accessed on 27th June 2025).

PROCEDURAL SKILLS: IV ACCESS, LUMBAR PUNCTURE, ECG INTERPRETATION, ABG, AND THORACOCENTESIS

8

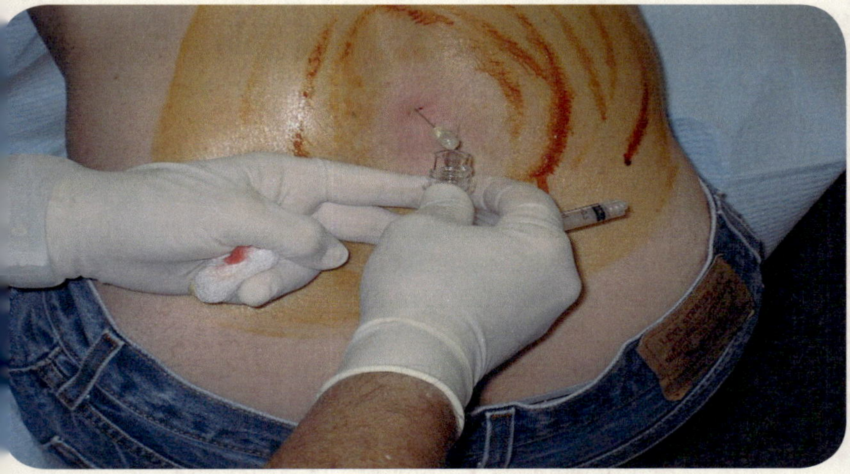

LEARNING OBJECTIVES

After studying this chapter, you will be able to:

1. Discuss intravenous (IV) access in clinical practice;
2. Understand the concept of lumbar puncture;
3. Explain the basic ECG interpretation;
4. Define arterial blood gas (ABG) analysis;
5. Describe the fundamentals of thoracocentesis.

Introduction

Achieving procedural skill proficiency in the clinical setting is the foundation of healthcare professionals, particularly in emergency medicine and critical care. Intravenous (IV) placement, lumbar puncture (LP), electrocardiogram (ECG) interpretation, ABG result, and thoracentesis are more than task-oriented activities but are integral aspects of patient care in a holistic sense. A clear concept of the anatomical foundation and related complications of each of these skills is a requirement. Expertise in these procedures has typically ensured improved patient outcomes, considering the need for prompt and accurate interventions in emergency environments. Furthermore, the significance of these procedural skills transcends individual practice; it further means the evolving nature of medical education and clinical competencies. As the provision of healthcare becomes increasingly complex, the creation of standardized protocols and competencies is necessary. Improved clinical ultrasound imaging, for instance, helps demonstrate the need for healthcare professionals to adopt new approaches and integrate them into competency profiles. Such advancements lend credence to the fact that clinical ultrasound should be considered a core competency across specialty areas with a view to enhanced patient assessment and intervention planning (Adhikari, 2014). Furthermore, patients' advocacy is crucial in order to promote the effective execution of these procedures. It should be crucial for nursing staff to work hand-in-hand with medical professionals during invasive procedures to ensure holistic patient care that focuses not only on the physiological but also on the emotional and psychological well-being of patients. Research emphasizes the significant role that thoughtful nursing care can play in helping to achieve patient outcomes in critical care settings, thereby reasserting the importance of interprofessional collaboration (Adhikari, 2014). As such, the integration of procedural skills into clinical practice necessitates continuous education, collaboration, and an uncompromising commitment to ensuring high standards of patient care across all medical specialties.

Definition of Procedural Skills in Clinical Practice

Procedural skills in clinical practice consist of a series of tangible actions that health practitioners must perform competently to ensure the effectiveness and safety of patient care. They possess cognitive and psychomotor components, and they are essential components in clinical evaluation and interventions. Central to procedural proficiency is the mandate for extensive training and education because the complexities of various procedures, i.e., IV access, LPs, and thoracentesis, require precise technical competence and critical thinking. Moreover, the successful execution of these procedures is often irretrievably entwined with patient outcomes, and it is incumbent on practitioners to upgrade their skill set on an ongoing basis. Findings from emerging research underscore considerable curricular shortcomings in procedural education, potentially impeding such basic skills' acquisition, particularly in the low and middle-income settings, further accentuating the call for an integrated approach to procedural training in clinical practice (Mtombeni, 2017). The usefulness of procedural competencies is further underscored by their direct impact on patient care and the efficiency of the health system. For instance, drug administration through IV routes depends on the proficiency of staff members in IV access to prevent complications such as thrombus formation or infection. Within ICUs, the complex task of dealing with several IV lines necessitates greater skills, i.e., the ability to work with incompatible solutions effectively (ESICM LIVES 2017, 2017). Therefore, procedural skills not only allow for immediate clinical action but also contribute significantly towards optimizing the use of resources in healthcare. In emergency situations, where action within a timely period can be lifesaving, acquiring these skills becomes all the more crucial, since delays or inaccuracies can lead to serious outcomes. Lastly, the acquisition of higher-order procedural skills is essential in mediating the bridge between practice and theory, converting medical training into practical advantages for patients. Ongoing assessment and refinement of procedural skills are essential to balance healthcare practice with evolving medical standards and technologies. The scenario of medical training in procedural skills reflects broader movements, including movement towards SBE to enhance hands-on training without sacrificing PS. Through the use of emerging training strategies, such as simulation and competence-based assessment, healthcare professionals can maximize their clinical performance while lowering the risks of interventional procedures. Curricula for schools must include sophisticated training strategies in order to provide a sound foundation for future professionals who will be able to confidently handle complex clinical cases. Core competency development, as seen in recent consensus studies, provides a blueprint for structuring practical education and guaranteeing ongoing learning and adaptation in procedural skills during clinical practice (Mtombeni, 2017). By emphasizing procedural skill definition and its importance, healthcare education is able to fulfill its mission of providing competent, capable professionals who are able to adapt to modern medicine.

Importance of Mastering Procedural Skills for Healthcare Professionals

Mastering procedural skills by health care providers is crucial as these skills directly influence PS and treatment outcomes. For example, the procedural skills of performing procedures such as IV access, LP, and thoracocentesis require not only technical skills but also complete anatomy and patient management knowledge. For example, a poorly executed LP can cause traumatic samples compromising diagnostic integrity and increasing pain to the patient, highlighting the necessity of procedural technique improvement (Derebe, 2017). Additionally, increasing complexities in patient cases require medical practitioners to stay competent at their procedural skills to adapt to individual clinical conditions and therefore enhance overall patient outcomes and satisfaction. In addition to the technical, effective pedagogy and practice settings also play a pivotal role in acquiring skills. Teaching quality, facility access, and commitment of the learner are determining factors in procedural skill acquisition. LP training research on the pedagogy considered significant variation in pass rates based on these factors and there needs to be a set curriculum and standardized instruments for measuring procedural skills competence (Derebe, 2017). Healthcare facilities must, therefore, accord high priority to resource planning and craft facilitative environments conducive to skill acquisition and, consequently, high-quality patient care. Additionally, the role of healthcare practitioners as professionals is not merely technical proficiency at procedures; it includes an essential element of patient care and communication as well. Mastery of procedural skills provides practitioners with confidence to communicate efficiently with patients in order to assure that they can explain the procedure, reassure, and calm fears. In addition, in life-threatening conditions like ICUs, where vigilant monitoring and quick intervention are the rule, the ability to interpret ECGs and analyze ABGs is a key element of effective rapid decision-making and management. , including proficiency in procedural skills in all forms of patient interaction accentuates the holistic nature of healthcare provision, further supporting the perception that technical skill and compassionate care are reciprocal elements of professional competence.

8.1. IV Access

Learning Outcome

1. Understand the indications for intravenous access;
2. Explain the techniques for successful IV insertion;
3. Focus on complications and management of IV access.

The clinical value of IV access cannot be overemphasized, as it continues to be an essential pathway for the administration of drugs, fluids, and nutrients directly into the venous system. IV access is especially useful in emergency clinical settings, where rapid therapeutic intervention can significantly affect outcomes in patients. The acquisition of established, timely and reliable IV access constitutes an essential procedural skill that healthcare workers must accomplish to meet the demands of acute care environments. As captured by Mtombeni (2017), the development of a core set of procedural competencies in emergency medicine highlighted the importance of IV access as an integral procedure among the mandatory prerequisites, acknowledging its core position in clinical education. Furthermore, clinical competency for the placement of an IV catheter is inextricably linked with the overall competency of emergency healthcare professionals, and it will continue to require systematic training and assessment. In planning for the facilitation of better clinical practices, choosing the appropriate IV access devices also plays a critical role. A number of considerations, including the condition of the patients and the type of therapy required, and how long IV therapy is predicted to last, dictate peripheral or central venous access. For instance, patients requiring prolonged drug infusion or with spastic peripheral veins will find central venous catheters beneficial.

As demonstrated by ESICM LIVES 2017 (2017), the choice of IV solutions and flushing regimens is also vital in preventing IV therapy-related complications such as infections or thrombosis. Such intensive training involving both technical skills of catheter placement and the choice of proper devices and solutions is essential in preparing healthcare providers for effective IV access. Moreover, the process of IV access is not just a procedural technique but also involves critical thinking and decision-making. Clinicians are required to assess various factors of the patient, including age, disease history, and current health condition, to determine the most suitable method for IV access. This intricate strategy is facilitated by new evidence revealing the impact of a person's skill level and procedural competence on PS and quality of care. Through the process of consensus-building proposed by Mtombeni (2017), nursing and medical curriculum programs should continue to evolve by integrating procedural skills training with evidence-based practices so as to maintain healthcare practitioners at all times in a position to deal effectively with IV access issues. Being grounded in these concerns will ultimately improve patient care and quality results across different clinical environments.

8.1.1. Indications for Intravenous (IV) Access

Intravenous (IV) access is a fundamental skill in the practice of medicine that permits clinicians to introduce fluids, drugs, and nutrients directly into the venous system. Indications for IV access have expanded enormously, driven by the imperative to effective resuscitation in critically ill patients and the delivery of emergency drugs, particularly in emergency medicine, quick IV access can be lifesaving, specifically in acute cases of cardiac arrest or uncontrolled hemorrhage in which expeditious fluid resuscitation is crucial. According to research highlighted in medical curricula, the necessity of obtaining IV access, especially in controlled environments, is an indicator of the importance of the skill to healthcare providers and an argument supporting the need for proficiency in IV procedures as part of undergraduate medical education (Mtombeni, 2017). IV access is also necessary for the care of patients with chronic conditions requiring long-term treatment regimens. For example, cancer patients receiving chemotherapy or needing multiple blood transfusions enjoy established IV lines that reduce the need for repeated needle sticks, thereby decreasing discomfort and risk of complications. Choosing an optimal venous access site, either peripheral or central, depends on the duration of therapy and the viscosity of the infusate. Anatomic barriers to patient, history of venous access complications, and clinical necessity must be considered. The growing nature of complexity of ICU and surgical patient care—in the guise of the requirement for multiple intravenous catheters—elicited by this problem invokes a familiar issue again, stressing the necessity of highest technique and IV access procedure training, as explained through research on core competencies in emergency medicine (ESICM LIVES 2017, 2017). Finally, competency in performing and sustaining IV access is a central aspect of effective competence in emergency and critical care healthcare professionals. Effective training in IV skills requires an understanding of indications, contraindications, and complications of IV therapy. Mastery in the clinical procedure of IV therapy not only results in enhanced patient outcomes but also in increased levels of care across all healthcare disciplines. , including IV training in undergraduate education, as proposed in some consensus-building research, addresses the curriculum shortfall in emergency medicine training. In turn, as healthcare evolves, continuing proficiency with IV access is essential to readying future clinicians for meeting the diverse requirements of their patients (Mtombeni, 2017) (Figure 8.1).

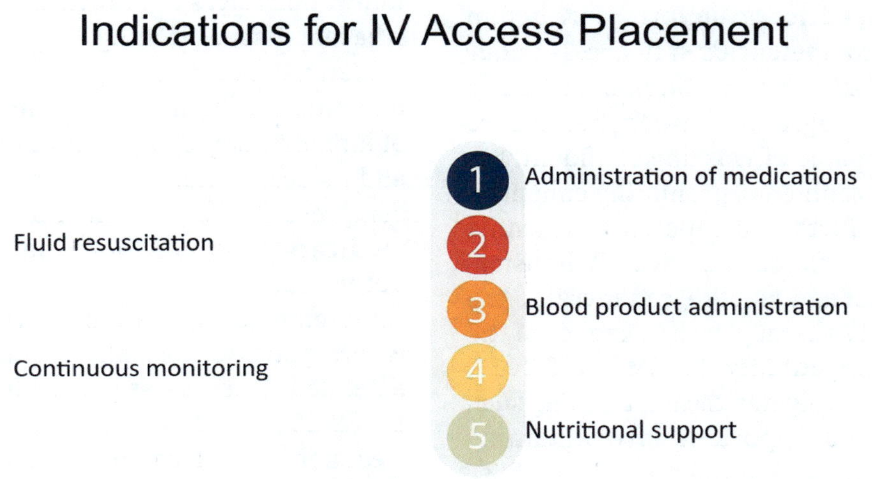

Figure 8.1. Indications for IV access placement.

Source: https://fastercapital.co/i/IV-Access--Ensuring-Smooth-Administration-of-Life-Saving-Treatments--Indications-for-IV-Access-Placement.webp.

8.1.2. Techniques for Successful IV Insertion

Proper IV placement is a required skill that supports patient care in a wide range of medical settings. To achieve optimal success with this intervention, the clinician must conduct an initial assessment of the patient's venous anatomy, hydration status, and clinical needs. Selecting the appropriate site of IV access, preferably the forearm or hand, is paramount because these sites will have superficial veins that are less difficult to access. The size of the catheter used is also crucial; low-gauge catheters are best suited for children or frail patients, while a higher gauge might be employed in adults where there is an urgent need for fluid resuscitation. This systematic approach not only makes the patient comfortable but also minimizes complications like infiltration and phlebitis, thereby allowing a successful IV insertion process. Apart from initial evaluation, certain methods can considerably increase the probability of successful IV placement. One of the most favored methods is the use of a tourniquet in an attempt to engorge veins, making them easier to see and feel. Warm compresses or the gravity method are also widely employed by therapists to engorge veins before insertion. Education of the patient promotes a cooperative environment, which reduces tension and increases cooperation during IV insertion. Moreover, maintaining the area clean is also important to avoid infection, and skilled practitioners are likely to adhere to the protocol in place, such as the use of sterile gloves and alcohol swabs. An orderly approach that incorporates these methods can greatly improve the procedural outcomes and patient satisfaction, highlighting the importance of competency in IV access. Furthermore, training and proficiency in IV insertion can make a significant contribution to healthcare outcomes in various settings, particularly emergency medicine. In accordance with a review of the literature, practice and simulation-based training can reinforce procedural skill development, with the emphasis being on the need for a uniform curriculum addressing key competencies in IV access under medical education programs (Mtombeni, 2017). Such training programs render healthcare professionals capable of working confidently in challenging environments, promoting enhanced patient care. A further competence, learning different separator fluids to apply in IV infusion, for instance, NaCl and glucose, can increase the effectiveness of IV therapy at the expense of the risk of drug incompatibility (ESICM LIVES 2017, 2017). With improving healthcare, building such skills will become important in maintaining high-standard patient-focused care (Figure 8.2).

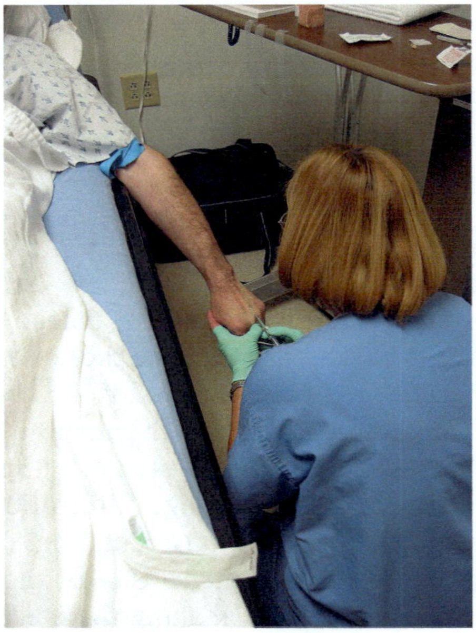

Figure 8.2. A nurse is inserting an 18-gauge IV needle with a cannula.

Source: https://upload.wikimedia.org/wikipedia/commons/thumb/f/ff/Intravenous_attempt.jpg/800px-Intravenous_attempt.jpg.

8.1.3. Complications and Management of IV Access

Positioning of IV access, while crucial in drug and fluid administration, is not without complications. Complications are infiltration, phlebitis, and catheter-related bloodstream infection (CRBSI), each with particular challenges to management. Infiltration refers to extravasation of IV fluid into adjacent tissue, leading to pain and swelling, sometimes necessitating catheter removal. But phlebitis can be manifested in the appearance of inflammatory symptoms at the insertion site, and its occurrence can require the use of warm compresses or the administration of antidiluent medication to alleviate pain and prevent deterioration. Moreover, CRBSIs carry life-threatening complications, particularly in ICUs, where patients normally require multiple and extended IV access, as per the literature (ESICM LIVES 2017, 2017). Thus, timely detection and treatment of such complications are essential for safeguarding PS and ensuring favorable health outcomes. Effective management methods for IV access complications are multifaceted, with prevention as well as treatment being the focus. Aseptic technique insertion can significantly reduce the incidence of CRBSIs. Furthermore, utilizing new catheter designs, such as antimicrobial surface catheters, can further help to protect against infection and prevent IV-line failure. The assessment of IV sites at regular time intervals for inflammation, infiltration, or other complications is equally important in facilitating early correction of problems. It has been shown that educational programs for healthcare personnel regarding the correct methods of catheter insertion and care can improve procedural skill and, by extension, patient outcomes (Mtombeni, 2017). Ongoing professional development, thus, is a crucial factor in reducing complications with IV access. When complications do arise, early detection and proper management are paramount in preventing negative consequences. For example, in the event of infiltration, cessation of IV infusion at once and raising the affected limb can reverse edema and prevent tissue damage. For phlebitis, one common recommendation is the application of warm or cold compresses, with the potential administration of non-steroidal anti-inflammatory drugs to relieve pain. In proven CRBSI, strict infection control policy adherence is recommended, together with the establishment of broad-spectrum antibiotics. These cases attest to the benefits of a protocol for IV access complication management that integrates immediate and longer-term responses to continued patient care. Each complication underscores the significance of procedural expertise by trained providers and the implementation of system-wide protocol for optimizing PS during their healthcare experience (Figure 8.3).

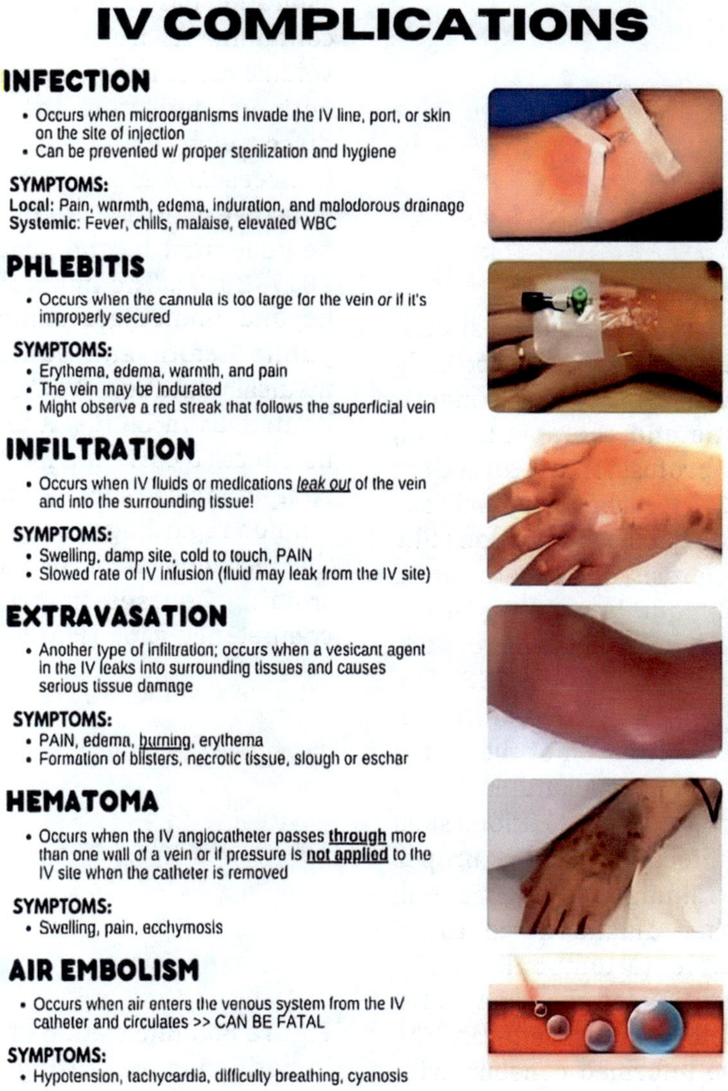

Figure 8.3. IV complication.

Source: https://media.licdn.com/dms/image/v2/D4E22AQEAlSdACqi_8A/feedshare-shrink_800/feedshare-shrink_800/0/1684144020084?e=2147483647&v=beta&t=GA8th3tTj54oeuvv6WcC6tsScsgDYPzO642QKekaYCU.

Test Your Knowledge

1. What are the primary indications for establishing intravenous (IV) access in clinical settings?
2. What are the key steps and techniques to ensure successful peripheral IV insertion?
3. What complications can arise from IV access and how can they be identified early?

8.2. Lumbar Puncture (LP)

Learning Outcome

1. Discuss the indications for performing a lumbar puncture;
2. Understand the step-by-step procedure for lumbar puncture;
3. Describe risks and complications associated with lumbar puncture.

The lumbar puncture (LP) is a foundational procedural skill in clinical practice, especially in the emergency and neurology departments. It is both a diagnostic and therapeutic tool, allowing the health professionals to collect cerebrospinal fluid (CSF) for laboratory analysis, hence facilitating the diagnosis of infections like meningitis, multiple sclerosis, and subarachnoid hemorrhage. The technique is needling of the spinal canal, typically at the L3-L4 or L4-L5 intervertebral levels, to obtain CSF. The procedure requires good knowledge of human anatomy, particularly the location of the spinal cord and pertinent anatomical landmarks, to minimize the risk of related complications such as nerve damage or infection. Because proper execution is so vital, training in LP is essential, especially where other diagnostic methods might not be available (Mtombeni, 2017). Preparation and execution of the LP involve strict adherence to detail and procedures. The patient must first give informed consent, with an explanation of the procedure and risks involved. Proper patient positioning, generally lateral decubitus with knees to the chest, has the effect of opening up the intervertebral spaces to allow needle placement. With the puncture site cleaned appropriately, the practitioner selects an appropriate size needle and approach angle. CSF aspiration has to be carried out with care so that contaminants are not introduced, and sufficient volume has to be retrieved for laboratory analysis without subjecting the patient to excessive discomfort. Follow-up after the procedure is necessary to identify any immediate side effects, e.g., headache or backache, which can be generated by the procedure (ESICM LIVES 2017, 2017). The implications of an LP extend beyond immediate clinical impacts to affect public health and educational outcomes of medical education. Where medical resources are limited, as in LMICs, it is important that there be effective curricula for significant procedural competencies, such as LP. Consensus expert opinion regarding procedural skills necessitates the inclusion of LP in undergraduate medical training courses in order to complete the competency gaps (Mtombeni, 2017).

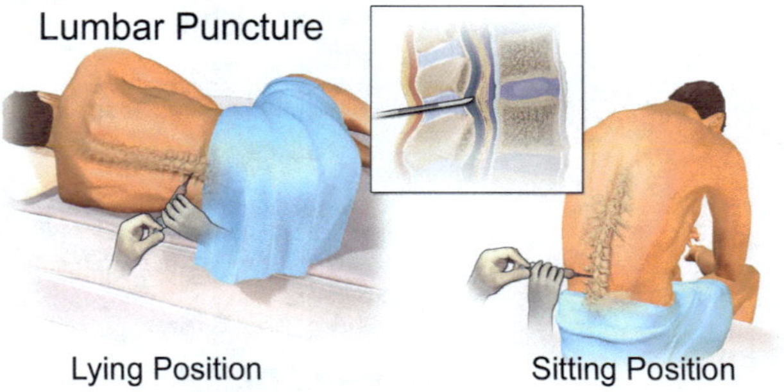

Figure 8.4. Illustration of lumbar puncture (LP) in both lying and sitting positions.

Source: https://images.squarespace-cdn.com/content/v1/53c1a2cce4b0e88e61f99b70/a3a1cd2e-683d-4dac-8441-ab00b0be6365/Blausen_0617_LumbarPuncture.png.

By focusing on instruction in proficient procedural skills, healthcare practitioners can optimize diagnostic function and patient care for the underserved by stressing the possibility of transformation through high-quality medical education. In the end, with healthcare system change, it will be essential that providers possess a robust skill set, including LP skill, to deliver high-quality and just care (ESICM LIVES 2017, 2017) (Figure 8.4).

8.2.1. Indications for Performing a Lumbar Puncture

The criteria for performing an LP are at the center of clinical practice, with neurology and emergency medicine being its principal domains. The procedure is primarily utilized to obtain CSF for diagnostic purposes, which enables clinicians to assess such conditions as infections, inflammatory disorders, and malignancies. As a case in point, an LP is generally requested if the patient is suspected of having meningitis or central nervous system (CNS) hemorrhage due to the fact that CSF analysis may reveal pathogens, white blood cells, and other critical parameters for the purpose of making an early diagnosis and initiating therapy. The use of LP in the evaluation of idiopathic intracranial hypertension and multiple sclerosis only adds to its pivotal position in formulating a prognosis and guiding therapeutic interventions. This is thus a technique that needs to be perfected by physicians dealing with neurologic emergencies and chronic diseases. The LPs also have therapeutic applications, particularly in the delivery of medications into the cerebrospinal compartment. Certain diseases such as acute compressive spinal cord injury may necessitate the intrathecal injection of chemotherapeutic agents or anesthetics, which requires mastering techniques performed in LP. Moreover, in the case of elevated intracranial pressures, an LP can also be therapeutic and diagnostic; fluid withdrawal from the CSF space decreases tension and averts complications. Dual-purpose use for LPs indicates the need for proper training and adherence to established practices in order to prevent PS and for effective results in therapeutic as well as diagnostic ends. Such procedural abilities are particularly emphasized in education curricula for the preparation of future healthcare providers with desirable emergency management capabilities, as certified by Mtombeni (2017). Although there exist numerous benefits of LPs, there are some important contraindications healthcare professionals should be aware of prior to performing the procedure. Underlying pathology, such as increased intracranial pressure due to a mass lesion, coagulopathy, or infection along the puncture track, may significantly raise the risk of complications such as brain herniation and infections. For this reason, a complete clinical assessment, including imaging, is valuable to exclude the potential for an LP in specific patient populations. The necessity to balance the diagnostic benefits with the potential risks encapsulates the subtlety of clinical decision-making. As highlighted in emerging education paradigms for procedural skill, understanding LP indications and contraindications further reinforces physicians' need to develop an accurate process to patient evaluation and procedural execution, and thus enhance patient care in emergency and critical care environments (ESICM LIVES 2017, 2017) (Figure 8.5).

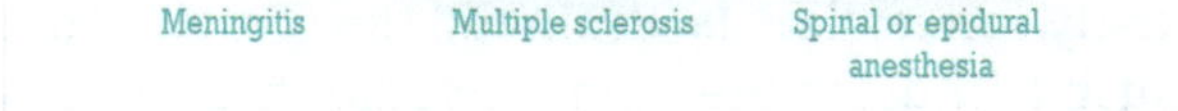

Figure 8.5. Indications for lumbar puncture.

Source: https://images.medindia.net/surgicalprocedures/450_237/indications-for-lumbar-puncture.jpg.

8.2.2. Step-by-Step Procedure for Lumbar Puncture

In the conduct of this LP, the process is followed by adequate patient evaluation and preparation. The patient should be informed about the procedure, its indications, and potential complications so that consent can be obtained. The patient is then positioned suitably in position, normally lateral recumbent or sitting bedside, forward leaning to provide easier access to intervertebral spaces. The practitioner should then proceed to administer a thorough antisepsis of the lower back to prevent infection. It is important to identify the correct lumbar interspace, often between L3-L4 or L4-L5, at which a needle shall be inserted. This preparation stage is essential in establishing a sterile environment and providing the patient with the utmost comfort and reassurance and therefore optimizing the procedure encounter. The second stage is the implementation of the LP itself, starting with the placement of a local anesthetic to prevent pain from needle penetration. The practitioner then slowly inserts the spinal needle, taking care to navigate between the spinous processes until the dural sac is entered. This requires not just hand skill but good knowledge of spinal anatomy to avoid frequent complications such as damage to nerves or hemorrhage. Following dural puncture, CSF should drain freely from the hub of the needle, indicating successful entry into the subarachnoid space. CSF can be obtained at this time for diagnostic testing, taking care to draw samples sequentially if more than one tube is needed. The best technique is needed to achieve maximum diagnostic yield with minimum patient discomfort and complication. Lastly, once CSF is drained, the practitioner must withdraw the spinal needle in a prompt manner with gentle pressure applied to the site of puncture to minimize post-procedure complications like headache or bleeding. The site must be dressed securely, aside from teaching the patient about post-procedure care, which may involve hydration and bed rest to reverse potential CSF leakage. There should be a strict monitoring protocol to observe any post-LP side effects, e.g., pain in the back or neurological. Teaching warning signs, e.g., headache or change in sensation, will allow the patient to report if urgent action is required. Collectively, LP technique proficiency is essential to clinicians, bolstering their procedural repertoire in the treatment of various neurological conditions in practice effectively (ESICM LIVES 2017, 2017) (Figure 8.6).

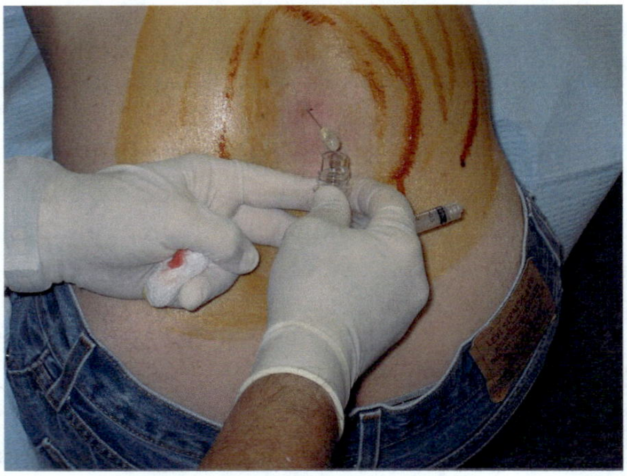

Figure 8.6. A lumbar puncture is being performed. The needle is in place, and the CSF is being collected in a small tube. The operator is wearing gloves to prevent infection. A large area on the back has been washed with an iodine-based disinfectant, leaving the back a brown/yellow color.

Source: https://upload.wikimedia.org/wikipedia/commons/thumb/f/fe/Wikipedian_getting_a_lumbar_puncture_%282006%29.jpg/800px-Wikipedian_getting_a_lumbar_puncture_%282006%29.jpg.

8.2.3. Risks and Complications Associated with Lumbar Puncture

The LP process, while invaluable in the diagnosis and treatment of most neurological diseases, carries risks and complications inherent to it that must be balanced with the greatest care. These are the potential occurrences of post-lumbar puncture headache (PLPH), observed in a significant percentage of patients, particularly when the larger needle is employed. This headache is typically characterized as position-dependent, with worsening with an erect posture and improvement while recumbent.

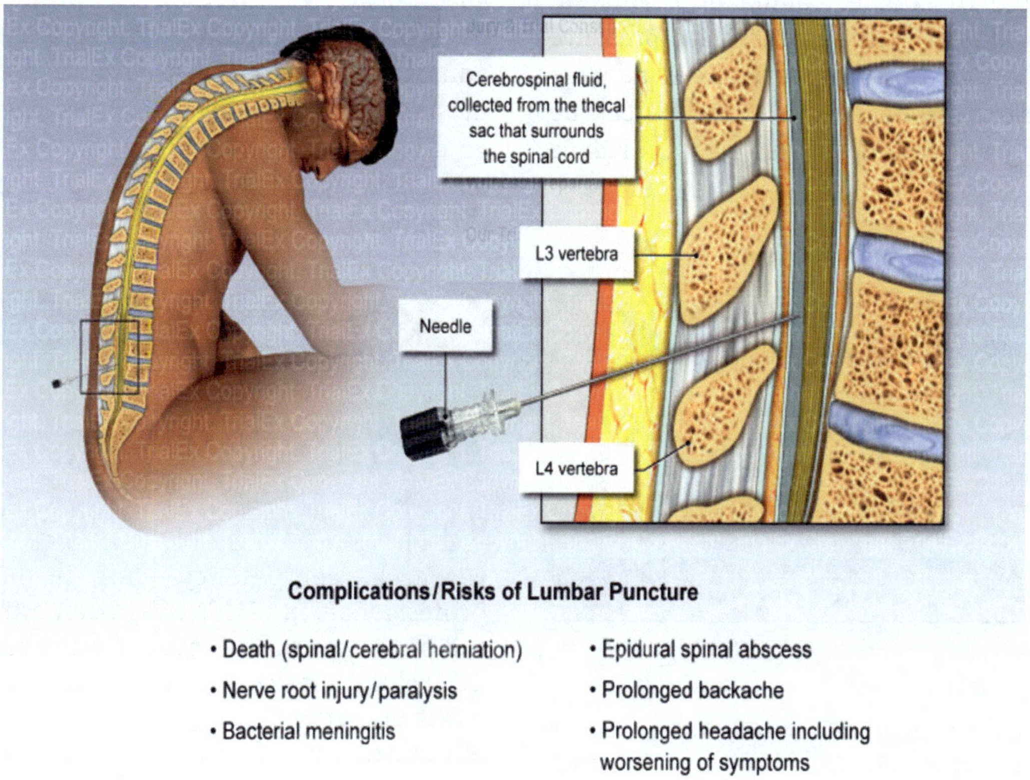

Figure 8.7. Complications/risks of lumbar puncture.

Source: https://cdn.trialex.com/library_media/production/5229d8196492346e8c788286a6f2a81a/c/SP_C_1201-library_medium.jpg.

The pathophysiology is believed to be secondary to the leak of CSF through the puncture site, resulting in decreased intracranial pressure. Furthermore, the occurrence of PLPH may be influenced by patient age, hydration, and the technique utilized during the procedure, so utmost care must be exercised to prevent risk and educate patients regarding potential complications (Mtombeni, 2017). Aside from PLPH, LP can lead to more severe complications like infection and hemorrhage. Intrathecal infection, or meningitis, is a consequence if sterile technique is not done very carefully or if the needle is inserted through an unintentional skin infection. The patients' overall medical status, including immunocompromised conditions, is a factor in this risk and the reason why pre-procedure assessment is essential. Hematoma formation, although less probable, is a consequence if the needle inadvertently enters a blood vessel during insertion. This risk is amplified in coagulopathic or weak patients. To counteract these risks, clinicians should be firm in following aseptic protocols, perform thorough evaluation, and weigh the procedure's advantages against the underlying conditions that may increase the likelihood of complications (ESICM LIVES 2017, 2017). Lastly, neurological complications, though rare, remain a prevalent issue associated with LP. These may manifest as reversible neurological deficits or, in the worst cases, permanent damage from nerve damage due to needle trauma or brainstem herniation due to acute intracranial pressure change. Though cases of permanent damage are very rare, the damage, if it occurs, can be devastating, and it underscores the importance of good patient selection and good familiarity with anatomy prior to the procedure. Patient education also plays a vital role; educating patients about possible symptoms and what goes on in the procedure can promote better outcomes and patient-provider trust. Finally, educating oneself with information regarding LP and taking the necessary precautions will go a long way in minimizing the risk involved and ensuring the procedure is a safer process (Mtombeni, 2017) (Figure 8.7).

Test Your Knowledge

1. What are the primary clinical indications for performing a lumbar puncture?
2. Describe the step-by-step procedure for performing a lumbar puncture, including patient positioning and needle insertion sites.
3. What are the common risks and complications associated with lumbar puncture?

8.3. ECG Interpretation

Learning Outcome

1. Understand the basics of electrocardiogram (ECG) and its significance;
2. Describe Common arrhythmias and their ECG characteristics;
3. Explain the importance of accurate ECG interpretation in clinical decision-making.

In the context of emergency medicine, interpretation of the ECG is a critical procedural skill that underscores the importance of timely diagnosis and treatment of patients who experience cardiac events. With cardiovascular disorders so prevalent, learning to accurately interpret the ECG can have a revolutionary impact on patient outcomes. Compared to other procedural skills that may be very technical, e.g., LP or IV access, interpretation of ECG involves a sensitive understanding of cardiac rhythm and the physiological significance of each abnormality. As evidenced through various research, competency gaps in healthcare professionals in LMICs have been attributed to the poor exposure to procedural training (like ECG) at the undergraduate level, with a cascading effect on patient care (Mtombeni, 2017). Thus, enhancement of the teaching mechanism pertaining to ECG competencies is needed to develop proficient healthcare professionals able to make real-time decisions. Reading ECG entails several levels of learning, beginning from the identification of normal sinus rhythm up to the identification of pathologies such as arrhythmias, ischemia changes, and conduction. Learners and practitioners adopt systematic approaches to interpretation that include the utilization of mnemonics and algorithmic aids to assist in the reading of the complex details of the ECG. Moreover, the significance of differentiating between a single waveform and another and between intervals should not be overestimated because they can have ruinous clinical impacts if interpreted wrongly. It has been demonstrated that augmenting the curriculum and emphasizing key competencies in the interpretation of ECG can fill knowledge gaps in medical trainees (ESICM LIVES 2017, 2017). By establishing a strong educational framework, the health care systems are then positioned to train up-coming professionals such that they can interpret ECG data in a competent way. Positioning ECG interpretation among the entire content of procedural skills calls for an innovative medical education approach in emergency medicine. It entails technical proficiency in ECG interpretation as well as integration of clinical contexts in which these interpretations would alter patient management. For example, the capacity to distinguish between ST-elevation myocardial infarction and non-ST-elevation myocardial infarction is most important in the acute treatment protocols. Also, repeated review by simulation and peer teaching can maximize skill and confidence levels among the learners. As has been shown, the educational needs are pressing, particularly where there are limited healthcare resources, highlighting the need for a wide-ranging curriculum focusing not just on procedural knowledge, but also critical thinking to deal with complex clinical situations (Mtombeni, 2017). A true focus on developing ECG interpretation skills as part of emergency medicine training is ultimately essential to enhance overall patient safety and care.

8.3.1. Basics of Electrocardiogram (ECG) and Its Significance

The ECG is an essential tool in modern medical practice that provides a graphic representation of the electrical activity of the heart. This test measures the rhythm, rate, and overall electrical conduction of the heart and is literally worth its weight in gold for the identification of an enormous variety of cardiac disorders, including arrhythmias, myocardial infarctions, and electrolyte imbalances.

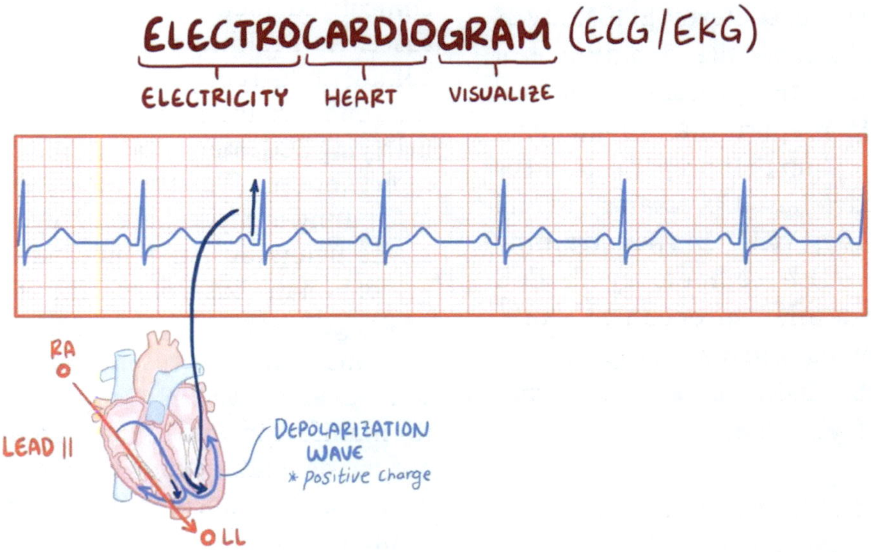

Figure 8.8. Electrocardiogram (ECG).

Source: https://d16qt3wv6xm098.cloudfront.net/K4zwYlFjRDmFLIrJ65Ge0Qq7T3uF2pEY/_.jpg.

By placing electrodes on the patient's skin, health care providers can capture precise electrical signals that reflect the workings of the heart. The value of ECG not only lies in its diagnostic utility but also in its expanded applications for monitoring response to therapy and guiding future clinical decisions. It is a matter of profound understanding of the fundamentals of an ECG, that is, the P wave,

QRS complex, and T wave, and the various phases of cardiac activity they symbolize. Each element of the waveform holds valuable information regarding atrial and ventricular depolarization and repolarization, giving clinicians real-time insight into heart function. Understanding of these elements allows medical professionals to identify deviations from the norm immediately, which could indicate emergent health issues, thus enhancing PS and outcomes. In clinical practice, initial ECG interpretation can be crucial, especially in the case of emergencies where immediate decision-making is essential in a patient's outcome. Furthermore, providing procedural skills training with ECG interpretation, among others, like IV access and LP, helps to reinforce the fact that patient care is not a one-dimensional process. As is pointed out in existing literature, clinical competencies, such as those related to POCUS, must be transferred among medical specialties so they can be made to fit into various clinical contexts (ESICM LIVES 2017, 2017). Emphasizing the significance of ECG interpretation in the process of medical education can help prepare the ground for a wide-ranging curriculum that prepares trainees to deal with practice-based problems (ESICM LIVES 2017, 2017). With proper training of students to acquire competency in ECG interpretation and other procedural skills, medical professionals will be well-placed to provide top-notch quality care in different medical settings (Figure 8.8).

8.3.2. Common Arrhythmias and Their ECG Characteristics

Understanding common arrhythmias and the corresponding ECG characteristics is essential to successful clinical practice and procedural skills, particularly in those settings in which proficiency in ECG interpretation is necessary. Arrhythmias, or irregular heart rhythms, can occur in various forms, including atrial fibrillation, ventricular tachycardia (VT), and bradycardia. Each of these has unique ECG characteristics of importance for diagnosis and management. For instance, atrial fibrillation is characterized by the absence of P waves and an irregular rhythm and can lead to inadequate cardiac output as well as increased risk of thromboembolic complications. Knowledge of these patterns not only helps in the proper interpretation of the ECG but also directs the intervention needed in stabilizing patients facing these potentially fatal states. VT represents a more advanced challenge, typically with wide and ridiculous QRS complexes, at a greater than 100 beats per minute. The rapid rhythm can compromise left ventricular function and cause major hemodynamic instability. ECG profiles for VT may be very varied from time to time, sometimes presenting as a normal sinus rhythm or other arrhythmias, so it is important to investigate the patient's history and clinical background for interpretation. These are not only demanding exact ECG reading, but also instant clinical judgment, often called upon in acute cases. As healthcare practitioners grow more comfortable recognizing such patterns, they thus enhance their procedural skills, eventually marrying ECG interpretation and relevant clinical interventions (Thierry et al., 2013). Another fascinating arrhythmia is bradycardia, which is a rate below 60 per minute and is frequently evident on the basis of specific ECG features like prolonged PR intervals or prominent junctional rhythms. Clinical presentation of bradycardia can be vastly varied, ranging from nil at all to manifestations of compromised cardiac output, depending upon the cause and extent of deviation from normal rhythm. Comprehension of the nature of bradycardia is not only crucial for diagnosis but also for deciding when to treat, whether this can be achieved through pacing or with medication. The integration of improved techniques, such as deep learning, into reading ECGs is likely to help improve both accuracy and efficiency of diagnosis and thereby potentially achieve positive results for bradycardic patients (Bizopoulos & Koutsouris, 2019). By acquiring the ECG characteristics of these common arrhythmias, physicians are able to greatly enhance their procedural expertise in the context of current medical practice (Figure 8.9).

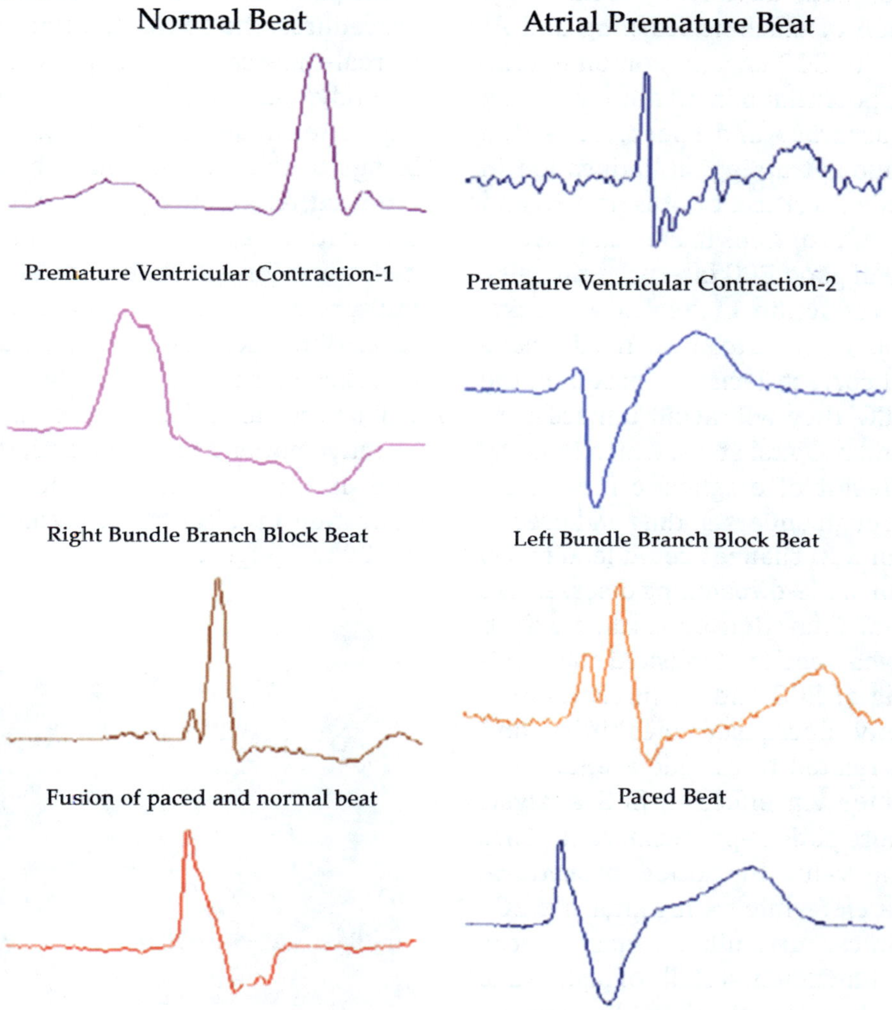

Figure 8.9. Typical arrhythmia heartbeats in time domain (lead II signal).

Source: https://www.researchgate.net/profile/Chia-Hung-Lin-6/publication/222821372/figure/fig9/AS:668554609315858@1536407248823/Typical-arrhythmia-heartbeats-in-time-domain-Lead-II-signal.png.

8.3.3. Importance of Accurate ECG Interpretation in Clinical Decision-Making

Accurate interpretation of ECGs is the cornerstone of clinical decision-making, allowing for early diagnosis and treatment of cardiovascular diseases. ECG is the initial method for the identification of arrhythmias, myocardial ischemia, and other cardiac defects and thereby determines clinical interventions. Accuracy in ECG interpretation is paramount; interpretation mistakes will result in mismanagement, which might have adverse effects on the patient. As observed in several studies, under-recognition as well as over-recognition of ECG alterations can go a long way in influencing a patient's clinical course, hence the need for properly trained healthcare providers. Also, with advancing technology, the incorporation of machine learning and AI into the analysis of ECG is gaining momentum, which can have potential benefits of improving interpretation accuracy and speed. Thus, the need for continuous training and education in interpreting ECGs is critical to preserve PS and optimize therapeutic options in clinical practice. The importance of good ECG interpretation also resides in the reduction of healthcare costs and improved patient outcomes. If clinicians make rapid and correct decisions based on the results of an ECG, they will avoid unnecessary interventions and hospital stays, which in many cases are the result of diagnostic indecision. Moreover, a thorough understanding and precise interpretation of ECG changes could lead to the early recognition of life-threatening diseases like acute myocardial infarction or cardiac arrest. For instance, it has been established that real-time monitoring of ECG and its interpretation has significantly decreased morbidity and mortality rates related to cardiac events. Also, positive outcomes via effective ECG analysis contribute to more patient-physician confidence that fosters the value of skilled procedural procedures. Therefore, integrating intensive ECG training into clinical curriculum is most critical, highlighting the fundamental skills of high-grade patient care. At last, the relationship between effective ECG interpretation and procedural skill highlights the intricate aspects of successful clinical practice. Though these interventions, such as IV access, LP, and thoracentesis, require technical skill, knowledge of the cardiac implications reflected in ECG readings can supplement the clinician's overall assessment of the patient's condition. For example, in urgent procedures, the ability to interpret ECG signals in real-time can alert healthcare providers to hemodynamic instability, enabling them to adjust technique accordingly. This divergence brings to the fore not only the technical facts required to conduct procedural skills but also the critical and analytical thinking abilities necessary for effective clinical judgment, and interpretation skills that directly impact patient care. With increasing sophistication in health care, acquiring these mutually supporting skills will be crucial in delivering comprehensive and effective patient-centered care, thereby making ECG literacy a core component of clinical education in all areas of medicine (Thierry et al., 2013) (Figure 8.10).

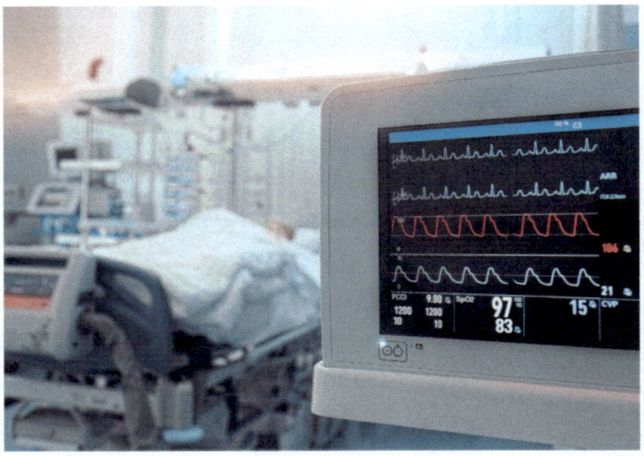

Figure 8.10. Presenting accurate-ECG-data in clinical decisions.

Source: https://www.noravmedical.com/wp-content/uploads/2024/07/Essential-Role-of-Accurate-ECG-Data-in-Clinical-Decisions.png.

Test Your Knowledge

1. What is the basic principle of an electrocardiogram (ECG) and why is it important in clinical practice?
2. How does accurate ECG interpretation impact clinical decision-making and patient management?

8.4. Arterial Blood Gas (ABG) Analysis

Learning Outcome

1. Understand the purpose and indications for ABG analysis;
2. Discuss the procedure for obtaining and analyzing ABG samples;
3. Deal with interpretation of ABG results and clinical implications.

Arterial blood gas (ABG) measurement is one of the major diagnostic tools of clinical medicine, particularly in assessing the respiratory and metabolic state of a patient. From the assessment of oxygen, carbon dioxide, and arterial blood pH, medical practitioners are able to determine whether a patient is able to perform homeostasis. The measurement is most important in handling diseases such as COPD, kidney impairment, and metabolic disorders. The process of the procedure is to get a blood sample from the radial artery, and it needs to understand arterial structures to prevent complications like hematoma or arterial occlusion. Additionally, knowledge of the use of ABG analyzer and result interpretation helps to play a key role in determining the therapeutic maneuvers that restore proper gas exchange and acid-base balance in patients. It is crucial to understand the underlying physiology in order to properly interpret ABG. The parameters that are measured—oxygen tension (PaO_2), carbon dioxide tension ($PaCO_2$), and pH—are indicative of a patient's respiratory and metabolic status. Reduced levels of PaO_2 indicate hypoxemia, suggesting inadequate oxygenation, while elevated levels of $PaCO_2$ suggest respiratory acidosis, which can be due to ventilatory impairment. On the other hand, metabolic acidosis can also present in a normal or low PaCO2 because the body is already compensated by hyperventilation. Clinicians should also be skilled in mixed acid-base disorders in which two or more pathologies can interact with each other, making the clinical situation complicated. Therefore, expertise in ABG analysis not only contributes to clinical judgment but also strengthens patient care outcomes by guiding timely and appropriate interventions (Mahadevan & Garmel, 2012). The inclusion of ABG testing in daily clinical practice underscores the significance of procedural skill in health care professionals. Skill in this regard involves not only the performance of the arterial puncture but also the analysis and interpretation of results after the puncture in the context of a comprehensive clinical assessment. Training on ABG procedures should involve proper methods, including site selection, asepsis, and minimizing patient discomfort. Simulation training and continuing education programs could improve the proficiency of healthcare professionals to conduct these critical procedures proficiently. Furthermore, the ability to communicate ABG results and meaning to patients and inter-professional teams facilitates inter-professional treatment planning decision-making, ultimately leading to better PS and quality of care (Mahadevan & Garmel, 2012) (Figure 8.11).

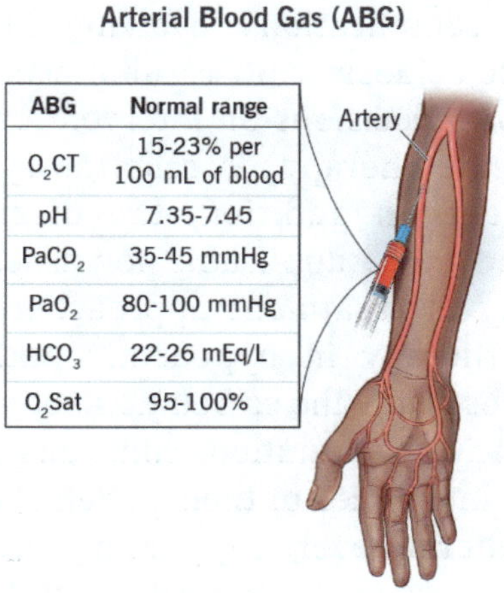

ABG	Normal range
O_2CT	15-23% per 100 mL of blood
pH	7.35-7.45
$PaCO_2$	35-45 mmHg
PaO_2	80-100 mmHg
HCO_3	22-26 mEq/L
O_2Sat	95-100%

Figure 8.11. Arterial blood gas (ABG).

Source: https://my.clevelandclinic.org/-/scassets/images/org/health/articles/22409-arterial-blood-gas.

8.4.1. Purpose and Indications for ABG Analysis

In clinical medicine, the interpretation of ABG is critically diagnostic in nature. It evaluates the patient's respiratory and metabolic condition, providing very valuable information about oxygenation, acid-base status, and carbon dioxide levels. The test is particularly indicated in situations of respiratory distress, with base conditions of acute exacerbations of COPD, pneumonia, or asthma attack having the potential to cause severe gas exchange abnormalities. Additionally, ABGs are useful when monitoring patients under sedation or anesthesia, in which ventilation could be compromised. Taking precise measurements of the arterial gases, medical personnel can readily identify and treat life-threatening scenarios, ultimately optimizing patient outcome within the emergency and critical care setting. Competency in interpreting ABG is fundamental in making therapeutic intervention in the acute care setting. The indications for ABG assessment exceed acute care scenarios since it is also important in the care of chronic conditions. For instance, renal failure, diabetes, or metabolic disease patients often require regular acid-base status checks to avoid complications involving alkalosis or metabolic acidosis. ABG results in these cases may inform decisions on intervention, such as bicarbonate therapy or respiratory support adjustment. In addition, the discussion is more and more applicable for assessing the efficiency of treatment approaches, such as oxygen therapy in hypoxemic patients. By closely observing the correlation between ABGs and clinical presentation, clinicians may deal with the intricacies of their patients' condition on a general level, supporting the holistic approach essential for successful medical practice. Interestingly, ABG analysis education is mandatory for all healthcare professionals, including not only emergency medicine clinicians but also nurses and respiratory therapists. Uniform protocols must be developed both for obtaining and interpreting ABG values to ensure consistency and accuracy in clinical use. Such institutions can benefit from initiatives like the ones proposed by the Academic College of Emergency Experts in India, which encourage the development of full-fledged training programs for developing procedural skills in emergency medicine. These advances can go a great distance in improving patient care by empowering healthcare professionals to carry out ABG analyses confidently and accurately. Therefore, encouraging a culture of academic excellence in this field is critical to improve PS and treatment effectiveness within acute clinical settings (Aggarwal et al., 2014; Adhikari, 2021) (Figure 8.12).

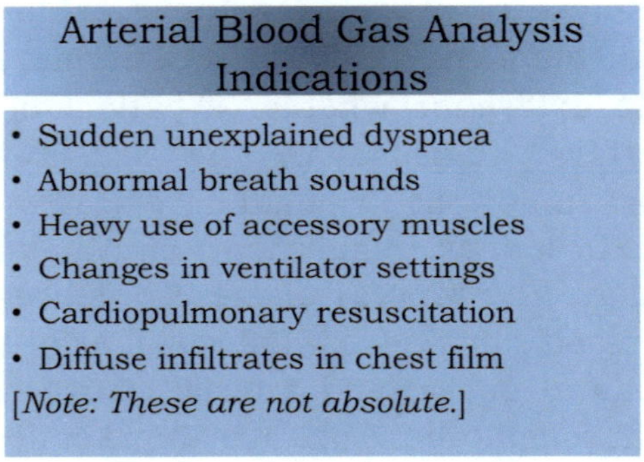

Figure 8.12. Indications for ABG analysis.

Source: https://mededu.blob.core.windows.net/public/assets/bloodgasAssets/Slide04.jpg.

8.4.2. Procedure for Obtaining and Analyzing ABG Samples

The collection of pulse-oximetric and ABG samples is essential to clinical management, facilitating accurate assessment of the patient's respiratory and metabolic function. The radial artery is preferred owing to its accessibility and collateral blood supply provided by the ulnar artery. Positioning of the patient is important; the wrist needs to be extended and maintained in an antiseptic-free area to ensure there are no infections. When feeling for the pulse to determine the same, a hemostatic technique is initiated, most commonly the Allen test, to determine adequate collateral circulation. The thorough preparatory process guarantees that the sample achieved will portray the physiological state of the patient, thus enhancing the validity of subsequent analyses and guiding principal intervention measures in emergencies, as noted in the procedural competency literature on emergency medical training (Mtombeni, 2017). Once the site is appropriately prepared, the clinician proceeds with arterial puncture through the use of a prefilled heparin syringe to prevent clot formation. The needle should be inserted at 30 degrees in relation to the direction of the pulse, with firm aspiration as it goes through the wall of the artery. A successful harvest is indicated by sufficient return into the syringe, and reposition or use of an alternative site is performed if return is poor. Following withdrawal, pressure is applied firmly to the area of puncture in a bid to minimize bleeding, and the sample must be capped and transported without delay to the laboratory for assessment. Notably, proper handling of ABG samples is required; delays may result in degraded results by means of gas diffusion, invalidating their diagnostic accuracy. This technical stringency not only testifies to the importance of technical expertise but also reflects the subtle appreciation of patient care present within clinical settings (ESICM LIVES 2017, 2017). Analysis of ABG samples requires sophisticated biochemical testing that discloses information regarding the state of the patient's respiratory system, metabolic function, and overall acid-base homeostasis. The interpretation most often entails consideration of significant parameters: pH, partial oxygen (PaO_2) and carbon dioxide ($PaCO_2$) pressures, and bicarbonate (HCO_3^-) level, all of which together determine clinical management. Correct interpretation entails understanding the underlying pathological phenomena resulting in abnormal measurements. For example, low pH with elevated PaCO2 may indicate respiratory acidosis, requiring clinical intervention at once. Therefore, doctors not only have to be skilled in taking ABG sample procedures but also skilled in reading results correctly. Regular training, as the medical trainers' consensus has put forward, is necessary in order to bridge gaps in procedural competencies needed in delivering high-quality emergency care in diverse clinical environments (Mtombeni, 2017) (Figure 8.13).

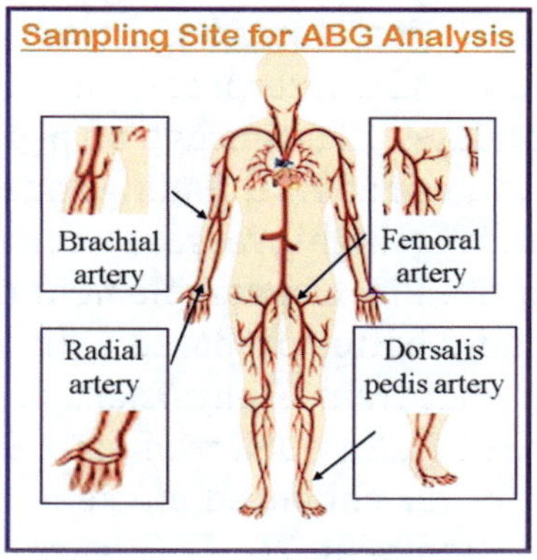

Figure 8.13. Sampling site for arterial blood gas (ABG) analysis.

Source: https://wecaregolp.com/wp-content/uploads/2023/05/Sampling-Site-for-Arterial-Blood-Gas-ABG-Analysis.jpg.

8.4.3. Interpretation of ABG Results and Clinical Implications

The interpretation of ABG is a crucial procedural skill in practice, particularly in emergency and critical care. ABGs provide basic information regarding a patient's acid-base status, oxygenation, and carbon dioxide, all of which are basic in diagnosing respiratory or metabolic derangement. For instance, elevated carbon dioxide can indicate respiratory failure, and low pH can indicate metabolic acidosis. Good interpretation entails not only familiarity with normal physiological ranges but also the ability to correlate these results with clinical presentation and other information to make a diagnosis. These abilities are most crucial in low- and middle-income countries, where clinical education and resource availability can vary extensively, making training in ABG core competencies by highly skilled individuals very vital (Mtombeni, 2017). The therapeutic implications of ABG results are extensive, affecting patient management and prognosis. A patient with acute respiratory failure, for instance, will have hypoxemia and hypercapnia by ABG, which will necessitate emergent measures such as supplemental oxygen or ventilation. On the other hand, metabolic disturbances like lactic acidosis need emergent identification and treatment of the causative etiology. A thorough understanding of these implications enhances the triage skills of clinicians and allows for early therapeutic interventions. Procedural skill deficits, as evidenced in the literature, in ABG interpretation can detract from patient care. Closing these deficits through systematic training is therefore necessary to enhance clinical outcomes across different healthcare settings (ESICM LIVES 2017, 2017). Integration of ABG interpretation into medical education programs addresses these concerns and consolidates the concept of procedural expertise in emergency medicine. The ability to interpret and utilize ABG findings adequately enhances clinical skill as well as promotes critical thinking during high-pressure scenarios. Furthermore, educational programs incorporating simulation training can complement traditional didactic methods, thereby making future health care providers better prepared with resources for effective ABG interpretation. Such a strategy guarantees that trainee physicians are adequately prepared for intricate clinical issues, leading to improved PS and quality of care. Such a focus on procedural skills can make the healthcare system strive for enhanced efficiency in managing acute and chronic cases where ABG analysis is crucial (Mtombeni, 2017) (Figure 8.14).

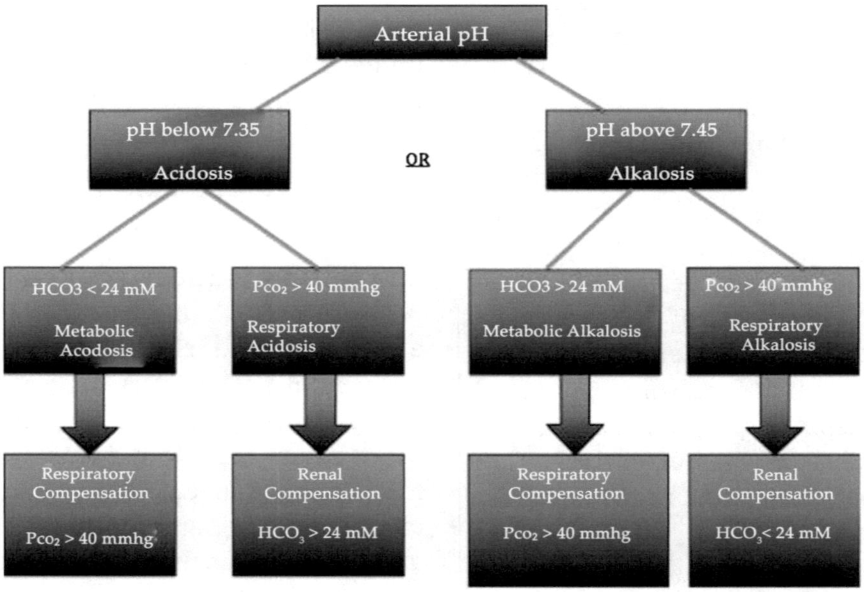

Figure 8.14. Stepwise approach to interpreting ABGs starting with pH.

Source: https://www.researchgate.net/publication/287359911/figure/fig6/AS:308569103716377@1450580015502/Stepwise-approach-to-interpreting-ABGs-starting-with-pH.png.

Test Your Knowledge

1. What are the main clinical indications for performing an arterial blood gas (ABG) analysis?
2. What clinical conditions can be diagnosed or monitored effectively using ABG analysis?

8.5. Thoracocentesis

Learning Outcome

1. Understand the indications for performing thoracocentesis;
2. Describe the technique and equipment used in thoracocentesis;
3. Focus on potential complications and post-procedure care.

Thoracocentesis is an important procedural skill in emergency medicine practice as a life-saving intervention for patients presenting with pleural effusions, pneumothorax, or other conditions that may compromise respiratory function. Thoracocentesis is performed by inserting a needle into the pleural space to withdraw a diagnostic or therapeutic amount of excess fluid or air. Skill with thoracocentesis is essential because incorrect technique will lead to complications of pneumothorax or damage to vital structures within the thorax. With the increasing frequency of conditions that produce pleural effusions, competence to undertake this timely procedure is increasingly being advanced as an essential skill among health practitioners, especially within intensive care and emergency settings. Anatomical landmark knowledge and adherence to sterile techniques are critical variables that optimize the safety and efficacy of thoracocentesis. In addition to the technical expertise of conducting thoracocentesis safely, medical professionals must also conduct proper assessment and preparation of the patient before instituting the procedure. This involves taking a thorough medical history, performing a physical exam, and using imaging tests like ultrasound or chest X-rays to precisely identify the location of the effusion or pneumothorax. With knowledge of the underlying cause of the patient's symptoms, healthcare professionals can make well-informed decisions about whether thoracocentesis is necessary and how urgently it must be performed. Ideally, the procedure would be performed within a controlled environment, e.g., a hospital with real-time backup available in the event of unexpected complications. By incorporating clinical judgment into the procedural pathway, practitioners are able to maximize patient outcomes and reduce the risk of adverse events.

The acquisition of procedural expertise in thoracocentesis, particularly in teaching institutions, remains crucial for enhancing the general skill level of prospective healthcare providers. Current literature emphasizes the need for formal training courses with both theoretical practice and practical experience within safe environments. As reiterated in the modern curricula of medical education, faculty consensus can allow for identification of essential procedural competencies, thereby enabling alignment of training programs with contemporary clinical requirements (Mtombeni, 2017). This ensures that future medical practitioners simply learn the procedural maneuvers but are also cognizant of the rationale behind every step of thoracocentesis. As a result, this extended training can significantly improve the quality and confidence of clinical professionals in performing vital procedures, ultimately improving patient outcomes in settings where thoracocentesis is commonly required (ESICM LIVES 2017, 2017) (Figure 8.15).

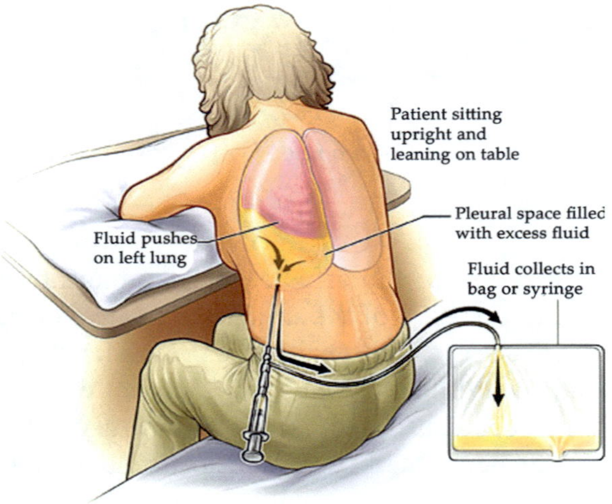

Figure 8.15. The illustration shows a person undergoing thoracentesis. The person sits upright and leans on a table. Excess fluid from the pleural space is drained into a bag.

Source: https://upload.wikimedia.org/wikipedia/commons/f/f5/Thoracentesis.jpg.

8.5.1. Indications for Performing Thoracocentesis

Thoracocentesis is a valuable intervention used both for diagnostic and therapeutic purposes in patients with pleural effusions. The primary indication for this type of intervention is when there is an accumulation of excess fluid in the pleural space that leads to dyspnea or pleuritic chest pain. Pleural fluid analysis not only helps establish the underlying etiology of the effusion—either infectious, malignant, or inflammatory but also contributes to the direction of further therapy. For instance, if the pleural fluid study reveals an exudative profile, infections like tuberculosis or malignancies could be involved and hence need directed therapeutics. In the acute context, swift resolution of respiratory distress through fluid drainage can significantly enhance patient comfort and clinical outcome. Therefore, knowledge of the indications for thoracocentesis is important for clinicians managing patients with pleural disease. Apart from symptomatic relief, thoracocentesis plays an important role in the management of patients diagnosed with underlying pulmonary conditions, such as congestive heart failure or pneumonia. These conditions are likely to be the cause of parapneumonic effusion formation, with fluid collection secondary to the pneumonia. For such cases, thoracocentesis allows physicians to assess the nature of the fluid and determine whether it is uncomplicated or complicated, thereby directing respective treatments—e.g., infection by antibiotics or hospitalization for intensive observation.

Moreover, malignancy patients usually present with pleural involvement, and thoracocentesis can allow cytologic examination for the elimination or confirmation of cancer. By recognizing the complex indications of thoracocentesis, clinicians can, in a positive manner, make a contribution to the overall management of patients with respiratory distress due to pleural pathologies. The second crucial indication for performing thoracocentesis is the evaluation of hemothorax, where the pleural space becomes filled with blood, generally due to trauma or cancer. Early treatment and diagnosis of hemothorax must take place to prevent complications such as airway obstruction or respiratory failure. Thoracocentesis in this scenario not only allows evacuation of the hematoma but also ensures that the etiology of the bleed is determined, with the aim of intervention being made at an early point. Furthermore, when other imaging techniques are not sufficiently informative or when the patient is unstable, a thoracocentesis can both diagnose and treat. Under these conditions, the process demonstrates the integration of procedural proficiency with clinical acumen, hence the relevance in the practice of critical care and emergency medicine to optimize patient outcomes and guide logical care planning (Adhikari, 2021).

8.5.2. Technique and Equipment Used in Thoracocentesis

The technique of thoracocentesis involves several critical steps and materials required for safe execution. To begin with, there is a need for patient positioning; typically, the patient sits up with arms resting comfortably on a table. Positioning assists in achieving maximum exposure of the pleural space. The sterile site must be duly prepared using an antiseptic solution to decrease infection risks. The equipment required consists of a thoracocentesis kit, which is generally a sterile cannula and needle, a container for collecting pleural fluid, and a syringe. In addition, ultrasound can be utilized to guide needle placement when fluid accumulation is not easily seen, to enhance further procedural safety and accuracy. Correct identification of the intercostal space during the process is important, often performed at the posterior axillary line on the 7th or 8th intercostal space. Local anesthetic is administered once the correct site is identified to reduce patient discomfort. Insertion of the needle slowly above the rib to avoid nerve and vessel damage. As the pleura is entered by the needle, the practitioner will feel a pop, which would verify entry into the space. Second, pleural fluid may be aspirated into the syringe and discarded for diagnostic analysis or for relief of a therapeutic drain. The art of being capable of mastering these technical aspects is crucial in both providing PS and realizing the desired clinical advantage. After the procedure, strict monitoring and documentation are crucial components of thoracocentesis. After the procedure, patients are usually asked to stay in bed for a couple of hours to monitor for any complications, e.g., pneumothorax or hemorrhage. Imaging studies, e.g., chest X-rays, may be done to ensure that there has been no complication. Additionally, the aspirated pleural fluid is commonly sent for laboratory analysis to assist in diagnosis, i.e., cytological study and biochemical study. Precise communication with the patient regarding possible risks and post-procedure care is essential in managing the patient's expectations and ensuring a smooth recovery process. The above holistic overview reflects the importance of technique and equipment in thoracocentesis and highlights its role in enhancing procedural success and PS (ESICM LIVES 2017, 2017; Mtombeni, 2017) (Figure 8.16).

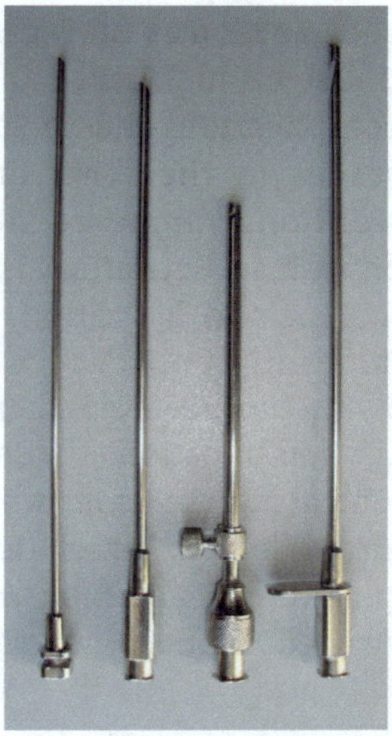

Figure 8.16. Instruments for thoracocentesis and needle biopsy of the pleura.

Source: https://upload.wikimedia.org/wikipedia/commons/thumb/f/f8/Needle_biopsy_of_the_pleura.PNG/320px-Needle_biopsy_of_the_pleura.PNG.

8.5.3. Potential Complications and Post-Procedure Care

In procedural skills, awareness of potential complications plays a crucial role in ensuring PS and quality care. For instance, when IV access is present, there are complications such as infiltration, phlebitis, and thrombosis that lead to pain, swelling, and possible progression to more severe conditions such as venous thrombosis. Additionally, as anatomical abnormalities are present in this condition, such as in Paget-

Schroetter Syndrome, the upper extremity deep vein thrombosis is much more susceptible and thus it is crucial that health care providers are vigilant while carrying out IV insertions and observe carefully for signs of complication (Amin et al., 2019). Identification of potential risks is a part of the entire clinical practice, which enables on-time intervention and decreases the incidence of adverse outcomes. Post-procedure care is an important feature following procedures such as LP and thoracentesis. After LP, patients must be monitored for headache, a common complication due to leaks of CSF. This can present in the form of PLPH, for which interventions might be necessary to enhance symptoms. Patients also must be instructed on rest and hydration, an element that will significantly impact recovery. In like manner, following thoracentesis, hemothorax or pneumothorax, complications that may warrant additional medical intervention, must be closely observed and monitored. Timely identification of such complications, combined with relevant post-procedure guidelines, can contribute to enhanced recovery and patient satisfaction. Incorporating the introduction of new technologies into procedural care, as underscored by medical education curricula, is also essential in avoiding a high rate of complications as well as improving patient outcomes after procedures. For example, recent advances such as ultrasound guidance for IV access and thoracentesis have been found to reduce the incidence of complications arising from these procedures. In making sure the practitioners are well acquainted with the technical aspects and tools at their command, they are more equipped to navigate through and circumvent potential complications. In addition, incorporation of substantial training in professional ethics and the law ensures that practitioners maintain high standards of care with regard to PS and informed consent in their practice (Adhikari, 2021). Lastly, the multi-dimensional approach to complication management and post-procedure care significantly enhances patients' overall procedural experience.

Test Your Knowledge

1. What are the common clinical indications for performing a thoracocentesis?
2. Describe the technique and necessary equipment used to safely perform a thoracocentesis.
3. What are the potential complications of thoracocentesis, and how can they be prevented or managed?

8.6. Comparison of Procedural Skills

Learning Outcome

1. Understand the similarities in preparation and patient care across procedures;
2. Explain the differences in techniques and equipment used;
3. Understand the impact of procedural skills on patient outcomes.

A critical examination of procedural proficiency in clinical practice illustrates significant differences among multiple techniques, particularly in the method of application and education. IV access is one of the most frequently performed procedures in acute care settings because of its central function in the delivery of medications and fluid resuscitation. Skillful practice of IV has been noted in the literature as critical, particularly in ICUs where patients can have multiple lines due to the complexity of their therapeutic plan. Simulation training has been a breakthrough approach in learning the skill, where clinicians can develop confidence and reduce patient discomfort and complications due to IV insertion (Mtombeni, 2017). These instructional methods emphasize the importance of standardized training protocols in order to offer competency, particularly in areas where procedural exposure may be reduced. Conversely, LP is a technically demanding procedure with both accuracy and anatomical data demands, typically employed for diagnostic and therapeutic purposes in neurology. The difficulty of skills is further compounded by patient anatomy, positioning, and potential complications, including infection and nerve damage. Successful pedagogical practice often utilizes cadaveric training and supervised learning experience to enhance competency amongst medical students and residents. A groundbreaking study identified that agreement on LP competencies needed would have the potential to profoundly improve training outcomes, paralleling endeavors amongst other procedural specialties (Mtombeni, 2017).

By prioritizing inquiry-based learning and continual feedback, faculty can maximize their curricula to lower their learning curve, thus enhancing PS and practitioner confidence in the performance of this critical procedure. Additionally, interpretation of ECGs and ABGs presents unique challenges due to the complexity of cardiac and respiratory physiology. The skills are of highest significance in the expeditious diagnosis of potentially life-altering conditions. While skill acquisition for both approaches can be realized using traditional lectures, innovative models such as interactive case studies and web modules optimize learner engagement and retention. Literature supports the application of technology in ECG training, ensuring improved understanding of arrhythmias and myocardial infarctions among trainees. Furthermore, as knowledge of ABG analysis keeps expanding, establishing a clear procedural competency in this area can bridge knowledge gaps in much the same way it was seen in IV access and LP training (ESICM LIVES 2017, 2017). As those procedural skills continue to evolve, ongoing evaluation of instruction methods will remain crucial to optimizing clinical outcomes.

8.6.1. Similarities in Preparation and Patient Care Across Procedures

In procedural skills, the significance of vigilant preparation and patient vigilance emphasizes the role of healthcare providers using a systematic strategy. In all procedures, such as IV access, LP, and ECG interpretation, vigilant preparation is crucial to ensure PS and procedural success. For example, in preparing for an IV access, the healthcare providers should choose the correct catheter size and site, as for ensuring the accurate anatomical landmarks before conducting an LP. Both procedures require patient anatomy knowledge and proper technique to avoid complications. This systematic preparation provides an environment that optimizes the likelihood of good results and minimizes the patient's discomfort, synchronizing procedural goals among a range of medical procedures. No less essential to procedural success, however, is attention to patient care, which ranges beyond specific techniques. Regardless of whether the procedure is ABG sampling or thoracentesis, practitioners must communicate with patients to explain the procedure, thus minimizing anxiety and eliciting informed consent. Establishing confidence through open communication is one of the cornerstones of high-quality care that operates across various procedures. In ECG interpretation, for instance, explicit descriptions in terms of electrode position and the purpose of the test help de-mystify the process to patients, following the patient-centered strategy adopted in LPs and other invasive interventions. By putting patient comfort and comprehension first in these encounters, clinicians achieve the twin objectives of technical skill and empathetic care. Use of standardized processes in preparation and patient care throughout these procedural competencies not only maximizes procedural effectiveness but also encourages a safety culture. On procedures like IV access and thoracentesis, the implementation of particular protocols can improve workflows and minimize the potential for complications. Evidence indicates that applying standardized procedures improves the level of predictability in results, such as in the research assessing separator fluid for IV lines, where standardized methodologies improved the process (ESICM LIVES 2017, 2017).

Similarly indicated through the greater application of data analysis, as exemplified in machine learning techniques in assessing patient risk for ICU readmission, is the necessity for ongoing improvement in practices according to standardized interpretations of information (ESICM LIVES 2017, 2017). Therefore, developing a culture of consistency in preparation and patient care raises procedural practice to the highest level of excellence to ensure that patients are given superior quality care in different medical procedures.

8.6.2. Differences in Techniques and Equipment Used

The wide variety of procedure skills required in clinical practice necessitates a singular set of intervention-specific methods and tools. For example, IV access is quite different from LPs in the techniques employed. IV access tends to utilize flexible catheters and appropriate venipuncture practices to facilitate quick and efficient administration of drugs and fluids. Unlike that, LPs require special spinal needles specifically designed for precise penetration of the subarachnoid space, emphasizing the crucial differences in the technique and equipment. Sensitivity to such differences minimizes complications and optimizes patient outcomes because poor technique or application of improper equipment can result in deleterious effects in terms of bleeding or infection. Thus, how a procedural skill is acquired is imperative to healthcare practitioners in the promotion of PS and effective treatment procedures. In addition, equipment used for each procedure, such as ECG reading and ABG interpretation, reflects clinical medicine's technical developments. ECGs rely on electrodes placed at strategic points on a patient's body to pick up electrical signals of the heart through devices that interpret the signals into readable formats. On the other hand, ABG is done on special analyzers and syringes that test specimens of blood to establish the effectiveness of gas exchange and acid-base balance. The differences in calibration and procedure inherent in both techniques speak to the fact that clinicians must not only be skilled at operating equipment but also at effectively interpreting results.

A comprehensive understanding of these devices enhances diagnostic accuracy and clinical judgment, ultimately enhancing patient care. Finally, the contrast between procedural techniques also exists for procedures such as thoracocentesis, which is the removal of fluid from the pleural space. Practitioners need to apply an aseptic technique, specific needle design, and correct patient positioning in order to obtain maximum safety and effectiveness. The selection of devices, e.g., needles and collection vessels, is also significant in the context of risk of complications such as pneumothorax or infection in case of noncompliance with conventional practice. The same is the case with implications of machine learning on clinical predictive models covered in research work incorporating advanced computing techniques that evince a shifting perspective of procedural results and evaluations of risk. The incorporation of advanced machine learning techniques into routine practice is able to facilitate improved management of patients, conveying details on procedural variation in line with individual physiological patterns, as illustrated through a research study (ESICM LIVES 2017, 2017). Overall, the diversity in methods and materials applied under various procedures emphasizes the importance of specialized training and continuous learning within the healthcare sector.

8.6.3. Impact of Procedural Skills on Patient Outcomes

The competence of medical practitioners in procedural skills directly influences patient outcomes in most medical conditions. Essential procedures such as IV access, LP, and thoracentesis are essential to effective patient management, particularly in the acute environment. A proficient practitioner can perform these interventions with greater efficiency and accuracy, therefore, lowering patient discomfort and procedural complications. Inability to perform procedures can translate to increased incidence of complications such as infection or procedural failure, which worsens a patient's health and contributes to longer hospitalization stays. Hence, ongoing training and examination of procedural skills are necessary, as seen through systematic core competencies identification for safe practice in emergency care (Mtombeni, 2017). The procedural skill is best observed in procedures such as ECG interpretation and ABG analysis, whereby the effect of timely and accurate results can mean everything in the way of treating a patient. These professionals must have not only the technical ability to conduct these procedures but also interpretive skill to properly estimate the ramifications of their results. For instance, improper placement of ECG leads or compromised blood sample handling results in misdiagnosis and leads to delay in life-saving treatment. By enabling proficient competence among doctors with these skills, healthcare systems can enhance predictive diagnosis and PS. Furthermore, the education curricula should focus on the development of such skills to fill existing loopholes in medical students' education, which consequently will lead to enhanced clinical outcomes (ESICM LIVES 2017, 2017). Finally, the cumulative impact of procedural skills extends beyond individual patient contacts, influencing healthcare efficiency and resource utilization as a whole. In high-risk environments, such as ICUs in which patients may require multiple IV therapies, possessing the ability to deal with procedural complications is the paramount concern. Research has also highlighted the role of procedural expertise in ensuring complex medication regimens, observing that inefficient practice may lead to unnecessary utilization of healthcare resources and patient distress from serial invasive procedures (ESICM LIVES 2017, 2017). Therefore, the clear linkage between proficient procedural skill and effective patient outcomes supports the imperative for effective training systems and ongoing evaluation of medical staff competence. By putting these skills into the limelight of medical training, healthcare organizations can foster a culture conducive to outstanding patient care.

Test Your Knowledge

1. What are the common steps in preparation and patient care that apply to invasive procedures?
2. How do the techniques and equipment differ between procedures?

SUMMARY

Procedural skill proficiency in areas such as IV access, LP, ECG interpretation, ABG analysis, and thoracentesis is central to the practice of modern medicine. Each of these interventions entails distinct techniques, clinical uses, and possible complications that must be treated by healthcare providers with expertise. As demonstrated by comprehensive educational models, integration of theoretical knowledge and experiential practice prepares medical practitioners to perform these interventions safely and effectively. Systematic understanding of these procedures not only improves patient care but also enhances the overall efficiency of healthcare delivery systems. Additionally, a strong emphasis on procedural training enables lifelong learning, as practitioners master a constantly evolving clinical landscape. Lastly, the applicability of these procedural skills goes beyond technical performance to encompass critical thinking and decision-making in practice. The ability to interpret outcomes from ECGs or ABG testing, for instance, is valuable for proper early diagnosis and treatment of numerous conditions. Similarly, successful IV access can be a critical determinant of patients' outcomes, especially in emergency cases where time matters. Constant exposure to real-life material of such procedures, coupled with concrete methods of assessment, is valuable in developing confidence and competency required in high-risk settings. Successful training protocols presented in academic literature emphasize the importance of a balanced mix of didactic education and experience, by which procedural skill acquisition is an integration. Finally, ongoing research and scholarship, as shown by institutions like The George Washington University School of Medicine and Health Sciences, is essential to refining procedural techniques and educational approaches. By engaging in research into these procedural competencies themselves, students and clinicians can contribute to an increasingly robust body of evidence that informs best practice and standardizes care across different clinical settings. The synergy between education, research, and practice generates a culture where continuous improvement is the shared objective for all professionals within healthcare. In this fast-evolving field, the commitment to honing procedural competence through study and practice ultimately corresponds to improved PS, satisfaction, and results in healthcare delivery, thereby meeting the fundamental objectives of medicine.

Procedural skills are crucial to providing quality patient care and optimal outcomes in healthcare. Procedural skills range from the straightforward to the extremely complex and are crucial across all healthcare facilities, but more so in ICUs. Procedural skills competency in methods such as IV access, LP, and interpretation of ECG directly affect the ability of healthcare professionals to manage acute medical conditions. For instance, IV access is not only a routine procedure; it is the gateway to medication administration, fluid resuscitation, and blood transfusion, which are all lifesaving in emergency situations. Inability to perform IV procedures can lead to complications like patient discomfort, heightened infection risks, and prolonged hospital stays, leading to a compelling need for comprehensive training in such skills. Outside of the immediate application to clinical practice, technical skill can enhance diagnostic refinement and treatment efficacy. Thoracocentesis or sampling for ABG, for instance, are not merely technical maneuvers; they provide crucial data regarding the patient's physiological state. ABG analysis, for instance, makes possible appraisal of acid-base status and oxygenation, facilitating immediate correction of respiratory or metabolic imbalances. Thoracocentesis similarly may relieve killer pleural effusions, significantly improving patient outcome. The importance of training in these procedures cannot be exaggerated because proficiency has an impact both on PS and on the quality of care provided. It is essential to ensure that healthcare professionals are skilled in these required procedures to prevent complications and optimize overall healthcare efficiency. Lastly, the inclusion of procedural skills training in healthcare education is vital in preparing upcoming practitioners to deal with the challenges of clinical practice. As the technology in healthcare keeps evolving and the patients become more and more complex, continuous education on procedural skills becomes more essential. Practice models such as cross-disciplinary education and simulation training can promote confidence and skill retention in healthcare workers. Furthermore, studies show that improving procedural ability not only improves patient management but also enhances teamwork within the healthcare setting, building a culture of excellence and collaboration. Thus, emphasizing the significance of procedural skill development among health professionals is paramount, as evident from studies that illustrate the connection between skill competence and improved PS outcomes, such as reduced readmissions and overall care effectiveness (ESICM LIVES 2017, 2017ESICM LIVES 2017, 2017).

KEY TERMS FROM THIS CHAPTER

Arrhythmias
Arterial occlusion
Carbon dioxide (PaCO2) pressures
Diagnostic methods
ECG interpretation
Electrolyte imbalances
Emergency medicine training
Human anatomy
Intravenous catheters
IV access
Arterial blood gas (ABG)
Bradycardia
Collect cerebrospinal fluid (CSF)
ECG competencies
Electrocardiogram (ECG)
Emergency management capabilities
Health system
Imaging tests
Irregular heart rhythms
IV-line failure

CRITICAL THINKING QUESTIONS

1. **Which of the following veins is most commonly used for peripheral intravenous (IV) access in adults?**
   a. Basilic vein
   b. Cephalic vein
   c. Median cubital vein
   d. Femoral vein
2. **What is the most appropriate intervertebral space for performing a lumbar puncture in an adult?**
   a. L1-L2
   b. L3-L4
   c. L2-L3
   d. T12-L1
3. **Which ECG finding is characteristic of an acute anterior myocardial infarction?**
   a. ST elevation in leads II, III, aVF
   b. ST elevation in leads V1-V4
   c. Deep Q waves in leads I and aVL
   d. Peaked T waves in leads V5-V6
4. **Which of the following ABG results is indicative of respiratory acidosis?**
   a. pH 7.25, $PaCO_2$ 60 mmHg
   b. pH 7.50, $PaCO_2$ 30 mmHg
   c. pH 7.35, $PaCO_2$ 40 mmHg
   d. pH 7.45, $PaCO_2$ 50 mmHg
5. **Which of the following is the safest site for performing thoracocentesis to drain pleural fluid?**
   a. Midclavicular line, 2nd intercostal space
   b. Posterior axillary line, 8th intercostal space
   c. Paravertebral line, 3rd intercostal space
   d. Midaxillary line, 4th or 5th intercostal space

Short Answer Questions

1. What are the key indications and contraindications for establishing intravenous (IV) access?
2. Describe the step-by-step procedure for performing a lumbar puncture, including patient positioning and the needle insertion site.
3. What are the main components of a normal ECG, and how do you identify common arrhythmias on the ECG tracing?
4. Outline the proper technique for obtaining an arterial blood gas (ABG) sample and the precautions to minimize complications.
5. What equipment is required for thoracocentesis, and how is the procedure performed safely?
6. List common complications associated with IV access, lumbar puncture, and thoracocentesis, and explain how to prevent them.
7. How does accurate interpretation of ECG and ABG results influence clinical management decisions?

Answers to Critical Thinking Questions

1. (c); 2. (b); 3. (b); 4. (a); 5. (d)

REFERENCES

1. Adhikari CL. Curriculum for Masters in General Practice - Bhutan. *J Family Med Prim Care.* 2021;10(6):2061-2119. doi:10.4103/jfmpc.jfmpc_1727_20(accessed on 27th June 2025).
2. Aggarwal, P., Galwankar, S., Kalra, O. P., Bhalla, A., Bhoi, S., & Sundarakumar, S. (2014). The 2014 Academic College of Emergency Experts in India's Education Development Committee (EDC) white paper on establishing an academic department of emergency medicine in India–Guidelines for staffing, infrastructure, resources, curriculum and training. *Journal of Emergencies, Trauma, and Shock, 7*(3). http://acee-india.org/acee-emtox/downloads/JETS_128_14_DOI_PDF.pdf (accessed on 27th June 2025).
3. Amin, A., Epstein, J., Lacayo, M., & Morakinyo, E. (2019). A series of unfortunate events – A rare presentation of thoracic outlet syndrome. https://www.nyacp.org/files/Final%20Book(3).pdf (accessed on 27th June 2025).
4. Bizopoulos, P., & Koutsouris, D. (2019). Deep Learning in Cardiology. *IEEE reviews in biomedical engineering, 12*, 168–193. https://doi.org/10.1109/RBME.2018.2885714(accessed on 27th June 2025).
5. ESICM LIVES 2017 : 30th ESICM Annual Congress. September 23-27, 2017. (2017). *Intensive care medicine experimental, 5*(Suppl 2), 44. https://doi.org/10.1186/s40635-017-0151-4(accessed on 27th June 2025).
6. Derebe, A. (2017). Teaching lumbar puncture procedures at Yekatit 12 Hospital Medical College Pediatrics Department–An exploratory and descriptive study. https://nadre.ethernet.edu.et/record/458/files/f1037814632.pdf (accessed on 27th June 2025).
7. George Washington University. (2024). *2024 Medical Student Research Day abstracts.* https://core.ac.uk/download/617786065.pdf (accessed on 27th June 2025).
8. Kawaguchi, I., & Saucedo, C. (2025). *WestJEM Full-Text Issue.* https://core.ac.uk/download/656118287.pdf (accessed on 27th June 2025).
9. Mahadevan, S. V., & Garmel, G. M. (2012). *An Introduction to Clinical Emergency Medicine.* Cambridge University Press. ISBN 978-0-521-74776-9 (pbk.)(accessed on 27th June 2025).
10. Mtombeni, S. (2017). Identifying procedural core competencies for undergraduate emergency medicine education at the University of Zimbabwe College of Health Sciences. https://core.ac.uk/download/188741950.pdf (accessed on 27th June 2025).
11. Singh, J., Matern, L. H., Bittner, E. A., & Chang, M. G. (2022). Characteristics of simulation-based point-of-care ultrasound education: A systematic review of MedEdPORTAL curricula. *Cureus, 14*(2), e22249. https://www.cureus.com/articles/83834-characteristics-of-simulation-based-point-of-care-ultrasound-education-a-systematic-review-of-mededportal-curricula.pdf (accessed on 27th June 2025).

CRITICAL CARE PRINCIPLES

9

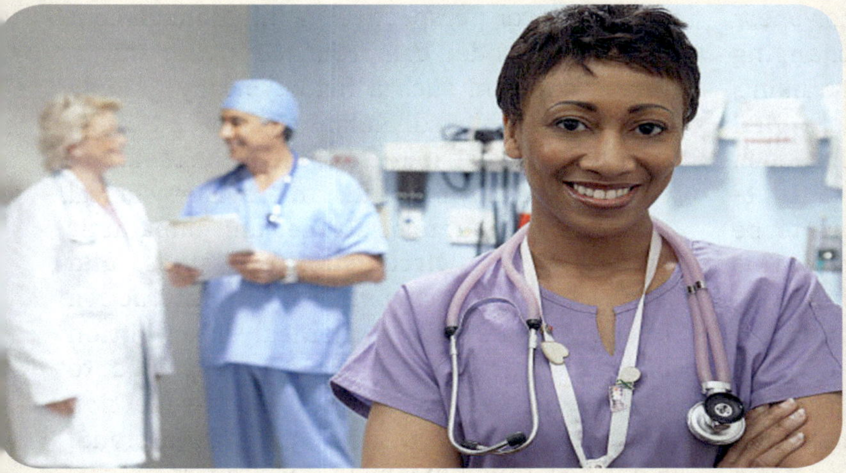

Introduction

Learning about its underpinning principles is of paramount importance in critical care for students and practitioners alike in the healthcare sector. Critical care principles are a unifying principle that guides clinical decision-making, with PS and quality of care always at the forefront of healthcare delivery. Understanding and appreciation of these principles allows healthcare professionals to better navigate the complexities of critical conditions, finally leading to better patient outcomes. As Contreras et al. (2020) point out, the importance of efficient training and preparedness can be promoted by proactively oriented education that prepares for health crises such as the COVID-19 pandemic. The development of a solid knowledge base of key principles of critical care will allow healthcare workers to establish the resilience needed to face novel challenges in practice. Moreover, simulation-based training is important in the education of healthcare professionals who work in critical care. As Contreras et al. (2020) describes the development of interprofessional simulation programs reflects the way in which

LEARNING OBJECTIVES

After studying this chapter, you will be able to:

1. Discuss patient assessment in the realm of critical care;
2. Understand communication in critical care;
3. Focus on ethical considerations in critical care;
4. Describe the advanced life support (ALS) techniques;
5. Deal with infection control measures;
6. Understand family involvement in critical care.

experiential training prepares staff members for the high-stakes nature of healthcare during crisis events. Simulation allows for practicing clinical scenarios, through which healthcare professionals can learn to establish critical skills like crisis resource management and infection control. Such a proactive stance not only increases the technical skills of practitioners but also makes them psychologically ready to handle actual-life crises. Incorporation of these pedagogical practices in critical care education reflects how preparedness and responsiveness are necessary even in a rapidly changing healthcare environment. Besides clinical training, knowledge about population health is a vital aspect of critical care disciplines. As has been outlined, the shift from fee-for-service to value-based care compels healthcare leaders to be familiar with population health principles. This is important for fostering effective initiatives that resonate with the needs of populations as well as strengthening healthcare delivery systems. By incorporating population health into the curriculum of health administration students, emerging leaders can better construct bridges between public health and healthcare systems. This emphasis on total comprehension is not only to equip students with the capability to face the challenges they will face but also to align with the great principle of delivering broad-spectrum and patient-centered care in critical care settings.

Definition of Critical Care

Critical care is a specialized area of medical care designed for the management and care of patients with life-threatening diseases needing rigorous monitoring and intervention. Critical care functions predominantly in ICUs, where health professionals employ advanced technologies and therapeutic modalities for patients with critical illness or surgical complications. The discipline depends on the blending of several fields, where it takes cooperation among doctors, nurses, and other health professionals to coordinate multifaceted treatment regimens. At the heart of the critical care definition is acknowledgment of the dynamic, largely unpredictable character of critical illness, necessitating ongoing evaluation and speedy interventions to stabilize patients and forestall further deterioration. Therefore, the essential character of critical care is embedded in its real-time and responsiveness, compelling clinicians to shift and refine treatment strategies in real time. A second essential component of defining critical care is the ethical perspective in the management of patients under compromised health status. Practitioners in such a field typically grapple with highly ethical dilemmas such as end-of-life care and the distribution of medical resources. Not only are they mandated to provide technical interventions, but to be attuned and empathetic to the unique circumstances, values, and preferences of each patient. This interaction is more than just a medical intervention because practitioners are also expected to subject themselves to critical self-reflection regarding their cultural and professional identities, thus humanizing healthcare. In this way, they can form therapeutic relationships that empower patients and families to become active participants in treatment decisions. This ethical perspective of clinical practice and psychology broadens the conversation about what is referred to as critical care beyond a set of procedures to an all-encompassing philosophy of addressing complex patient needs (Bury & Strauss, 2006). Furthermore, the importance of effective communication in critical care cannot be overstated, particularly when interacting with multi-ethnic patient populations. With the healthcare setting becoming increasingly multicultural, clinicians must manage complex cultural dynamics that influence patients' understanding of their disease and the treatment offered. Employing a tailored clinical approach to communication taking these complexities into consideration, can enhance healthcare delivery and ensure equitable interactions. These models, being grounded in extensive literature on communication practice, center on content, process, and relational dynamics within the environment. Emphasis on open communication and common understanding enables health practitioners to transcend boundaries and hence provide better health outcomes for patients from diverse backgrounds, particularly marginalized populations (McKivett et al., 2018). Finally, this perspective reimagines critical care as a sophisticated dance between medical expertise and compassionate engagement, solidifying its position as an integral pillar to modern healthcare systems (Figure 9.1).

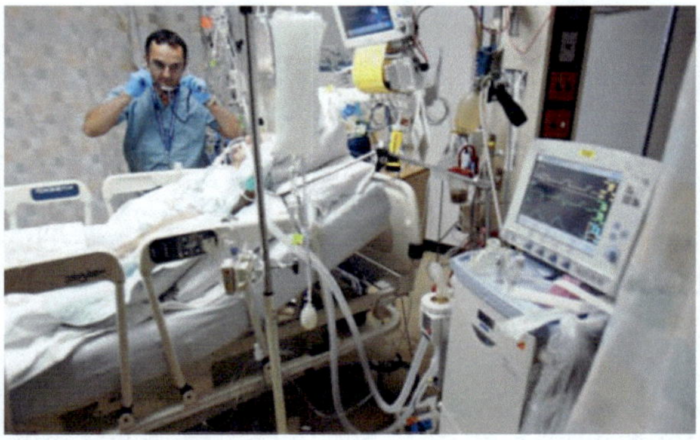

Figure 9.1. A patient being managed in an intensive care unit.

Source: https://upload.wikimedia.org/wikipedia/commons/a/a7/Respiratory_therapist.jpg.

Importance of Critical Care in Healthcare

Critical care is a critical component of modern healthcare, particularly for the treatment of severe and life-changing illnesses. The ICU denotes the acute need for sophisticated medical care, with the ability to treat patients who are under extreme physiological stress. Beyond merely treating acute illnesses, this intense degree of medical intervention restores patients through comprehensive rehabilitation processes tailored to individual needs. For instance, obesity, which is becoming more prevalent in the ICU setting, brings unique challenges to be addressed with a coordinated approach to treatment. A proper understanding of metabolic support, ventilator management, and multidisciplinary coordination becomes essential in delivering effective outcomes. Ultimately, critical care principles re-emphasize the application of a tailored approach, maximizing the chances of survival and recovery for patients with critical illnesses (McKivett et al., 2019). In addition, the integration of advanced technologies in intensive care has transformed patient management and can redefine healthcare narratives. AI, telemedicine, and other digital health technologies are a paradigm shift in how health professionals can monitor, assess, and communicate with patients. However, the ethical issues encompassed within these technologies must be taken seriously, particularly on matters of patient autonomy and informed consent. The ethical principles of beneficence and non-maleficence, both based in bioethics, are central to evaluating the impact of such innovations on patient experience and patient engagement. As practitioners of critical care move through these developments, an ethical framework will continue to be central to optimizing patient outcomes while minimizing technology-related risks (Burr et al., 2019). Thus, the worth of critical care extends beyond timely intervention, such as ethical aspects of a global nature in modern medical care. Finally, the worth of critical care is identified through its facilitation of safeguarding healthcare systems in the event of public health crises. The COVID-19 pandemic revealed the robustness of critical care services in adapting and responding to tremendous patient demands under unprecedented circumstances. During periods of such crises, the ability of healthcare facilities to offer efficient triage measures, optimize utilization of resources, and ensure quality care is most crucial. Moreover, coordination among agencies involving critical care physicians and public health agencies results in a multi-pronged response with a focus on patient health and population health. This collaborative effort confirms the fundamental importance of critical care as being not merely a clinical necessity, but as an important ingredient in fortifying healthcare infrastructures against adversity. Above all, the principles governing critical care address a far-reaching applicability, emphasizing its value in protecting individual patients and public health at large (Figure 9.2).

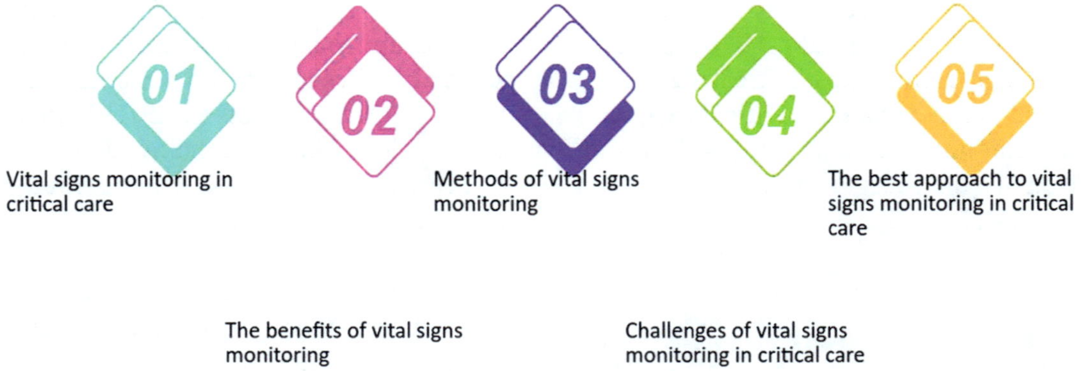

Figure 9.2. Monitoring vital signs in critical care.

Source: https://fastercapital.co/i/Life-support--Life-Support-in-the-ICU--Providing-Vital-Care--The-Importance-of-Monitoring-Vital-Signs-in-Critical-Care.webp.

Overview of Critical Care Principles

In medicine, critical care principles underpin the management of patients with life-threatening illnesses. Critical care principles are instrumental in directing health professionals toward making timely and effective interventions that essentially affect patient outcomes. An essential part includes rapid patient assessment and stabilization of the physiological condition, such as monitoring vital parameters, ensuring protection of adequate airway, and initiating proper resuscitative measures. By understanding these principles, clinicians will be able to make decisions that will set priorities for interventions to alleviate immediate threats to life, thereby enhancing the chances of recovery. This systematic approach not only guides clinical practice but also enforces teamwork and the importance of communication among multidisciplinary teams, including concerted effort in intensive care units. At the heart of effective critical care is patient-centered care, which emphasizes the incorporation of patients' values and needs into clinical choices. This idea supports collaborative engagement with patients and families, fostering an atmosphere of partnership that optimizes emotional support for challenging medical situations. Research indicates that when patients are engaged in their care activities, it can lead to improved satisfaction and adherence to treatment protocols. In addition, the potential barriers to participation must be addressed; for instance, in cancer survivors' needs management, healthcare providers must consider barriers as indicated by systematic user reporting, which captures issues such as fatigue and adequacy of support during clinic visits (Bradbury et al., 2019). By utilizing these findings, critical care guidelines can be optimized to offer holistic patient care. Moreover, critical care implementation goes beyond short-term medical interventions to address long-term effects, particularly for vulnerable populations. For youth with serious socioeconomic barriers, such as those in the justice system or homeless, moving into secure employment becomes key to recovery and rehabilitation. Principles aimed to aid this group recognize the complex problems they face, stressing the need for customized, intensive interventions to help secure not only employment, but also retention in the labor force. With the addition of statistics gathered from successful job programs, health practitioners can refine their strategies for successfully addressing such issues, so that these opportunity youth are not left out of their search for stability and success (Bradbury et al., 2019). With the extensive utilization of critical care terminology, immediate health issues alongside more prolonged support structures become most important.

9.1. Patient Assessment

Learning Outcome

1. Describe initial evaluation techniques;
2. Focus on continuous monitoring of vital signs;
3. Understand the use of diagnostic tools in critical care.

In the critical care setting, patient assessment is the foundation of providing adequate treatment and favorable health outcomes. Comprehensive assessment of the state of the patient is the outcome of systematic approaches that incorporate both clinical observations and patient history. Clinicians must have the capability to interpret vital signs, laboratory results, and symptoms reported by the patients as well as psychosocial factors likely to affect health behaviors. The role of motivational interviewing (MI) becomes important here since it allows clinicians to talk with patients more effectively about their treatment barriers and health behaviors. With emphases in recent research, incorporating MI in medical education underscores the need to build an empathetic environment where patients feel supported to be active participants of their treatment choices (Halbach & Keller, 2017). Consequently, patient assessment skills are improved using techniques like MI, which not only improves communication but also affects favorable health outcomes. Patient assessment is not a one-time initial process but a recurring process that needs to be watched and reevaluated, particularly in critical care. A key component of this recurrent assessment is the implementation of evidence-based practices to ensure that interventions remain sensitive to alterations in the patient's condition. Consultation with stakeholders and systems thinking are methods that are particularly effective for the understanding of patient needs in the context of health complex environments. By studying interdependencies between various elements of healthcare and how they influence the delivery of care, clinicians can make their assessments more appropriate so that they can respond to specific gaps in care (Marshall-Ponting et al., 2012). This combined understanding is essential, especially in urgent care environments, where abrupt changes in a patient's condition necessitate immediate and reflective action. The effectiveness of patient assessment is also significantly enhanced by the use of new techniques that focus on the engagement of the patient and goal-directed interventions. Simulation and analytic visual modeling are techniques that can be essential in training healthcare professionals to operate in these dynamic decision-making environments. Through such a culture that promotes role-playing and scenario training, clinicians are able to practice delivering multidimensional care that aligns with best practices in patient assessment. Individual competence is not only increased but also provides an opportunity to hone skills that benefit the entire patient experience. Identification and satisfaction of the personal needs of patients through comprehensive assessment and advanced training methods ultimately facilitate medical professionals to provide timely and effective treatment in emergency situations, thereby advancing principles of critical care (Marshall-Ponting et al., 2012).

9.1.1. Initial Evaluation Techniques

The first assessment processes perform a crucial role in optimizing the best patient outcomes in the context of critical care. These measures are meant to assess the patients' status methodically upon presentation in ICUs or EDs. Through detailed assessment tools, healthcare practitioners are capable of gaining invaluable data regarding vital signs, history, and presenting complaints. This baseline information gives the healthcare teams a true picture of the state of the patients' health, enabling timely and knowledgeable clinical decisions. The application of standard assessment tools not only assists in the identification of immediate threats to life but also assists in developing individualized care plans tailored to every patient's specific needs and conditions, thus establishing a framework for subsequent therapeutic interventions.

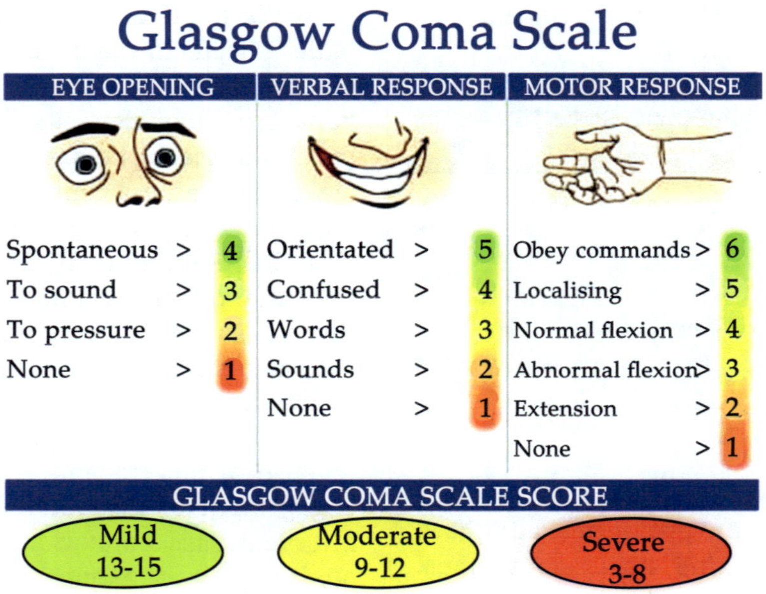

Figure 9.3. Glasgow Coma Scale.

Source: https://s3.us-east-2.amazonaws.com/medictests-production/ckeditor_assets/pictures/637/content_gcs_%281%29.jpg.

Moreover, initial evaluation techniques involve qualitative and quantitative measures, enhancing the precision and efficiency of the evaluation process. Observational tests combined with physiological measurements can provide an evidence-based foundation for decision-making. For instance, tools such as the Glasgow Coma Scale and severity scoring systems (e.g., APACHE II) provide standardized procedures for evaluating neurological status and general severity of health. The use of clinical performance indicators, as emphasized in the strategies for ambulance services, ensures that evaluation is not just possible but also in accordance with the best practice in patient care, and in the end, aids in improved clinical performance. The holistic approach forces health professionals to engage effectively with patients, hence increasing the likelihood that life-threatening conditions will be identified early and addressed properly, thus ensuring PS. Furthermore, the need to develop better early evaluation techniques to meet the particular demands of critical care cannot be overstated. Lean principles, traditionally associated with manufacturing, have begun to show promise in the provision of health care, suggesting that optimization techniques can improve emergency responsiveness within health care organizations. The integration of lean techniques in framework evaluation can rationalize processes, remove waste, and maximize patient throughput, enhancing critical care efficiency. Consistent application of such concepts, as outlined by the Health and Care Infrastructure Research and Innovation Centre, demonstrates that sticking to such guidelines allows organizations to experience radical productivity and service quality gains. In critical care, where minutes often count, making sure that methods of appraisal are effective and efficient can have a direct impact on survival rates for patients and overall care quality (Figure 9.3).

9.1.2. Continuous Monitoring of Vital Signs

The practice of continuous monitoring of vital signs is revolutionizing the critical care setting by providing real-time feedback of patient status, thereby enhancing clinical judgment. Traditional monitoring would entail periodic manual observations that expose patients to unanticipated deteriorations in their condition. It has been evidenced that such gaps can be significantly impactful; hence, real-time continuous monitoring systems can detect changes in heart and breathing rates in real time, allowing the interventions to occur before they cause damage. For instance, a study that evaluated a wireless and wearable monitoring system demonstrated its capacity to provide accurate heart rate data in a high percentage of patients and showed its capacity to augment existing clinical procedures and workflows (Hernandez-Silveira et al., 2015). As the healthcare systems adopt these technologies, there will be a shift towards more active patient management, founded on the values of critical care, where timely responsiveness is the foremost consideration. The greatest benefits of continuous monitoring are not only in early detection but also in automatic invalid data management, which is highly critical in critical care settings where accuracy would not be sacrificed.

The said research proved that the new digital patch system was successful in rejecting invalid physiological data, enabling healthcare professionals to focus on valid readings that are most relevant to patient care. This level of accuracy is critical because identifying patients in critical situations correctly makes it possible to take fast action and interventions that can make a significant difference in patient outcomes. Moreover, technology application in patient monitoring constructs a comprehensive care model, whereby teams of health professionals can react based on firm facts backed by ongoing monitoring rather than sporadically acquired assessments, fundamentally reconstituting the practice of critical care (Hernandez-Silveira et al., 2015). Further, the multidisciplinary nature of critical care leads to better patient administration when constant monitoring is employed. In individual cases, as in the case of MPS VI patients, continuous data gathering allows for the establishment of tailored management programs by multidisciplinary teams. Consensus guidelines for managing diseases like MPS VI acknowledge the requirement for intense monitoring protocols, consistent with a larger trend in which ongoing monitoring is key to successful therapeutic practice. With progressing healthcare, the adoption of continuous vital sign monitoring is expected to be a determining factor in enhanced quality of life and clinical outcomes, demonstrating a movement towards more integrated and responsive care systems within critical settings. The incorporation of advanced technologies, thus, demonstrates a necessary aspect of contemporary critical care principles (Figure 9.4).

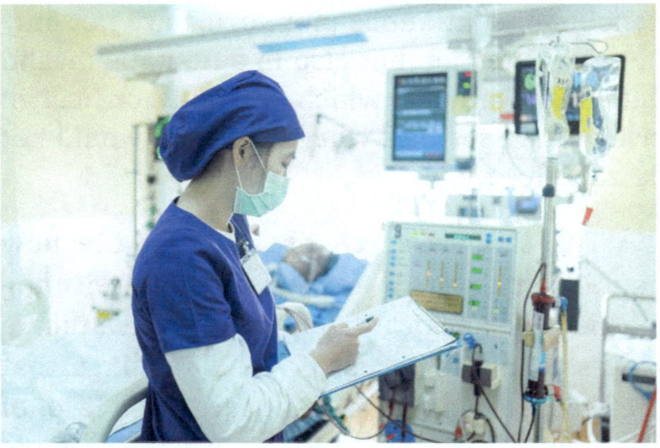

Figure 9.4. Physician at the critical care monitoring of vital signs.

Source: https://www.jeffersonhealth.org/content/dam/health2021/images/photos/stock/people/clinical/physician-at-the-critical-care-monitoring-the-patient.png.

9.1.3. Use of Diagnostic Tools in Critical Care

Diagnostic equipment in critical care is key to the successful management of acutely sick patients. Diagnostic equipment enhances the accuracy of patient examination, aiding clinicians in the rapid identification of life-threatening illnesses. For instance, the use of histidine-rich protein-2 (HRP2) based rapid diagnostic tests (RDT) to identify malaria in Zanzibar shows how diagnostic equipment can affect the treatment process significantly. Even with HRP2 sensitivity for *Plasmodium falciparum* being very low at 76.5%, the high specificity of the test at 99.9% ensures that healthcare providers are assured of diagnosing malaria cases, facilitating timely and correct treatment. This adherence to test outcomes underscores the diagnostic instrument's function in facilitating conformity with care rituals as well as in facilitating the prevention of the risks associated with uncontrolled diseases, an issue of utmost importance within critical care units where time itself is literally of the essence (Shakely et al., 2013). Additionally, the utility of diagnostic instruments is their integration within prevailing healthcare protocols, including the integrated management of childhood illness (IMCI). By incorporating RDTs into febrile patient management guidelines, clinicians can make decision-making less complicated, reducing the number of misdiagnoses. In Zanzibar, evidence showed the RDTs' good performance among various groups, particularly among children below five years. This specificity of population allows for targeted interventions and enhances the overall quality of patient care in acute facilities. Such integration is essential in achieving improved health outcomes, as evidenced by the high compliance rates of the test results and follow-up treatment protocols, which validate diagnostic instruments as not only effective but integral components of well-rounded critical care interventions (Shakely et al., 2013).

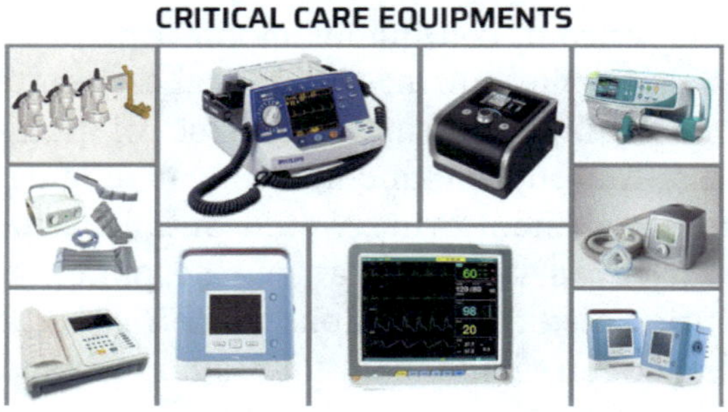

Figure 9.5. Critical care equipment.

Source: https://porvootransitioncare.com/assets/img/new-page-danish/CRITICAL-CARE-EQUIPMENTS.jpg.

At the same time, the diagnostic tool environment is evolving to address the challenges of outpatient care, particularly where inpatient diagnostics are not feasible. Research has increased to call attention to the ambulatory care environment, which treats a significant proportion of medical cases. By imposing tight diagnostic and safety standards in such an environment, physicians can better enhance the quality of care provided outside hospital walls. The focus on PS and quality enhancement highlights the systemic benefits of integrating high-tech diagnostic machinery for real-time decision-making. As evidenced in the literature, managing the broad range of factors that influence the delivery of patient care among outpatients can lead to the establishment of stable health care systems centered on PS while enhancing critical care practices in a wide range of environments (Figure 9.5).

Test Your Knowledge

1. What are the key components of the initial evaluation of a critically ill patient?
2. What vital signs and parameters are continuously monitored in critical care, and what changes might indicate clinical deterioration?

9.2. Communication in Critical Care

Learning Outcome

1. Discuss about interdisciplinary team collaboration;
2. Deal with effective communication with patients and families;
3. Focus on documentation and reporting standards.

Effective communication is a vital element of critical care that plays an important role in influencing patient outcomes and the functioning of healthcare teams. Under conditions of high pressure in settings such as ICUs, the ability to transfer information effectively and efficiently can make all the difference between life or death. Research places particular emphasis on the role of interpersonal skills during handovers in conveying important patient information between providers without omission or error. The findings of Scott et al. (2012) acknowledge that even though evidence-based medicine has been coping with standardized care for a long time, handover in critical care requires a nuanced understanding of communication to address complex clinical cases. Therefore, building a culture that promotes open lines of communication can lead to enhanced teamwork and ultimately to PS and quality of care in critical care. Moreover, the application of standard communication protocols has proven to enhance the effective flow of information among multidisciplinary teams. With the application of structured handover techniques, such as SBAR (situation, background, assessment, recommendation), health professionals are in a position to better structure discussions and reduce ambiguity while taking care of patients. This is particularly helpful in critical care, where rapid decision-making is essential. The evidence considered by Scott et al. (2012) encourages such best practices to be used to a greater extent, emphasizing that concurrent evaluations of such instruments will lead to continuous improvement. As healthcare settings continue to evolve, the use of such systematic instruments will lead to greater clarity and improved understanding among team members, thus underlining the importance of communication in high-stakes environments. Also, the greater complexity in patients' needs in critical care necessitates a planned communication strategy that is in line with the principles of a patient-centered approach. For instance, integrating a medical home model can significantly improve coordination of care by ensuring that communication is targeted to particular patient needs and desires. The results derived from the study reveal that effective communication strategies prioritize patients' involvement in their care processes. This model not only points to the importance of information sharing between providers but also to the necessity of dealing with individual patients' situations and priorities. In this way, healthcare professionals are able to create an open space that upholds patient autonomy while promoting working together through decision-making, thus leading to better health outcomes in critical care settings.

9.2.1. Interdisciplinary Team Collaboration

Interprofessional collaboration between teams is a cornerstone of great critical care practice because it provides an environment in which different professional perspectives can enhance the patient's outcome. In high-stress settings such as a neonatal intensive care unit (NICU), the integration of diversified skill sets allows for a more holistic approach to treating the patient. As emphasized by the American Academy of Pediatrics, communication and collaboration are essential not just to improve clinical results but also to provide emotionally supportive care environments for families. With this integration, there is a need to have formal communication procedures and regular interdisciplinary meetings that allow team members to share patient progress and information exchange to improve the quality of care delivered. Application of such interprofessional practice is even more important in end-of-life care scenarios, where the sensitivity of the matter requires increased support and precision among healthcare workers and families (Keith-Chancy, 2024). In order to apply interdisciplinary collaboration in critical care settings effectively, there is a requirement to have common knowledge about team roles and responsibilities. All of these professions bring unique expertise to an integrated patient care encounter, but without a definition of these roles, confusion can lead to inefficiency and even error. Training programs that enforce collaboration can assist in making teams more functional and the delivery of care more efficient. Also, in a bid to rationalize procedures for care, feedback mechanisms have to be used so that team members are able to articulate their experiences and suggestions for change. Results of surveys for interdisciplinary improvement teams can inform such development by providing snapshots of communication dynamics and the effectiveness of teamwork practices in acute care environments (Keith-Chancy, 2024).

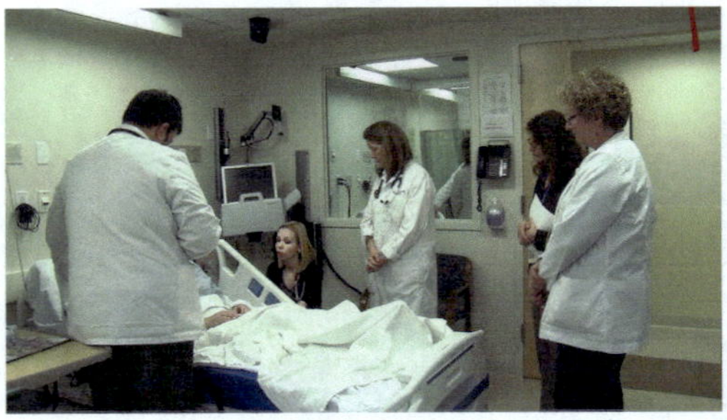

Figure 9.6. Interdisciplinary team collaboration in critical care.

Source: vhttps://i.ytimg.com/vi/Si722OAe3HA/hq720.jpg?sqp=-oaymwE7CK4FEIIDSFryq4qpAy0IARUAAAAAGAElAADIQj0AgKJD8AEB-AH-CYAC0AWKAgwIABABGF4gZShRMA8=&rs=AOn4CLDzkJtoSeUmVk66kFpTqlhktio5kg.

Routine review and updating of these frameworks ensure responsiveness and adaptability to the needs of complex patients. Interdisciplinary teamwork must also transcend direct clinical practice to embrace elements of trauma-informed care, which addresses the emotional and psychological needs of patients and families. Establishing a supportive culture of empathy and shared responsibility among team members can go far in reducing stress associated with critical care environments. Trauma-informed practices involve ongoing training and self-evaluation of team dynamics, leading to enhanced resilience for healthcare professionals. As demonstrated in most case studies, the integration of supportive structures and collaborative strategies can enhance positive outcomes and establish a resilient care network for marginalized communities. By fostering a culture of collaboration, the challenges of critical care can be met more effectively by healthcare teams, such that care of the patient is holistic and compassionate (Figure 9.6).

9.2.2. Effective Communication with Patients and Families

Clear communication with families and patients is a cornerstone of critical care practices that influences not only the delivery of healthcare but also the patient experience. Open communication creates a culture of trust that forces patients and families to take an active role in their own care decision-making. This process is especially important in critical circumstances where patients are incapacitated. They most often take the lead role as the primary decision-makers, thus compelling healthcare professionals to relay complex medical information in a simpler form. The challenge lies in bridging the gap between medical terminologies and patient comprehension that can directly impact patient outcomes and satisfaction. Effective strategies, such as adopting an empathetic style and employing various visual aids, can significantly enhance understanding as well as stimulate dialogue-based participative decision-making, hence serving the needs of both patient and family in challenging situations. Effective communication is also essential in providing palliative care, notably for those suffering from incurable diseases such as dementia. Research further highlights the different challenges facing healthcare workers in addressing communication in end-of-life situations. Certain of these patients may have a problem communicating their wishes or feelings, which would subsequently create more anxiety for families. Under such circumstances, as the literature has noted, it is essential to have open talk about the anticipatory needs of the patients and families (Birch & Draper, 2008). Through opening doors to begin respectful conversations that honor the patient's own wishes, medical professionals' needs are not only fulfilled on a physical level but also on an emotional and psychological. This holistic method brings about a culture of care to ensure that patients receive the dignity and compassion they deserve as they make their way towards the end of life. In addition to the challenges of communication in health care settings, the provision of creative therapies offers promising avenues to enhancing patient and family engagement.

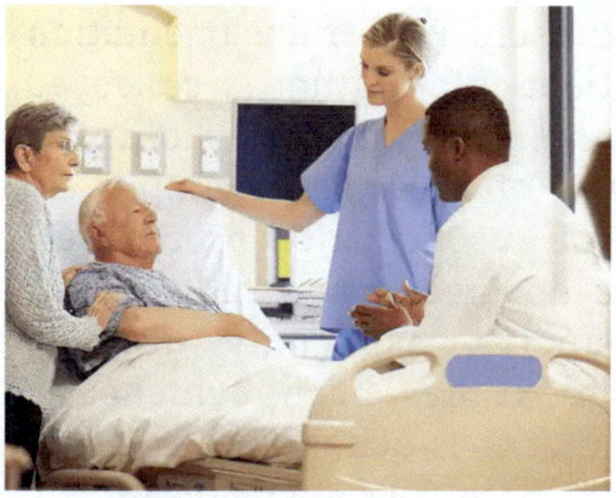

Figure 9.7. Effective communication with patients and their families.

Source: https://tutorcare.co.uk/wp-content/uploads/2021/11/course_content_image_end_of_life.webp.

The arts traditionally woven into health care have shown potential in facilitating communication and emotional expression, particularly in the military medical system. The National Initiative for Arts and Health in the Military elucidates that arts interventions reinforce traditional medical practice, not just healing body sickness but also addressing the mind and emotional issues of patients and families (The Stern Center for Evidence-Based Policy, 2015). With the curative powers of the arts, medical practitioners are in a position to develop a more integrated model of communication that engages patients on a personalized level. This not only accelerates healing and health but can also strengthen the relationships between patients, families, and healthcare professionals, and therefore highlight the importance of effective communication in critical care settings (Figure 9.7).

9.2.3. Documentation and Reporting Standards

In critical care, the importance of documentation and reporting standards cannot be overemphasized. The standards form the foundation of sound communication between healthcare providers and between providers and consumers. Proper documentation ensures that patient information is conveyed clearly, hence minimizing the possibility of errors at change of care. For example, enhancing medication reconciliation procedures through rigorous documentation reduces prescribing discrepancies, especially during patient discharge. It has been evidenced through studies that it is achievable to experience an improvement in the right medication lists when implementing an organized team-based method in documentation. Such an enhancement is necessary since poor or incorrect documentation has been documented to lead to adverse events, which consequently influence PS and care quality, thereby requiring strict standards for optimum best practice in critical care settings (Marvin et al., 2016). On top of that, the flexibility of standards of documentation is most important in critical care due to the dynamic change in patient conditions. Clinical performance indicator integration is a central aspect in such cases. Through the development of these indicators based on best evidence and engaging service users and clinicians, healthcare systems make it possible for the process of documentation to be meaningful and user-friendly. Putting in place performance monitoring procedures makes it easier for the development of meaningful benchmarks that address not only clinical effectiveness but also patient-centered care. Well-designed indicators enhance safe and equitable healthcare, thus creating a platform where continuous quality improvement can thrive. This allows health professionals to reduce variations in the provision of care systematically, maintaining optimal levels of documentation and reporting throughout critical care processes (Siriwardena, 2007). Moreover, the consequences of documentation and reporting standards filter down below the level of individual patient care to the overall healthcare system. Proper documentation not only increases PS and continuity of care but also provides valuable insights to feed back into quality improvement initiatives. When healthcare organizations put a greater emphasis on accurate and complete reporting, they foster an environment of responsibility and ongoing learning. This is particularly relevant within critical care units, where decisions frequently hinge on volumes of clinical data. By utilizing systematic documentation processes, organizations are better able to gauge performance indicators to monitor trends and make data-driven decisions, ultimately leading to improved patient outcomes. Therefore, structured documentation processes are integrated into the direct care of patients as well as systemic improvements over the long term in healthcare environments (Siriwardena, 2007; Marvin et al., 2016).

Test Your Knowledge

1. How does effective interdisciplinary team collaboration impact patient outcomes in a critical care setting?
2. What strategies can healthcare providers use to communicate clearly and compassionately with critically ill patients and their families?

9.3. Ethical Considerations

Learning Outcome

1. Discuss informed consent in critical care;
2. Understand end-of-life decisions and palliative care;
3. Deal with resource allocation in healthcare.

In the case of critical care, ethical principles come first since healthcare professionals are frequently faced with conflicts that undermine the very essence of beneficence, non-maleficence, autonomy, and justice. These ethical principles offer a framework for guiding medical decisions, which are particularly needed in risky cases where patients are unable to communicate in their own interest. The inherent subtlety of such ethical dilemmas calls for a careful balancing act between the unique needs of the patient and the general ramifications for the health system as a whole. The allocation of limited resources, for instance, must be balanced against this, especially when aggressive therapies could be extremely costly with no likely benefit. Through the careful assessment of patient and organizational ability, medical staff are then free to move forward with ethical decision-making that upholds the integrity of the practice but strives to maximize patient results, as postulated in current literature (Farías-Yapur, 2023). The fluid complexities of ethical decision-making are further augmented when adding vulnerable groups, i.e., children or those unable to make informed decisions. Ethical frameworks must prioritize the interests of such patients while exercising caution in considering the effects of costly treatments not just on the patient but also on the health care system. It is important to have a code of practice that establishes objective management standards so as to guide clinicians in their decision-making efforts. This reflects a broader ethical responsibility, whereby personal biases are stripped from patient treatment to preserve the dignity and rights of all, regardless of circumstances or background. This makes ethical standards universal and rational and preserves both patient health and social integrity in complex clinical scenarios (Montalto, 2014). Furthermore, the ethics of critical care also find their way in the field of medical research, particularly when interacting with vulnerable populations. Autonomy and informed consent are even more important in cases where the subjects may not fully be able to value the impact of their involvement in clinical trials. The moral questions surrounding research practices, particularly in vulnerable groups, are a delicate balancing act that needs to meticulously guarantee safety and welfare as well as advances in medical understanding. The ethical principles must be pliable, however, to the special challenges within each group of research conditions without compromising the core fundamental ethical principles. While healthcare professionals address such intricacies, they must at the same time demand the implementation of rigorous ethical practices that protect both the rights of individual patients and the broader mandate of enhancing patient care under critical care principles (Farías-Yapur, 2023).

9.3.1. Informed Consent in Critical Care

Informed consent in critical care is an essential process that provides the foundation for ethical medical practice, attempting to balance respect for patient autonomy with the ability to make informed decisions in the event of medical emergencies. The condition of critical care is such that informed consent may be more complicated since patients are incapacitated or have life-threatening conditions where immediate medical intervention is required. In such circumstances, healthcare workers are confronted with a conflict between their requirement to ensure urgency and their moral obligation to advise patients clearly on what decision is being presented to them, along with its potential consequences. Such a conflict illustrates the need for critical care professionals to develop guidelines that consider patients' capacity to make decisions, and also look into surrogate decision-makers as authoritative proxies when the patient cannot articulate his or her desires. Besides, the informed consent doctrine in intensive care transcends procedural compliance to involve effective communication and shared decision-making between healthcare providers and patients. The healthcare providers must guarantee patients, where possible, sufficient information regarding the nature of their medical condition, proposed interventions, and available options. There is a need to adopt simple language, avoid medical jargon, and ensure that patients understand the consequences of their choices. Involving caregivers and family members in the process can further improve the process to a larger degree, as it may give a better insight into the patient's values and preferences. Finally, this process not only satisfies ethical needs but also maximizes trust and cooperative dynamics in the clinician-patient relationship and, therefore, overall satisfaction in the critical care setting. Despite the ethical requirements regarding informed consent, there are still significant challenges involved in its use. Critical care situations demand rapid decision-making not only from the medical fraternity but also from the patients or their representatives, at times in pathetic circumstances. Emotional stress that the families undergo when undergoing such critical moments can cause them to face difficulties in understanding the information provided and also in communicating their wishes. Furthermore, religious beliefs impact healthcare decision-making and may compound the complexity, for example, in the intersection of religious dogma and medical ethics (Petrova & Clifford, 2009). Moreover, evolving legal standards and regulations for informed consent necessitate ongoing education for healthcare professionals to guarantee that they are equipped to navigate these complexities. Overcoming these challenges is essential to build upon the ethical foundation of informed consent in critical care, ultimately safeguarding patients' rights and improving care outcomes (Figure 9.8).

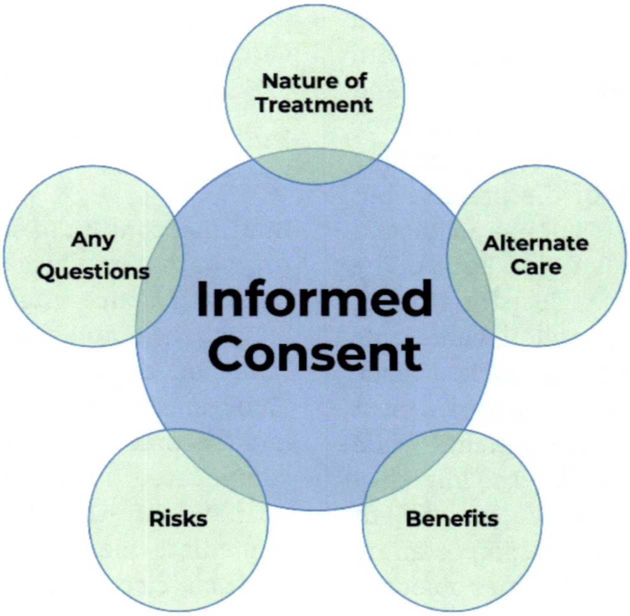

Figure 9.8. Informed consent.

Source: https://postgraddc.com/wp-content/uploads/2022/08/Informed-Consent.png.

9.3.2. End-of-Life Decisions and Palliative Care

The landscape of end-of-life decisions is intertwined with the palliative care ethos, where the primary focus is alleviation of suffering and improvement in the quality of life for dying patients. Palliative care emphasizes patient autonomy, allowing patients to be involved participants in decision-making for their treatment. But this independence becomes dangerous when pitted against more paternalistic approaches in the medical care context, as in the case of Belgium's euthanasia regime. Critics have been concerned that, even as patients are theoretically in charge, there is a culture of pervasive paternalism that undermines actual consent, especially in vulnerable populations, such as those with cognitive impairment or existential conflicts. This tension between paternalism and autonomy requires a rethinking of the end-of-life decision structure in the model of healthcare such that the patient's voice remains paramount in every stage of care (Cohen-Almagor, 2016).

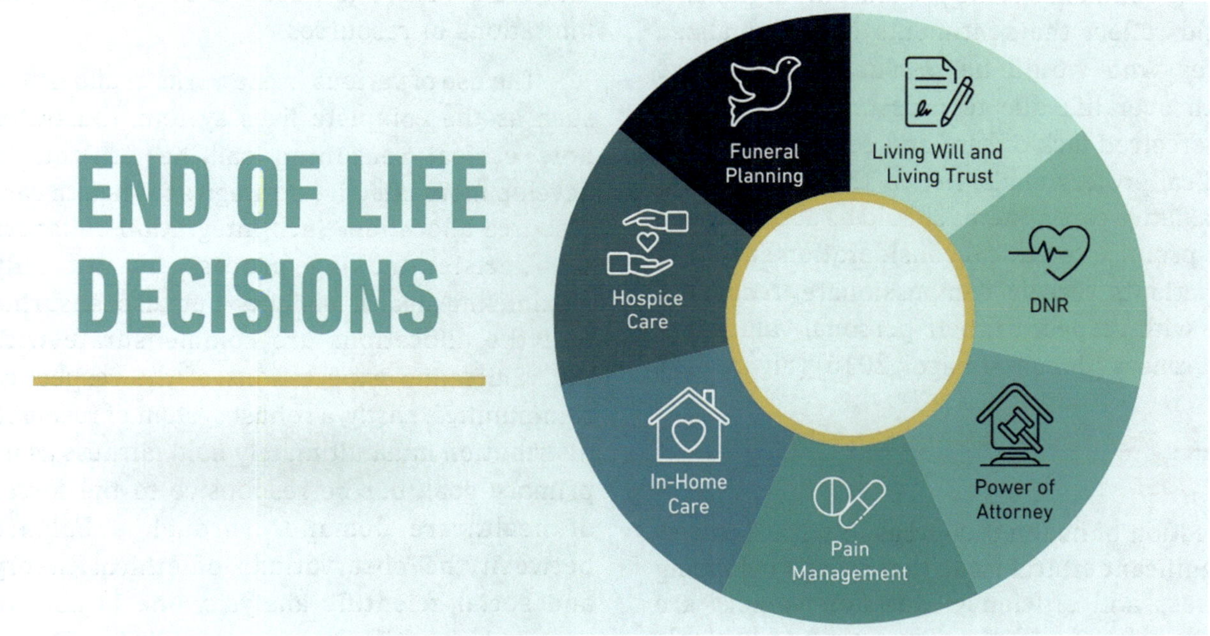

Figure 9.9. End of life decisions.

Source: https://www.mesotheliomahub.com/app/uploads/2024/06/End-of-Life-Decisions.jpg.

Primary care has a vital but too often overlooked function in the delivery of palliative care. Since most people wish to die at home, PCPs are generally the focal points in providing adequate end-of-life care that respects patient choices. Nonetheless, systematic barriers often impede these providers from delivering the integral care needed to function optimally in this role. Issues such as constrained resources, shortages of palliative methodology training, and weak coordinated care pathways can significantly restrict the optimal potential of primary care practitioners to maximize terminal care. In addition, the traditional hospital-based paradigm of death unfairly imposes on families and health teams as well, for instance, with the necessity to empower primary care practitioners to enable discussions and interventions about end-of-life preferences (Munday & Dale, 2007). In opposition to these challenges, the closing of gaps in primary care is central to enhancing the quality of dying for patients and their families. With society's continued evolution, the controversy surrounding end-of-life options must also address not just the clinical necessities of care but even the ethical implications of making such choices. The increasing rate of euthanasia and assisted dying controversies reveals intimate social tensions around autonomy, suffering, and definitions of quality of life. It is necessary to address these debates with respect and tolerance, ensuring that all types of various viewpoints are entered into policy and practice. Also, as observed from reported experiences in countries that have legalized euthanasia, the pro and anti-arguments would reflect the sentiments of marginalized voices who would be persuaded to choose death over life due to pressure from society or perceived lack of care and compassion from medical professionals. Hence, the development of palliative care systems should be accompanied by a promise to ethical consideration such that all patients receive compassionate, respectful care with respect to their personal values and preferences (Cohen-Almagor, 2016) (Figure 9.9).

9.3.3. Resource Allocation and Fairness

Allocation of health resources in critical care is a significant ethical issue that entails balancing fairness and efficiency. Decision makers are generally faced with the distribution of available health resources among various needs, leading to implications for the health system and patients. An investigation of healthcare decision criteria reveals a multi-dimensional interaction of factors informing resource allocation, of which fairness is a dominant concern. Equity and justice, according to Guindo et al. (2012), were identified as necessary criteria that emerged again and again in discussions on healthcare decision-making.

These present a challenge to policymakers both in terms of normative strategies and the pragmatic visages of their choices, stressing the need for a profound understanding of the application of equitable healthcare practice. An effective resource allocation strategy involves the intermingling of both ethical foundations and empirical foundations. By analyzing social scientific studies alongside ethical premises, decision-makers are able to more comprehensively understand the public's wishes concerning the allocation of limited medical resources. As set out by Persad (2017), this dynamic between ethics and social science is essential towards constructing mechanisms that are sensitive to public values yet face the limitations of resources.

The use of various frameworks of allocation, such as the complete lives system, illustrates how ethical reasoning can be utilized to develop more effective strategies for health care resource allocation. Such integration enhances the decision-making process by not only maximizing health benefits but also ensuring that the allocations are commensurate with the values and expectations of the respective communities. Lastly, a robust system of resource distribution must ultimately hold fairness as its primary goal, but be responsive to the forces of healthcare demand. Through a balance between the observations of ethical theory and social scientific analysis, one is able to engage in healthcare decision-making with an appreciation for the complexity involved in these practices. Policymakers and practitioners are encouraged to regularly exchange views on the pressing ethical issues they face, as brought to light by the variety of factors they take into consideration in their decisions, for instance, the overarching themes of efficacy, equity, and patient needs outlined by Guindo et al. (2012). Through the formulation of this discourse, health systems can move toward establishing allocation practices that are both effective and fair, paving the way toward improved patient outcomes within intensive care settings.

Test Your Knowledge

1. How can informed consent be ethically obtained from critically ill patients who may lack decision-making capacity?
2. What ethical principles should guide decisions about withholding or withdrawing life-sustaining treatment in critically ill patients?

9.4. Advanced Life Support (ALS) Techniques

Learning Outcome

1. Understand cardiopulmonary resuscitation (CPR) protocols;
2. Explain the use of mechanical ventilation;
3. Deal with the administration of medications in emergencies.

In critical care, advanced life support (ALS) techniques are a vital component in the treatment of life-threatening illnesses. ALS techniques include advanced airway management, pharmacologic therapy, and mechanical device utilization, such as extracorporeal membrane oxygenation (ECMO). Advanced as a complex intervention, ECMO has transformed the intensive care approach to patients with severe cardiac or respiratory failure. By providing short-term support, ALS techniques not only stabilize patients but also give them time to recover or undergo further medical care. Thus, familiarity with these techniques allows clinicians to act rapidly and efficiently, taking the best possible care of severely distressed patients, ultimately shaping outcomes in a favorable way. A key component of ALS is extracorporeal life support (ECLS), consisting of ECMO and associated technology. The innovations of ECLS have pushed the limits of critical management care for non-responder patients. Specifically, venovenous ECMO supports complete respiratory support, while venoarterial ECMO is able to sustain circulation with acute cardiac failure effectively. Such newer modalities enable healthcare professionals to have critical intervention, such as bridging patients to heart transplantation or a mechanical assist device. While enormously valuable, one must accept that the best practices for these new treatments have yet to be determined using quality evidence, an essential area of future clinical practice and research (Shekar et al., 2014). Additional training and preparedness in the use of ALS techniques, such as ECMO, are essential to ensuring that health care teams are adequately prepared to meet difficult circumstances. SBE has become a crucial component of clinician training in the critical care environment. Through exposure to high-stakes, realistic scenarios, SBE enhances collaborative work and technical skills necessary for effective patient management. New developments in ECMO simulation technology have attempted to close gaps between theoretical understanding and true practice by establishing a realistic, contrived environment that closely resembles the patient scenario. These training programs not only build individual skills but also foster a culture of readiness and adaptability in care teams working in high-risk environments (Alinier et al., 2018).

9.4.1. Cardiopulmonary Resuscitation (CPR) Protocols

Cardiopulmonary resuscitation (CPR) protocols are a central component of emergency medical protocols to resuscitate cardiac arrest victims through restoration of circulation and respiration. CPR protocols entail a series of systematic steps that have to be performed by medical staff and trained laypeople in order to guarantee the likelihood of a successful attempt at resuscitation. The American Heart

Association promotes the immediate activation of CPR, believing that the application of chest compressions at a specific rate and depth to make sure the perfusion of crucial organs should be maintained. This knowledge is important not only for the medical practitioners but also for members of the general public, as CPR by bystanders has been found to lead to significant improvement in survival rates in cases of out-of-hospital cardiac arrests. The harmonization of standardized methods in CPR processes is a basic concept of critical care that attaches importance to the need for immediate intervention and coordination of all the players within an emergency setting. In dealing with the CPR protocol nuances, it is of prime importance to recognize the need to harmonize these processes with various environments and situations. For instance, research on CPR in microgravity highlights the need to learn about how fundamental procedures can need to be modified when done in unique environments, such as in space (Billica et al., 1991). The administration of CPR protocols needs to take into account not just the physiological mechanics of resuscitation but also the environmental influences that can potentially impact their efficacy. This involves lengthy training and simulation of protocols based on specific situational scenarios, especially in high-stakes environments where traditional approaches might need to be reevaluated. In addition, continuous research and optimization of these protocols enable medical staff to remain current with evolving best practices and advances in resuscitation science. Another critical element of CPR protocols is taking into account the psychosocial dimensions of resuscitation, and specifically, family presence during such high-stakes episodes. Research has shown that the lack of standardized policies for family witnessed resuscitation contributes to inconsistent practice among medical professionals (Njoku, 2005). Such inconsistencies make it difficult for nurses to decide on allowing family members to witness the process during resuscitative attempts, making it imperative for hospitals to develop complete guidelines that take into account these ethical matters. The assertion of the inherent emotional burden of an attempt to resuscitate impacts the patient and the medical team, together with the present family. Instituting a direct protocol that aligns with clinical effectiveness as well as compassionate care is needed to create a whole approach of critical care concepts, therefore ensuring the dignity of the patient and the solidarity of the medical family are integrated into the practice (Figure 9.10).

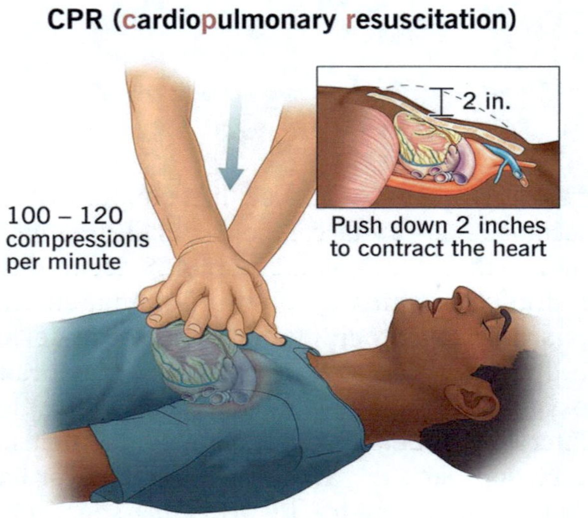

Figure 9.10. Illustration of cardiopulmonary resuscitation (CPR).

Source: https://my.clevelandclinic.org/-/scassets/images/org/health/articles/cpr.

9.4.2. Use of Mechanical Ventilation

Mechanical ventilation is a crucial intervention in the management of patients with respiratory failure. Artificial ventilation by this method is required when the patient's capacity to ventilate is compromised by diseases of the respiratory system, neurological diseases, or as a result of drug side effects. Head trauma or asthma exacerbation may lead to inadequate ventilation, and the patient must be mechanically supported. These conditions emphasize the necessity of determining indicators of mechanical ventilation in critical care conditions. Early intervention is important to avoid worsening of the respiratory status of the patient, since it has the potential to maximize outcomes and minimize the risks associated with prolonged hypoxemia or hypercapnia (Hill, 2020).

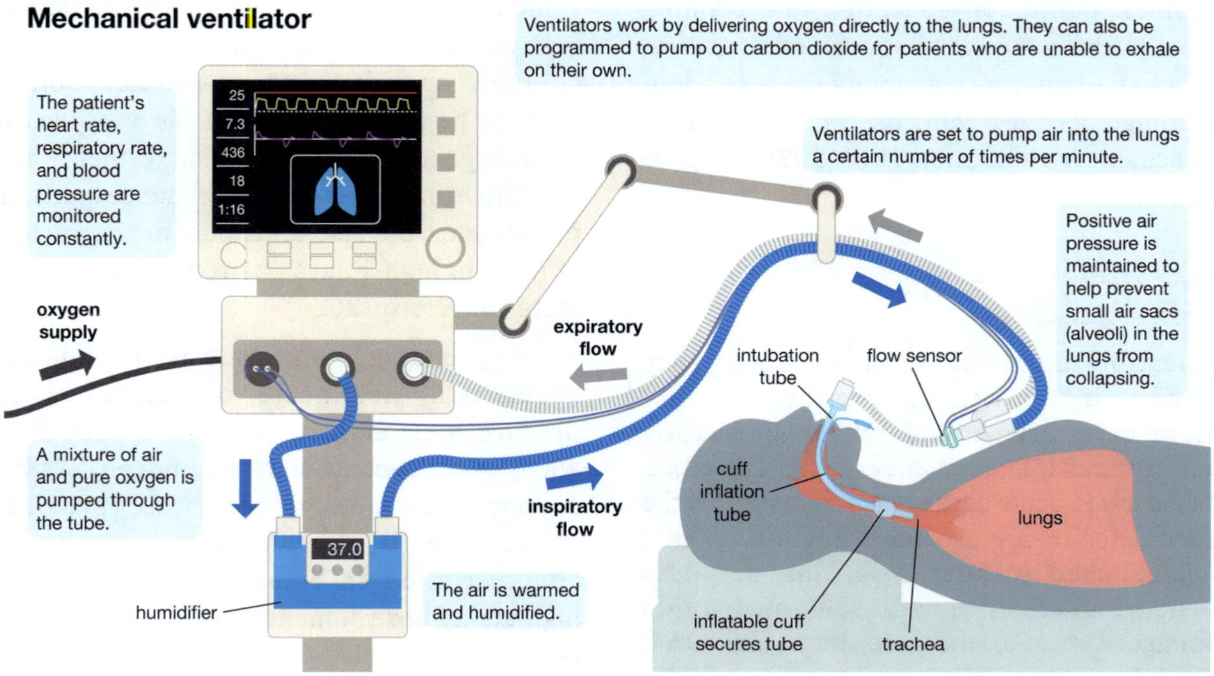

Figure 9.11. Mechanical ventilator illustration.

Source: https://cdn.britannica.com/37/270837-050-DFE276FE/mechanical-ventilator-parts-and-operation-illustration.jpg.

A clear understanding of the physiological principles of mechanical ventilation is at the center of successful patient care. Modern mechanical ventilators can support or fully control ventilation in various modes and adapt to the patient's requirements in a manner that ensures adequate oxygenation and carbon dioxide removal. Individually adapted application of the correct ventilation technique, e.g., volume-controlled or pressure-controlled mode, is founded on individual patient parameters, e.g., lung mechanics and underlying cause of respiratory failure. Further, technological advances in monitoring, such as thoracic electrical impedance tomography (EIT), have enhanced the clinician's ability to visualize lung function and adjust ventilator settings in real-time and have significantly influenced patient management during mechanical ventilation (Denaï et al., 2010). Through these measures, clinicians are able to maximize mechanical support to match the physiological realities of the patient's breathing patterns. Also, mechanical ventilation is not merely a matter of having the capability to ventilate but involves a strategy that maintains the lung in a state of protection and minimizes the risk of ventilator-induced lung injury (VILI). Reduced tidal volumes and the limitation of plateau pressures are now routine measures of protective lung ventilation. Monitoring of airway pressures and oxygenation indices closely allows the clinician to come to a decision regarding the manipulation of the ventilator and on weaning protocols. With advancing mechanical ventilation, integration of emerging technologies and evidence into clinical practice guidelines will be essential to improve patient outcomes. Continued education and training of healthcare professionals involved in critical care will be important, enabling them to adapt accordingly as they confront the complexities of mechanical ventilation (Hill, 2020) (Figure 9.11).

9.4.3. Administration of Medications in Emergencies

Medication administration in emergency situations is a critical component of quality patient care. Proper and timely medication administration influences the patients' outcomes, particularly in acute settings where time is of the essence. Healthcare providers ought to adhere to established standards for the purposes of ensuring effective and safe medication administration. For instance, implementation of standard procedures has been proved to enhance drug safety and reduce the incidence of errors, which, as evidenced by recent studies, is higher in stressful situations prevalent in emergency care settings.

Organizational personnel have managed to drive innovative approaches to addressing such issues, as documented in various case studies that attest to the effectiveness of systematic improvement in emergency drug administration (McCarthy & Blumenthal, 2006). Therefore, strong knowledge of these principles is essential to all critical care medical personnel. Preparation and training are also essential in the effective administration of medication in emergency cases. Medical professionals must be trained with theoretical data as well as practical knowledge so that they can effectively respond in emergency cases. That includes being well-versed with pharmacological principles, feeling appropriate dosing, and being aware of potential drug interactions. Moreover, simulation-based training has been recognized as a productive avenue for the enhancement of clinical skills in emergent cases to build both confidence and competence among providers. By integrating real-world clinical simulations into training courses, organizations are better able to prepare their employees for the complexities of emergency medication management. Such preventive measures not only enhance individual performance but also contribute to general team efficacy in high-stakes environments (San Jose State University, 2020).

By focusing on education and skill acquisition, healthcare organizations can prepare their staff to respond appropriately when every second matters. Interprofessional collaboration among healthcare providers is necessary to provide optimal medication administration in emergency situations. In high-stakes environments, clear communication between multidisciplinary teams can go a long way towards improving patient care outcomes. Establishing explicit communication pathways and medication delivery protocols for the team helps to streamline efforts so that members of the team are aware of their roles and responsibilities in emergency situations. Systematic debriefing following large-scale incidents may also foster interchange of insights and lessons learned and help create a culture of continuous improvement. Such teamwork not only helps to enable individual competency but also team relationships and operational effectiveness in crises. As affirmed by medication administration practice innovations in many healthcare organizations, focus on team-working during emergency medication administration leads to better PS outcomes and an overall healthier healthcare system (McCarthy & Blumenthal, 2006).

Test Your Knowledge

1. How do current CPR guidelines balance the need for rapid intervention with considerations for patient-specific factors?
2. What clinical criteria should guide the initiation and weaning of mechanical ventilation in critically ill patients?

9.5. Infection Control Measures

Learning Outcome

1. Understand the importance of hand hygiene;
2. Explain the use of personal protective equipment (PPE);
3. Focus on protocols for preventing hospital-acquired infections.

Infection control measures are a central component in the critical care setting, where the patients are most vulnerable due to compromised immune systems. These protocols should integrate a myriad of strategies that limit the risk of healthcare-associated infections (HAIs). These include rigorous hand hygiene practices among health workers, the use of personal protective equipment (PPE), and the sterilization of medical equipment. Research has established that systematic approaches such as these have the ability to significantly reduce infection rates, subsequently enhancing patient outcomes (Zumla et al., 2012). Moreover, continued education and training of health care workers regarding the latest infection control practices are required in maintaining excellent standards of care and ensuring compliance with guidelines set. Therefore, adequate understanding of the infection prevention dynamics should be prioritized significantly in critical care settings so that the patients and workers can be safeguarded against harm. Another strong challenge of infection control is the management of multidrug-resistant organisms (MDROs), which complicate patient treatment and recovery. As discussed, the emergence of microorganisms such as multidrug-resistant tuberculosis (MDR-TB) is an immediate hazard to public health across the world due to inadequate diagnostic centers and surveillance, particularly in low-income settings. At this juncture, the importance of interaction between antibiotic stewardship (AS) and infection control and prevention (IPC) programs is felt, where interdependent intervention tactics are needed to check the transmission of MDROs effectively. Tackling these issues relies on strong health systems able to offer early treatment and diagnosis to prevent healthcare facility transmission of resistant infections (Manning et al., 2018). A multidisciplinary approach is critical, as it is capable of bringing efforts together in coordinating patient care and ensuring the efficacy of antibiotic treatments in the future. Lastly, the institutional protocols' function cannot be overstated in relation to infection control practices in critical care. The protocols are the key strategies that guide the actions of healthcare workers and influence institutions' culture of safety. Integrating effective infection control practices, i.e., continuous HAIs surveillance, and establishing fast response teams in case of outbreaks, is revealed to be essential in intervening at the appropriate time. Those facilities in which there is a culture that emphasizes preventing infections show improved PS outcomes and reduce the occurrence of HAIs significantly (Zumla et al., 2012). In addition, enhancing interprofessional communication and teamwork among health care groups can help disseminate best practices, increasing the general standard of care across the department. Lastly, the continued sustainability of good infection control practices lies in the capacity to continuously improve and adapt to emerging challenges within the critical care environment.

9.5.1. Importance of Hand Hygiene

Hand washing is a fundamental component of infection prevention, particularly in the critical care setting where patients are compromised and HAIs pose a significant risk. Proper hand hygiene regularly has a dramatic impact on the occurrence of HAIs, which pose enormous morbidity and mortality in healthcare settings. With the application of alcohol-based hand rub or proper hand washing with soap and water, healthcare professionals render a protective barrier against pathogens, thereby improving patient health. The preventive measure not only curtails infection transmission but also enhances patient outcomes in total by facilitating a sterile environment required for healing. Hand hygiene is thus an imperative practice that signifies the commitment to quality care in critical care units. Furthermore, the implications of hand hygiene extend beyond a single PS; they also have an influence on broader public health outcomes. As healthcare systems struggle with the increasing threat of antimicrobial resistance, adherence to hand hygiene practices becomes increasingly essential. Effective IPC practice stops the spread of antimicrobial resistance and prevents outbreaks of highly transmissible diseases, as evidenced by the World Health Organization's recent emphasis on the establishment of core elements of IPC programs. Implementation of stringent hand hygiene protocols in these facilities is essential in the containment of both HAIs and the global problems posed by rising levels of resistance to antimicrobial agents. In this regard, the responsibility of training programs for healthcare workers cannot be overemphasized, as these cemented the implementation of routine hand hygiene to counter these significant health issues (Storr et al., 2017). Apart from enhancing the efficiency of infection control measures, hand hygiene also has a very significant role in creating trust among patients and healthcare professionals. Witnessing the healthcare staff maintaining rigorous hand hygiene measures instills confidence among the patients in the standards of safety within the facility. It is such trust that is very crucial in intensive care settings, where patients and their relatives are typically in a position of vulnerability. Furthermore, hand hygiene adherence plays a significant role in enhancing the quality of care rendered, as reflected in home-based care programs that make arrangements for the intermeshing of sanitation and patient care (The Stern Center for Evidence-Based Policy, 2015). Through the provision of a setting where hand hygiene takes precedence, healthcare institutions are capable of enhancing PS, reducing instances of HAIs, and improving the overall healthcare experience, ultimately as guided by the very nature of critical care (Figure 9.12).

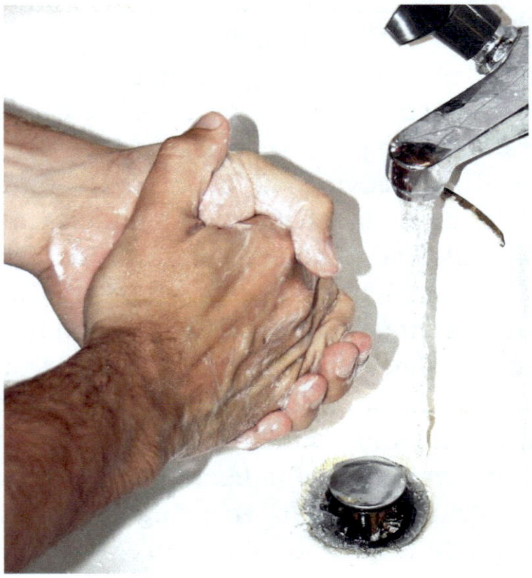

Figure 9.12. Hand washing with soap and water at a sink.

Source: https://upload.wikimedia.org/wikipedia/commons/thumb/1/1b/OCD_handwash.jpg/800px-OCD_handwash.jpg.

9.5.2. Use of Personal Protective Equipment (PPE)

Utilization of PPE is of utmost significance in intensive care, particularly in the management of patients during outbreaks of infectious diseases such as the COVID-19 pandemic. PPE functions as a barrier to protect against the spread of pathogens, preventing both healthcare professionals and patients from exposure to harmful microorganisms. With the double obligations of maintaining personal safety and promoting patient care, adherence to PPE guidelines has become a cornerstone of infection control practices. Allocation of resources, like adequate PPE stocks, is paramount in guaranteeing the effectiveness of operations within the healthcare systems. As observed during the pandemic, efficient efforts can enhance the supply of PPE, which has a direct impact on healthcare outcomes and the effectiveness of critical care services at large (Lancaster et al., 2020). Furthermore, the psychological impacts of wearing PPE must not be overlooked. Whereas PPE is meant to protect, it may create a psychological shield between caregiver and patient, possibly making communication harder and trust-building a challenge. The visual opacity of PPE makes patients feel isolated and isolate their caregivers as less accessible. Within high-anxiety environments, self-contained as EDs are in the face of overwhelming patient surges, immediacy of treatment necessitates not only mitigation of risk but also provision of a nurturing environment (Wong et al., 2020). Strategies for optimizing engagement under PPE wearing are needed, balancing protection needs with the emotional and relational aspects of care. The ongoing evolution of PPE standards underscores the need for regular training and awareness of healthcare professionals. Ongoing monitoring of PPE effectiveness, as well as real-time feedback mechanisms, is required to check maximum compliance and usage. In addition, establishing effective supply chains is important to ensure smooth availability of PPE in emergency situations. The COVID-19 pandemic highlighted the vulnerabilities in supply chains, prompting healthcare systems to explore innovative solutions, such as local manufacturing and international collaboration, to secure necessary resources (Lancaster et al., 2020). Ultimately, reinforcing a culture of safety and preparedness around PPE use fosters resilience among healthcare providers, allowing them to deliver high-quality care even in the face of unprecedented challenges (Figure 9.13).

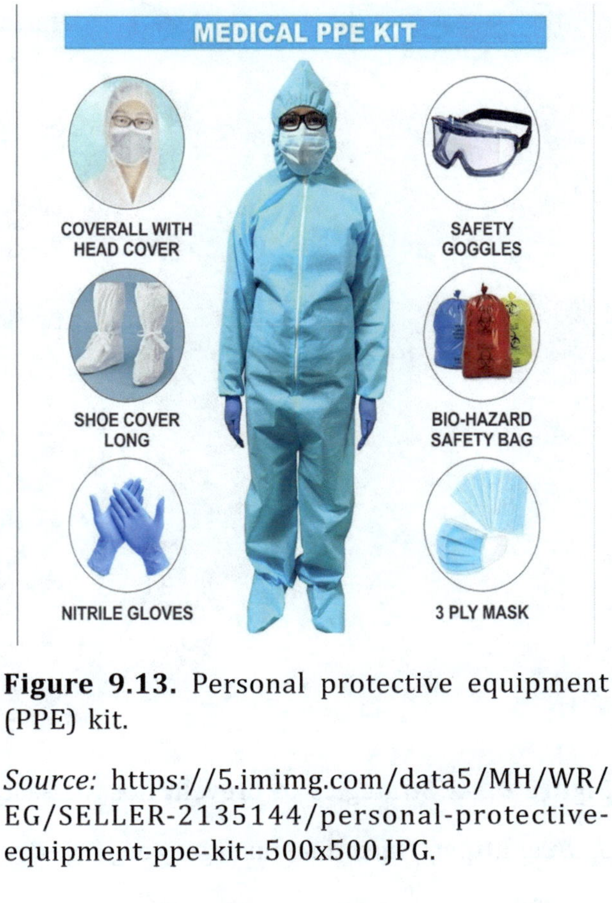

Figure 9.13. Personal protective equipment (PPE) kit.

Source: https://5.imimg.com/data5/MH/WR/EG/SELLER-2135144/personal-protective-equipment-ppe-kit--500x500.JPG.

9.5.3. Protocols for Preventing Hospital-Acquired Infections (HAIs)

Incidence of hospital-acquired infections (HAIs) is a gigantic challenge in critical care settings, requiring the development of standardized guidelines to combat their incidence. A good approach against prevention of HAIs encompasses several elements, from stringent hand hygiene procedures, invasive device management with utmost care, and the use of effective sterilization. Hand hygiene, for instance, is one of the simplest yet best practices that healthcare workers can adopt. Through continued observance of proper hand washing protocols, healthcare providers can safely minimize the transmission of pathogens and thereby safeguard patient outcomes. Furthermore, the integration of evidence-based education modules can foster a culture of safety among medical staff, enacting active engagement in the prevention of HAIs.

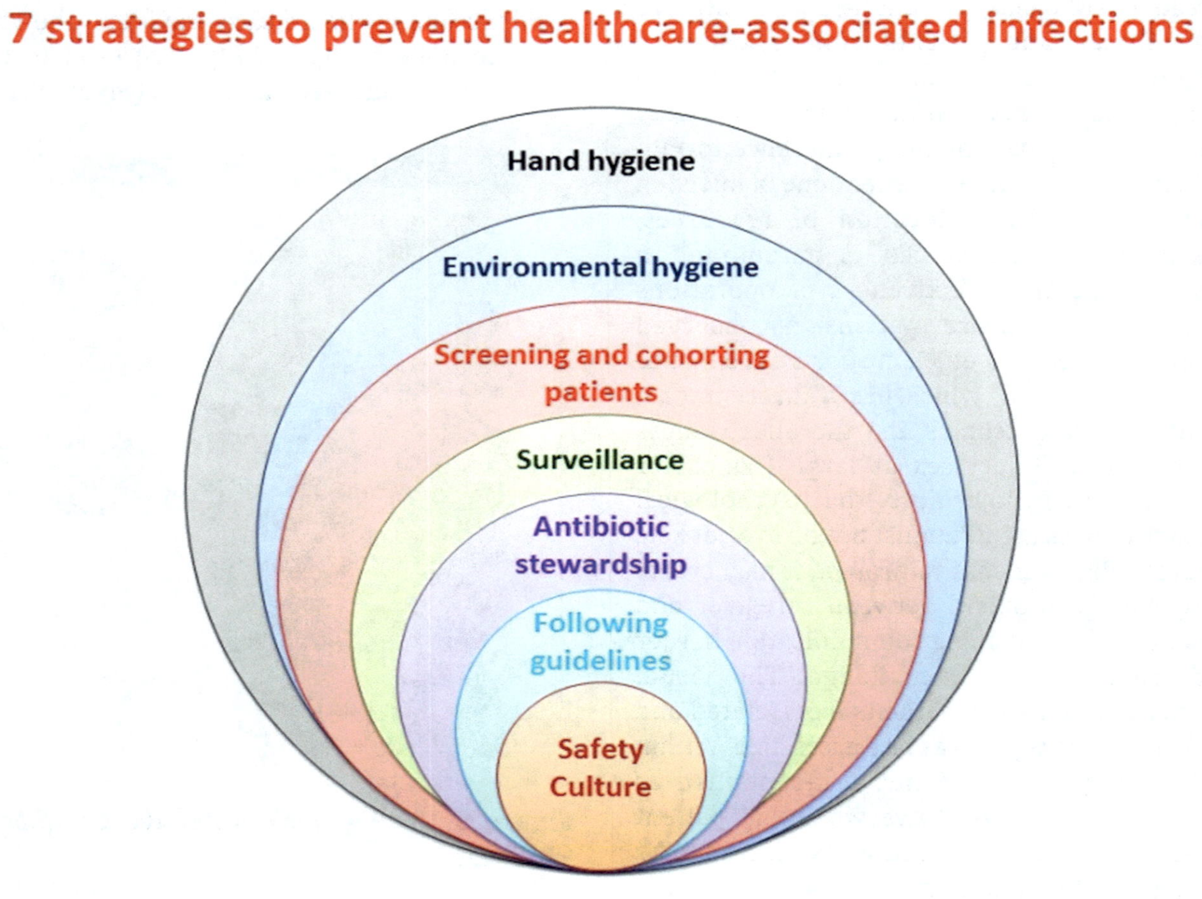

Figure 9.14. Strategies to prevent hospital-acquired infections (HAIs).

Source: https://infectionsinsurgery.org/wp-content/uploads/2019/02/prevention-1.jpg?w=863.

This is consistent with the cultural values advocated by Burke et al. (2008), highlighting the importance of a culture of safety in healthcare facilities. Besides hand hygiene measures, adherence to insertion and retention guidelines of invasive devices is important in the prevention. Central venous catheters, urinary catheters, and surgical site procedures are among the most common infection entry points, thus requiring stringent protocols. Utilization of checklists in these procedures may enhance best practice compliance, consequently reducing infection risk. Further, the protocols need to take into account timely catheter removal and management of the sterile field during surgery. Hospitals that strictly adhere to these protocols have lower HAIs, demonstrating the actual payoffs of systematic processes, corroborated by healthcare case studies by McCarthy & Blumenthal (2006). Through prioritizing these protocols, healthcare organizations can significantly enhance PS and quality of care. Finally, active monitoring and quantification of infection rates are an integral component of successful HAI prevention. Data measurement and analysis help to inform the efficacy of implemented protocols as well as identify areas for change. Hospitals that adopt a culture of transparency and accountability are able to utilize this information to enhance their infection prevention strategies. Regular feedback systems and audit mechanisms allow for an adaptive learning system where best practices can be shared and spread. The evidence from the European Federation of Nurses Associations, quoted by Burke et al. (2008), illustrates the need for systematic information gathering and sharing in establishing a culture of openness against HAIs. Thus, such a strategy not only enhances the quality of care accessible to patients but also improves the overall safety of the health environment (Figure 9.14).

Test Your Knowledge

1. Why is hand hygiene considered the single most effective method of preventing hospital-acquired infections?
2. How should the selection and proper use of PPE vary depending on the type of patient interaction or level of infection risk in critical care settings?

9.6. Family Involvement in Care

Learning Outcome

1. Explain the role of family in patient recovery;
2. Understand support systems for families of critical patients;
3. Focus on communication strategies for family engagement.

Involvement of family in care is being increasingly viewed as one of the most important aspects of effective patient-focused health care practice, particularly in intensive care settings. With increasing complexity in patients' needs, family involvement not only improves care experience but also results in improved health outcomes. Involvement could be in terms of being part of care planning, decision-making, and ongoing communication with health care professionals. A review observed that relatives tend to move from acting as passive witnesses to acting as active supporters, emphasizing their desire to collaborate with care teams (Hayward et al., 2021). This indicates a common awareness of families' potential role in the healthcare process, especially in environments such as ICUs where patients may be unable to express their desires. Hence, building productive relationships between health providers and families can help optimize the total care quality delivered. Furthermore, family involvement dynamics are contextualized by numerous factors influencing the extent to which families are engaged in the care system. Research indicates that aspects such as prior experience of family members with the healthcare system, quality of communication between staff and families, and availability of support programs have the capacity to influence levels of involvement. Interventions for engaging families may lead to increased patient and family satisfaction and better well-being (Inglis et al., 2024). It is the duty of the health professionals to identify these determinants and change practice accordingly so that families are empowered and better informed throughout the process of care.

By being proactively interested in identifying and responding to the unique needs of every family, critical care teams can build a more responsive healthcare environment that is respectful of and sensitive to family members' preferences and knowledge. In summary, integrating family involvement into critical care practice is not only a beneficial practice but a necessary step to optimal health outcomes. As highlighted in recent studies, quality family involvement can enhance patient experiences and a partnership agreement between families and caregivers. Improvement measures encompass maximizing communication, providing access to family members, and an admission of their role within the care continuum (Inglis et al., 2024). All future research must aim to build on these results by determining systemic ways of implementing these ideals effectively in a way that both patients and families receive the participation and care they require during challenging times. By prioritizing family involvement, healthcare professionals can fill the gap between clinical care and the psychological, emotional, and practical demands of families and patients.

9.6.1. Role of Family in Patient Recovery

The role of family healing in a patient is a critical factor in the healing process, particularly in the dynamics of critical care. The family is usually the initial support system for the patient, providing both psychological and emotional stability during the course of a medical emergency. Research confirms that families incorporated in the care process result in improved outcomes in patients, including shorter stays in the hospital and enhanced emotional stability. This participation can take many different forms, from entering into discussions with doctors and nurses to assisting with treatment schedules. Additionally, family involvement creates a support system where patients feel safer and supported, important for healing, particularly in high-stress situations common to intensive care units. Moreover, the family's impact on patient recovery extends beyond emotional encouragement; it includes functional assistance in decision-making and collaboration with treatment plans. When patients struggle to grasp complex medical information, family members can intervene and interpret such information into concrete actions.

This collaborative process not only diminishes the feeling of loneliness but also creates a shared vision for the health journey of the patients. With healthcare now digitalized in the means of telehealth and EHRs, the families are faced with the challenge of utilizing these technologies effectively, thereby further enhancing their engagement. Such a multifaceted engagement is consistent with the move towards whole-person practices in healthcare, according to the broader discussion of patient care principles (Burr et al., 2020). Family dynamics also significantly determine the recovery pathway of patients, particularly in mental health. For instance, the management of individuals with disorders such as schizophrenia has in the past strongly emphasized medication as the primary treatment, often overlooking the therapeutic potential of supportive psychosocial interventions.

In more recent years, there has been a strong focus on holistic, family-based treatments that are focused on enhancing the health of the individual as a whole, as opposed to pharmacological-based solutions. Engaging family members as partners in care has the potential for more targeted and useful treatment plans because they are most likely to be aware of the patient's needs and preferences. Such partnerships not only enhance treatment compliance but can also contribute towards improved overall mental health outcomes, orienting healthcare practice towards a more integrative model (Aderhold et al., 2009) (Figure 9.15).

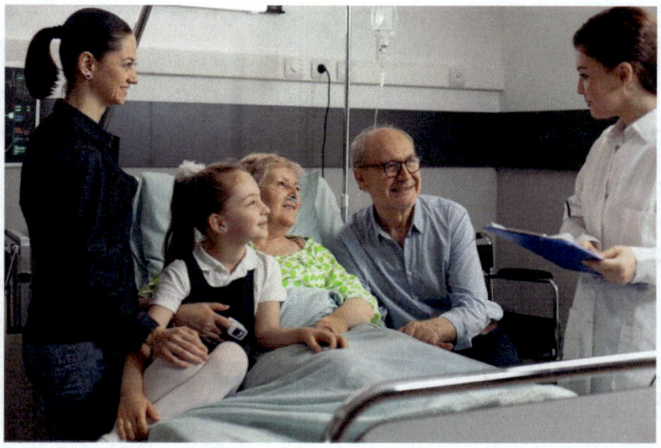

Figure 9.15. Family involvement in patient recovery.

Source: https://evokewellnessoh.com/wp-content/uploads/2025/03/Inpatient-Rehab-1024x682.jpg.

9.6.2. Support Systems for Families of Critical Patients

It is an extremely stressful and overwhelming experience having a family member in critical care. Not only are families exposed to emotional disturbance but also to actual-life adversity, including dealing with healthcare systems and rendering major medical decisions in times of stress. Establishing robust support systems is the most important strategy for overcoming the psychological impacts on families and maintaining their well-being in adverse situations. These support systems can be promoted within hospitals through concerted efforts, like building family-centered care practices that focus on communication and involvement. Support systems can even have professional counselors, social workers, and peer support groups who offer emotional and practical assistance. By incorporating these elements into critical care, healthcare facilities can develop a condition that honors the needs of family members, thereby enhancing their capacity to cope during an emergency. The integration of systematic change can significantly improve family care delivered to critical patients. Active leadership within healthcare organizations is one of the most significant aspects of this, and it can facilitate the adoption of family-centered policies. By adopting quality improvement strategies, healthcare teams can create programs that not only focus on outcomes of the patient but also on the psychological and emotional well-being of the families. It is critical to encourage continuous, team-based healing relationships that not only comprise medical staff but also social services and psychological counseling. This combined strategy minimizes loneliness and ensures a sense of belonging among families, thus enhancing the general experience of taking care of their loved ones in critical care settings (Wagner et al., 2012). Furthermore, research into ICUs' varying capabilities can inform the best approach to support families in critical care. Outcomes of research into ICUs' readiness to execute clinical trials reveal vast variability in resources and organization, impacting the family experience of those receiving treatment. The overall concept of Normalizing Research is to incorporate research into the day-to-day care and produce a culture that values clinical practice, as well as family care. With an understanding of the driving forces affecting care dynamics, health professionals can tailor individualized approaches that meet both patient and family needs, ultimately enhancing the experience through what can be a traumatic event. These settings not only enhance resilience within the family but also in the clinical setting, a culture of care and support (Pattison et al., 2019).

9.6.3. Communication Strategies for Family Engagement

Effective family participation in intensive care settings requires the use of good communication techniques that are focused on clarity and empathy. One of the keyways is creating a culture of openness, whereby the families are invited to ask their questions and express their concerns. This entails being listened to and heard by their needs and making healthcare professionals available and open to discussion. The early childhood leader advisory group of The David and Lucile Packard Foundation reinforces the importance of such engagement activities in fostering healthy relationships, ultimately resulting in better care and decision-making (The Stern Center for Evidence-Based Policy, 2015). In situations when patients' families struggle with the intricacies of critical care, tailored communication strategies, including interpretive services and visual aids, can bridge gaps in understanding, thus enhancing the whole experience for both families and healthcare providers. The diversity in family structure and cultural background calls attention to the necessity for individualized communication methods within critical care environments. Methods need to be sensitive to the unique requirements and desires of each family, including cultural expertise and enhancing cross-cultural communication. The research on Indigenous palliative care preferences illustrates this necessity, as culturally safe care enhances involvement and best results (Shahid et al., 2018). For example, involving family members in care planning and taking into account cultural customs can significantly influence the effectiveness of healthcare delivery. Such culturally responsive practices not only honor the identity of families but also improve trust, thereby supporting their continued engagement and collaboration in the care process. On another note, feedback loops constantly between families and healthcare teams are essential in evaluating and refining communication strategies. Having regular intervals to update family members and discuss care plans makes it possible to include family observations and desires, and there is a sense of collaboration in care. The communication strategies promoted by organizations, as explained in the book authored by The David and Lucile Packard Foundation, support the idea that ongoing conversation enhances family engagement, resulting in enhanced child and family health within healthcare systems (The Stern Center for Evidence-Based Policy, 2015). Similarly, effective palliative care models have shown that ongoing communication produces greater family comprehension of the nature of available care options offered to them and reinforces commitment to utilize such services (Shahid et al., 2018). By focusing on dynamic relations, healthcare providers can attain a more responsive and humane critical care environment for families.

Test Your Knowledge

1. How can the presence and involvement of family members influence the psychological and physical recovery of critically ill patients?
2. What communication approaches are most effective in engaging families during a patient's critical illness?

SUMMARY

In synthesizing the critical care principles presented throughout this essay, the value of efficient resource allocation as a cornerstone to quality healthcare is achieved. The challenges faced by decision-makers in health policy are contingent upon a profound understanding of intricate standards that comprise patient outcomes and healthcare equity. As well-documented in recent literature, the definition of decision criteria, ranging from health outcomes to economic impacts, provides a structured process for prioritization of interventions. The study highlighted by Guindo et al. (2012) applauds diversity in terminology and the need for a unifying framework, showing that clarity in decision-making truly makes a difference in equitable distribution of healthcare resources. This extensive review paves the way for the development of robust multicriteria decision-making tools that will be able to aid care systems worldwide. The effective application of these principles also demands a shift toward patient-centered care models. For this purpose, integration of active leadership and continuous quality improvement initiatives becomes essential to transform healthcare practice. Such notions of transformation, explained by Wagner et al. (2012), foster interactive settings that emphasize therapeutic relationships and increased access to care. By prioritizing patient engagement and rationally addressing their needs, health systems can improve satisfaction and health outcomes. The far-reaching consequences, consequently, are gigantic, as they improve patient satisfaction along with streamlining the usage of resources, thereby addressing the core paradigm shift of critical care. Ultimately, as we conclude this essay, the central integration of the aforementioned principles within healthcare paradigms offers a lead to maximize decision-making in critical care centers. The emphasis on equity, effectiveness, and partnership between stakeholders, highlighted in Guindo et al. (2012), provides a comprehensive view with which policymakers can evaluate and enhance health care interventions. It is essential in the future that the stakeholders remain committed to the application of evidence-based approaches and expand efforts focused on the diminution of health care inequities. By doing so, the above-mentioned principles can go a long way in developing a stronger healthcare system that holds both quality and access in high regard in highly critical care environments.

In critical care, the clinical practice is guided by principles that are most important to ensure ideal patient outcomes. The most basic among these guiding principles is the understanding of the patient conditions' complexity and variability. Critical care professionals have to continuously assess and monitor because the status of patients may change quickly, and intervention should be initiated in good time. This consistent attentiveness requires not just technical proficiency but also the ability to comprehend and enact evidence-based practice with direct influence on patient care. Further, the incorporation of a multidisciplinary strategy into critical care teams demonstrates the collaborative strategy behind successful treatment, in which specialists across disciplines collaborate towards common goals. This holistic approach is the essence of critical care in focusing on the human experience rather than clinical indicators, ultimately translating into improved outcomes and satisfaction for patients in a high-risk environment. Another fundamental aspect of critical care is communication and decision-making between medical practitioners. Having all of the members at one level of comprehension can contribute significantly to patient care during emergencies, where quick decision-making is required. Communication results in an environment where the members feel free to voice concerns, provide insights, and contribute to collective problem-solving. Moreover, knowing the importance of family involvement in decision-making of care can make the patient's support system more robust, both medicinally and emotionally, during their moment of need. Institutions increasingly understand that the integration of family and caregiver input enhances care strategies and synchronizes treatment with patient values and preferences. To enable these exchanges, clinical models that place interdisciplinary collaboration at the forefront provide healthcare teams with the instruments necessary to deliver evidence-based and empathetic care. Lastly, education and ongoing professional development are crucial in reinforcing salient critical care principles. As the healthcare landscape evolves, so too do the critical care professionals' competencies. The training programs must address not only clinical know-how but also population health concepts, which emphasize models of care delivery that benefit through value as opposed to volume. Healthcare organization administrators and educators strive to reshape curricula to accommodate these necessary practice changes so that future leaders can grapple with the complexities of today's healthcare landscape. Through a focus on adaptive learning and integration of concepts from related fields like public health, programs can build a staff that can manage the multifaceted challenges of critical care settings effectively. This proactive approach offers a platform for sustaining maximum standards of care and improving patient outcomes in the long term, as clearly spelled out by root objectives in health administration education (The Stern Center for Evidence-Based Policy, 2015; Caron et al., 2018).

KEY TERMS FROM THIS CHAPTER

Advanced life support (ALS) techniques
Belgium's euthanasia regime
COVID-19 pandemic
Critical care
Digital patch system
End-of-life decisions
Extracorporeal life support (ECLS)
Family dynamics
Glasgow Coma Scale
Hand washing
Healthcare experience
Healthcare infrastructures
Healthcare-associated infections (HAIs)
Infection rates
Intensive care settings
Medication administration
Modern healthcare
Motivational interviewing (MI)
Multidrug-resistant organisms (MDROs)
Patient experience

CRITICAL THINKING QUESTIONS

1. **Which of the following tools is commonly used to assess the level of consciousness in critically ill patients?**
   a. Braden Scale
   b. Glasgow Coma Scale
   c. Morse Fall Scale
   d. APACHE II Score
2. **Effective communication in critical care settings primarily aims to:**
   a. Reduce the length of hospital stay
   b. Satisfy hospital administrative requirements
   c. Prevent medical errors and enhance patient outcomes
   d. Improve hospital infrastructure
3. **Which of the following is a key ethical principle in critical care decision-making?**
   a. Autonomy
   b. Profitability
   c. Expediency
   d. Popularity
4. **What is the recommended compression-to-ventilation ratio for a single rescuer performing CPR on an adult?**
   a. 5:1
   b. 15:2
   c. 30:2
   d. 50:2
5. **What is the most effective method for preventing the spread of infections in critical care units?**
   a. Daily bathing with antiseptics
   b. Routine use of prophylactic antibiotics
   c. Wearing N95 masks at all times
   d. Strict hand hygiene compliance

Short Answer Questions

1. What are the essential components of a comprehensive patient assessment in critical care, and how do these guide prioritization and intervention?
2. How can critical care teams ensure clear, accurate, and empathetic communication among multidisciplinary staff and with patients and families, especially under high-stress conditions?
3. What ethical dilemmas commonly arise in critical care settings, and how can principles such as autonomy, beneficence, and justice guide clinical decisions?
4. How should informed consent be managed in critical care when patients are incapacitated, and what role do surrogate decision-makers play in this process?
5. What are the current standards for performing high-quality CPR and administering emergency medications during a cardiac arrest in the ICU?
6. How does strict adherence to hand hygiene and appropriate use of PPE reduce the incidence of hospital-acquired infections in critical care units?

Answers to Critical Thinking Questions

1. (b); 2. (c); 3. (a); 4. (c); 5. (d)

REFERENCES

1. Zumla, A., Abubakar, I., Raviglione, M., Hoelscher, M., Ditiu, L., McHugh, T. D., Squire, S. B., Cox, H., Ford, N., McNerney, R., Marais, B., Grobusch, M., Lawn, S. D., Migliori, G. B., Mwaba, P., O'Grady, J., Pletschette, M., Ramsay, A., Chakaya, J., Schito, M., ... Atun, R. (2012). Drug-resistant tuberculosis--current dilemmas, unanswered questions, challenges, and priority needs. *The Journal of infectious diseases, 205 Suppl 2*, S228–S240. https://doi.org/10.1093/infdis/jir858(accessed on 27th June 2025).
2. Aderhold, V., Agar-Jacomb, T., Barnes, A., Bennett, L., Burston, C., Calton, T., Carpenter, L., et al. (2009). Minimal-medication approaches to treating schizophrenia. https://core.ac.uk/download/107296.pdf (accessed on 27th June 2025).
3. Inglis, R., Leaver, M., Pell, C., Ahmad, S., Akter, S., Bhuia, F. I. A., Ansary, M., B S, S., Begum, M., Chakraborty, S. R., Chowdhury, H., Chowdhury, M. A. R., Deb, P., Akhter Farzana, N., Ghose, A., Harun Or Roshid, M., Hoque Tipu, M. R., Hosain, S., Hossain, M. M., Moinul Islam, M., ... Faiz, M. A. (2024). Understanding patient and family experiences of critical care in Bangladesh and India: What are the priority actions to promote person-centred care?. *PLOS global public health*, *4*(6), e0003372. https://doi.org/10.1371/journal.pgph.0003372(accessed on 27th June 2025).
4. Hernandez-Silveira, M., Ahmed, K., Ang, S. S., Zandari, F., Mehta, T., Weir, R., Burdett, A., Toumazou, C., & Brett, S. J. (2015). Assessment of the feasibility of an ultra-low power, wireless digital patch for the continuous ambulatory monitoring of vital signs. *BMJ open*, *5*(5), e006606. https://doi.org/10.1136/bmjopen-2014-006606(accessed on 27th June 2025).
5. Alinier, G., Hassan, I. F., Alsalemi, A., Al Disi, M., Ait Hssain, A., Labib, A., Alhomsi, Y., Bensaali, F., Amira, A., & Ibrahim, A. S. (2018). Addressing the challenges of ECMO simulation. *Perfusion*, *33*(7), 568–576. https://doi.org/10.1177/0267659118777194(accessed on 27th June 2025).
6. Akyol, M. U., Alden, T. D., Amartino, H., Ashworth, J. L., et al. (2019). Recommendations for the management of MPS VI: Systematic evidence- and consensus-based guidance. https://core.ac.uk/download/323074857.pdf (accessed on 27th June 2025).
7. Alderson, P., & Morrow, V. (2006). Multi-disciplinary research ethics review: Is it feasible? https://core.ac.uk/download/pdf/82794.pdf (accessed on 27th June 2025).
8. Pattison, N., Arulkumaran, N., O'Gara, G., Connolly, B., Humphreys, S., Walsh, T., Hopkins, P., & Dark, P. (2019). Synthesis of qualitative research studies regarding the factors surrounding UK critical care trial infrastructure. *BMJ open*, *9*(12), e030815. https://doi.org/10.1136/bmjopen-2019-030815(accessed on 27th June 2025).
9. Manning, M. L., Septimus, E. J., Ashley, E. S. D., Cosgrove, S. E., Fakih, M. G., Schweon, S. J., Myers, F. E., & Moody, J. A. (2018). Antimicrobial stewardship and infection prevention-leveraging the synergy: A position paper update. *American journal of infection control*, *46*(4), 364–368. https://doi.org/10.1016/j.ajic.2018.01.001 (accessed on 27th June 2025).
10. Attard Montalto, S. (2014). Ethical principles in pediatric practice. https://core.ac.uk/download/46603075.pdf (accessed on 27th June 2025).
11. Guindo, L. A., Wagner, M., Baltussen, R., Rindress, D., van Til, J., Kind, P., & Goetghebeur, M. M. (2012). From efficacy to equity: Literature review of decision criteria for resource allocation

and healthcare decisionmaking. *Cost effectiveness and resource allocation : C/E, 10*(1), 9. https://doi.org/10.1186/1478-7547-10-9(accessed on 27th June 2025).

12. Marvin, V., Kuo, S., Poots, A. J., Woodcock, T., Vaughan, L., & Bell, D. (2016). Applying quality improvement methods to address gaps in medicines reconciliation at transfers of care from an acute UK hospital. *BMJ open, 6*(6), e010230. https://doi.org/10.1136/bmjopen-2015-010230 (accessed on 27th June 2025).

13. Shakely, D., Elfving, K., Aydin-Schmidt, B., Msellem, M. I., Morris, U., Omar, R., Weiping, X., Petzold, M., Greenhouse, B., Baltzell, K. A., Ali, A. S., Björkman, A., & Mårtensson, A. (2013). The usefulness of rapid diagnostic tests in the new context of low malaria transmission in Zanzibar. *PloS one, 8*(9), e72912. https://doi.org/10.1371/journal.pone.0072912(accessed on 27th June 2025).

14. Billica, R., Gosbee, J., & Krupa, D. T. (1991). Evaluation of cardiopulmonary resuscitation techniques in microgravity. https://core.ac.uk/download/pdf/42816255.pdf (accessed on 27th June 2025).

15. Birch, D., & Draper, J. (2008). A critical literature review exploring the challenges of delivering effective palliative care to older people with dementia in the acute hospital setting. https://core.ac.uk/download/82906952.pdf (accessed on 27th June 2025).

16. McCarthy, D., & Blumenthal, D.(2006). Committed to safety: Ten case studies on reducing harm to patients. [New York, N.Y.] : Commonwealth Fund, April 2006 https://core.ac.uk/download/71350251.pdf (accessed on 27th June 2025).

17. Contreras, M., Curran, E., Ross, M., Moran, P., Sheehan, A., Brennan, A. M., Cosgrave, D., McElwain, J., Lavelle, C., & Lynch, B. (2020). Rapid development of interprofessional in situ simulation-based training in response to the COVID-19 outbreak in a tertiary-level hospital in Ireland: initial response and lessons for future disaster preparation. *BMJ simulation & technology enhanced learning, 7*(3), 159–162. https://doi.org/10.1136/bmjstel-2020-000679 (accessed on 27th June 2025).

18. Denaï, M. A., Mahfouf, M., Mohamad-Samuri, S., Panoutsos, G., Brown, B. H., & Mills, G. H. (2010). Absolute electrical impedance tomography (aEIT) guided ventilation therapy in critical care patients: simulations and future trends. *IEEE transactions on information technology in biomedicine : a publication of the IEEE Engineering in Medicine and Biology Society, 14*(3), 641–649. https://doi.org/10.1109/TITB.2009.2036010(accessed on 27th June 2025).

19. Burke, J., Smith, L. N., Sveinsdóttir, H., Willman, A., et al. (2008). Patient safety in Europe: Medication errors and hospital-acquired infections. https://core.ac.uk/download/90014.pdf (accessed on 27th June 2025).

20. Bury, D., & Strauss, S. M. (2006). The scientist-practitioner in a counselling psychology setting. https://core.ac.uk/download/2708189.pdf (accessed on 27th June 2025).

21. Caron, R. M., Hewitt, A., Carmalt, J. H., & Hooker, E. A. (2018). Teaching Population Health: Innovations in the Integration of the Healthcare and Public Health Systems. Journal of Health Administration Education, 35(4), 527-550.(accessed on 27th June 2025).

22. Wong AH, Roppolo LP, Chang BP, et al. Management of Agitation During the COVID-19 Pandemic. *West J Emerg Med*. 2020;21(4):795-800. Published 2020 May 22. doi:10.5811/westjem.2020.5.47789(accessed on 27th June 2025).

23. Petrova, D., & Clifford, J.(2009). Religion and healthcare in the European Union: Policy issues and trends. https://core.ac.uk/download/214315351.pdf (accessed on 27th June 2025).
24. Cohen-Almagor, R. (2016). Patient's autonomy, physician's convictions and euthanasia in Belgium. https://core.ac.uk/download/151161696.pdf (accessed on 27th June 2025).
25. Lancaster, E. M., Sosa, J. A., Sammann, A., Pierce, L., Shen, W., Conte, M. C., & Wick, E. C. (2020). Rapid Response of an Academic Surgical Department to the COVID-19 Pandemic: Implications for Patients, Surgeons, and the Community. *Journal of the American College of Surgeons*, *230*(6), 1064–1073. https://doi.org/10.1016/j.jamcollsurg.2020.04.007(accessed on 27th June 2025).
26. Munday D, Dale J. Palliative care in the community. *BMJ*. 2007;334(7598):809-810. doi:10.1136/bmj.39174.605081.80(accessed on 27th June 2025).
27. Farías-Yapur, A. (2023). Defining success and ethical decision-making in vascularized composite allotransplantation: A bioethical deliberation model. https://core.ac.uk/download/578750035.pdf (accessed on 27th June 2025).
28. Shekar, K., Mullany, D. V., Thomson, B., Ziegenfuss, M., Platts, D. G., & Fraser, J. F. (2014). Extracorporeal life support devices and strategies for management of acute cardiorespiratory failure in adult patients: a comprehensive review. *Critical care (London, England)*, *18*(3), 219. https://doi.org/10.1186/cc13865(accessed on 27th June 2025).
29. Friedlander, D. (2014). Student-centered learning: Dozier-Libbey Medical High School. https://core.ac.uk/download/71364835.pdf (accessed on 27th June 2025).
30. Hayward, J. K., Gould, C., Palluotto, E., Kitson, E. C., & Spector, A. (2023). Family involvement with care homes following placement of a relative living with dementia: a review. *Ageing and Society*, *43*(7), 1530–1575. doi:10.1017/S0144686X21000957(accessed on 27th June 2025).
31. Halbach, P., & Keller, A. O. (2017). Evaluating motivational interviewing in the physician assistant curriculum. https://core.ac.uk/download/213073350.pdf (accessed on 27th June 2025).
32. Storr, J., Twyman, A., Zingg, W., Damani, N., Kilpatrick, C., Reilly, J., Price, L., Egger, M., Grayson, M. L., Kelley, E., Allegranzi, B., & WHO Guidelines Development Group (2017). Core components for effective infection prevention and control programmes: new WHO evidence-based recommendations. *Antimicrobial resistance and infection control*, *6*, 6. https://doi.org/10.1186/s13756-016-0149-9(accessed on 27th June 2025).
33. Hill, B. (2020). Principles of mechanical ventilation for non-critical care nurses. https://core.ac.uk/download/390062517.pdf (accessed on 27th June 2025).
34. McKivett, A., Paul, D., & Hudson, N. (2019). Healing Conversations: Developing a Practical Framework for Clinical Communication Between Aboriginal Communities and Healthcare Practitioners. *Journal of immigrant and minority health*, *21*(3), 596–605. https://doi.org/10.1007/s10903-018-0793-7(accessed on 27th June 2025).
35. Amanda Jane Marshall-Ponting, Khairy A.H. Kobbacy, Stelios Sapountzis, and Michail Kagioglou
36. (2012). A multi-faceted approach to optimizing a complex unplanned healthcare system. International Journal of Logistics Systems and Management 2013 15:2-3, 239-248 https://core.ac.uk/download/5225387.pdf (accessed on 27th June 2025).

37. Keith-Chancy, E. (2024). Integration of trauma-informed practices for end-of-life care in the NICU. https://core.ac.uk/download/614448191.pdf (accessed on 27th June 2025).

38. Shahid, S., Taylor, E.V., Cheetham, S. *et al.* Key features of palliative care service delivery to Indigenous peoples in Australia, New Zealand, Canada and the United States: a comprehensive review. *BMC Palliat Care* **17**, 72 (2018). https://doi.org/10.1186/s12904-018-0325-1(accessed on 27th June 2025).

39. Burr, Christopher and Burr, Christopher and Morley, Jessica, Empowerment or Engagement? Digital Health Technologies for Mental Healthcare (May 24, 2019). Available at SSRN: https://ssrn.com/abstract=3393534 or http://dx.doi.org/10.2139/ssrn.3393534(accessed on 27th June 2025).

40. Njoku, J. (2005). Nurses' perception of family presence during resuscitation. https://core.ac.uk/download/223074368.pdf (accessed on 27th June 2025).

41. Bradbury, K., Steele, M., Corbett, T., Geraghty, A. W. A., Krusche, A., Heber, E., Easton, S., Cheetham-Blake, T., Slodkowska-Barabasz, J., Müller, A. M., Smith, K., Wilde, L. J., Payne, L., Singh, K., Bacon, R., Burford, T., Summers, K., Turner, L., Richardson, A., Watson, E., ... Yardley, L. (2019). Developing a digital intervention for cancer survivors: an evidence-, theory- and person-based approach. *NPJ digital medicine, 2,* 85. https://doi.org/10.1038/s41746-019-0163-4(accessed on 27th June 2025).

42. Scott P, Ross P, Prytherch D (2012), "Evidence-based inpatient handovers: a literature review and research agenda". Clinical Governance: An International Journal, Vol. 17 No. 1 pp. 14–27, doi: https://doi.org/10.1108/14777271211200710(accessed on 27th June 2025).

43. San Jose State University. (2020). Dietz, Elizabeth "Liz" Oshry. https://core.ac.uk/download/301583385.pdf (accessed on 27th June 2025).

44. Siriwardena, A. N. (2007). Development and use of clinical performance indicators for ambulance services and prehospital care: A discussion paper for a clinical quality improvement framework for ambulance services. https://core.ac.uk/download/16498419.pdf (accessed on 27th June 2025).

45. Wagner, E., Sugarman, J. R., Phillips, K., Coleman, K., & Reid, R. J. (2012). Guiding transformation: How medical practices can become patient-centered medical homes. https://core.ac.uk/download/71358341.pdf (accessed on 27th June 2025).

GENERAL MEDICINE APPROACH IN PAIN MANAGEMENT

10

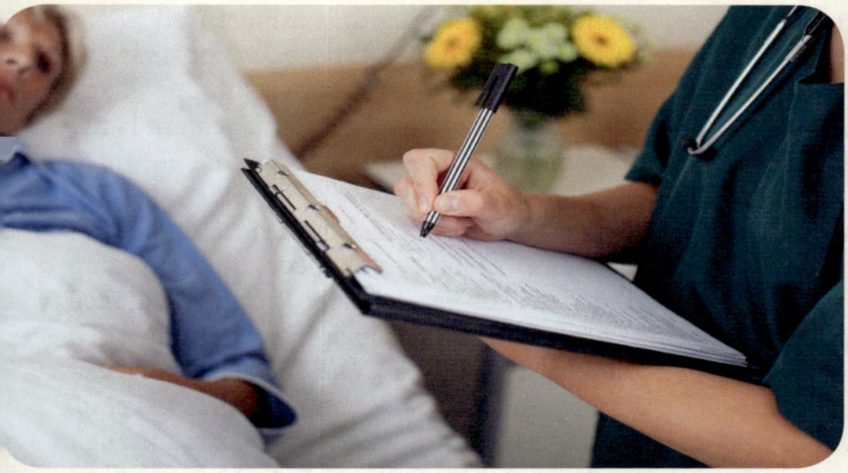

LEARNING OBJECTIVES

After studying this chapter, you will be able to:

1. Understand pain;
2. Discuss the assessment of pain for effective pain management;
3. Focus on pharmacological and non-pharmacological interventions for effective pain management;
4. Explain the role of general practitioners (GPs) in pain management;
5. Describe the challenges in pain management.

Introduction

In pain management, efficient interventions play a crucial role in patient outcomes and quality of life improvement. Pain is an acute or chronic state that entails a multifaceted set of physiological, psychological, and social factors. A generalized medical strategy should be adopted to confront this multidimensional state to allow healthcare professionals to use an integrated treatment program. This approach aims not just to alleviate pain but also to eliminate its causes, so patients can benefit from an interdisciplinary model of care. There are numerous practices, both pharmacological and non-pharmacological, that may be employed to achieve relief from pain, promote functionality, and stimulate healing. One must understand the intricacies of each approach, setting the stage for a tailored pain management program that is sensitive to the individual patient's requirements. As medicine reacts to the opioid crisis, it has become more and more important to look to other analgesics that minimize risks associated with opioid use. The utilization of nonsteroidal anti-inflammatory medications (NSAIDs) in pain treatment is one of the best examples of this movement. While NSAIDs are used extensively for their ability to minimize pain in a wide variety of contexts, particularly in sports medicine, their implications and possible side effects must be critically examined. Research cites the short-term benefits of NSAIDs in relation to effective pain relief and enhancement of recovery for athletes, yet also reveals long-term risks that may hinder spontaneous tissue healing and overall health outcomes. Therefore, there is an urgent need for clinicians to adopt a balanced approach, employing NSAIDs responsibly while seeking out other pain mechanisms to enable PS and optimize recovery (Urbański et al., 2024). Secondarily, the pain management landscape itself continues to shift in response to public health issues like the growing prevalence of prescription opioid use disorders. Experts point to the necessity of changes in physician training, prescribing practices, and addiction treatment to address this critical issue directly. Multistakeholder initiatives by members of the medical profession attempt to steer policies toward ensuring proper pain management. Recommendations call for the establishment of prescribing standards, operational prescription drug monitoring programs (PDMPs), and education on overdose prevention as important. These more comprehensive measures seek not only to address immediate pain management but also the long-term ramifications of uncontrolled pain and substance abuse (Alexander et al., 2015). Collectively, these efforts are part of a comprehensive medicine strategy aimed at managing pain with a focus on maximizing patient outcomes while preserving safety and efficacy.

Definition of Pain Management

The philosophy of pain management is a comprehensive collection of interventions aimed at minimizing pain and enhancing the overall quality of life in individuals suffering from all types of pain. Pain occurs in numerous forms—acute, chronic, or in connection with specific medical conditions—and thus pain management needs to be individualized and multidisciplinary. In general medicine, health professionals are eager to emphasize that intervention must be sensitive to the pain causes as well as to psychosocial processes that may enhance the people's experience of distress. This treatment method aligns with recent evidence that shows that the success of pain management programs is increased where both biological and psychosocial processes are addressed actively (Burton et al., 2009). A key component of effective pain management is the utilization of the biopsychosocial model, which recognizes that pain is not just a biological entity. It includes biological, psychological, and social factors and therefore enhances understanding of the patient's experience. Present evidence indicates that psychosocial interventions, such as emotional well-being and social support, can have a significant impact on outcomes for pain. For instance, studies have shown that although some relief may be obtained through biomedical intervention alone, they are not effective in giving optimal outcomes when psychosocial aspects are neglected (Rankin et al., 2018). Thus, pain management procedures that involve this broader approach are likely to result in long-term sustainable benefits for patients, promoting enhanced recovery and functionality. Moreover, the environment of pain management is ever-evolving, so healthcare professionals must be aware of the latest evidence-based care. With changes in the paradigm of medical education, emphasis is increasingly placed on training future healthcare professionals in pharmacological as well as non-pharmacological pain management techniques. This includes increasing awareness of interdisciplinary teamwork and patient-centered care (Rankin et al., 2018). Lastly, a complete definition of pain management would have to encompass the mandate to educate those who deal with pain, imparting an intrinsic philosophy of a reverence for the significance of ongoing learning and adaptability in clinical practice. By such culture, providers will be assured they are adequately equipped to meet patients' many-sided needs for pain (Figure 10.1).

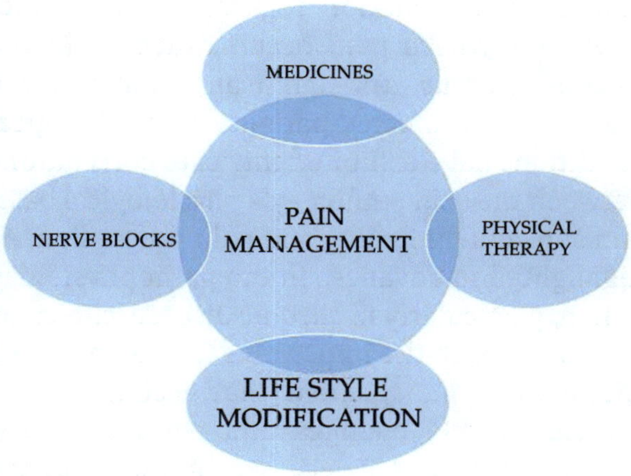

Figure 10.1. Pain management.

Source: https://www.kauveryhospital.com/wp-content/uploads/2023/12/154-1.jpg.

Importance of a General Medicine Approach

The general approach in general medicine is essential in the management of pain because it lays down an overall system of comprehending and managing the complicated nature of pain. Chronic pain is a prevalent disorder that significantly influences patients' quality of life and the healthcare system as well. Medical education, on the other hand, barely meets the needs of pain management. Evidence from the literature indicates disproportionate focus on pain education, where the majority of medical schools offer it just marginally within their curricula. For instance, a UK and USA systematic review indicates that 96% of medical schools lack compulsory, specialized teaching in pain medicine (Shipton et al., 2018). Therefore, physicians may be poorly equipped to detect and treat pain suitably, and hence indicate the critical need for a general medicine orientation with an emphasis on intensive training of medical students in pain treatment. Secondly, having a general medicine orientation allows physicians to consider the international aspects of patient treatment in responding to pain. This approach promotes the inclusion of biological, psychological, and social determinants that improve a patient's pain experience. Determinant analysis of chronic pain management in medical students and GPs reveals that while patients' reports of pain are given prominence, other determinant elements, for instance, social support and patient preferences, are often overlooked (Rankin et al., 2019).

By building a broader understanding of pain management, the practice of general medicine is able to maximize clinical decision-making into more personalized and effective therapy. This integrated practice is crucial in building a deeper understanding of the unique condition of each patient and ultimately improving outcomes and satisfaction in pain management practice. Last but not least, the strength of a general medicine approach is that it serves to foster collaboration among various specialties involved in pain management. Effective pain management is often a multidisciplinary process, and this can be attained by having a good understanding of general medicine concepts. Through the provision of medical professionals with a strong foundation in general medicine, they will be in a position to speak more clearly and collaborate better with specialists such as anesthesiologists, physiotherapists, and psychologists, thus setting an integrated plan for pain management. The systematic review gives momentum to the reevaluation of medical curricula such that pain medicine is dealt with properly and is included in medical education (Shipton et al., 2018). Such collaboration not only improves student learning but can also revolutionize patient care by providing a concerted effort to address the multimodal demands of pain management across disciplines.

10.1. Understanding Pain

Learning Outcome

1. Explain the types of pain: acute versus chronic;
2. Discuss the physiological mechanisms of pain;
3. Focus on psychological aspects of pain perception.

Pain management is closely related to the holistic understanding of pain, where it consists of multiple interactions between sensory, emotional, and cognitive processes. Pain is greater than the body experience; it is personal experience and also susceptible to psychological states such as depression and anxiety, and cultural beliefs. This multifaceted character needs a biopsychosocial treatment approach that integrates biological, psychological, and social dimensions in the explanation and treatment of pain. Employing this type of approach enables clinicians to deliver interventions that are sensitive to the unique experiences of individual patients and thereby optimize the efficacy of pain intervention practice. Current research highlights the importance of evidence-based care extending beyond symptomatic relief to encompass systematic assessment of the emotional and psychological status of patients, paving the way for more holistic pain care. Educational outreach programs like "academic detailing" have played a critical role in bridging the gap between clinical evidence and day-to-day practice in pain care. As observed in previous research, such programs offer clinicians current, rigorously tested information, ultimately looking to improve the quality of care. These programs promote an interactive dialogue, where healthcare professionals are given information on the most recent treatment options and evidence-based practices directed at particular patient requirements. For instance, through targeted education programs, clinicians can gain effective pain management techniques that are not misprescribing, reducing the prescribing of potentially harmful medication. The success of this model, as demonstrated through reductions in inappropriate prescribing behavior, shows how far-reaching the impact of education and continuous dialogue can be on pain management in diverse healthcare settings (Avorn, 2017). Moreover, information regarding the distinct situations where pain occurs, such as in the case of pruritus, can significantly improve the treatment for affected patients. Dermatological conditions have exhibited intricate correlations between the skin pathology's physiological basis and subsequent itching and pain perception. As highlighted in advances in the pathophysiology of itch, particularly in chronic disease, clinicians must recognize the imperative for personalized therapeutic management that accommodates individual skin changes and overall factors. Such appreciation is necessary not only for the best assessment and management but also to facilitate alleviation of generalized consequences of chronic pain and associated diseases on the quality of life in patients. The findings of both mainstream and complementary treatments seek to further build on the understanding of treatment modalities available, emphasizing the necessity of an integrated approach in pain management plans (Yosipovitch, 2013).

10.1.1. Types of Pain: Acute versus Chronic

It is important to comprehend the distinction between acute and chronic pain to ensure appropriate pain management in general medicine. Acute pain is usually an immediate response to a discernible injury or illness and is a physiological response in the form of a protective one. It most often arises suddenly and is related to some tissue damage, signaling to the body to respond to injury. This type of pain usually subsides with the healing process and may only last a finite amount of time, generally not exceeding three to six months, and may be more easily detected and treated by health care providers. The predictable onset and cessation of acute pain most commonly allow for specific treatment, such as pharmacologic or physical therapy intervention, thereby facilitating recovery and preventing chronic pain syndromes with their attendant complications. Alternatively, chronic pain presents a far more challenging problem in pain control. Chronic pain is unlike acute pain because it continues after the healing period, oftentimes persisting for months or years. It can arise from a variety of reasons, including ongoing medical conditions, abnormal healing injuries, or may even occur without a diagnosable cause. Chronic pain is characterized by its maladaptive nature, where the messages of pain may persist despite the absence of ongoing injury. Patients with chronic pain themselves describe a clear decrease in their quality of life that affects their physical function and emotional well-being. Therefore, chronic pain is controllable via a multidisciplinary strategy through the integration of pharmacological treatments, psychological therapy, and other ancillary interventions to address the multifaceted impact of the condition (Kirchhof et al., 2016). The management of acute and chronic pain reflects their contrast in nature as well as causation mechanisms. For acute pain, treatment is often directed to the direct treatment of distress and recovery via approaches such as analgesics, anti-inflammatory drugs, and, in certain instances, surgery. On the other hand, management of chronic pain demands a more holistic and individualized process, not merely with drugs but with physical therapy and psychological counseling to help repair the emotional toll of enduring pain. As the medical field continues to simplify the knowledge of both types of pain, rigid compliance with clinical protocols and personalized treatment programs remains critical (Kirchhof et al., 2016). This ensures that specialists will address the issues of acute and chronic pain in a manner that is in keeping with the best general medicine standards (Figure 10.2).

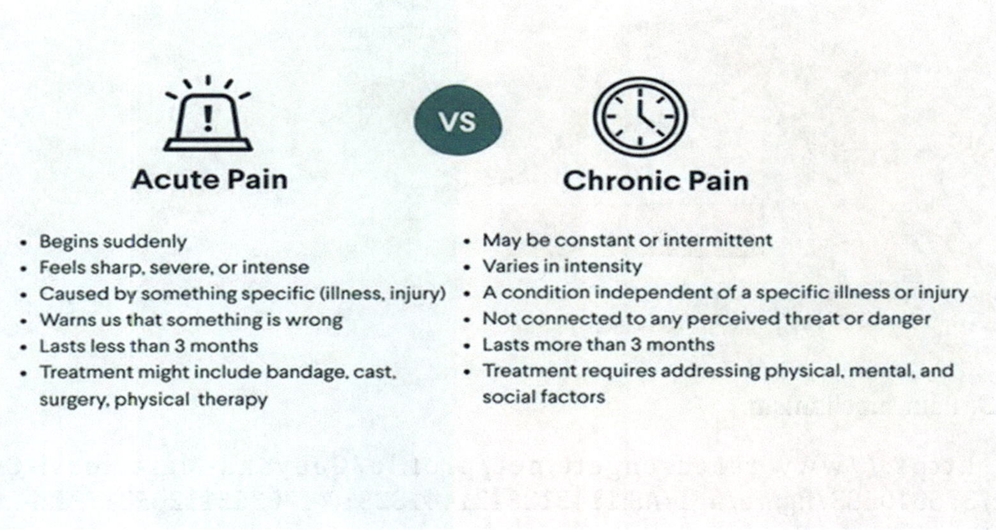

Figure 10.2. Acute versus chronic pain.

Source: https://www.fernhealth.com/wp-content/uploads/2022/04/acuteVsChronic3.jpg.

10.1.2. Physiological Mechanisms of Pain

The physiological mechanisms of pain are complex entities that are subject to both biochemical and neural mechanisms. At the most elementary, pain perception begins with nociceptors—sensory nerve cells that are specialized to react to potentially damaging stimuli. The receptors translate signals of damage, inflammation, or injury into electrical signals that travel along peripheral nerves to the spinal cord and ultimately to the brain. Once the signals enter the CNS, the brain interprets them, and a pain sensation is experienced. An aspect that plays a crucial role here is the adaptability of the nervous system. Maladaptive adjustments such as neuroplasticity can occur in chronic pain, leading to amplification of pain signals and sensitivity levels, making it hard to manage (Coluzzi et al., 2017).

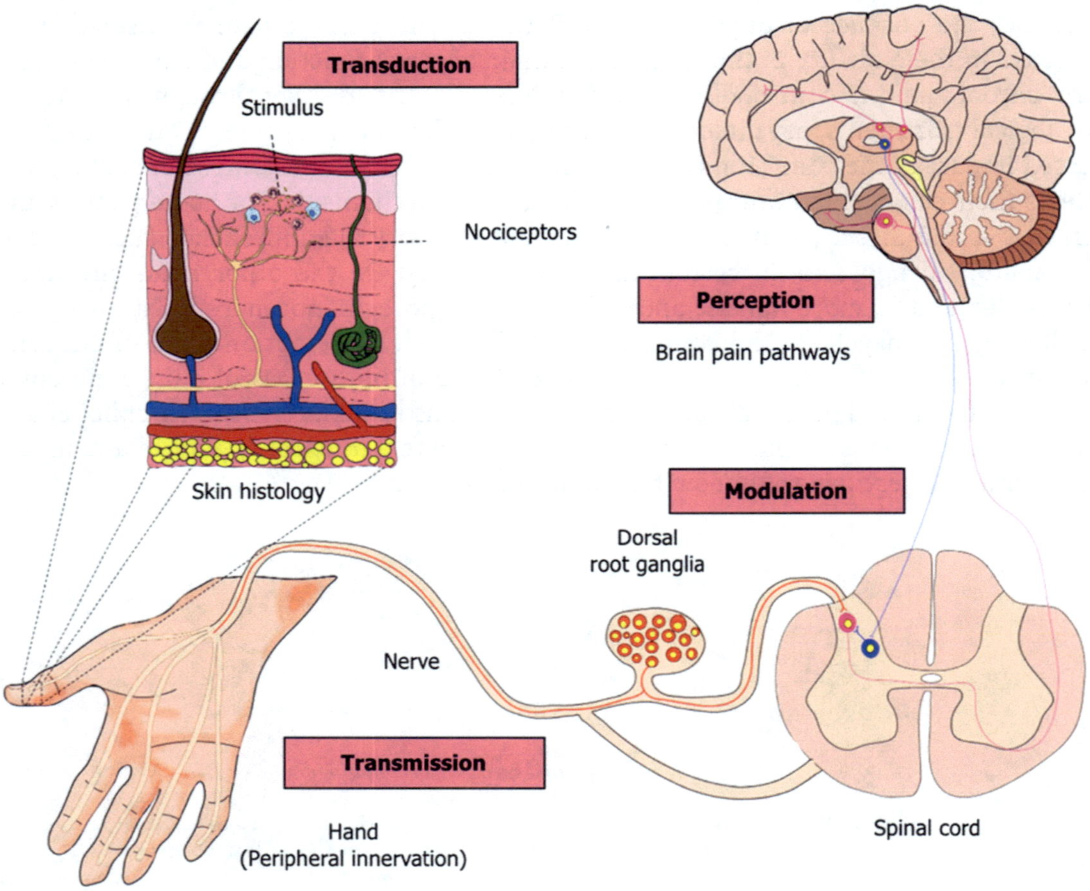

Figure 10.3. Pain mechanism.

Source: https://www.researchgate.net/profile/Geovana-Martelossi-Cebinelli/publication/376810683/figure/fig1/AS:11431281214418281@1703561126521/Pain-mechanism-Representative-diagram-of-anatomical-levels-involved-in-the-steps-of-pain.ppm.

The state of chronic pain creates a special pathophysiological state, where pain transforms from an ordinary symptom to a disease in itself. Chronic pain syndromes—osteoarthritis, chronic back pain, and fibromyalgia—are distinguished by alterations in functional and structural characteristics of the nervous system. Long-term pain, for instance, may shift neurotransmitter levels, receptor density, and neuronal connections, all of which have important impacts on one's pain threshold and sensitivity. This indicates the necessity of identifying such underlying mechanisms in formulating treatment approaches. A pain management plan specifically tailored to a patient, considering the specific pathophysiological features of a patient's condition, is essential to maximize outcomes as well as prevent further complications of pain chronification (Morton et al., 2017). Incorporation of drugs with multimechanistic action can also be significant in maximizing pain management. Tapentadol, for example, is an opioid agonist and also blocks the reuptake of norepinephrine, both centrally and peripherally. The dual action creates a therapeutic avenue for treating pain associated with neural or structural adaptation. Proper diagnosis and early treatment are essential as they may delay the transition from acute to chronic pain and thus avert long-term alteration of pain pathways. As research advances, information regarding the physiological intricacies of pain will remain of utmost significance to develop effective and efficacious interventions, imperative to improve the quality of life in patients with chronic pain (Coluzzi et al., 2017) (Figure 10.3).

10.1.3. Psychological Aspects of Pain Perception

An understanding of the psychological determinants of pain perception is of crucial significance within general medicine approaches to pain management. Pain is not solely a physiological experience; it also exists with a powerful psychological component mediated by anxiety, depression, and prior histories of pain. Cognitive and emotional functioning have been seen to boost or inhibit pain perception, leading to a complex relationship between body and mind. Patients also often report that stress and negative emotions can exacerbate their pain, while positive distractions can alleviate it. Identification of such psychological factors allows clinicians to tailor pain management interventions aimed at influencing both the sensory and affective components of pain, which in turn enhances treatment outcomes and patient satisfaction. A combination of psychological therapies, such as cognitive behavioral therapy (CBT) and mindfulness-based stress reduction (MBSR), has also been found to be quite effective in managing pain. These therapies aim to shift the attitudes of patients towards pain, utilizing mechanisms that improve relaxation, enhance coping strategies, and promote a positive attitude.

There is evidence to suggest that CBT decreases the intensity of pain and improves quality of life through its influence on maladaptive cognitions and pain-related behavior. Mindfulness training also helps to create an awareness of the present moment by allowing the patient to de-attune from unhelpful rumination about pain. By integrating psychological factors into pain treatment regimens, healthcare providers are better able to provide patients with an integrative picture of pain relief, ultimately allowing patients to take an active role in their recovery. Furthermore, the intersection between psychological factors and pain is supported by emerging neuroscientific discoveries that illustrate the way the brain structures pain.

EEG-based experiments show significant differences in brain activity when subjected to painful stimulation, which correlate highly with psychological states. N2-P2 complex waveforms found in EEG traces are representative of neural correlates of pain experience that are conditioned by affective and cognitive contexts, suggesting that psychological distress can augment pain responses in the CNS. As discussed in recent research, integration of neurophysiological measures such as EEG and facial EMG into pain therapy can introduce a multi-dimensional approach to treating such psychological factors. The multidimensionality acknowledges the complex nature of pain, facilitating treatment programs that treat both psychological and physiological factors (Kim, 2025; Ma et al., 2025) (Figure 10.4).

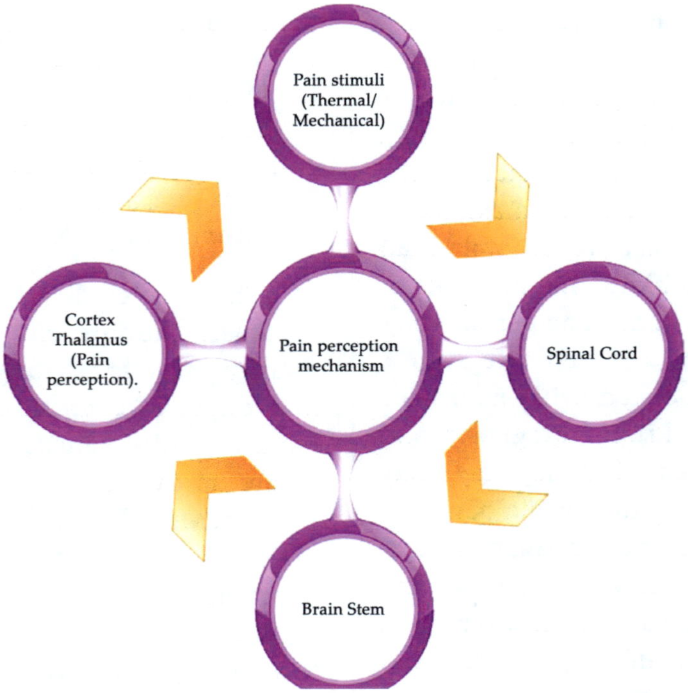

Figure 10.4. Diagram showing pain perception mechanism.

Source: https://www.researchgate.net/profile/Armando-Zarrelli-2/publication/233847740/figure/fig1/AS:601696036220935@1520466922456/Fig-1-Diagram-showing-Pain-perception-mechanism.png.

Test Your Knowledge

1. What are the main differences between acute and chronic pain?
2. Which key neurotransmitters are involved in pain perception?

10.2. Assessment of Pain

Learning Outcome

1. Discuss patient history and symptom evaluation;
2. Explain the use of pain scales and assessment tools;
3. Understand the importance of a multidisciplinary approach in the assessment of pain.

Pain assessment is a key component of effective pain management in primary care. Pain assessment involves multimodal assessment with various instruments and techniques to measure the patient's subjective experience as well as the pain mechanisms. Pain intensity, quality, and duration are identified by the clinicians through subjective as well as objective measures, such as pain rating scales, physical examination, and patient history. This combined model enables the health care providers to differentiate between acute and chronic pain, a necessity to tailor appropriate interventions. A detailed insight into the cause of the pain and its impact on the day-to-day life of the patient can often influence the treatment plan significantly, bringing it in line with the overall pain management goals outlined in the general medicine paradigm. Secondly, specific pain mechanisms must be identified to develop targeted treatment interventions. For instance, the assessment process might involve biomechanical evaluations to determine muscular tightness or dysfunction that generates pain in patients presenting with musculoskeletal complaints. A good example of this is the activities of the pectoralis minor muscle (PMm), which, upon contraction, can alter scapular alignment and motion and result in pain and restricted range of motion in the shoulder region. Through direct measurement of the tightness of PMm, clinical practitioners can implement accurate methods of rehabilitation for pain relief through stretching the muscle and enhancing arm elevation mechanics. Such specific attention, highlighted in recent studies, emphasizes the importance of individualized assessment and intervention strategies in addressing impairments with movement and associated pain, thereby allowing for an integrated understanding of the condition and needs of the patients (Morais & Cruz, 2016). In addition to physical findings, psychological factors also affect a patient's pain experience. Pain is not solely a bodily symptom; it is often influenced by emotional and cognitive factors such as anxiety, depression, and patient expectation. Pain measurement also should include assessment of these psychosocial factors, as they can enhance or decrease the pain experience. This multidisciplinary approach recognizes that ideal pain management involves collaboration among physical and mental health care providers. Understanding the connection between emotion and pain helps deepen the assessment process and inform holistic treatment strategies that consider the patient's overall well-being. Incorporating psychological testing and physical examination, clinicians can move towards a more empathic and effective pain model with positive overall patient outcomes in general medicine (Schlotz & Powell, 2014).

10.2.1. Patient History and Symptom Evaluation

An effective pain management plan in general medicine is dependent on careful patient history and symptom evaluation. The process of obtaining appropriate and accurate medical history allows physicians to differentiate the multifaceted character of pain, particularly in chronic non-cancer pain conditions. The assessment process should include evaluation of the physical status of the patient, psychosocial factors, and a history of response to treatment. As became clear from research, chronic pain is most frequently linked with psychiatric comorbidities like depression, which can complicate the treatment (Chelminski et al., 2005). Knowing the background of the patient enables health professionals to adjust therapeutic techniques to more effectively treat physical and psychological components of pain, thereby creating more positive outcomes for patients and greater satisfaction with the treatment process. Symptom evaluation is also critical in directing clinical decisions on treating pain. The employment of standardized measuring tools enables clinicians to quantify pain severity, functional impairment, and mood disturbance in a systematic approach. For instance, the brief pain inventory (BPI), Center for Epidemiological Studies-Depression Scale (CESD), and pain disability index (PDI) have been identified as useful measures in quantifying the progress in patients over time (Chelminski et al., 2005). Regular follow-up and symptom monitoring over time help clinicians identify potential problems such as drug abuse, reducing the efficacy of the treatment and PS. Additionally, these tests enhance patient-care provider communication, enabling therapeutic trust and empathy-based relationships—the key ingredients in chronic pain management. Finally, new methods, such as telephone triage, can augment patient history and symptom evaluation in primary care. These activities involve sophisticated communication and clinical competence to properly record critical patient data in interaction with decision-support technology. Nurses and medical professionals must negotiate the subtleties of patient communication against the formal structure of the technology used. Empathetic appreciation of a patient's pain and symptoms is paramount, as it measures the success of triage processes and successful pain management in general. Balancing people's care with technology needs is key to enhancing the patient experience, leading to enhanced pain management programs tailored to individualized needs (Figure 10.5).

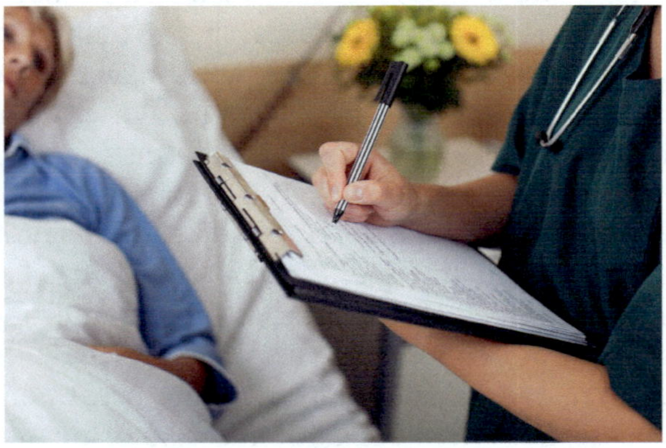

Figure 10.5. Obtaining the case history of a patient.

Source: https://www.vascularwellness.com/wp-content/uploads/2021/05/shutterstock_141478693-scaled.jpg.

10.2.2. Use of Pain Scales and Assessment Tools

Application of pain scales and assessment tools is a critical component of pain management in a clinical setting. They are designed to quantify the subjective experience of pain to bridge the communication gap between patients and healthcare providers. Pain rating scales range from simple numeric scales, in which patients are rated on a zero-to-ten scale for pain, to more sophisticated multidimensional scales, which rate physical, emotional, and social aspects of pain. These types of scales are particularly valuable for populations such as the elderly, where adequate pain control can have a marked effect on quality of life. Nonetheless, the interindividual variation in pain perception requires a discriminating approach to the choice and use of tools so that healthcare providers adapt assessment to the unique needs of each patient. Furthermore, the problems built into proper assessment of pain point to the need to use validated tools, especially when working with vulnerable populations such as patients with cognitive impairment. Research shows high levels of under-detection of pain in these groups, which is most likely to be due to communication difficulties or behavioral changes that mask signs of pain. Special equipment for patients with dementia, for example, has been introduced to enable carers to detect the degree of pain through observation of behavior and measurement criteria. The systematic reviews employed to evaluate such tools, though they identify an abundance of choice, also indicate deficits in their clinician utility. Most tools are not entirely validated for application in diverse clinical environments (Lichtner et al., 2014). This means that ongoing efforts to validate these assessment tools must be made to improve the advancement of pain management plans. Finally, while pharmacological measures dominate pain management, the acknowledgment of the role of non-pharmacological approaches is growing, pioneered by emerging research recognizing a wide range of interventions that are effective. The inclusion of behavioral assessment models and complementary therapies in addition to standard medication offers a more holistic approach to pain management, particularly among aged patients residing in nursing homes. Studies have shown that non-pharmacologic interventions can produce considerable improvements in outcomes for patients, and therefore, health care practitioners need to be instructed regarding these modalities (Schofield

& Reid, 2006). This holistic approach not only enhances clinicians' capacity to deliver customized care but also justifies continuing education and guideline adaptation to support continued enhancements in pain assessment practice (Figure 10.6).

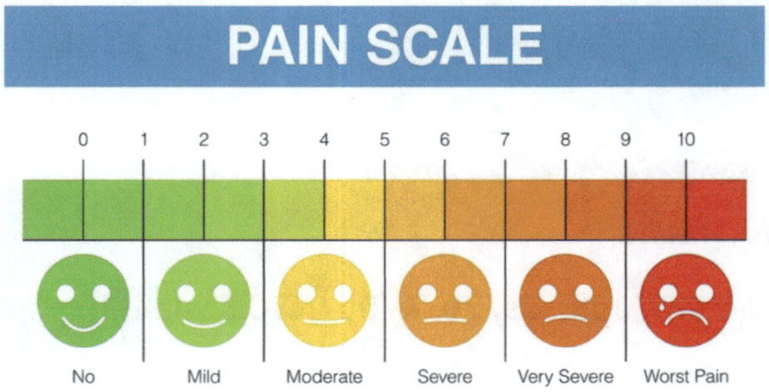

Figure 10.6. Pain scale.

Source: https://www.kauveryhospital.com/blog/wp-content/uploads/2020/09/ThinkstockPhotos-539684888-1280x640-1-1.jpg.

10.2.3. Importance of a Multidisciplinary Approach in Assessment

Multidisciplinary evaluation is critical to the understanding and treatment of pain in general medicine. It integrates diverse viewpoints of various medical practitioners—physicians, psychologists, and physical therapists—and as a result, is a more comprehensive way of assessing patient needs. Pain is a complex phenomenon that is not only rooted in physiology but also possesses psychological and social underpinnings.

When physicians of different specialties collaborate, they are best placed to assess the holistic aspects of a patient's pain so that no critical component is overlooked. This holistic process is used to guide individual treatment plans that take into account not just the expression of pain but also the cause, with the patient as a whole being at the center of the management process. Such comprehensive assessments can lead to improved intervention and improved results for pain individuals. Multidisciplinary assessments are not only significant for overall pain disorders but also for specific health disorders, such as women's sexual pain disorders, where integrating biological, psychological, and sociocultural factors comes particularly useful. Numerous studies have established that comprehensive assessments, such as full medical and psychosocial histories, are essential for accurate diagnosis and treatment of these disorders.

The group of experts who convened at the 3rd International Consultation on Sexual Medicine underscored the significance of multidisciplinary approaches in examining complex issues like these, which are not possible to understand completely through a singular lens (Laramee, 2011). Then, the involvement of specialists from various fields enables clinicians to create more evidence-based treatment plans that cover all dimensions of a patient's distress, once again validating the usefulness of interdisciplinary practice in medicine. Lastly, the application of patient-centered care as a pillar of integrated pain management services is fated to fall short in practice. Although policy guidelines call for patient feedback to be included in assessment, practice in reality often excludes this important aspect. Evaluations focus on clinical signs of pain rather than the patient's experience per se, and therefore, there is a gap between policy and practice (Howarth & Haigh, 2007). By developing a multidisciplinary environment that takes into account patient experience and integrates these into the processes of treatment, healthcare professionals can render their pain management more effective. This not only guarantees a more satisfying patient result but also aligns clinical practice with the ultimate aim of generating care responsive to unique needs and improving the overall quality of healthcare delivery (Figure 10.7).

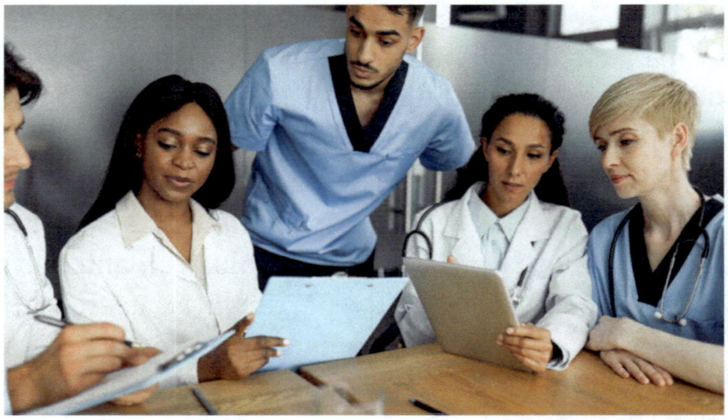

Figure 10.7. Multidisciplinary approach to pain assessment.

Source: https://integrativespineandsports.com/wp-content/uploads/2024/01/NYCISS-Jan-26.png.

Test Your Knowledge

1. What key elements should be included when taking a patient's pain history to accurately characterize the pain management?
2. How does involving a multidisciplinary team improve the accuracy and effectiveness of pain assessment and management?

10.3. Pharmacological Interventions

Learning Outcome

1. Understand non-opioid analgesics;
2. Describe opioid medications and their risks;
3. Discuss adjuvant therapies in pain management.

Pharmacological management is a major component of pain management in the context of general medicine. They constitute a group of medicines designed to alleviate pain and enhance the health of patients. Non-opioid analgesics such as NSAIDs and acetaminophen are commonly the first line of treatment for mild to moderate pain. Their ease of availability and efficiency make them a standard part of clinical practice. But the complexity of pain syndromes necessitates multidimensional analgesic therapy, frequently with adjunctive use of opioids for severe pain control. Increasingly, the medical literature has enlightened us as to the risks of opioid administration and how to achieve optimal pain control without risking abuse and addiction. In addition, the pain treatment setting is evolving, with an increased emphasis on non-pharmacologic interventions to augment pharmacologic interventions. Recent studies suggest that adding multidisciplinary treatment approaches—like CBT, exercise, and mindfulness—can enhance pain management success while reducing medication reliance. For instance, research evidence indicates that non-pharmacological interventions can be highly beneficial in pain management for vulnerable populations, e.g., newborns undergoing painful medical procedures, since such interventions can reverse the long-term impact of unrelieved pain on their behavior and physiological functioning (Hills et al., 2020). Therefore, it is imperative that physicians not only consider pharmacological measures but also efficiently integrate non-pharmacological therapies within pain management measures. While multimodal combinations can have various advantages, numerous barriers still hinder the efficient implementation of non-pharmacological pain management strategies. The application of opioids has been a norm in the treatment of long-term pain, but rising awareness of opioid use and subsequent mortality has led national organizations to urge a reduction in dependence on the substances (Swezey, 2018). The shift indicates the necessity for doctors to undergo education and training in effective pain management using alternative interventions. By establishing an environment that allows for the exploration and application of many pain relief methods, experts are better able to cure patient needs more holistically, which ultimately results in a more effective and ethical way of treating patients for medicine as a whole.

10.3.1. Non-Opioid Analgesics

In the setting of pain management, the non-opioid analgesics are an integral option compared to opioid medications, being effective pain relief agents while suppressing the potential for abuse as well as undesired side effects. Non-opioid analgesics like NSAIDs and acetaminophen are widely used in the management of mild to moderate pain that stems from ailments such as arthritis, muscle injury, and post-surgery pain. The benefit of these medications is that they inhibit the production of prostaglandins—substances which enhance the inflammatory response and sensitize pain receptors—in such a way that pain perception is lessened without the CNS effects typical of opioids. Moreover, as the global medical community grapples with the epidemic of opioid crisis, advocating for non-opioid analgesics is not merely a clinical necessity but a public health necessity that speaks to the need for ongoing research and clinician education about effective pain management strategies. While non-opioid analgesics are generally rated as first-line drugs, how effective these are will vary greatly with a patient's particular condition and with what type of pain. For instance, NSAIDs are particularly indicated for inflammatory process pain because they are anti-inflammatory. However, the potential for untoward effects such as gastrointestinal bleeding and renal impairment necessitates careful selection and management of patients. Acetaminophen, which is also safer but could endanger liver toxicity, especially in chronic users or drinkers, is a suitable alternative. Physicians need to work through a careful review of every patient's risk factors and medical history to maximize pain management strategies that responsibly include non-opioid analgesics while reducing harm, ultimately developing a balanced strategy in the context of pain relief options overall in general medicine.

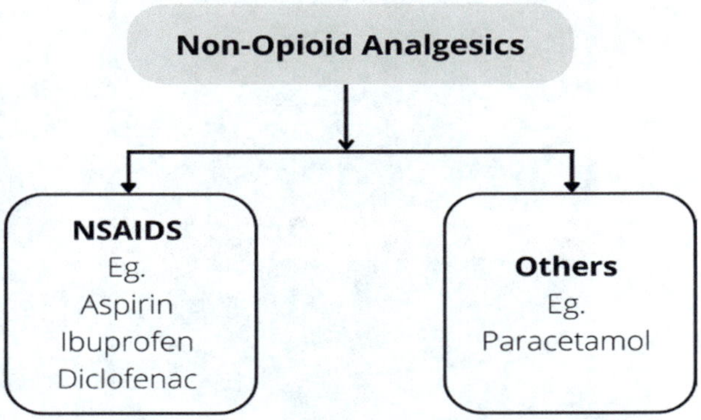

Figure 10.8. Non-opioid analgesics.

Source: https://s3-us-west-2.amazonaws.com/typeset-prod-media-server/f69a9424-9bd4-4927-b0fb-00e5b187a6d6image1.jpeg.

Though non-opioid analgesics have their benefits, difficulties persist in their use and the larger context of pain management. International variation in the availability of these medications may also result in insufficient relief from pain for patients in certain regions, particularly in low-resource environments, thus exacerbating the global healthcare crisis of unrelieved pain (Coluzzi et al., 2015). While non-opioid analgesics pose less risk for drug dependency compared to opioids, their misuse is not entirely nonexistent either. New evidence indicates potential risks related to analgesic long-term use, such as increased rates of fracture, particularly in long-term users (Coluzzi et al., 2015). As the medical profession continues to deal with the dilemma of pain management, accessibility, safety, and efficacy should be balanced while encouraging research into present available and novel non-opioid analgesic treatments (Figure 10.8).

10.3.2. Opioid Medications and Their Risks

The use of opioid medications has become a double-edged sword in the realm of pain management, helping millions of individuals while also culminating in significant risks simultaneously. Opioids were first celebrated for their strength as agents for the management of both acute and chronic pain, which made them freely prescribed in the heterogeneous medical setting. The spread of opioid misuse and overdose reflects the darker aspect of this drug intervention.

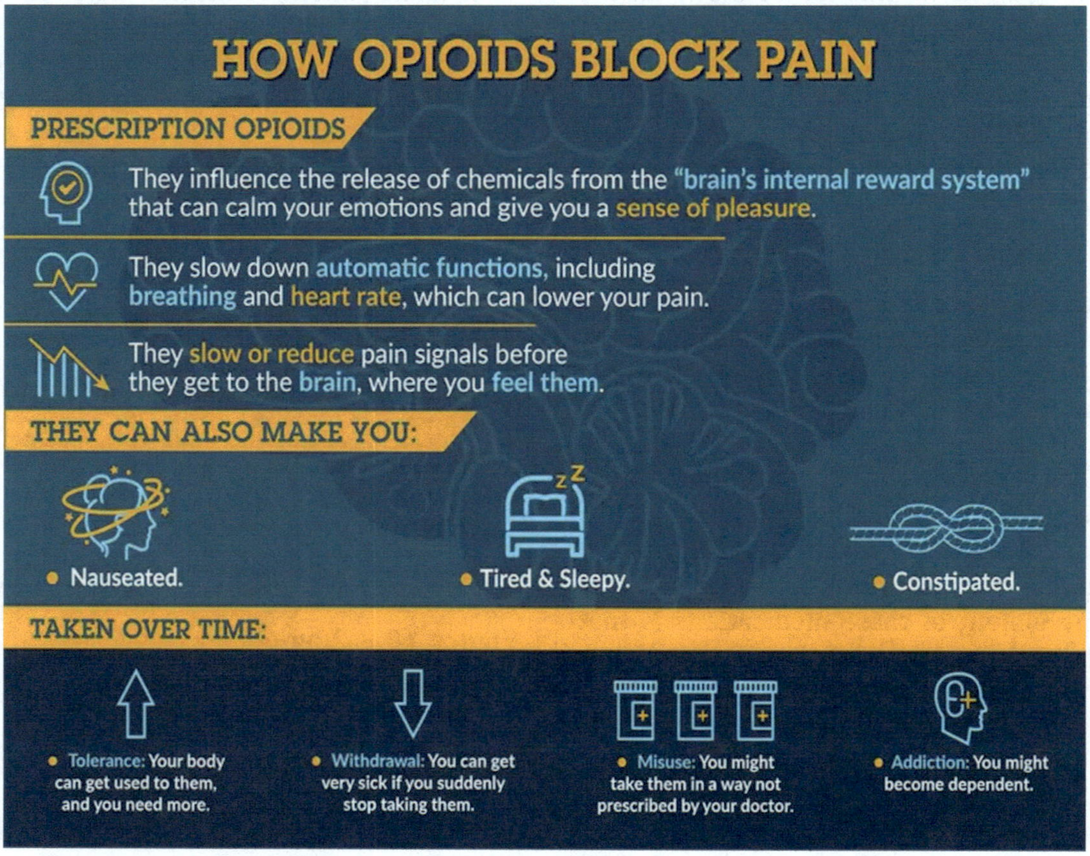

Figure 10.9. Representation of how opioids block pain.

Source: https://img.lb.wbmdstatic.com/vim/live/webmd/consumer_assets/site_images/article_thumbnails/reference_guide/opioid_narcotic_pain_medications_ref_guide/Opioids.png?resize=750px:*&output-quality=75.

According to recent reports, many patients have become addicted, resulting in a subsequent public health epidemic that demands a pressing reevaluation of prescribing practices and modes of pain relief. This contradictory consequence is a call for medical professionals to weigh the alleviation of suffering against the avoidance of the dangers involved with opioid medications to ultimately encourage a more prudent practice of pain management that prioritizes PS. In the context of the opioid crisis, societies at a national level have urged a change in paradigms of pain management. Emphasizing the importance of nonpharmacologic interventions, the national societies urge practitioners to embrace other methods that can reduce pain effectively but with the lower risks of opioid addiction and overdose that follow. Despite this trend, several barriers exist between such practices being implemented; examples are the entrenched practice of using medication to ease pain by both providers and patients. Additional barriers are to be found in unfamiliarity with nonpharmacologic methods, reimbursement issues, and limited access to multidisciplinary teams that can offer multifaceted solutions for pain management. Battling these challenges becomes imperative in enhancing patient outcomes and reducing opioid dependence, thereby promoting a comprehensive vision of pain management within primary care (Swezey, 2018). Further, expert viewpoints stress the importance of systemic interventions in significantly curbing the opioid epidemic. Medical education programs focus on equipping clinicians with the power to implement comprehensive strategies of pain management with minimal use of opioid prescriptions. Reports have emphasized the requirement to enforce rigorous prescribing protocols and intensify PDMPs to curb probable abuse. Furthermore, overdose education and naloxone distribution programs with integration offer individuals at risk access to lifesaving interventions. By encouraging a culture of collaboration between medical experts, policymakers, and members of the community, these programs aim not only to reduce opioid-related morbidity and mortality but also enhance greater awareness of pain management that identifies with the complexity of the patient's needs (Alexander et al., 2015) (Figure 10.9).

10.3.3. Adjuvant Therapies in Pain Management

Adjuvant therapies are invaluable for overall pain management, especially in chronic conditions when conventional analgesics fail. Therapies such as acupuncture, massage, and yoga not only complement pharmacotherapy but also empower patients to become active participants in their recovery. Such modalities have also become increasingly popular during the last decade, with healthcare professionals recognizing the multidimensionality of pain and its psychosocial factors. Research has shown that these unconventional therapies can significantly reduce perception of pain and associated symptoms such as depression and anxiety, enhancing patients' quality of life. The incorporation of these adjuvant therapies into an overall medicine system provides an integrated approach, utilizing both the physical and the psychological components of pain management. Complementary therapy also involves psychological therapy such as CBT, which can help patients alter their own perceptions of pain. CBT can teach patients coping techniques and overcome distorted patterns of thinking, allowing for better control of pain. A cranial electrical stimulation (CES) trial was conducted to assess its effect on various symptoms, including pain, in women undergoing chemotherapy for breast cancer. The trial, though unable to identify any statistically significant difference between the CES and sham treatments, acknowledged the importance of testing multiple modalities for addressing the extensive spectrum of symptoms of chronic pain management. This underscores the necessity for ongoing research into a range of adjuvant therapies since patients have complex clinical profiles presenting individualized management protocols (Lyon et al., 2015). Implementation of this array of adjuvant therapies within pain management regimens needs an interdisciplinary approach, combining expertise from disparate fields such as complementary medicine, psychology, and standard pharmacotherapy. The long-term aim is to create personalized pain treatment regimens that not only alleviate pain but also enhance patients' psychological and emotional well-being. A coordinated model comprising physicians, psychologists, and unconventional practitioners can maximize the effectiveness of treatment protocols. While studies like the CES study identify evidence gaps for certain approaches, it also points to the need for new, innovative research on promising therapies (Boehm, 2006). As pain care evolves, the integration of adjuvant therapies represents a significant development toward comprehensive, patient-centered treatment.

Test Your Knowledge

1. What are the primary classes of non-opioid analgesics used in pain management?
2. In what clinical scenarios are non-opioid analgesics preferred over opioids?
3. What role do adjuvant medications play in managing pain, particularly neuropathic or chronic pain?

10.4. Non-Pharmacological Interventions

Learning Outcome

1. Explain the role of physical therapy and rehabilitation in pain management;
2. Describe psychological therapies: CBT and mindfulness;
3. Deal with complementary and alternative medicine (CAM) approaches in pain management.

In the field of pain management, non-pharmacological interventions have emerged as core strategies that augment the traditional pharmacological interventions. These interventions encompass a wide spectrum of techniques, including physical treatments, cognitive-behavioral strategies, and complementary treatments, to treat not only the physiological but also the psychological aspects of pain. The efficacy of these interventions is particularly pertinent in populations who may be prone to medication side effects, such as newborns and the elderly. For instance, Hills et al. note the importance of such non-invasive interventions in pain relief in newborns and emphasize the impact of suboptimal pain control on having significant implications on an infant's behavior and physiological development. By combining such strategies, healthcare professionals can enhance overall pain control, with improved patient outcomes and quality of life. The integration of non-pharmacological interventions in pain control is also in line with the growing trend of individualized patient care. Recent research has shown that the majority of healthcare providers still insist on using pharmacological interventions, which can lead to poor pain control in select populations. A systematic review noted that although many studies have centered on non-pharmacologic interventions, the traditional assumption among healthcare professionals is that such interventions are adjunct or second-best to medication. However, the evidence presented in the literature identifies a variety of effective strategies, including CBT and education-based programs, which can have a significant impact on the management of chronic pain among care home residents. These results underpin an argument to expand education among healthcare providers to include a broader spectrum of treatment modalities in practice, enabling more pervasive pain management through a more holistic approach. In addition to better patient outcomes on an individual level, the use of non-pharmacologic therapy also has the promise to enable a more proactive healthcare system. These interventions not only reduce reliance on drugs, which have adverse effects or lead to dependency, but also enable patients to become active stakeholders in managing pain. By implementing interventions such as mindfulness, relaxation techniques, and exercise, patients are able to acquire coping skills that promote resilience and autonomy in managing pain. Moreover, as the Burdett Trust for Nursing highlights, there is a need for more research on the non-pharmacological methods in overcoming myths and obstacles prevalent in healthcare settings. The shift towards an interdisciplinary approach to pain management, addressing both pharmacological and non-pharmacological aspects, is a paradigm shift aligned with current evidence-based practices in overall medicine.

10.4.1. Physical Therapy and Rehabilitation

In rehabilitation and physical therapy, pain management is a key part of an interdisciplinary treatment regimen. These interventions are designed to minimize pain, enhance function, and optimize quality of life for patients with a variety of musculoskeletal disorders. By integrating manual therapies, therapeutic exercises, and modalities such as heat or cold, physical therapists attempt to treat causative mechanisms and promote healing. This approach not only allows for physical recovery but also addresses the psychological aspects of pain that can reduce anxiety and improve mood. The multifactorial nature of pain necessitates individualized rehabilitation protocols that meet the requirements of each patient, underscoring the importance of patient-based care in maximizing outcomes. Physical therapy is also optimized through its efficacy by interdisciplinary collaboration, which is pivotal in developing global rehabilitation plans. Bringing together concepts of multidisciplinary healthcare professionals like doctors, occupational therapists, and even psychologists encourages a deeper understanding of the multidimensional nature of pain. Making sure that rehabilitative efforts are not only effective in curing physical injuries but are also healthy for patients' emotional and social well-being is the advantage of multidisciplinary approaches. For example, the inclusion of mental health practitioners in a rehabilitation team can help overcome the psychological hurdles to body recovery, thereby enhancing therapy compliance. Furthermore, this interdisciplinary approach is consistent with contemporary medical trends that focus on the need to treat patients as holistic entities and not isolated physical cases. As research continues to progress, new innovative techniques and methods of physical rehabilitation and therapy continue to be created, greatly improving paradigms of pain management. Evidence has shown that tactics such as art therapy intervention can prove useful additional support in the rehabilitation process, particularly for hurt athletes. Empirical evidence indicates that art therapy can potentially provide a more holistic healing process by attending to athletes physical, affective, and relational needs to optimize not just recovery but pain management outcomes as well. Additionally, the application of technology, such as virtual reality and biofeedback equipment, holds promise in enabling enhanced patient engagement and outcomes. These advances show the shift toward more efficient and tailored rehabilitation methods, further detailing the significance of combining different healing modalities in general medicine practice for pain treatment (Hodea et al., 2024; Semelng, 2024) (Figure 10.10).

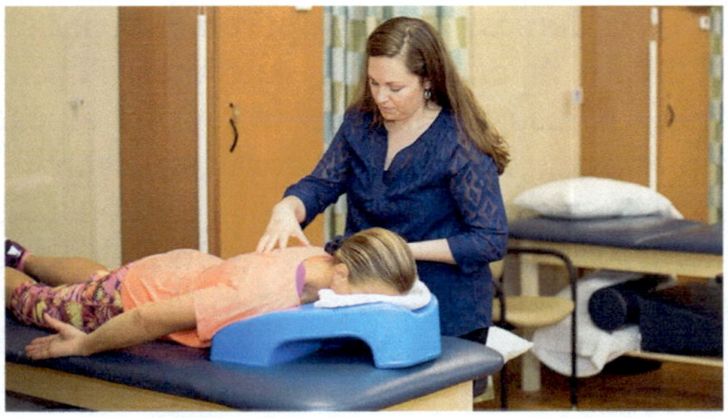

Figure 10.10. Physical therapist managing pain.

Source: https://www.choosept.com/globalassets/choosept/assets/spotlight-images/physical-therapy-treatment-table_750x419.jpg.

10.4.2. Psychological Therapies: CBT and Mindfulness

Psychological interventions, particularly CBT and mindfulness, have emerged as significant components of the management of chronic pain in the general medical environment. Interventions target the psychological underpinning of pain, which can have the effect of magnifying the physical pain experience. CBT targets learning to become familiar with and modify distorted pain cognitions and pain behaviors so that individuals regain control over their experience and response to pain stimuli. Practice aims at developing skills, endowing patients with coping strategies that reduce distress regarding pain. In accordance with studies, the combination of CBT and physical rehabilitation has been shown to lead to improved results since patients can cope with pain challenges more effectively as well as maintain involvement in treatment programs (Malfliet, A., Ickmans, K., Huysmans, E., Coppieters, I., Willaert, W., Bogaert, W. V., Rheel, E., Bilterys, T., Wilgen, P. V., & Nijs, J. (2019). Best Evidence Rehabilitation for Chronic Pain Part 3: Low Back Pain. *Journal of clinical medicine*, *8*(7), 1063. https://doi.org/10.3390/jcm8071063 et al., 2019). Mindfulness offers a different approach by developing a non-judgmental acceptance of the moment in spite of pain experience. This treatment method asks individuals to stand back from their feelings and thoughts in a place of aversion or nonattachment, cultivating an experience of acceptance. MBSR classes have been shown to decrease reported pain and increase overall well-being in the chronically painful. It relies on the principle that altering the individuals' relationship to pain can result in a decrease in perceived suffering. Psychological flexibility, a central component in the therapy of mindfulness, can lead to better emotional regulation and less anxiety and, in the end, offer a means of more effective coping with chronic pain syndromes (Whitinget al., 2018). A synergistic effect is created by combining the CBT and mindfulness interventions by enhancing each treatment's positive effect.

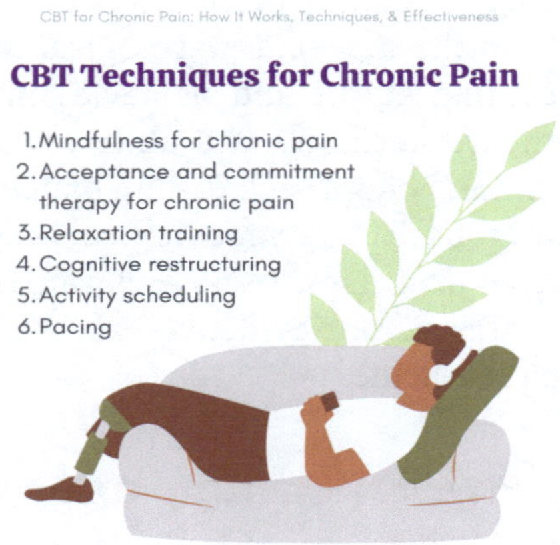

Figure 10.11. CBT techniques for chronic pain.

Source: https://www.choosingtherapy.com/wp-content/uploads/2022/05/3-8.png.

They implement the application of these therapies together to address both cognitive and affective components of pain and thereby offer an integrative means of controlling pain. These patients receiving this dual treatment protocol usually report more empowerment and resilience in coping with chronic pain conditions. Further, the long-term outcomes shown from these treatments suggest that they possess a phenomenon different from immediate relief, promoting improved long-term coping capacity and well-being. Thus, healthcare practitioners increasingly recognize the importance of incorporating such psychological treatments within holistic pain management regimens, thus suggesting a paradigm shift towards the overall treatment process for chronic pain (Whiting et al., 2018; Malfliet et al., 2019) (Figure 10.11).

10.4.3. Complementary and Alternative Medicine (CAM) Approaches

The incorporation of complementary and alternative medicine (CAM) protocols in the pain management paradigm has assumed significance as patients seek alternative care through holistic therapies rather than conventional therapies. This is in line with the growing acknowledgement of the multifaceted nature of pain, particularly chronic pain syndromes such as neuropathic pain. The patients get displeased with the conventional medicines due to their minor benefits and unwanted side effects, so they opt for CAM modalities. Closs et al. (2007) point out that patients often resort to other self-management strategies, including CAM, which responds to the individualized tastes of managing pain. This self-governed investigation demonstrates the importance of obtaining an understanding of and incorporating patients' preferences and values in their pain management treatment, like the incorporation of CAM as an adjuvant to traditional medical treatments. CAM is a broad group of therapeutic interventions, including acupuncture, herbal supplements, and cognitive-behavioral interventions. Among them, acupuncture is one of the most studied methods in the management of pain syndromes and has been the subject of systematic reviews because it is effective. Linde et al. (2001) present the point that although acupuncture is widely applied, clinical trials have produced inconclusive evidence, with a vast majority of them having methodological defects. However, acupuncture supporters argue about its perceived advantage in specific situations such as postoperative nausea and pain management. The differing findings underscore the necessity of stringent clinical trials to establish the efficacy of acupuncture in pain management conclusively. Hence, the integration of evidence-based CAM methods calls for a stringent analysis of available data to offer patients effective and safe treatments. Despite the superficial benefits of CAM approaches, additional studies are required to examine their effectiveness and the psychological, social, and emotional care that needs to accompany these therapies. Closs et al. (2007) capture the struggles of individuals with chronic pain, who do not necessarily have well-integrated care systems operating on their behalf that meet their multifaceted needs. While CAM interventions are the route that the majority of patients take, there is a glaring absence of organized psychological and social support that can actually help to augment their overall coping abilities. As such, future research needs to not only validate the efficacy of some CAM interventions, such as acupuncture and traditional herbs, but also examine the overall support situation for individuals to efficiently cope with their pain. A comprehensive plan for pain management, with evidence-based treatments and supportive systems as indicated, is a major innovation in maximizing quality of life in patients with chronic pain disorders.

Test Your Knowledge

1. How do physical therapy and rehabilitation techniques contribute to pain relief and functional improvement in patients with chronic pain?
2. In what ways does cognitive behavioral therapy help patients manage pain?
3. How can mindfulness-based stress reduction and relaxation techniques influence the perception of pain?

10.5. Role of General Practitioners (GPs)

Learning Outcome

1. Understand initial diagnosis in pain management for effective treatment planning;
2. Focus on coordination with specialists for effective pain management;
3. Deal with ongoing patient education and support in the effective management of pain.

The contribution of the general practitioners (GPs) to pain management is multifaceted and key because they are the initial professionals to encounter individuals in pain. The GPs possess a unique skill of conducting comprehensive assessments and creating patient-specific treatment plans that are required for effective pain management. Their holistic approach addresses not only the biological aspects of pain but also its social and psychological aspects. As demonstrated in studies, GPs prefer trusting patient explanations of pain and treatment histories, further emphasizing that a good grasp of each patient's experience is most important in decision-making processes for managing pain (Rankin et al., 2019). This baseline role provides room for the reality that patients are best directed through various treatments, their comprehension, as well as adherence to prescribed therapies. Consequently, GPs have a central role in optimizing patients' quality of life through pain control in a holistic manner. GPs also have a central function in making multidisciplinary care available for patients with chronic pain disorders. Effective pain control often requires the coordinated effort of specialists, therapists, and support services to handle the multifactorial interplay underlying a patient's perception of pain. Involvement of GPs in such an interprofessional environment enhances communication between health professionals as well as continuity of care, critical to the achievement of optimal results in pain relief. Evidence shows that patients value rapid access to their GP along with open and compassionate communication, particularly when dealing with complex pain syndromes (Johnson, et al., 2018). Through the facilitation of ACP and patient-centered discussions, GPs are capable of ensuring that treatment interventions remain focused on the evolving needs of their patients and thereby contribute to more effective pain management. Lastly, the role of education by GPs plays a fundamental role in shaping patients' perceptions and the overall strategy for pain management within the healthcare system. GPs not only prescribe treatment options but also serve as educators, educating patients on their conditions and the rationale behind different methods of pain control.

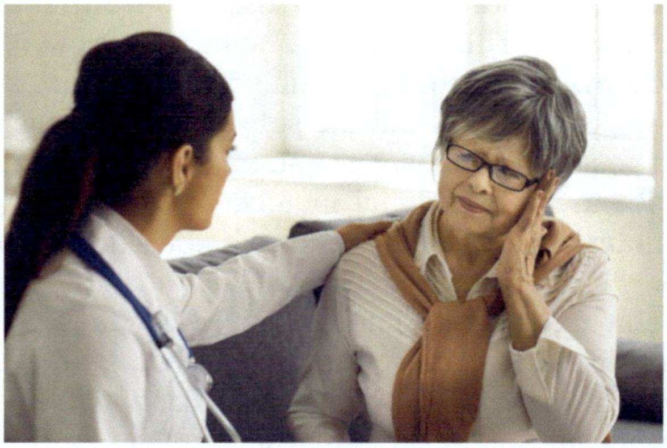

Figure 10.12. A general practitioner handling a patient to manage pain.

Source: https://westviewmedical.com.au/wp-content/uploads/2018/05/Untitled-design.png.

The implementation of improved curricula in medical education and continuing professional development will enhance the skills of GPs in pain management, particularly with the evolving health climate and emerging pain control options (Rankin et al., 2019). Through the delivery of knowledge and instruments to GPs to enable effective pain management, the healthcare profession will be able to ensure appropriate, informed care is provided to patients. By this continuous enhancement of competency in general practice, there is, in effect, the promotion of the reduction in the pain population burden, paving the way for improved health and patient satisfaction (Figure 10.12).

10.5.1. Initial Diagnosis and Treatment Planning

The initial diagnosis in pain management is a pivotal step that dictates the course of treatment planning. It is a comprehensive evaluation that incorporates a clear-cut medical history, physical examination, and, often, diagnostic tests. This multidimensional approach allows clinicians to identify the underlying etiology of pain, acute or chronic, and comorbidities. Appropriate diagnosis not only leads to the choice of curative treatment, but it also assists in setting realistic targets for the patient. For example, awareness of the psychosocial consequences of a specific condition, e.g., the stigma associated with STIs as reported by Duncan et al. (2001), can be significant in terms of how patients perceive and experience their pain and therapy. Thus, effective communication and patient education become critical components of this phase, as they lower anxiety levels and promote involvement in the management process. Treatment planning following an initial diagnosis is directed towards a patient-focused approach, striking a balance between clinical evidence and the patient's individual needs. Creating an integrated pain management plan involves not merely pharmaceutical interventions but also non-pharmacological treatments, depending on the individual clinical presentation and lifestyle of the patient. Clinicians have to consider the patient's preference, any probable obstacles to treatment, and the advantages and risks of the various treatment options. In the elderly, this is particularly essential as they are underrepresented in palliative care consultations despite their complicated medical conditions, as observed in The Stern Center for Evidence-Based Policy, 2015. The patients have to be empowered through shared decision-making, particularly in conditions such as chronic pain, where there are inter-individual differences in pain perception and response to therapy. This enables patients to be empowered. An individualized treatment plan can thus ensure better adherence and general patient satisfaction. Continual monitoring of the pain intensity and reappraisal of treatment efficacy are also an important part of the initial diagnosis and planning phase of treatment. The cyclical process allows time-efficient modifications to be incorporated in the treatment regimen, with patient feedback and clinical observation informing modifications. The routine follow-ups not only help in the recognition of any emergent complications or treatment side effects but also provide the opportunity for maintenance of the therapeutic relationship between patient and clinician. These sessions can be used by clinicians to educate patients on the natural history of their conditions and unlearn misconceptions or dread regarding diagnosis and prognosis, according to Duncan et al. (2001). Besides, this type of interaction is necessary in order to control expectations and make patients comfortable during the treatment process. Utilizing this proactive approach in controlling pain eventually results in enhanced health outcomes as well as enhancing patients' quality of life.

10.5.2. Coordination with Specialists

Effective pain management at times is a collaborative effort with experts whose insights may be a determining factor in the success of treatment. GPs, while skilled in handling every kind of health-related issue, at times are confronted with complex pain syndromes that require the expertise and knowledge of a specialist like a neurologist, rheumatologist, or pain management specialist. Not only does this broaden the options for treatment, but it also gives a clearer picture of what the patient is suffering from. For instance, specialists can provide information on advanced diagnostic techniques or novel therapeutic strategies to a GP who is not aware of them. Second, integrating the specialist's advice into a patient's pain management plan also aids in ensuring a multi-dimensional strategy for managing various needs of a patient's health. Coordination with specialists is thus pivotal in developing an efficient and integrated pain management plan. The effective coordination of specialist and GP care also rests on good communication, an absolute pillar in any collaborative healthcare model. Interdisciplinary meetings regularly and shared Electronic Health Records can make the process more efficient to ensure that everyone is informed and on the same page regarding the patient's goals of treatment. Such initiatives were documented by Mach et al. (2019), emphasizing not just coordination of care with specialists, but with community-based services as well as family members. Through open communication channels, healthcare professionals are able to be updated on the response of the patients to the treatments provided, as well as any emerging needs that might arise. This constant dialogue among specialists and generalists not only improves patient outcomes but also engages the patient by enrolling them in their own care and keeping them educated. Additionally, the structural model of pain management can be educated from models that have been developed in other aspects of medical care, including the palliative care model detailed by Bradford (2011). This plan prioritizes the imperative necessity of collaboration in maximizing the quality of life for patients coping with complex pain disorders. Through adherence to evidence-based practices from programs like the End-of-Life Care Strategy, general medicine can maximize its strategy for pain management through systematic coordination with experts. For instance, employing indicators of effective pain relief, such as patient comfort in the home environment, can provide valuable information on treatment efficacy. From learning from other specialties and liaising more effectively with experts, GPs are able to make their management strategies for pain more patient-centered and efficient with better final health results (Figure 10.13).

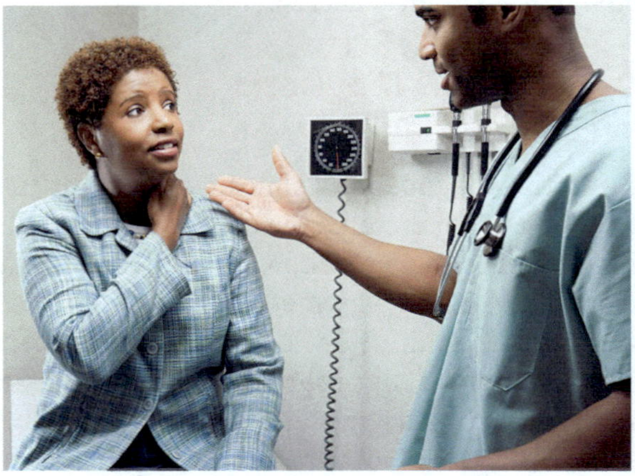

Figure 10.13. A patient coordinating with a pain management specialist.

Source: https://midsouthpain.com/wp-content/uploads/2020/08/shutterstock_381286129_2041e4f60afd374dcc1a6c2000e03d62_2000.jpg.

10.5.3. Ongoing Patient Education and Support

Ongoing education of patients and support are essential to effective pain management in general medicine. Through gaining insight into their conditions, their treatment and self-management plans, patients can become involved as responsible partners in their own care. This allows not only increased compliance with prescribed therapies but also enhanced patient-clinician communication. Educating patients about the nuances of pain treatment, both pharmacologic and non-pharmacologic, equips them with the information to make decisions. Furthermore, optimal education that can accommodate varied patient literacy levels and learning modes holds the potential to significantly improve outcomes. Of greatest concern to this task is the provider's ability to involve the patient in a manner that respects the patient's worldview and calls him or her into his or her care, thereby adhering to the entirety of the whole-person model of pain management that underlies general medicine. In the context of care on an ongoing basis, activities like phone triage and computer decision-support system (CDSS) usage richly complement patient interaction. These instruments allow clinicians to navigate complex clinical discussions while recording precisely the patients' stated needs and conditions. Problems, however, are built into these interactions, particularly in communication issues and diverse patient presentations. Nurses need to balance the technology-based demands of CDSS with the need for patient-centered care, calling for prudent communication skills. The use of technology in educating patients and in support highlights the importance of continuous training and the availability of resources to healthcare professionals. The complexity of these exchanges highlights the importance of maintaining strong support systems that are capable of addressing individual patient cases while being sensitive to clinical protocols, effectively improving the quality of care in pain management settings (Murdoch et al., 2014). In addition, clinical guideline development, such as the adaptation of overseas cancer pain management guidelines to Australian practice, demonstrates the need for continuous patient education. These guidelines offer the avenue of performing effective screening and assessment in a way that ensures patients are given individualized advice based on their own needs. By promoting evidence-based pain management strategies—ranging from widespread screening to creative pharmacologic management—health clinicians can enable patient comprehension of their treatment pathway. Public accessibility of these guidelines through media like the Cancer Council Australia Wiki ensures that patients and clinicians have access to current advice and best practice. Such dynamic adaptability, underscored by persistent patient education initiatives, serves as a critical pillar for improving pain management outcomes and a patient-centered approach-oriented manner for general medicine (Lovell et al., 2015).

Test Your Knowledge

1. What key steps should GPs take during the initial assessment of a patient presenting with pain to develop an effective treatment plan?
2. How can GPs determine when to refer patients to pain specialists or multidisciplinary teams?

10.6. Challenges in Pain Management

Learning Outcome

1. Discuss the opioid crisis and its implications;
2. Focus on variability in patient responses to treatment;
3. Understand ethical considerations in pain management.

For the management of pain, medical professionals face many difficulties that necessarily influence the success of treatment. Foremost among them is the variation in patients' response to pain medication depending on genetic factors, comorbidities, or mental illnesses. These pose a challenge to creating one standardized approach to pain relief, meaning that treatment will have to be individualized to the patient and potentially take time and money. In addition, the stigma of chronic pain is bound to create misunderstanding among patients and providers that results in inadequate pain control and poor quality of life. This divergence calls for adopting an integrative approach in developing ways to enhance patient-provider communication and integrated care in pain management, thereby facilitating a smoother treatment environment. Yet another central challenge is the reality of racial and ethnic disparities in pain practice. The evidence suggests that minority patients face various barriers when they receive maximum healthcare services, such as language difficulties and cultural misinterpretation (Alexander et al., 2015). These disparities not only undermine the quality of care delivered to such patients but also amplify their pain experiences. Moreover, the underrepresentation of other populations in clinical trials limits the generalizability of pain management outcomes, thus making the existing protocols ineffective in such populations.

In order to address such disparities, the health systems have to, as a collective effort, implement culturally competent practices and policies that ensure equitable access to pain management services, ensuring that all patients receive quality and adequate care depending on their unique needs. Besides disparities, the process of patients with different backgrounds also poses unique challenges in pain management. These types of patients are likely to experience difficulties in adapting to healthcare systems, thus limiting their access to important services (Betancourt et al., 2009). Moreover, the providers may also find it difficult to engage such patients in pain management conversations due to differences in language and beliefs. Trust-building is paramount, and this could require that healthcare providers understand the patients' migration history and its effect on patient safety and comfort. By realizing the pivotal role that family members play in making the care process easy, it becomes essential that patient-friendly settings be promoted to encourage effective communication and respect for individual values. Such interventions work towards enhancing the effectiveness of pain management interventions and, ipso facto, optimizing patient outcomes and satisfaction.

10.6.1. Opioid Crisis and Its Implications

The opioid epidemic is a serious public health issue that requires a systematic review of pain management strategies in general medicine. The steep climb in opioid prescribing in the past two decades has contributed to widespread addiction and abuse, burdening not just individuals but also their families and communities. These issues have brought into focus the central place of stigma concerning opioid use and addiction, which Alexander Tsai and associates define as the social forces propelling the crisis. The stigma is apt to dissuade individuals from seeking help, which makes it even harder for there to be good intervention in managing pain as well as preventing addiction. The intersection of the need for pain control and the opioid crisis necessitates a shifting of medical paradigms to allow for services to serve contemporary needs, in a way that both the patients' pain and the likelihood of abuse of opioids are adequately addressed. An enhancement of postoperative pain management practice is one of the most significant things to address in managing the problem of the opioid crisis. These need to be investigated as a risk factor for long-term opioid use following surgery, as emphasized in the literature. Preoperative opioid use, anxiety, and a history of substance abuse are major risk factors that immensely enhance the likelihood of long-term opioid dependence. The intervention window to prevent persistent use is narrow, which makes interdisciplinary collaborative care between surgical and anesthesiology services a crucial issue. By incorporating multimodal analgesia protocols and regional anesthesia techniques, doctors can effectively reduce the use of opioids, thereby decreasing exposure and abuse risk. The innovative approach allows recovery to be maximized while complications for opioid dependence are reduced, thereby negating a severe problem in the big picture of the opioid epidemic. Other implications of the opioid epidemic have to do with policies governing prescription practices and patient training in pain management. General medicine also urgently needs to update its own protocols to favor safer alternatives over opioids. Improved recovery pathways are helpful paradigms for maximizing patient benefits without eliminating the advantages of opioid treatment. Moreover, education matters; patients must be educated on the dangers of the use of opioids as well as the alternatives of non-opioid pain management options. The inclusion of educational programs in the patient care continuum can assist in the process of making informed decisions and, therefore, reduce the stigma of seeking help for pain management issues. With the use of such strategies, there is an opportunity to redirect the pain management arena in general medicine towards a more cautious approach to opioid prescribing and consumption, as well as dampen the current crisis (Lovell et al., 2015) (Figure 10.14).

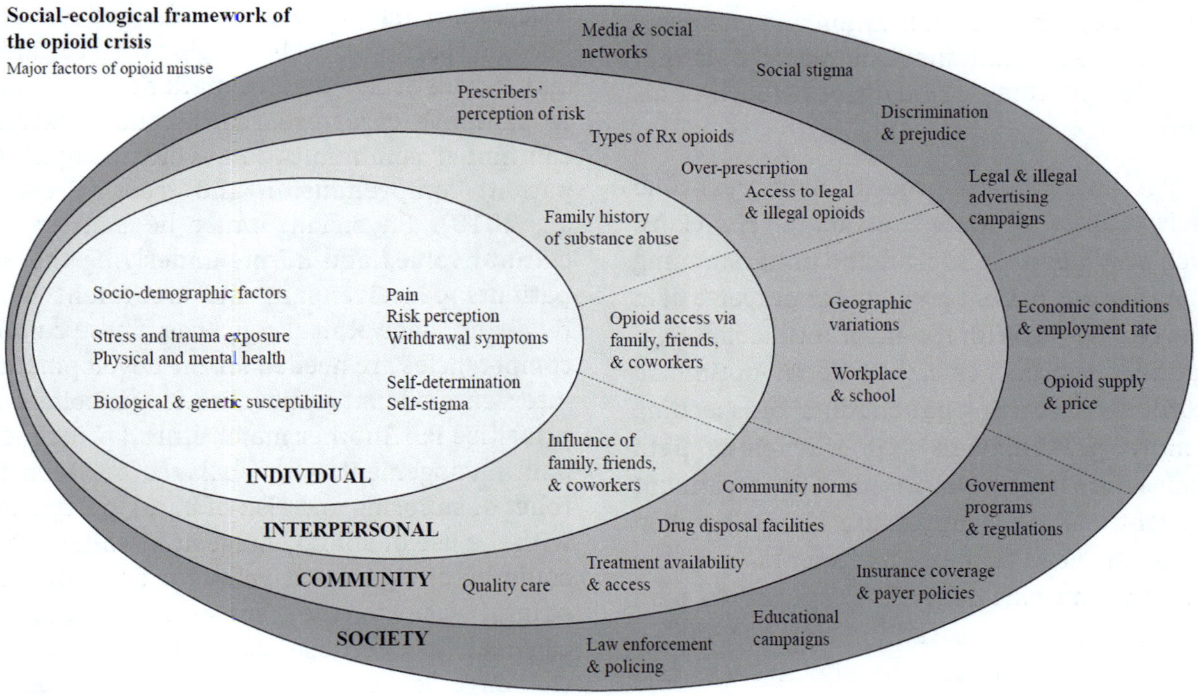

Figure 10.14. The social-ecological framework of the opioid crisis: socio-demographic status consists of age, race, gender, ethnicity, education, income, and unemployment factors.

Source: https://www.researchgate.net/profile/Mohammad-S-Jalali/publication/333031985/figure/fig1/AS:757591697281026@1557635344906/Social-ecological-framework-of-the-opioid-crisis-Socio-demographic-status-consists-of.ppm.

10.6.2. Variability in Patient Responses to Treatment

A significant challenge with the general medicine approach to pain treatment is natural variation between patients in the response to treatment. This can be attributed to a variety of factors, including genetic status, mood status, and comorbid disease. To illustrate, patients can have variations in drug metabolism secondary to genetic polymorphisms, which can lead to different therapeutic effects from an identical drug dose. Psychological conditions of depression and anxiety can enhance the experience of pain, creating complexity in the effectiveness of treatment. Understanding these complexities is important for medical professionals to make interventions that treat individual patient characteristics, ultimately maximizing patient satisfaction and treatment success. Technology has also begun to address the complexities of pain management by providing and monitoring improved data. For example, a wireless pain-drawing solution conserves patient time since they can note the spatial location and character of the pain but simultaneously record data that will reflect its time-varying aspect (Serif et al., 2005).

The innovative approach allows real-time observation of treatment results for clinicians, which provides a more profound understanding of how various patient populations perceive pain in the real world. With the aid of such technology, treatment approaches can be better optimized according to changing patient data, thus leading to more personalized and efficacious pain management regimens. In addition, treatment interventions like acupressure have also shed light on the need for more treatment modalities in controlling variability in response to pain management. In one randomized controlled trial, researchers tested the effectiveness and feasibility of acupressure in children undergoing cancer therapy and showed the ways in which diverse therapeutic approaches can be tailored to accommodate diverse symptom profiles (Lown et al., 2019). Such research points to the benefits of integrating comprehensive approaches to therapeutic intervention, acknowledging that there is only one approach that might adequately address the multifactorial process of pain. With ongoing developments in medicine, being able to identify variability in patient response and accepting alternative, patient-specific treatment approaches will be essential to achieving the best outcomes in controlling pain.

10.6.3. Ethical Considerations in Pain Management

In pain management, ethical issues must always take the driver's seat as the physician performs the fine ballet between pain relief and medical protocols. Patient autonomy is a fundamental principle in these cases, where the patient must be fully knowledgeable about what procedures he or she can have, including the potential risks involved. This process of informed consent becomes particularly challenging with culturally and linguistically diverse patients. According to palliative care research, language barriers can hinder communication, which complicates patient comprehension and trust (Green et al., 2018). Physicians must be sensitive to cultural values and norms underlying the way patients perceive pain and treatment while resolving these ethical concerns. These cultural competencies are needed for the development of interventions that respect individual beliefs but prioritize PS. Another major ethical principle in pain management is the balance between the relief of suffering and risk of harm, particularly with the use of opioid analgesics. While opioids could be of significant value for clinically very painful patients, they are also addictive and can lead to overdose, constituting an ethical challenge to health workers. Ethics does not only require clinicians to consider how effective such interventions are, but also that they weigh the impact their prescribing has on broad public health problems. As demonstrated in GP training, there is a need for systematic education on the benefits and ethical implications of opioid use within palliative and chronic care environments. Current training courses, while aimed at the medical management of pain, also fall short in regard to readiness regarding the ethical component, hence the imperative of curriculum reforms dealing with these matters of prime importance (Abela & Mallia, 2010). The role of the family in pain management creates additional ethical issues, as their involvement has a significant bearing on the plan of care and the experience of the patients as a whole. In most cultures, families are considered a part of the patient's care and need to be included in discussions about pain management and end-of-life care by providers. It becomes moral when patient autonomy clashes with family wishes because medical caregivers must maneuver such sensitive encounters skillfully. The research topics evoked in the study with palliative care clinicians emphasize the importance of understanding patients' and families' migration histories, facilitating trust and allowing for dialogue regarding pain management goals (Green et al., 2018). Ultimately, the holistic strategy that recognizes the complexities of family dynamics and culture profiles is the secret to ethical practice in pain management and most closely supports the goal of providing compassionate, patient-specific care for each patient.

Test Your Knowledge

1. How has the opioid epidemic influenced current pain management practices?
2. What factors contribute to the variability in patients' responses to pain treatments?
3. How do healthcare providers navigate ethical dilemmas related to undertreatment versus overtreatment of pain?

SUMMARY

In evaluating a general medicine approach to pain treatment, it is known that the use of various treatment modalities together will foster more positive patient outcomes for those who endure chronic pain. One example includes the combining of therapies such as high-intensity light amplification by stimulated emission of radiation (LASER) therapy (HILT) and exercise therapy. The evidence also shows that HILT not just reduces pain but also enhances the efficacy of therapeutic exercise, hence facilitating more rehabilitation activity. The review of comprehensive literature mirrors that low back pain patients greatly benefited by this integrated approach and emphasizes the recovery-maximizing capability of this approach as well as overall quality-of-life enhancement (Chauhan et al., 2024). Consequently, the findings of evidence from this analysis affirm the validity of multidisciplinary treatment protocols in controlling pain. Additionally, the topic of new and evolving analgesic techniques highlights the evolving character of postoperative pain management. Specifically, the application of regional analgesic techniques such as the modified perichondral approach to thoracoabdominal nerve block (M-TAPA) has been promising in resolving postoperative pain following laparoscopic cholecystectomy. A study documented significant decreases in opioid consumption and postoperative ratings of pain in subjects receiving M-TAPA, and regional approaches are a paradigm shift in perioperative pain management (Castillo-Dávila et al., 2024). The ability to suppress pain while decreasing opioid dependence not only meets the demand for immediate pain relief but contributes to the overall objective of curbing opioid-related issues in the healthcare system. In conclusion, the broader medicine strategy of pain management is the emphasis on individualized, evidence-based treatments that are adapted to meet the specific needs of individual patients. The combination of numerous therapeutic approaches, including HILT in conjunction with exercise therapy and innovation in regional analgesic techniques, equips healthcare practitioners to provide better and safer pain relief solutions. With an increasingly dynamic discipline with strong research supporting such multidimensional approaches, one would hope that clinicians would adopt such strategies for optimum patient results in pain management. The success of pain management, in the end, lies in following through on the development and evolution of these strategies on an ongoing basis as new evidence emerges, so that the call remains on continuous education and inter-professional communication.

Pain management in general medicine is a multifaceted problem, with a requirement to grasp both the psychosocial and the biological aspects of pain in an integrated context. Key to effective pain management is the recognition that low back pain, as characterized in The Lancet Low Back Pain Series, remains the most disabling condition globally, affecting individuals across all socioeconomic groups and producing individual and societal harms. The trend towards inappropriately treating patients—e.g., unwarranted imaging and opioids—undermines the success of pain management. Accordingly, evidence-based practice is crucial to avoid the repeated burden of pain among various populations, especially in low-resource environments where the dichotomy between evidence and clinical practice is glaringly obvious (Avorn, 2017). Systematic reviews and guidelines are essential in directing clinical practice towards evidence-based interventions for effective pain management. The PRISMA guidelines, for example, emphasize the requirement of open reporting of systematic reviews that can facilitate informed decision-making among healthcare professionals using the best available evidence. Such a framework not only enhances the validity of research evidence but also aids policy and clinical practice settings to encourage non-pharmacological management and multimodal pain management strategies. Overreliance on pharmacological treatments, particularly opioids, has been found to be counterproductive, and recent controversy over their benefits demonstrates an immediate need for more research on safer and effective alternatives (Buchbinder et al., 2020). Finally, the intricacies of pain management call for an integrated design that focuses on patient-centered care. Solutions need to involve education in the biology of pain and blend this with novel and context-specific interventions targeting physical, emotional, and psychological dimensions of pain. The team-based strategy entails the engagement of patients and medical professionals in collaborating to create an atmosphere where continuous enhancement of pain management is under review and calibration. With the changing global context of pain management, recognition of the ongoing issues—such as excessive use of low-value care—will be paramount in formulating approaches to optimize care provision and reduce the high human and economic costs associated with unmanaged or ineffectively managed pain (Avorn, 2017).

KEY TERMS FROM THIS CHAPTER

- Anti-inflammatory drugs
- Biomedical intervention
- Biopsychosocial model
- Biopsychosocial treatment approach
- Chronic pain
- Chronic pain management
- Chronic pain syndromes
- Cognitive behavioral therapy (CBT)
- Comprehensive assessments
- Coping strategies
- EEG-based experiments
- General practitioners (GPs)
- Integrated treatment program
- Mindfulness-based stress reduction (MBSR)
- N2-P2 complex waveforms
- Non-pharmacologic interventions
- Opioid medications
- Pain assessment
- Pain control
- Pain disability index (PDI)

CRITICAL THINKING QUESTIONS

1. **Which of the following is considered the most reliable method for assessing a patient's pain?**
   a. Blood pressure measurement
   b. Patient self-report using pain scales
   c. Physical examination alone
   d. MRI imaging
2. **Which of the following is an example of a non-pharmacological intervention in pain management?**
   a. NSAIDs
   b. Opioids
   c. Cognitive Behavioral Therapy (CBT)
   d. Antidepressants
3. **What is the primary role of General Practitioners (GPs) in pain management?**
   a. Provide initial assessment, diagnosis, and coordinate multidisciplinary care
   b. Perform surgical interventions for pain relief
   c. Prescribe only opioid medications
   d. Refer all pain patients directly to pain specialists
4. **Which of the following is a common challenge faced in effective pain management?**
   a. Accurate diagnosis of pain cause
   b. Patient reluctance to communicate pain
   c. Availability of both pharmacological and non-pharmacological treatments
   d. All of the above
5. **Which pharmacological class of drugs is most appropriate for initial management of mild to moderate acute pain?**
   a. Opioids
   b. NSAIDs (Non-Steroidal Anti-Inflammatory Drugs)
   c. Antidepressants
   d. Anticonvulsants

Short Answer Questions

1. What are the different types of pain, and why is it important to distinguish between them in clinical practice?
2. What are the key components of a thorough pain assessment, and how do they influence the development of an effective pain management plan?
3. What are the main classes of pharmacological treatments for pain, and how are they selected based on the type and severity of pain?
4. How do non-pharmacological treatments complement medication-based approaches, and what evidence supports their use in pain management?
5. How can general practitioners effectively manage pain in primary care, and when should they consider referral to specialists or multidisciplinary teams?
6. What strategies should GPs use to educate patients about pain management options, expectations, and potential risks?

Answers to Critical Thinking Questions

1. (b); 2. (c); 3. (a); 4. (d); 5. (b)

REFERENCES

1. Abela, J. C., & Mallia, P. (2010). An evaluation of palliative care education in the specialist training programmed in family medicine. https://core.ac.uk/download/46602275.pdf (accessed on 27th June 2025).
2. R. S. Laramee, "How to Read a Visualization Research Paper: Extracting the Essentials," in IEEE Computer Graphics and Applications, vol. 31, no. 3, pp. 78-82, May-June 2011, doi: 10.1109/MCG.2011.44. (accessed on 27th June 2025).
3. Lown, E. A., Banerjee, A., Vittinghoff, E., Dvorak, C. C., Hartogensis, W., Melton, A., Mangurian, C., Hu, H., Shear, D., Adcock, R., Morgan, M., Golden, C., & Hecht, F. M. (2019). Acupressure to Reduce Treatment-Related Symptoms for Children With Cancer and Recipients of Hematopoietic Stem Cell Transplant: Protocol for a Randomized Controlled Trial. *Global advances in health and medicine*, *8*, 2164956119870444. https://doi.org/10.1177/2164956119870444(access ed on 27th June 2025).
4. Alexander GC, Frattaroli S, Gielen AC, eds. The Prescription Opioid Epidemic: An Evidence-Based Approach. Johns Hopkins Bloomberg School of Public Health, Baltimore, Maryland: 2015(accessed on 27th June 2025).
5. Johnson, C. E., McVey, P., Rhee, J. J., Senior, H., Monterosso, L., Williams, B., Fallon-Ferguson, J., Grant, M., Nwachukwu, H., Aubin, M., Yates, P., & Mitchell, G. (2018). General practice palliative care: patient and carer expectations, advance care plans and place of death-a systematic review. *BMJ supportive & palliative care*, bmjspcare-2018-001549. Advance online publication. https://doi.org/10.1136/bmjspcare-2018-001549(accessed on 27th June 2025).
6. Avorn, J. (2017). Academic detailing: "Marketing" the best evidence to clinicians. *JAMA, 317*(4), 361–362. https://www.semanticscholar.org/paper/bc3ceb87e5a53aef265f692cab986a441fa3441d (accessed on 27th June 2025).
7. Urbański, W., Dolata, N., Balcer, B., Kruczkowska, A., Bulzacki, E., Cebula, A., ... Liszka, P. (2024). NSAIDs in Sports Medicine: Balancing Quick Relief with Long-Term Health Impacts. *Quality in Sport, 36*, 56892. https://doi.org/10.12775/QS.2024.36.56892(accessed on 27th June 2025).
8. Hills, E., Rosenberg, J., Banfield, N. (2020). A multidisciplinary approach to the implementation of non-pharmacological strategies to manage infant pain. Infant, 16(2), pp. 78-81.(accessed on 27th June 2025).
9. Murdoch, J., Barnes, R., Pooler, J., Lattimer, V., Fletcher, E., & Campbell, J. L. (2015). The impact of using computer decision-support software in primary care nurse-led telephone triage: interactional dilemmas and conversational consequences. *Social science & medicine (1982), 126*, 36–47. https://doi.org/10.1016/j.socscimed.2014.12.013(accessed on 27th June 2025).
10. Shipton, E. E., Bate, F., Garrick, R., Steketee, C., Shipton, E. A., & Visser, E. J. (2018). Systematic Review of Pain Medicine Content, Teaching, and Assessment in Medical School Curricula Internationally. *Pain and therapy*, *7*(2), 139–161. https://doi.org/10.1007/s40122-018-0103-z(accessed on 27th June 2025).
11. Lyon, D., Kelly, D., Walter, J., Bear, H., Thacker, L., & Elswick, R. K. (2015). Randomized sham controlled trial of cranial microcurrent stimulation for symptoms of depression, anxiety, pain, fatigue and sleep disturbances in women receiving chemotherapy for early-stage breast

cancer. *SpringerPlus, 4*, 369. https://doi.org/10.1186/s40064-015-1151-zf (accessed on 27th June 2025).

12. Lovell, M., Luckett, T., Boyle, F., Stubbs, J., Phillips, J., Davidson, P. M., Olver, I., von Dincklage, J., & Agar, M. (2015). Adaptation of international guidelines on assessment and management of cancer pain for the Australian context. *Asia-Pacific journal of clinical oncology, 11*(2), 170–177. https://doi.org/10.1111/ajco.12352 (accessed on 27th June 2025).
13. Closs, S. J., Staples, V., Reid, I., Bennett, M. I., & Briggs, M. (2007). Managing the symptoms of neuropathic pain: an exploration of patients' experiences. *Journal of pain and symptom management, 34*(4), 422–433. https://doi.org/10.1016/j.jpainsymman.2006.12.004(accessed on 27th June 2025).
14. Duncan, B., Hart, G., Scoular, A., & Bigrigg, A. (2001). Qualitative analysis of psychosocial impact of diagnosis of Chlamydia trachomatis: implications for screening. *BMJ (Clinical research ed.), 322*(7280), 195–199. https://doi.org/10.1136/bmj.322.7280.195(accessed on 27th June 2025).
15. Malfliet, A., Ickmans, K., Huysmans, E., Coppieters, I., Willaert, W., Bogaert, W. V., Rheel, E., Bilterys, T., Wilgen, P. V., & Nijs, J. (2019). Best Evidence Rehabilitation for Chronic Pain Part 3: Low Back Pain. *Journal of clinical medicine, 8*(7), 1063. https://doi.org/10.3390/jcm8071063 (accessed on 27th June 2025).
16. Boehm, K. (2006). Acquisition, distribution and perspectives of healthcare information in complementary and alternative medicines (CAM). https://core.ac.uk/download/29816899.pdf (accessed on 27th June 2025).
17. Buchbinder, R., Underwood, M., Hartvigsen, J., & Maher, C. G. (2020). The *Lancet* series call to action to reduce low value care for low back pain: An update. *Pain, 161*, S57–S64. https://doi.org/10.1097/j.pain.0000000000001869 (accessed on 27th June 2025).
18. Morton, L., Elliott, A., Cleland, J., Deary, V., & Burton, C. (2017). A taxonomy of explanations in a general practitioner clinic for patients with persistent "medically unexplained" physical symptoms. *Patient education and counseling, 100*(2), 224–230. https://doi.org/10.1016/j.pec.2016.08.015(accessed on 27th June 2025).
19. Burton, A. K., Kendall, N. A., Pearce, B. G., Birrell, L. N., & Bainbridge, L. C. (2009). Management of work-relevant upper limb disorders: a review. *Occupational medicine (Oxford, England), 59*(1), 44–52. https://doi.org/10.1093/occmed/kqn151(accessed on 27th June 2025).
20. Castillo-Dávila, L. F., Torres-Anaya, C. J., Vazquez-Apodaca, R., Borboa-Olivares, H., Espino-Y-Sosa, S., & Torres-Torres, J. (2024). Modified thoracoabdominal nerve block via perichondral approach: An alternative for perioperative pain management in laparoscopic cholecystectomy in a middle-income country. *BMC Anesthesiology, 24*. https://www.semanticscholar.org/paper/969136e06b24f5315173bc1a5788bac088734d8d (accessed on 27th June 2025).
21. Chauhan, D., Sharma, S., & Jangra, M. (2024). A literature review on maximizing pain management in low back pain: A combined approach of high-intensity LASER therapy and exercise therapy. *Journal of Clinical and Diagnostic Research.* https://www.semanticscholar.org/paper/c6a048988ee2bdd8ca8ed0b2305428f81d6495a8 (accessed on 27th June 2025).
22. Whiting, D. L., Deane, F. P., Simpson, G. K., Ciarrochi, J., & Mcleod, H. J. (2018). Acceptance and Commitment Therapy delivered in a dyad after a severe traumatic brain injury: A feasibility

study. Clinical Psychologist, 22(2), 230–240. https://doi.org/10.1111/cp.12118c(accessed on 27th June 2025).

23. Coluzzi, F., Fornasari, D., Pergolizzi, J., & Romualdi, P. (2017). From acute to chronic pain: tapentadol in the progressive stages of this disease entity. *European review for medical and pharmacological sciences, 21*(7), 1672–1683.(accessed on 27th June 2025).

24. Coluzzi F, Pergolizzi J, Raffa RB, Mattia C. The unsolved case of "bone-impairing analgesics": the endocrine effects of opioids on bone metabolism. *Ther Clin Risk Manag*. 2015;11:515-523. Published 2015 Mar 31. doi:10.2147/TCRM.S79409 (accessed on 27th June 2025).

25. Lichtner V, Dowding D, Esterhuizen P, et al. Pain assessment for people with dementia: a systematic review of systematic reviews of pain assessment tools. *BMC Geriatr*. 2014;14:138. Published 2014 Dec 17. doi:10.1186/1471-2318-14-138 (accessed on 27th June 2025).

26. Morais, N., & Cruz, J. (2016). The pectoralis minor muscle and shoulder movement-related impairments and pain: Rationale, assessment and management. *Physical therapy in sport : official journal of the Association of Chartered Physiotherapists in Sports Medicine, 17*, 1–13. https://doi.org/10.1016/j.ptsp.2015.10.003(accessed on 27th June 2025).

27. Rankin, L., Stålnacke, B. M., Fowler, C. J., & Gallego, G. (2018). Differences in Swedish and Australian medical student attitudes and beliefs about chronic pain, its management, and the way it is taught. *Scandinavian journal of pain, 18*(3), 533–544. https://doi.org/10.1515/sjpain-2018-0039(accessed on 27th June 2025).

28. Rankin, L., Fowler, C. J., Stålnacke, B. M., & Gallego, G. (2019). What influences chronic pain management? A best-worst scaling experiment with final year medical students and general practitioners. *British journal of pain, 13*(4), 214–225. https://doi.org/10.1177/2049463719832331(accessed on 27th June 2025).

29. Tacha Serif, Gheorghita Ghinea, and Andrew O. Frank. 2005. Visualizing pain data for wheelchair users: a ubiquitous approach. J. Mob. Multimed. 1, 2 (June 2005), 161–177. (accessed on 27th June 2025).

30. Betancourt, J. R., King, R. R., & Green, A. R. (2009). Improving quality and achieving equity: A guide for hospital leaders. The Disparities Solutions Center, Massachusetts General Hospital. https://core.ac.uk/download/71352207.pdf (accessed on 27th June 2025).

31. Green, A., Green, M., Jerzmanowska, N., Lobb, E., et al. (2018). 'Death is difficult in any language': A qualitative study of palliative care professionals' experiences when providing end-of-life care to patients from culturally and linguistically diverse backgrounds. https://core.ac.uk/download/213607752.pdf (accessed on 27th June 2025).

32. Louise Howarth, M., & Haigh, C. (2007). The myth of patient centrality in integrated care: the case of back pain services. *International journal of integrated care, 7*, e27. https://doi.org/10.5334/ijic.203(accessed on 27th June 2025).

33. Hodea, F., Hariga, C., Bordeanu-Diaconescu, E. M., Cretu, A., Dumitru, C. Ş., Ratoiu, V. A., Lascar, I., et al. (2024). Assessing donor site morbidity and impact on quality of life in free flap microsurgery: An overview. *Life, 15.* https://www.semanticscholar.org/paper/df845de07c783f5164b54fac741b74f1b0f3d551 (accessed on 27th June 2025).

34. Kim, H. (2025). Neuroscience-based approaches in chronic pain management: Integration of mind-body interventions in rehabilitation. *Exploration of Medicine.* https://www.

semanticscholar.org/paper/7dceaa55f8a9115d9731228ab63cb89d7cf1a66b (accessed on 27th June 2025).

35. Kirchhof, P., Benussi, S., Kotecha, D., Ahlsson, A., Atar, D., Casadei, B., Castellá, M., et al. (2016). 2016 ESC guidelines for the management of atrial fibrillation developed in collaboration with EACTS. *European Heart Journal, 37,* 2893–2962. https://doi.org/10.1093/eurheartj/ehw210 (accessed on 27th June 2025).

36. Linde, K., Vickers, A., Hondras, M., ter Riet, G., Thormählen, J., Berman, B., & Melchart, D. (2001). Systematic reviews of complementary therapies - an annotated bibliography. Part 1: acupuncture. *BMC complementary and alternative medicine, 1,* 3. https://doi.org/10.1186/1472-6882-1-3(accessed on 27th June 2025).

37. Ma, C., Wang, C., Zhu, D., Chen, M., Zhang, M., & He, J. (2025). The investigation of the relationship between individual pain perception, brain electrical activity, and facial expression based on combined EEG and facial EMG analysis. *Journal of Pain Research, 18,* 21–32. https://www.semanticscholar.org/paper/6653cabf503583b3f5378f1b5739d693776aa91c (accessed on 27th June 2025).

38. Mach, F., Baigent, C., Catapano, A. L., Koskinas, K. C., Casula, M., Badimón, L., Chapman, M. J., et al. (2019). 2019 ESC/EAS guidelines for the management of dyslipidemias: Lipid modification to reduce cardiovascular risk. *European Heart Journal, 41,* 111–188. https://doi.org/10.1093/eurheartj/ehz455 (accessed on 27th June 2025).

39. The Stern Center for Evidence-Based Policy (2015). Addressing the health needs of an aging America: New opportunities for evidence-based policy solutions. University of Pittsburgh. https://core.ac.uk/download/75783019.pdf

40. Page, M. J., Moher, D., Bossuyt, P. M., Boutron, I., Hoffmann, T., Mulrow, C. D., Shamseer, L., et al. (2021). PRISMA 2020 explanation and elaboration: Updated guidance and exemplars for reporting systematic reviews. *BMJ.* https://doi.org/10.1136/bmj.n160 (accessed on 27th June 2025).

41. Schlotz, W., & Powell, D. J. H. (2014). Ambulatory assessment in neuropsychology: Applications in multiple sclerosis research. Zeitschrift für Neuropsychologie, 25(4), 239–251. https://doi.org/10.1024/1016-264X/a000140

42. (accessed on 27th June 2025).

43. Schofield, P. & Reid, D. M. (2006). The assessment and management of pain in older people: A systematic review of the literature. https://core.ac.uk/download/177013.pdf (accessed on 27th June 2025).

44. Chelminski, P. R., Ives, T. J., Felix, K. M., Prakken, S. D., Miller, T. M., Perhac, J. S., Malone, R. M., Bryant, M. E., DeWalt, D. A., & Pignone, M. P. (2005). A primary care, multi-disciplinary disease management program for opioid-treated patients with chronic non-cancer pain and a high burden of psychiatric comorbidity. *BMC health services research, 5*(1), 3. https://doi.org/10.1186/1472-6963-5-3(accessed on 27th June 2025).

45. Semelng'o, P. (2024). Effectiveness of art therapy programs in enhancing recovery and rehabilitation in sports medicine. *International Journal of Arts, Recreation and Sports.* https://www.semanticscholar.org/paper/e3e1e4bc0b9e911b1e0e47d802af45ac2a44352d (accessed on 27th June 2025).

CLINICAL DOCUMENTATION AND MEDICAL RECORDS

11

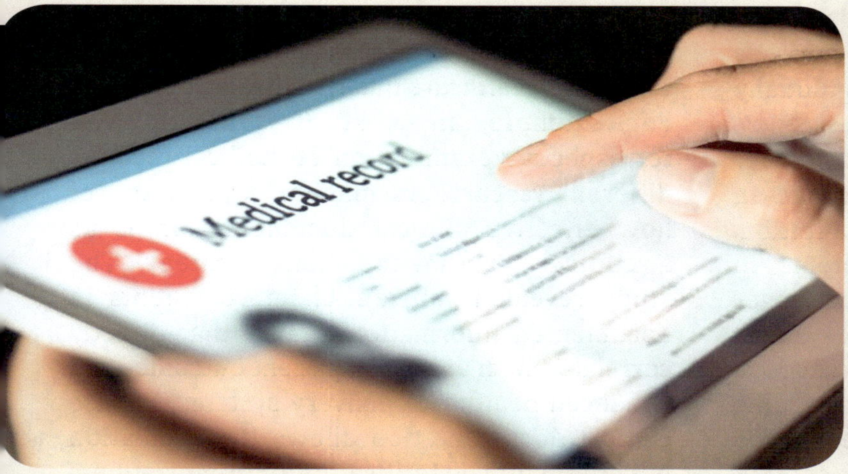

LEARNING OBJECTIVES

After studying this chapter, you will be able to:

1. Understand the historical context of clinical documentation and medical records;
2. Explain the types of medical records;
3. Describe legal and ethical considerations in the realm of clinical documentation;
4. Discuss best practices in clinical documentation;
5. Deal with challenges in clinical documentation;
6. Focus on future trends in medical records.

Introduction

Medical documentation and clinical records have evolved as a central component of healthcare delivery in this era. Care of patients is becoming increasingly complicated, and efficient systems that allow the coordination of communications among health professionals, control the workflow, and ensure quality patient outcomes are in demand in these days. Paper records to electronic medical records (EMRs) is a transition that represents a significant step forward in terms of technology that is part of greater initiatives towards digitization across the board. Initiatives in favor of this shift, such as those backed by medical practitioners, underscore the potential benefits of EMR implementation, including fewer medical errors and improved cost control in the healthcare setting (Lee et al., 2018). With further evolution of healthcare settings, understanding the fundamentals of clinical documentation is essential for practitioners who desire to meet the demands of contemporary healthcare settings. In addition to supporting coordination between medical professionals, effective clinical documentation contributes to greater PS and quality care. Clinical records are not just a legal document but a comprehensive repository of patient information, offering medical history, treatment, and outcomes. The process of documentation is part and parcel of accurate diagnoses and effective treatment plans, thus supporting better communication between patients and caregivers. For instance, education programs for health professionals on the proper utilization of EHRs have the goal of augmenting patient-centered communication, a quality aspect of optimal health delivery (Lee et al., 2018). As the clinical setting is gradually heading towards technology dependency, having the capability to document and transfer information correctly gains significance in achieving optimal health outcomes. In addition, the introduction of electronic systems in clinical documentation tests offers challenges to healthcare professionals. While EMR systems ensure effective processes and precision in data, some reports show mixed evidence regarding the actual impact on patient outcomes. Based on research, it is the sheer success of EMR implementations that can vary greatly with respect to the strategic goals set by healthcare administrators. Therefore, a reflective effort is necessary while implementing EMR systems; it is not enough to simply digitize the records (Lee et al., 2018). Attention must be given beyond simple implementation towards comprehensive training of the healthcare professionals in the use of such systems for effective functioning, so that the benefits of electronic records are reflected in actual improvements in the quality and safety of patient care.

Definition of Clinical Documentation

The clinical documentation principle forms the foundation of effective management of medical records within health institutions. Clinical documentation is essentially the uniform and accurate recording of patient information, treatment processes, and clinical encounters, all of which form a comprehensive report of a patient's journey through the healthcare system. This documentation is not only an administrative routine but a critical tool that directs clinical decision-making and maximizes communication among health care providers. Through extensive documentation of patient encounters, providers create a source of information that is essential to continuity of care, particularly in complex cases where numerous health care professionals are caring for the patient. Moreover, the role of clinical documentation extends not only to direct patient care but also to affecting broader aspects of healthcare quality and accountability. For example, in a study that involved retrospective examination of medical records, different researchers made a comparison of how effective clinical documentation is as a clinical risk management strategy. The study revealed substantial improvements in documented information quality that directly correlated with enhanced patient outcomes and enhanced healthcare delivery systems. Precise clinical documentation allows the evaluation of care quality, identification of organizational weaknesses, and is the foundation for evidence-based practice, ultimately improving the overall level of healthcare services to patients (Guzzo et al., 2017).

Continuity of care shows yet another critical element of clinical documentation because proper records offer a seamless experience to the patient when being transferred from one level of care to the next. In primary care, for instance, continuity of clinical records facilitates promotion of an integrated approach towards patient health. A study in the setting of a GP consultation environment established the degree of documentation provided to patients during consultations. The findings indicated that a large percentage of patients were not provided with medical records, and this raised questions about the potential suboptimal care caused by the disjointed documentation practices (Bugeja

& Abela, 2014). The definition of clinical documentation thus not only involves writing down information but also encompasses its role in informing integrated and uninterrupted patient care through consistent and accessible medical records (Figure 11.1).

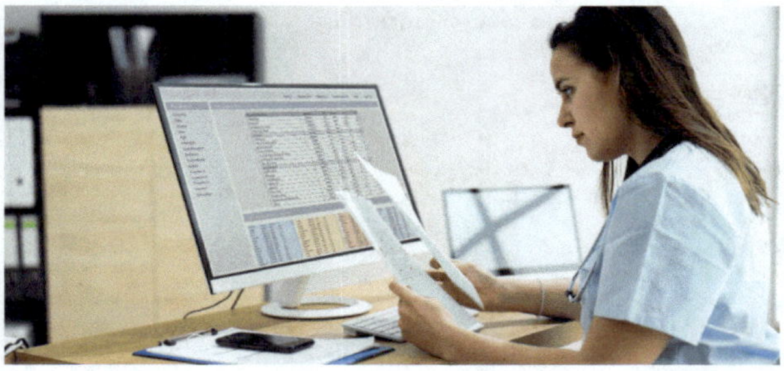

Figure 11.1. Specialist analyzing clinical documents.

Source: https://media.licdn.com/dms/image/sync/v2/D4E27AQEP8xqChx0EZQ/articleshare-shrink_800/articleshare-shrink_800/0/1746636180323?e=2147483647&v=beta&t=znNnOLSfG5j88mfFei54upKRvjWLkf_7qj2nqpoWrFc.

Importance of Medical Records in Healthcare

Medical records are the foundation of healthcare practice, holding a patient's entire medical history and allowing for good clinical decision-making. By meticulous documentation of critical information such as diagnoses, treatments, and patient response, healthcare providers are able to ensure continuity of care while averting errors. When computerized hospital information systems are effectively utilized, as evidenced by feedback from nurses' views, they enhance the clinical process and result in better patient outcomes. In this regard, the influence of medical records extends beyond the mere documentation to directly affect the quality of care delivered. Understanding how electronic systems determine nursing practice can shed light on the broader importance of medical documentation, highlighting its ability to establish a logical and efficient healthcare environment (Oroviogoicoechea & Watson, 2009). In addition to facilitating communication among healthcare professionals, medical records are critical in quality assurance and risk management. Detailed records allow for monitoring of trends in patient care, which can be utilized to create policies that will enhance standards of healthcare delivery. Furthermore, accurate documentation is important during legal cases, as evidence against accusations of malpractice. In the event of something going amiss, particularly in high-risk environments like ICUs, the accuracy and detail of medical records help establish adherence to professional standards." For instance, research identifies suboptimal end-of-life care, often well-documented in one way or another or not documented at all, which brings about discomfort and dissatisfaction in patients. Therefore, maintaining complete medical records is not just a legal responsibility but also an ethical requirement that promotes high-quality patient care (Ghabeljoo, 2017).

The value of medical records extends to the realm of public health and epidemiologic research. They provide a rich data source required to identify population health trends and can be utilized to guide the formulation of targeted health interventions. Researchers can identify common health issues, assess the effectiveness of treatment, and identify areas to intervene using aggregate medical record data. The ability to track health outcomes across various populations also assists in addressing disparities in healthcare delivery. While healthcare development is speeding up, its application for the use of public and individual health focuses on its core role in healthcare system development towards a more efficient system. Finally, the significance of precise, accessible, and comprehensive medical records is straightforward, being part of healthcare systems (Ghabeljoo, 2017) (Figure 11.2).

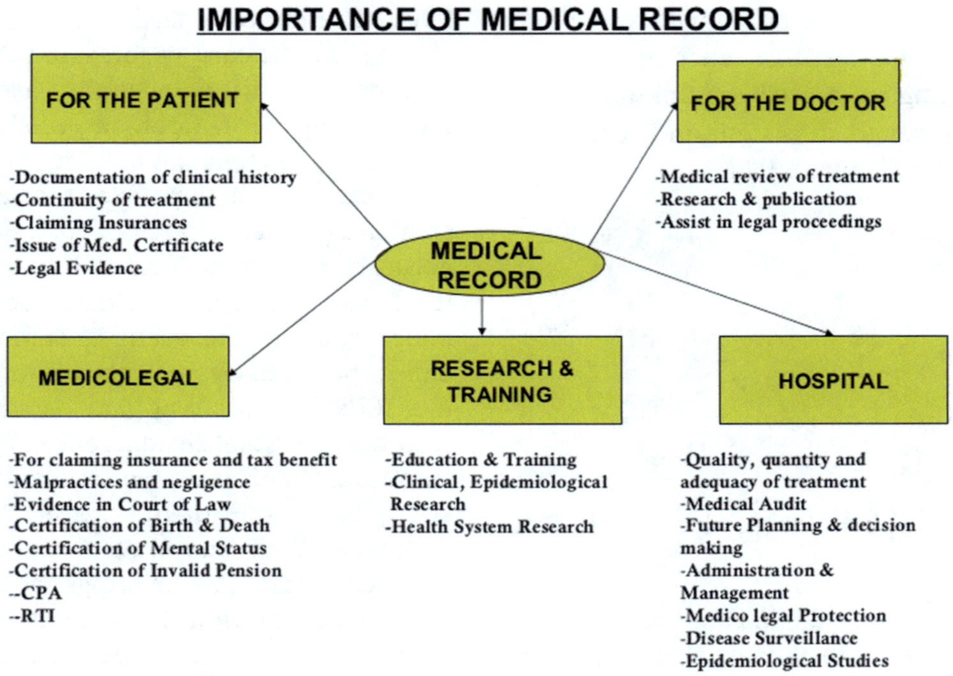

Figure 11.2. Importance of medical records.

Source: https://media.licdn.com/dms/image/v2/C5622AQEsWC4NPq34Vg/feedshare-shrink_800/feedshare-shrink_800/0/1662988838245?e=2147483647&v=beta&t=mAWtBBDmfPTMRlwXWKJ0U6Et0nlHucvWtARnwWK8KC8.

11.1. Historical Context

Learning Outcome

1. Understand the evolution of medical record-keeping;
2. Discuss key milestones in clinical documentation;
3. Explain the impact of technology on medical records.

Clinical documentation and medical records have a historical context that is deeply rooted in the evolution of health practice and technological advancements. Historically, medical records were maintained in paper form, which had issues with data availability, accuracy, and speed. As medical knowledge expanded, it was understood that there existed a necessity for standardized documentation practices. This transition was precipitated by the use of EHRs, which altered patient data procurement, storage, and retrieval. As is evidenced by contemporary research, this shift towards digitization significantly enhances the arrangement and sharing of health information, enabling more efficient clinical processes. The ongoing innovation and use of self-tracking technology and mobile health programs speak to the importance of understanding health information, toward a course of preventive medicine driven by knowledge gained through patient records and their effect on public health (Ledesma et al., 2016). Furthermore, the drive for standardized documentation is a pivotal move in clinical practice towards optimizing care delivery in multi-dimensional healthcare settings. The integration of standardized dental diagnostic terminology into EHRs is exemplary of this trend and reflects a larger movement toward diagnosis-centered care. Within a medium-sized dental group practice, the implementation of standardized documentation practices was facilitated more effectively by applying change management models, which established the need for new training and revised policies in sustaining consistent application. Results from this activity indicated that there was a significant increase in compliance, at 97% reported usage for the EHR and Dental Diagnostic Code.

The case illustrates how the transition to organized documentation within the clinical environment not only ensures improved patient care but also instills a culture of accountability and precision, which is pivotal in contemporary healthcare practices (Kalenderian et al., 2016). Clinical documentation transformation reflects broader transformations within healthcare philosophies such that emphasis on quality and patient-centered practices necessitates meticulous and reliable records. Historical perspective indicates that record-keeping within the healthcare industry has never been an ancillary factor in maintaining patient health and facilitating communications between the health care providers. As technology improves, the devices and frameworks employed for capturing clinical details have also evolved, with additional capabilities for data visualization and comprehension. Such devices allow health care providers to monitor health trends effectively, as they also enhance active health care management practices among the patients. The future demands of data privacy, security, and interoperability remain relevant but emphasize the continued relevance of previous development to inform current practice in medical records and clinical documentation (Ledesma et al., 2016).

11.1.1. Evolution of Medical Record-Keeping

The evolution of medical record-keeping has seen very progressive phases, from simple hand-written entries to sophisticated EHRs. Historically, medical record-keeping was very much a man-driven process, with paper records that not only slowed down access but also posed greater possibilities of misinterpretation and loss of important information.

The shift from these paper records into electronic systems was not just a technological advance but also a paradigm shift in practice and policy. Utilization of electronic records has resulted in improved communication among healthcare providers, enhancing patient care coordination and effectiveness. Besides, the technological changeover is preceded by an increasing demand for quality healthcare, which demands systems that support effective data handling as well as allow providers to meet regulatory needs efficiently. As the health care environment was transforming, so was the function and functionality of medical record systems. An open-source EHR system breakthrough came about, where medical facilities could customize their documentation procedures according to stated needs. These systems, such as OpenEMR and VistA, have been subjected to performance tests against functional standards, and studies have established that OpenEMR met all 32 standards available, making it an exceedingly effective system (Purkayastha et al., 2019). The transition to open-source solutions is only part of a greater movement towards simplifying the user experience and making it more interoperable across multiple healthcare systems. These developments not only demonstrate further evolution of medical record-keeping but also identify a need for ongoing review and refinement of health information technology (HIT) in response to changing needs in clinical documentation. The importance of quality in clinical documentation has been more widely adopted as a basis for effective healthcare provision. Current incentive programs aimed at improving the quality of documentation show a sensitivity to this necessity, as they aim to improve the overall care quality (Johnson, 2011). These programs generally incentivize caregivers to implement best practice record-keeping and evidence-based best practices, therefore inducing higher accuracy in patient files. Therefore, medical record-keeping evolution is not only technological but also integrative, embracing quality improvement processes that support patient-focused approaches. Accordingly, medical documentation continues to be dynamic in nature, responding to complex interdependencies between technological innovations, regulatory settings, and the needs of quality care, ultimately enhancing the clinical setting for healthcare providers and patients alike (Figure 11.3).

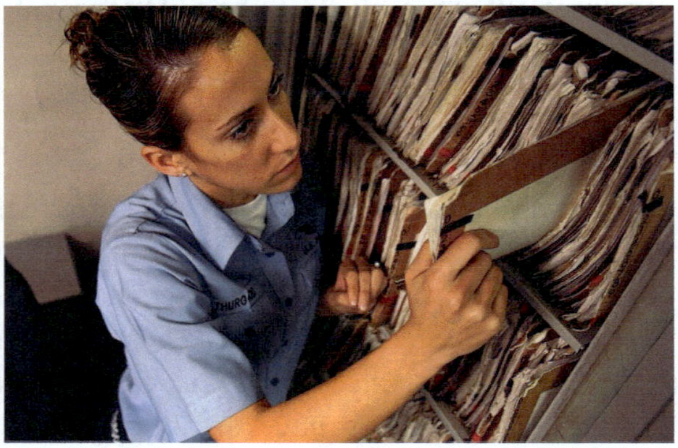

Figure 11.3. A medical record folder being pulled from the records.

Source: https://upload.wikimedia.org/wikipedia/commons/thumb/9/90/US_Navy_041019-N-5821P-019_Airman_Lauren_Thurgood_of_Las_Vegas%2C_Nev.%2C_pulls_patient_medical_records_in_the_inpatient_ward_aboard_the_conventionally_powered_aircraft_carrier_USS_Kitty_Hawk.jpg/1024px-thumbnail.jpg.

11.1.2. Key Milestones in Clinical Documentation

The history of clinical documentation has been characterized by some important milestones that radically altered the way that patient information is documented, stored, and retrieved. One of the most important milestones was the development of EHRs in the late 20th century. This technology revolutionized the process of documentation by enabling real-time data entry and retrieval, which improved accuracy and accessibility. The email integration of EHRs facilitated better communication among medical professionals, creating more coordinated and less expensive care. As noted, patients enrolled in an intensive care management program for public assistance recipients struggling with substance abuse were slightly more likely to receive treatment, demonstrating the benefit of comprehensive documentation in optimizing treatment outcomes (Martinez et al., 2009). These clinical documentation advances not only optimized record-keeping but also paved the way for further advances in health informatics and quality improvement initiatives. Standardization of medical records through established guidelines and best practices is yet another milestone in the history of clinical documentation. The application of standards, such as those given by the Health Insurance Portability and Accountability Act (HIPAA), facilitates uniformity and normalization of clinical documentation in healthcare facilities. The legislation has served to underpin patient confidentiality and ensure health records are comprehensive and easy to understand. Besides, initiatives like the Engaging Stakeholders in Identifying Priority Evidence-Practice Gaps and Strategies for Improvement in primary health care (ESP) Project further emphasized the necessity of applying quality improvement data to enhance healthcare. The stakeholders for this process were also able to review CQI data for 132 health centers and subsequently identify barriers and enablers of closing top-priority evidence-practice gaps (Dossetor et al., 2023). This collaborative work reflects the necessity of possessing robust clinical documentation systems to facilitate ongoing quality improvement. Another landmark in clinical documentation was the recognition of the importance of patient-centered documentation practices, with the focus of incorporating patient feedback into health records. This paradigm shift has inspired healthcare workers to engage patients more actively in their care activities, which has led to better communication and enhanced outcomes in health. By documenting patients' experiences, preferences, and concerns, clinicians can more effectively make interventions person-centered and individualized. Additionally, this collaborative approach is also in harmony with the overall aims of PCC, facilitating a therapeutic relationship between patients and providers. As the healthcare setting continues to evolve, the appreciation that fine clinical documentation relies not only on technical accuracy but also on successful patient participation is a significant improvement in how medical records are conceived. Ongoing evolution of these significant milestones drives clinical documentation quality and success alongside the provision of healthcare overall (Figure 11.4).

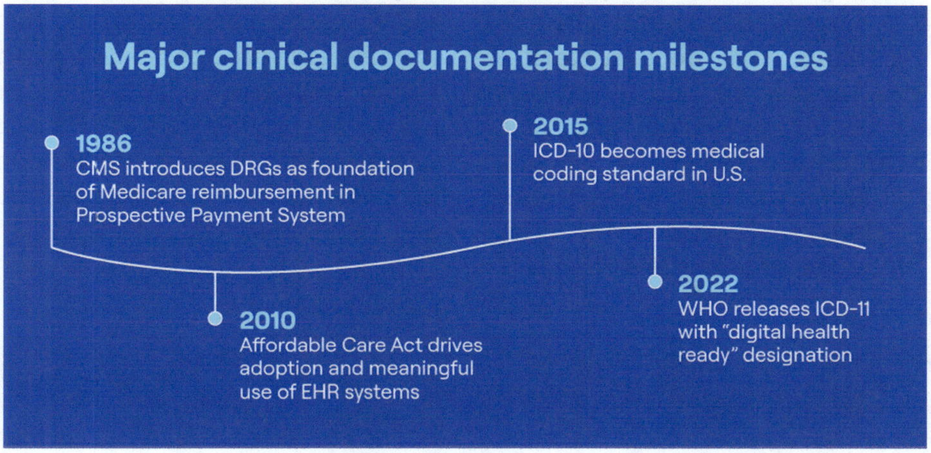

Figure 11.4. Major clinical documentation milestones.

Source: https://www.r1rcm.com/wp-content/uploads/2023/10/Image-Article-CDIIodine-Milestones-950x460-1.png.

11.1.3. Impact of Technology on Medical Records

The incorporation of technology into medical records has revolutionized clinical documentation processes significantly, with increased accuracy and efficiency being the result. EHRs have become the bedrock of this shift, making it easy to collect, store, and retrieve patient information. In contrast to paper-based systems, EHRs permit healthcare practitioners to immediately retrieve in-depth patient histories, making it easier to make more informed clinical decisions. This shift not only streamlines administrative work but also enhances PS by minimizing the likelihood of error through illegible handwriting or loss of documents. However, the implementation of EHR systems also has challenges, including that it requires extensive training and may experience system failures, which may lead to delays in patient care. But the benefits of greater accessibility and improved coordination between health care teams underscore the significant impact technology has had on today's medical records. Moreover, collaborative documentation is revolutionizing the way health care professionals engage their patients in consultation. The new approach allows for real-time interaction between clinicians and patients to enable a shared decision-making process. The law-making and technological advances in the delivery of healthcare have created an environment in which open communication and patient participation are necessary. By using collaborative documentation, professionals are able to capture patient contributions not only efficiently but also authenticate their experiences, with the outcome being a more patient-focused clinical consultation. Research confirms the efficacy of the method, with results demonstrating both increased provider satisfaction and improved patients' health outcomes. As collaborative documentation emerges in healthcare, so too does the realization that technology is not simply a mechanism for capturing data but also a means of reframing clinician-patient interactions to emphasize collaborative care (Maniss & Pruit., 2018). Moreover, training of healthcare professionals in patient-centered EHR use is imperative to ensure effective translation of these technological advancements into clinical practice. Despite the speedy deployment of EHR systems, providers are generally inadequately trained in technology-mediated patient communication. Training initiatives, such as those introduced at the Cleveland Clinic and the University of Chicago, have promise in equipping clinicians with skills to better engage patients. The participants indicated that they had a significant improvement in their ability to utilize EHRs in a patient-centered method, implying that personal effort may counter the disparity between diagnosing technology use and successful communication. This emphasis on training activities points towards the necessity for the preparation of healthcare professionals to handle the complexities of EHR systems in order to ensure that they operate harmoniously as key instruments for enhancing patient engagement and satisfaction (Lee et al., 2018).

Test Your Knowledge

1. How has the purpose and structure of medical records evolved from early handwritten notes to modern electronic health records (EHRs)?
2. What were some key milestones in the history of clinical documentation?

11.2. Types of Medical Records

Learning Outcome

1. Understand electronic health records (EHR);
2. Describe paper-based medical records;
3. Explain hybrid systems of documentation.

Medical records constitute the backbone of clinical documentation, providing an organized method of storing, retrieving, and dealing with patient information required for effective healthcare delivery. The types of medical records can be broadly categorized under a number of categories, including EMRs, EHRs, and paper-based charts. EMRs are electronic records that allow the exchange of real-time data among healthcare providers, facilitating care coordination and minimizing the risk of medical errors. On the other hand, EHRs summarize a broader scope of information by enabling interoperability between different healthcare centers, thus providing a broader perspective to a patient's history. This move towards digital forms also aligns with the government initiatives to modernize healthcare facilities and leverage technology for enhancing patient care outcomes, ultimately encouraging an optimal healthcare system. Paper medical records, though being gradually replaced by their electronic versions, are still valuable for clinical documentation. They have long been the standard in health care settings, containing invaluable treatment histories, laboratory results, and health care provider documentation. But the limitations of paper records become apparent as far as accessibility and time spent in retrieving them, which ultimately prove to be a source of hindrance for clinical decision-making. In the majority of cases, document practices associated with paper-based records can lead to inconsistency and loss of essential data. With healthcare organizations increasingly turning to electronic systems, information on various categories of medical records is essential to know exactly how they influence clinical workflows and patient outcomes.

This change underscores the necessity of intensive training in electronic record-keeping to minimize interoperability problems and maximize overall efficiency when documenting patient care. EMR adoption has been at the forefront of healthcare reform in the United States, driven by both advances in technology and an ever-growing need to improve the quality of healthcare. As emphasized by the findings of many research studies, the use of EMRs holds the potential to greatly enhance clinical outcomes, subject to the requirement that they be applied judiciously and strategically by health professionals and managers. For instance, the effectiveness of EMRs in controlling medical mistakes and healthcare costs is highly dependent on the objectives and management styles of healthcare institutions. Adopting a model to diagnose interoperability issues, as demonstrated in the case of hospital systems, can assist practitioners in addressing issues on a systemic level and thus obtain streamlined processes and better patient care (Binobaid et al., 2016). Not only do such models streamline processes, but they also provide an avenue for healthcare workers to make the most out of technology to realize improved outcomes (Lee et al., 2018).

11.2.1. Electronic Health Records (EHR)

Integration of EHRs into clinical practice is a paradigm shift in how healthcare providers document and manage patient information. Traditionally under the control of paper-based records, clinical documentation has increasingly found electronic alternatives that increase patient data accuracy and accessibility. EHR systems facilitate real-time modifications within clinical encounters to ensure enhanced provider communication and initiate better-coordinated care. As highlighted in recent efforts, the deployment of EHRs is less an innovation in technology than a healthcare environment culture shift that allows providers and patients to embrace this new mode of interaction. This shift aims to improve patient outcomes by offering settings where healthcare professionals can effectively talk to one another, boosting patient satisfaction as well as clinical performance (Leamon, 2016). But the move towards computerized records also poses significant questions about training and ease of use among users by healthcare providers. Despite the initiation of EHRs based on an aim to curtail medical mistakes and enhance service quality, several users cite dissatisfaction due to poor training and ergonomics of the systems. Pursuing these challenges is necessary, since how effectively the EHRs operate greatly depends upon the ability of the users to interact with the technology flawlessly. Without sound training and continuous support, the expected advantages of going for EHR systems may not reach their complete capacity. This brings into focus the necessity for educational interventions targeted at the aim of enhancing the capability of healthcare professionals to make effective use of EHRs so that they are better able to benefit from such systems in offering quality care (Simpson & Struchen-Shellhorn, 2008). In addition to this, the importance of policymaking in the facilitation of the right use of EHRs cannot be overstated, particularly where certain groups of people, like children, are involved. Public and private policy initiatives need to put in place interventions that facilitate the adoption of HIT among pediatric patients' providers. By recognizing the unique issues of children's health when it comes to EHR adoption, stakeholders are in a position to craft solutions that enhance the usability and functionality of such systems. These attempts are imperative, as they not only aim to correct existing disparities in healthcare technology but also serve as a catalyst for radical transformation in patient care overall. As healthcare infrastructures continue to evolve, it is essential that policymakers approach unique needs and exploit the application of EHRs in diverse patient groups, including vulnerable populations (Simpson & Struchen-Shellhorn, 2008) (Figure 11.5).

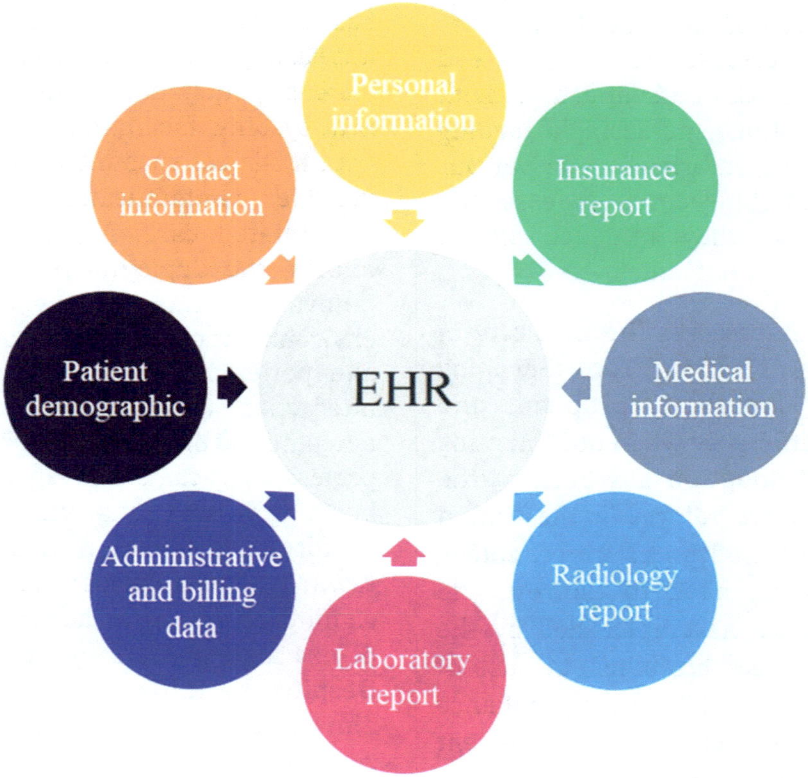

Figure 11.5. Electronic health record (EHR) model.

Source: https://www.researchgate.net/profile/Karim-Zarour/publication/359211436/figure/fig1/AS:1144722450067459@1649934508850/Electronic-health-record-EHR-model.png.

11.2.2. Paper-Based Medical Records

Throughout the evolution of healthcare documentation, paper-based records have been the central mode for storing, accumulating, and transferring patient information. Clinicians utilized physical charts as the medium for keeping accurate histories of patient encounters, diagnoses, and therapies for many decades. The records played a key role in the continuity of care and were crucial in providing adequate communication among clinicians. Paper systems, however, suffer from considerable drawbacks in the form of a higher probability of error due to illegible handwriting, missing documents, or a lack of immediate availability of critical information. Such drawbacks detract from the overall efficiency of healthcare provision, particularly in emergency situations where instant access to the patient's information is crucial. As the medical community increasingly recognizes the importance of accurate clinical documentation, a transition towards digitization and the utilization of EMR systems is developing strong momentum. From paperless to EMRs has emerged as a broad objective in the healthcare sector with several forces at its back, such as policy initiatives aimed at reducing medical errors and improving patient care. With significant investment in HIT, it is the expectation that EMR adoption will minimize most issues arising from paper records (Simpson & Struchen-Shellhorn, 2008). Despite the optimistic expectation, going electronic has its challenges. Data security issues, implementation costs, and worker training of providers are all formidable barriers that require a break. In addition to this, varying technological competence among employees can lead to unbalanced use patterns, which finally affect the quality of clinical documentation. Knowledge of these challenges therefore, is necessary for effective management of HIT integration into healthcare organizations. Despite the observed advantages of EMRs, paper-based systems persist as a legacy influencing clinical documentation activities. Paper charts are retained by most healthcare professionals, particularly in the case of facilities whose financial capabilities limit the adoption of novel technologies. Furthermore, the intricacy of patient data regularly necessitates a systematic method to document that has been readily facilitated by paper structures. Though the EMR proponents believe that digitization will facilitate smooth processes and enhance health care delivery, research presents incongruent evidence about the actual impact of the systems on patient outcomes and care effectiveness (Lee et al., 2018). This is a debate that highlights the need for broad-stroke strategies that not only facilitate the transition to electronic records but also ensure quality, priority and accuracy of clinical documentation. It becomes imperative for the stakeholders to converge and establish frameworks that bridge the gap between traditional methods and emerging technological innovations (Figure 11.6).

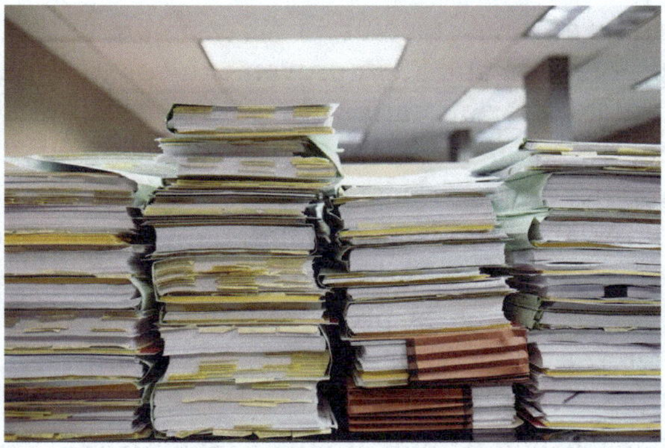

Figure 11.6. Illustration of paper-based medical records.

Source: https://www.isowire.com/wp-content/uploads/Disadvantages-of-Paper-Medical-Records.jpg.

11.2.3. Hybrid Systems of Documentation

As the medical practice further evolves, hybrid documentation systems are gaining more and more popularity since they integrate paper documentation with electronic documentation to enhance clinical workflows. This two-way approach allows healthcare professionals to leverage the strengths of both systems without necessarily having to endure the weaknesses of either. For instance, although EMRs can facilitate effective access and sharing of data, many clinicians value paper forms and handwritten notes, particularly in fast-paced environments such as emergency departments. Mixing these methods of documentation yields a merged record that can improve accuracy in patient care by facilitating the distinct needs of patients and the varying preferences of health care providers. Thus, hybrid documentation systems are a vital component in establishing a seamless balance between existing technology and long-standing procedures. Moreover, the use of hybrid documentation systems can lead to actual quality improvements in the provided care. Research suggests that both blended approaches of documentation, including EMRs and traditional structures, can promote process optimization and PS improvement. For example, studies of perioperative procedures determined that enhancing documentation through digital models of transformation not only reduced complexity but also facilitated patient-centered improvement across subprocesses (Ryan et al., 2019). This is proof that hybrid systems have the capacity to give room for continuous improvement while maintaining healthcare teams' flexibility and in tune with patient needs. As a result, hybrid documentation systems do not merely aim at raising efficiency but also facilitate a commitment to delivering high-quality care. Effective operation of hybrid systems depends significantly, however, on strategic utilization by healthcare administrators and practitioners. As attested by recent studies on EMR implementation, findings indicate that digital documentation results heavily depend on the authorities' intentions and management styles (Lee et al., 2018). This explains the importance of having hybrid system functioning goals align with overall organizational strategies to ensure integration is successful. Therefore, while hybrid documentation has the potential to strengthen clinical documentation quality, its success will be contingent on the design and facilitation of administrators in implementing it within their organizations. Training and support for staff personnel will be essential in making full use of hybrid documentation systems so that they can make meaningful contributions to overall health care quality and patient outcomes.

Test Your Knowledge

1. What are the key features and advantages of electronic health records (EHRs)?
2. In what clinical settings might paper-based medical records still be used, and what are their main limitations in modern healthcare?
3. What are hybrid medical record systems?

11.3. Legal and Ethical Considerations

Learning Outcome

1. Understand patient privacy and confidentiality;
2. Discuss legal requirements for documentation in clinical settings;
3. Focus on the ethical implications of record-keeping in clinical settings.

In the context of clinical documentation, legal and ethical concepts become paramount in shaping the practices that frame medical records. The legal requirement of healthcare professionals is to provide accurate, timely, and complete documentation, as failure to do so will translate into heinous malpractice claims. Besides, ethical principles such as beneficence and patient autonomy call for healthcare providers to prioritize the patient's welfare while handling documentation procedures. In occupationally mandated psychological assessments, for example, it is imperative that psychologists not only work within the framework of the law but also in accordance with ethics that guarantee respect and dignity in their evaluations. Thus, the convergence of these ethical and legal principles is crucial to ensure not only regulatory compliance but also the overall trust and quality of care provided to patients (American Psychological Association, 2018). Confidentiality remains one of the pillars of both legal and ethical principles in clinical documentation, particularly when dealing with sensitive patient information. As clinicians increasingly employ EHRs, the problem of juggling patient confidentiality with legal documentation needs becomes paramount. For instance, presymptomatic genetic testing centers often struggle to balance safeguarding patient confidentiality with legally required documentation of patient care procedures accurately. Evidence from a survey of Huntington disease centers demonstrates that while clinical care teams do their best to keep appointments and results confidential, many others rely on summary statements or simply fail to use the EHR altogether for documentation of sensitive information. This thin line emphasizes the ongoing need for revising policies that preserve patient privacy while ensuring that legal documentation is done effectively and ethically (American Psychological Association, 2018). With evolving times in the medical arena, especially with advancements in genetics and technology, legal and ethical considerations of clinical documentation need to keep up. Regular professional guidelines and advice are crucial for leading healthcare practice in documentation, particularly where new genetic data can influence patient care. The intersection of ethics and law in clinical documentation not only protects against malpractice but also fosters patient trust and informed decision-making. For instance, as patients demand more genetic testing that can give presymptomatic reports, open-ended policies will have to guide healthcare providers in reporting such delicate findings without compromising the ethical privacy rights of patients. Therefore, legal frameworks convergence and ethical standards will be important in establishing a responsible and humane clinical documentation strategy that addresses patient rights and quality of care.

11.3.1. Patient Privacy and Confidentiality

Patient privacy and confidentiality are essential tenets in healthcare, especially in the areas of medical records and clinical documentation. The HIPAA of 1996 plays a critical role in defining the era of patient privacy through the adoption of comprehensive regulations that mandate how personal health information is managed. The act defines roles for health care providers in the security of patient data and mandates them to adopt standardized practices in order to protect sensitive information. Therefore, the patients are assured with even more assurances that their medical records will be handled with the highest degree of confidentiality. With its culture of trust, HIPAA not only preserves confidentiality at the personal level but also ensures the overall integrity of the health system by ensuring patients feel secure about receiving care and sharing personal health information required for effective treatment. Besides, the overlap of nascent technology with healthcare practices also introduces new threats and prospects when it comes to patient confidentiality. Technologies such as telemental health and mobile health applications are effectively breaking down hindrances in the provision of services to patients who may face stigma, cost barriers, or physical location barriers when it comes to accessing mental health care. The rapid shift to digital solutions, however, poses severe concerns regarding the confidentiality of sensitive patient information. It should be noted that while such technologies are more convenient, they require robust privacy protections to give people the assurances they need in order to feel comfortable sharing personal health information. People are becoming less and less willing to adopt these new health solutions if they do not have clear guarantees about the security of their data. In this context, critical evaluation of current privacy legislation within the scope of health information, along with the integration of technology, is necessary in a bid to build patient trust and create a more diversified healthcare environment (Sherman, 2018). In contrast to the technical aspects of clinical record-keeping and documentation required in healthcare, the ethical obligation to maintain the confidentiality of patients is of great importance. Keeping private sensitive data not only supports legal compliance but also reflects the ethical practice of autonomy and patient respect. Enforcing HIPAA compliance standards and providing the highest regard for privacy procedures, healthcare organizations create a sanctuary for patient interactions, a critical component of successful treatment outcomes. Besides, this commitment to confidentiality provides a condition where patients feel comfortable sharing their medical concerns in depth, leading to enhanced diagnoses and more suitable treatment regimens. Lastly, patient privacy and confidentiality are not only legal mandates but also a cornerstone of excellent patient care that enhances the patient-provider therapeutic relationship and leads to healthier results (Nicholson & Smith, 2005) (Figure 11.7).

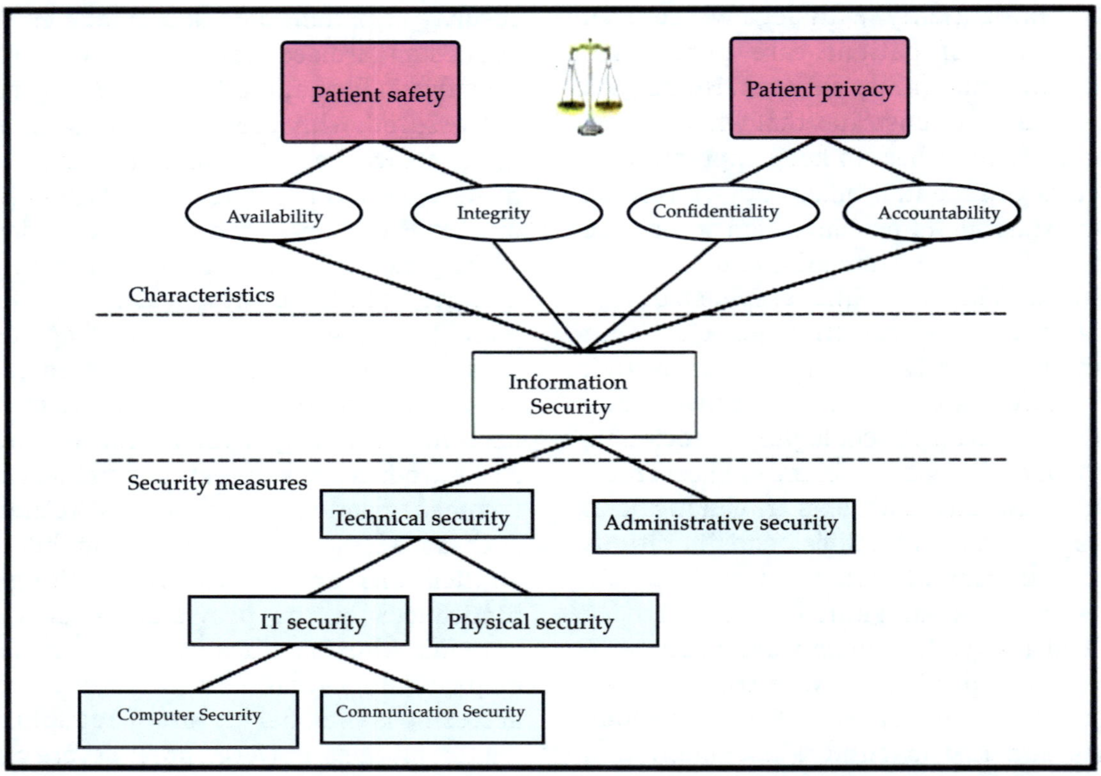

Figure 11.7. Patient safety and patient privacy and their relation to the information security model.

Source: https://www.researchgate.net/publication/285984258_Patient_Safety_and_Patient_Privacy_When_Patient_Reading_Their_Medical_Records.

11.3.2. Legal Requirements for Documentation

The legal requirements of clinical records are of utmost relevance to promote not only continuity of care but also compliance with the law. According to the law, medical professionals are legally obligated to maintain comprehensive and accurate medical records that depict the patient encounter. The records serve as critical legal documents in audits, investigations, and lawsuits, serving as proof of accountability for the delivery of health care. Failure to comply with these legal standards of documentation can result in severe consequences like financial penalties, loss of licensure, or even litigation against providers. Moreover, with the health care setting evolving further, documentation regulations keep on altering, and health professionals must be well aware of such legislation and standards in order to minimize risk due to non-compliance. Besides ensuring compliance, legal documentation also offers a basic mechanism to ensure such facilities uphold quality assurance and improvement within the healthcare setting. The medical record, as identified by the Italian Ministry of Health, is also an information tool documenting relevant demographic and clinical information throughout the course of a patient's care. Adequate documentation of this type is crucial for effective retrospective analysis and assists in determining these significant issues pertaining to organizational and technical matters of care delivery. By the critical evaluation of medical records, health facilities are capable of developing best practices while identifying where corrective action is required. The interplay of legal documentation with such evaluation processes not only points to the importance of having complete records but also to how they play a critical role in upholding a PS and quality improvement culture within the hospital (Guzzo et al., 2017). The confluence of healthcare and technology has also imposed more stringent legal demands on documentation, particularly in terms of the protection and privacy of data. The HIPAA rule imposes stringent regulations on the manner in which patient data must be documented, stored, and transmitted, safeguarding against misuse. As healthcare becomes digital, legal considerations surrounding documentation have increased, where proper security controls must be employed by healthcare practitioners. EMRs not only need to be correct but also adhere to the statutory requirements that guarantee patient confidentiality. Since the use of newer technologies is becoming increasingly common, innovation has to be balanced against legal standards for documentation to sustain patient trust and organizational integrity within the healthcare sector (Fair Labor Association, 2006).

11.3.3. Ethical Implications of Record-Keeping

The ethical application of record-keeping within healthcare settings is multifaceted, ranging from patient confidentiality and informed consent to medical records authenticity. As healthcare professionals strive to document patient interactions assiduously, it is important to acknowledge that the medical record is not only a storage for legal needs but also a symbol of the trust inherent in the patient-clinician relationship. Anonymity and secrecy are of prime concern; breaches of confidentiality can have serious repercussions, destroy patient confidence and endanger the individual to stigmatization. The moral implications of correct record-keeping are therefore of prime importance, as explained by initiatives seeking to ensure greater communication between the clinical and clerical staff, as defined by Gillies & Patel (2009). The multifaceted nature of ethical record-keeping serves to underscore its vital role in instilling accountability, transparency, and ultimately, enhanced healthcare outcomes. Furthermore, the use of advanced technologies in clinical documentation raises yet another ethical issue, that of the integrity of patient data. The presence of technology like voice recorders, the topic of debate by Pezaro & Lilley (2015), presents a possible solution for health professionals to break through challenges in creating contemporaneous records while having to provide instant care. Yet, it should be appropriately implemented with caution so that they do not inadvertently compromise the accuracy or security of patient data. Ethical considerations arise when weighing the balance between efficiency and the potential erosion of human interaction between patients and healthcare providers. This electronic transformation necessitates militant surveillance to defend against misuse and ensure that technological solutions actually enhance the quality of clinical documentation without sacrificing ethical standards. Finally, the integration of an ethical framework into clinical documentation practice is of ultimate importance to tackle problems created by record-keeping efficiently. Specialized education programs need to emphasize not merely the technicalities of documentation but also the ethical consequences of patient record-keeping. A well-balanced appreciation of the legal responsibilities and moral responsibilities of clinical documentation will instill a practice environment that enshrines patient care alongside effective record-keeping. As Gillies & Patel (2009) point out, the failure of current systems and the limitations of these systems to adhere to ethical standards can have serious consequences for patients and healthcare professionals alike. Hence, creating an environment that values ethical principles in record-keeping can reduce risk and support the essential role of reliable documentation in the provision of high-quality care with respect for patient rights and dignity (Figure 11.8).

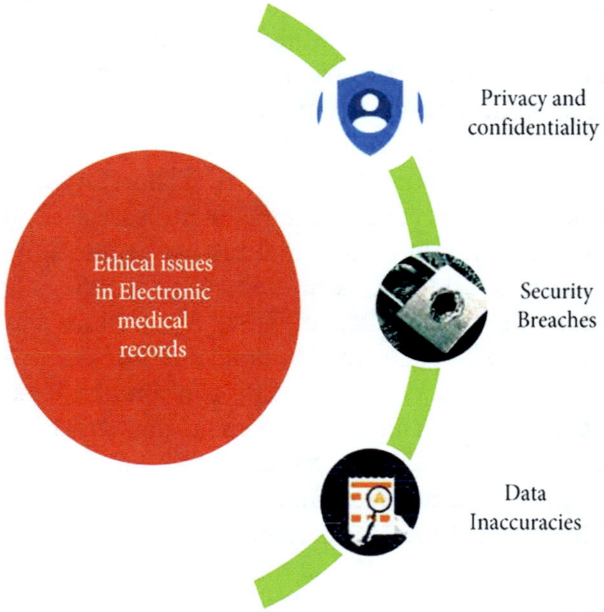

Figure 11.8. Ethical issues in electronic medical records.

Source: https://www.researchgate.net/publication/360769576/figure/fig3/AS:1158809535946868@1653293131829/Ethical-issues-in-electronic-medical-records.jpg.

Test Your Knowledge

1. How do clinical documentation practices uphold patient privacy and confidentiality?
2. What are the legal standards healthcare providers must follow when documenting clinical care?
3. Why is accurate, honest, and timely documentation considered an ethical obligation in clinical practice?

11.4. Best Practices in Clinical Documentation

Learning Outcome

1. Understand the basics of accuracy and completeness of medical records;
2. Focus on standardization of documentation practices in clinical settings;
3. Discuss training and education for healthcare professionals.

Clear and precise clinical documentation is the foundation of quality health care delivery, facilitated by demands for precision, simplicity, and conformity. Clinical documentation best practice requires the employment of concise language and consistent formats to facilitate clear communication among members of the healthcare team. This practice enhances continuity of care by presenting a degree of uniform and comprehensive information that is accessible to all team members. Secondly, adopting collaborative documentation approaches, particularly in behavioral healthcare, fosters a client-centered treatment climate that encourages patients to engage proactively in their treatment processes, which has been linked to improved therapeutic outcomes (Maniss et al., 2018). In addition, patient involvement in documentation is not only empowering but also strengthens the therapeutic relationship, and this enhances patient satisfaction and quality of care. Ongoing learning and adherence to legal and ethical standards form the essential components for effective clinical documentation. As healthcare regulations evolve, the process of documentation must be updated regularly to align with current practice and organizational standards. The practice minimizes chances of error, maintaining sensitive patient details well-documented and in secure storage. Adherence to EMRs is increasingly promoted as a best practice because it provides an orderly, systematic location for retaining and retrieving patient information (Lee et al., 2018). However, variations in policies of administration significantly influence how EMR systems are utilized and can even determine their success in enhancing care quality and cutting costs. It is thus of extreme significance to understand the relationship between documentation strategies and administrative styles to optimize EMR utilization. Finally, implementation of best practice in clinical documentation must also account for the importance of feedback and quality assurance processes. Continuous monitoring and assessment of documentation practice can identify areas for improvement, optimizing both individual and organizational practice. Regular audits and peer review enhance accountability and promote a culture of excellence among healthcare teams. In addition, providing positive feedback tests healthcare professionals to bind themselves to lifelong learning, having clinical documentation skills continuously reinforced and aligned with best practice. Lastly, stimulating a responsible approach to clinical documentation not only optimizes the value of medical records but also constitutes an essential contribution to PS and quality of care within the increasingly complex healthcare environment.

11.4.1. Accuracy and Completeness of Records

Precision and fullness of clinical records are of paramount significance in ensuring quality patient care as well as effective healthcare delivery. It is through precise records that clinicians can take well-informed decisions appropriate for individual patients' own unique medical histories, a necessity for proper treatment regimens. The link between diagnosis code correctness and medical information quality has been well-documented; higher quality medical information leads to more accurate and consistent diagnosis coding. In a study conducted at Dr. Moewardi Hospital, it was found that the proportion of patients with high-quality medical information and correct diagnosis codes was significantly higher, emphasizing the need for proper documentation practices in order to enhance patient outcomes (Maryati et al., 2019). The integrity of medical records not only affects patient care individually but also has practical implications beyond that, including healthcare costs and the sustainability of healthcare systems. Comprehensiveness in clinical documentation is also essential, as deficient records can lead to erroneous conclusions that compromise PS. The intrinsic nature of medical records calls for the capture of a wide spectrum of clinical data, demographic information, and care-related interactions during the treatment of a patient. A retrospective chart review of 1184 medical charts conducted at Teaching Hospital "Umberto I" highlights the importance of proper documentation in the determination of strengths and weaknesses in patient care. The findings indicate that systematic medical chart review is a useful tool for clinical practice assessment and can contribute to improved documentation standards (Guzzo et al., 2017). These evaluations also promote accountability and motivate medical professionals to adhere to best practices, further aiding the grand goal of enhancing PS and the quality of care. With the rapidly evolving nature of the healthcare industry, precise and thorough medical records have never been more critical. Thorough documentation makes it easier to provide continuity of care, particularly in transitional settings where patients shift between levels of healthcare services. Moreover, accurate records are crucial to policy development and research because they provide reliable data to assess healthcare quality and outcomes. Most findings underscore the patient prognosis and quality of clinical documentation, which indicates that good records are critical to effective clinical decision-making (Maryati et al., 2019). Where best practices in clinical documentation are sought to be applied in hospitals, ongoing education and training of medical personnel will become necessary to embed a culture of completeness and precision in medical documents and thus an overall quality improvement in healthcare.

11.4.2. Standardization of Documentation Practices

Standardization of documentation procedures in clinical settings is required to ensure the optimization of patient care quality and the global results of healthcare services. Standardized procedures for documenting and processing clinical information have the potential to assist healthcare providers in minimizing medical error and inconsistency, which are most often the causes of negative patient outcomes. Present initiatives reflect the importance of standardization as public and private sectors are now recognizing the need to implement full HIT systems. These systems can provide the capability to encourage systematic documentation, thereby making it feasible for all healthcare providers to be able to access proper and up-to-date patient information, particularly as it pertains to the unique needs of various populations, including children, who have been the focal point of most HIT initiatives (Simpson & Struchen-Shellhorn, 2008). In addition, the implementation of standardized documentation practices is essential in helping with improved communication among healthcare providers. When documentation habits are standardized, it enhances the ability of different specialists and departments to communicate well with each other, reducing the risk of miscommunication of patients on handoffs across care settings. Normalized computerized patient records can convey vital patient data explicitly, enabling healthcare teams to receive certain patient needs, thereby improving continuity of care. This HIT integration not only promotes coordination between care providers but also supports uniform clinical decision-making, thereby improving overall PS and satisfaction (Johnson, 2011). Despite the fact that standardization of documentation practices has numerous benefits, there are some challenges. Serious challenges have been encountered by healthcare systems, particularly in transitioning from paper records to electronic documentation. The publicly embarrassed failure of certain HIT implementations is a warning story; it raises issues about the potential for complexity in circumstances in which staff must resort to less complete, paper-based records when electronic systems are not working. These breakdowns tend to cause frustration and to discourage the efficiency benefits that standard practices are intended to provide. Therefore, future projects must incorporate lessons learned from previous implementations to design robust systems that not only improve documentation practices but also enhance the delivery of quality care across many healthcare environments (Johnson, 2011).

11.4.3. Training and Education for Healthcare Professionals

It is critical for proper training and education of clinical providers to be integral components in the delivery of high-quality clinical documentation and accurate medical records. With increasing patient care complexity, it is imperative that healthcare providers are informed about clinical documentation practices. This consists of awareness of compliance guidelines, i.e., those of the Centers for Medicare and Medicaid Services (CMS), and experience with EHR systems now prevalent in healthcare. Increased training that involves use of documentation standards not only increases accuracy but also benefits patient outcomes. Additionally, ongoing education is necessary to keep healthcare professionals up-to-date on evolving documentation requirements and technology. A knowledgeable workforce is required for ascertaining accurate and thorough medical records essential for quality patient care and continuity. In the care home and nursing contexts, the need for specialized training incorporating clinical documentation practices is increasingly acknowledged. Evidence indicates that nursing staff often find it challenging to document pressure ulcers and other skin integrity issues, and a high percentage of them are considered preventable (Kaye et al., 2016). Though the majority of the staff possess primary information on skin integrity care, there are gaps in training in terms of the usage of standardized grading scales and referral protocols to safeguard teams. This deficit indicates the necessity of training programs that heighten workers' expertise in patient health management documentation. By creating an understanding of clinical documentation and its role in safeguarding patients, healthcare organizations can improve the quality and reliability of medical records and ultimately improve care and safety. Moreover, incorporating behavioral health training in the overall education system of healthcare providers can go a long way in enhancing the efficiency of clinical documentation.

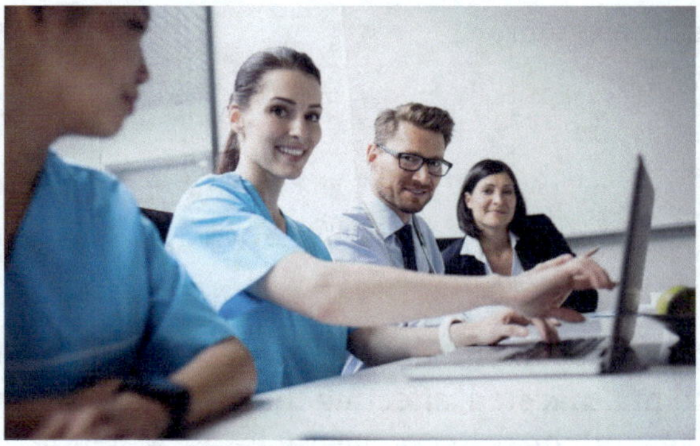

Figure 11.9. Training for healthcare professionals to ensure high-quality clinical documentation and accurate medical records.

Source: https://denclinical.com/public/upload/images/hizmetler/doctors-discussing-laptop-meeting-6183-1440x900.jpg.

The social worker integrated care competency scale (SWICCS) illustrates the need to equip social workers with competencies applicable in integrated care settings so that they can cater to both physical and behavioral health needs of patients (Davis et al., 2019). Whereas healthcare systems strive to provide holistic care, training programs must address a range of competencies related to holistic documentation practices. Establishing a sound educational framework not only facilitates tracing knowledge development but also empowers healthcare professionals to deliver culturally responsive and patient-centered care. This approach not only enhances the quality of clinical documentation but ultimately leads to enhanced patient outcomes and reduced health disparities across various populations (Figure 11.9).

Test Your Knowledge

1. Why is it essential for clinical documentation to be accurate, complete, and timely?
2. How does the use of standardized formats improve communication, continuity of care, and data analysis in clinical settings?

11.5. Challenges in Clinical Documentation

Learning Outcome

1. Discuss about common errors in medical records;
2. Explain the barriers to effective documentation;
3. Deal with the consequences of poor documentation.

Clinical documentation challenges are enormous and multifaceted, affecting the quality of patient care and healthcare systems as a whole to an enormous extent. One of the significant concerns is that various health information systems are not interoperable with each other. As is the situation with a case study of a complex healthcare provider in Saudi Arabia, interoperability problems can emerge from technical, semantic, and organizational barriers that hinder unhampered communication among different systems. The communication gap is not only making it difficult for information to be retrieved, but also creating opportunities for clinical errors and negative results for patients. Therefore, resolving these interoperability challenges becomes necessary in fostering a unified clinical documentation platform with the ability to facilitate precise and timely patient data exchange, ultimately contributing to improved healthcare. In addition, the value of clinical documentation is commonly devalued by shortcomings in medical record-keeping measures. One vivid illustration of this can be seen in a study assessing the quality of neonatal care in Tanzania's Kilimanjaro region, where the deficits in clinical records were reported to be very large. The study revealed that important information about the patients' health was frequently excluded from the records, such as maternal antenatal data and neonatal vital signs. This lack of comprehensive documentation not only disrupts PS but also prevents the delivery of evidence-based care by healthcare professionals. The inefficiencies indicate the necessity for standard documentation protocols and training for healthcare personnel such that all relevant clinical information is appropriately documented, resulting in improved patient outcomes. Finally, clinician workload contributes to the issues involved with clinical documentation. As the volume of patients grows and case complexity levels rise, clinicians tend to exhaust time to perform proper documentation activities. Urgency to complete administrative tasks within schedule constraints can lead to superficial or careless entries in clinical records, ultimately influencing the integrity of patient data. As appreciated during the evaluation of neonatal care in Kilimanjaro, staffing at some facilities was normally low, further hindering the quality of documentation. Optimization of clinician assistance by maximum staffing, effective processes of documentation, and the integration of newer technologies may reduce workload-related problems and foster an environment of meticulous clinical documentation, optimizing the efficacy of medical record management (Figure 11.10).

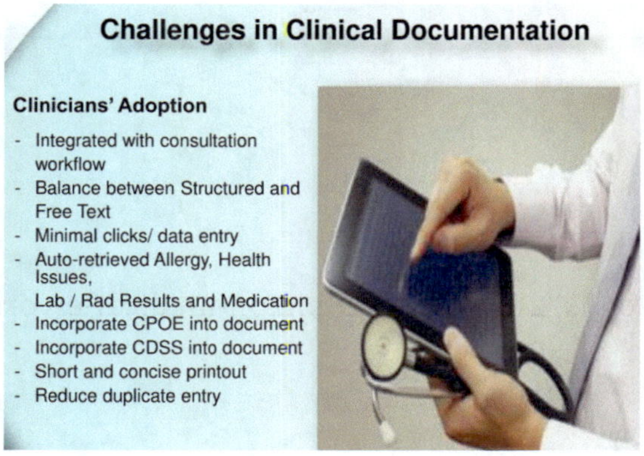

Figure 11.10. Challenges in clinical documentation.

Source:

11.5.1. Common Errors in Medical Records

Medical record errors significantly weaken the quality and safety of patient care. An example of a frequent occurrence is a result of documentation errors, due to various reasons like miscommunication among healthcare professionals and outdated systems that prevent real-time updates. A good example would be billing databases, widely used to track the quality of patient care, and can provide misleading reports if monitoring for errors is not done. Manual verification has also yielded discrepancies with positive predictive values of up to 96%; however, they also recorded a concerning 21% negative predictive value in certain cases. This highlights the need for rigorous validation protocols in medical record-keeping to ensure that clinical documentation is an accurate reflection of patient encounters and treatment outcomes, thereby safeguarding against potential adverse impacts on patient health and treatment efficacy (Tran, 2018). One of the significant categories of errors is technology implementation in clinical documentation, particularly in the EMS setting. Speech recognition (SR) programs have been launched with a promise of greater efficiency but without the ability to suppress inherent inaccuracies that can lead to reduced patient safety. Literature indicates that existing SR implementations are not always guaranteed to ensure the needed 99% accuracy, sometimes failing to detect similar sentences or eliminating background noise properly and, therefore, putting PS at risk. As a result, documentation errors introduced by SR systems could cause miscommunication, incorrect patient assessment, or inappropriate treatment regimens.

These shortages with improved algorithms, such as the bag-of-words post-processing method, may improve the accuracy of documentation in high-stakes settings (). The effects of erroneous medical records extend beyond individual patient visits to have a ripple effect on larger healthcare systems and quality metrics. Erroneous documentation can create a ripple effect of unfavorable consequences, which includes increased healthcare costs, liability, and diminished trust in healthcare providers. For instance, inaccuracies in recording patient screening rates will mislead health planning and resource allocation and yield suboptimal public health outcomes. The effects of these documentation errors not only undermine PS but also distort information being employed to measure population health. Therefore, the recognition of common errors in medical record-keeping and encouraging strict documentation standards is imperative to boost clinical performance and ensure responsibility within healthcare environments (Tran, 2018) (Figure 11.11).

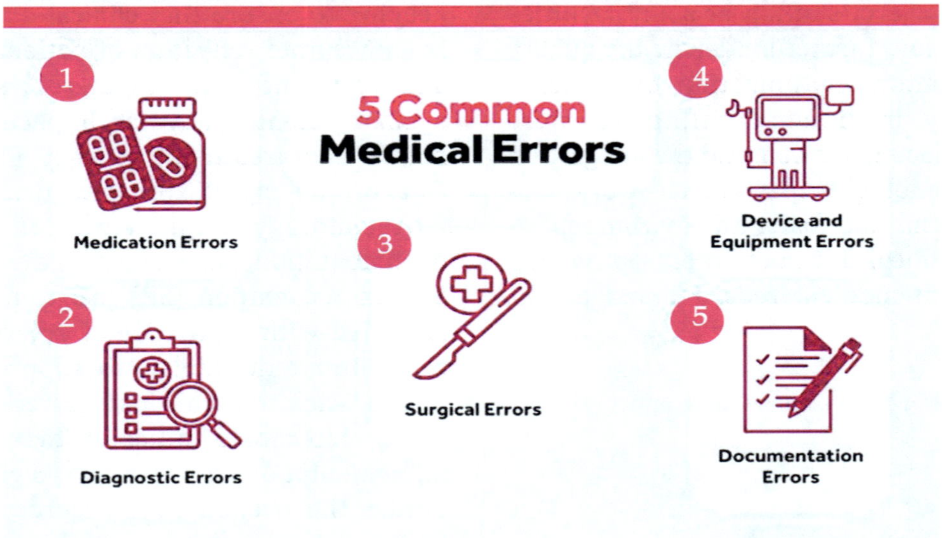

Figure 11.11. Five common medical errors.

Source: https://www.intelycare.com/wp-content/uploads/2024/07/5-common-medical-errors-infographic.png.

11.5.2. Barriers to Effective Documentation

The utility of clinical documentation is severely hindered by many challenges that health care practitioners encounter in practice. The sheer technical complexity of EHRs is probably the most significant challenge. While the transition to EHR systems was intended to automate documentation and improve patient care, it has tended to increase cognitive load for practitioners. This entanglement can result in incorrect data input culture and a lack of documentation, which ultimately impacts PS and continuity of care. In addition, as the recent assessments highlight, there could be poor communication skills among the health care providers that can escalate these issues and lead to misinterpretation of valuable information on EHR systems. Through the overcoming of these barriers, health care workers' competency can be increased and the quality of clinical documentation in general improved, with consequent more precise medical records (Leamon, 2016). A further key issue behind suboptimal documentation is brief training and education on optimal practices for using EHRs. Many providers, especially new professionals, report that they are not adequately prepared to work within EHR systems, leading to inconsistencies and inaccuracies in documentation. It is concerning that they lack training, and the integration of good documentation practices will be central to improving patient outcomes and adherence to clinical guidelines. For instance, recent studies have suggested that the inability to properly document postpartum depression screenings among women Veterans suggests an important need to enhance education and awareness of updated screening processes (Brown, 2017). Filling these knowledge gaps through the utilization of targeted training programs will help health care providers use EHRs appropriately, hence enhancing the validity of medical records and the quality of patient care. Lastly, environmental factors, such as administrative troubles and the culture of work, can limit good clinical documentation. Health care settings that have not prioritized documentation processes may lack adequate time or resources for the task, leading to rushed or inadequate documentation. Additionally, a disvalued culture that does not prioritize documentation can discourage providers from viewing it as an essential part of patient care. Previous endeavors have shown that developing a positive culture and supporting communications training can lead to improved use of EHRs, achieving a higher satisfaction rate of providers and patients (Leamon, 2016). By developing a work culture that emphasizes quality documentation and invests in training to support those efforts, health care organizations can work towards eradicating these obstacles and achieving more successful clinical documentation.

11.5.3. Consequences of Poor Documentation

Poor documentation in clinics can have a host of unintended effects that go beyond mere errors in record-keeping. Perhaps the most vital implication is the effect on patient care quality. When healthcare practitioners fail to document patient information clearly and comprehensively, significant facts regarding diagnosis and treatment regimens can be lost or distorted. This results in misdiagnosis and ineffective treatment regimens, ultimately compromising the well-being of patients. For instance, studies have indicated that precise medical information correlates with enhanced diagnosis coding precision. Where documentation is not precise, the likelihood of generating suboptimal diagnosis codes is increased considerably, disrupting maximal medical decision-making and possibly risking patient outcomes (Maryati et al., 2019). Inaccurate documentation can also incur a cost in finances for healthcare institutions. Hospitals and clinics depend on accurate billing codes from clinical documentation in order to receive appropriate reimbursement for services rendered. Incompleteness or inaccuracy in the documentation could have a direct effect on the billing process, either as lost revenues or inappropriate payment claims. These imbalances in finances could strain healthcare resources, impacting the overall quality of services rendered. An article put a spotlight on the importance of correct documentation processes, since billing disparities will distort quality metrics like rates of screening for colorectal cancer. Health care providers might misestimate their own measures in the absence of proper documentation, thereby complicating the problems of financial viability and quality of health care even further (Tran, 2018). Finally, poor documentation's fallout extends to the realm of legal remedy and ethical practice. Health care providers need up-to-date records not only for patient care but also for legal protection. Poor documentation may be a legal trap in a court of law, where missing or inconsistent medical records have the potential to discredit a provider's case against claims of malpractice. Lack of detailed records can lead to an unfavorable verdict in a court of law, which will end up harming professional reputations and careers. To that end, it also poses ethical concerns regarding patient rights and informed consent, as patients rely on meticulous documentation to obtain clarity in their medical care. By and large, the implications of poor documentation permeate many aspects of the healthcare system, highlighting the crucial necessity of sound clinical record-keeping protocols.

Test Your Knowledge

1. What are the most common types of errors found in clinical documentation?
2. What systemic or organizational barriers hinder effective clinical documentation?
3. What are the potential legal and ethical consequences of poor clinical documentation for both healthcare providers?

11.6. Future Trends in Medical Records

Learning Outcome

1. Understand integration of advancements in technology and artificial intelligence (AI) into clinical documentation and medical records;
2. Discuss the integration of telemedicine and documentation;
3. Explain the role of patient engagement in record-keeping.

With development in medicine, the use of EMRs is still a dominant trend shaping the future of the medical record. The adoption drive of EMRs has gained momentum because it can curb many inefficiencies experienced within healthcare systems. According to recent research, EMR can lead to a reduction in medical errors and the cost of healthcare as a whole, thereby enhancing the quality-of-care patients receive. This shift is not merely a technological leap; it demands a strategic vision of management to use these systems efficiently. Healthcare administrators' objectives have a significant contribution to EMR integration, and they determine the outcomes of using it (Lee et al., 2018). Hence, effective management practice is pivotal in realizing the ultimate benefits of EMR in improving patient outcomes, as well as streamlining medical documentation procedures. Another of the most important future trends in medical records is the evolution of interoperability standards between multiple healthcare systems. Interoperability allows seamless communication between different EMR systems and promotes coordinated care between multiple medical environments. Enhanced interoperability facilitates the seamless transfer of patient data so that the data can be freely available to providers in critical moments. This is increasingly vital as healthcare transitions towards value-based care, whereby patient satisfaction and outcomes dictate the levels of reimbursement. Also, as care further migrates into outpatient settings, the ability to exchange information across various platforms is crucial in treating chronic disease as well as ensuring continuity of care. Consequently, stakeholder collaborations designed to define and create interoperability standards will be of utmost priority in optimizing clinical documentation and overall healthcare delivery. One of the top concerns in medical record paths is patient privacy and data security. As health organizations migrate more and more to electronic records, they are vulnerable to cyberattacks and data breaches that put patient data at risk. Accordingly, upcoming trends will need to keep strong cybersecurity measures and strict compliance with privacy regulations, such as HIPAA, at the forefront. In addition to technical measures, information about the value of protecting data will also be critical in the creation of a security awareness culture. Based on continuing research, particularly in high-risk settings like ICUs, good practice in end-of-life documentation has been unsatisfactory, with heightened demands for improvement in clinical documentation and data protection quality (Ghabeljoo, 2017). Balancing the speed of technology evolution with strong data safety measures will be crucial in fostering trust and integrity in the future medical record environment.

11.6.1. Advancements in Technology and AI

The interplay of technology and AI innovation with clinical documentation and medical records is revolutionizing healthcare practice. Among the principal technological achievements is the development of advanced EHR systems, which automate the process of documentation, enabling healthcare professionals to efficiently document patient data. Not only do these systems enhance data collection, but they also increase the precision and completeness of medical records. AI-powered solutions amplify these benefits further by offering predictive analytics that assist clinicians in identifying likely health risks and facilitating anticipatory interventions. This revolution ultimately leads to improved patient outcomes, as clinical decision-making is aided by comprehensive and reliable information provided to healthcare professionals. In addition, the COVID-19 pandemic also catalyzed the adoption of digital health solutions at an accelerated pace. According to the new study, healthcare organizations have quickly integrated telehealth and remote monitoring technologies into their care models to achieve the capacity for long-term change in patient participation and clinical documentation practices. The changes to Medicare and federal guidelines had created an environment that supported speedy uptake of these technologies through enabling new virtual visit payment models. Therefore, healthcare professionals are able to offer more timely and effective care from a distance, thereby improving patient engagement and satisfaction as well as ensuring continuity of clinical documentation. Innovations such as these not only redefine the manner in which care is delivered but also enable clinicians to maintain accurate medical records regardless of physical boundaries. With future advancements in AI in the pipeline, their impact on clinical documentation is going to grow even more. There is evidence that AI technologies, such as natural language processing and machine learning, hold the capability of enhancing the documentation process through automating routine tasks and culling relevant information from disorganized notes. For instance, clinician notes can be processed by AI programs that summarize key information to create comprehensive patient summaries, aiding clinical assessments. Additionally, these technologies can identify patterns in medical records that inform treatment plans and improve risk stratification. In one of the studies comparing surgical procedures, it was noted that the application of AI-based insights leads to more accurate interventions and optimized clinical outcomes. Hence, greater research into such advancements can potentially redefine practice documentation, creating possibilities for a more responsive and efficient healthcare system.

11.6.2. Integration of Telemedicine and Documentation

With the integration of telemedicine into clinical documentation workflows, the way health providers interact with patients and manage records has evolved. Telemedicine, such as remote monitoring, patient consultations, and education, requires effective documentation to ensure regulatory compliance and deliver effective care. An important element in this integration is seamless data exchange between various telemedicine programs and EHR systems. Through the application of enterprise application integration (EAI) techniques, healthcare organizations are able to improve the level of service quality and streamline documentation operations, hence enhancing overall patient care outcomes (Khoumbati et al., 2008). The innovation in this technology not only provides timely access to patient records but also minimizes errors and fragmentation in treatment, ultimately leading to better clinical decision-making and PS. In addition, telemedicine encounters must be documented at the same high levels as in-person encounters. This includes thorough notes of patient interactions, diagnostic impressions, and treatment plans that are essential for ongoing patient care and continuity of care. The challenge is in standardizing the procedure for documenting different telemedicine services to offer the same consistency and accuracy. Furthermore, the conjoining of HIT and telemedicine can serve as an incentive to improve documentation competency. Increased attention to HIT implementation has been accompanied by many health policies aimed at minimizing medical errors and enhancing quality care (Simpson & Struchen-Shellhorn, 2008). Accurate documentation not only supports clinical decision-making but is also extremely crucial for billing, whereby providers are reimbursed correctly for the services they deliver. Finally, with the growth of telemedicine, the role of documentation also needs to change to accommodate new features that make remote care provision possible. This extends not only to textual comments but also to digital image recording, such as lab results and imaging studies that may be remotely received. With increasing usage of telehealth services, incorporating documentation tools into telemedicine software can simplify record-keeping and simplify information transfer between healthcare practitioners. As offered in models such as the MAESTRO model, a number of parameters that influence the adoption of EAI, which have a significant influence on enhancing the telemedicine documentation process, need to be considered by organizations (Khoumbati et al., 2008). Finally, the effective integration of telemedicine and documentation is required to facilitate quality patient care in combination with compliance with legal and ethical needs in the health care setting (Figure 11.12).

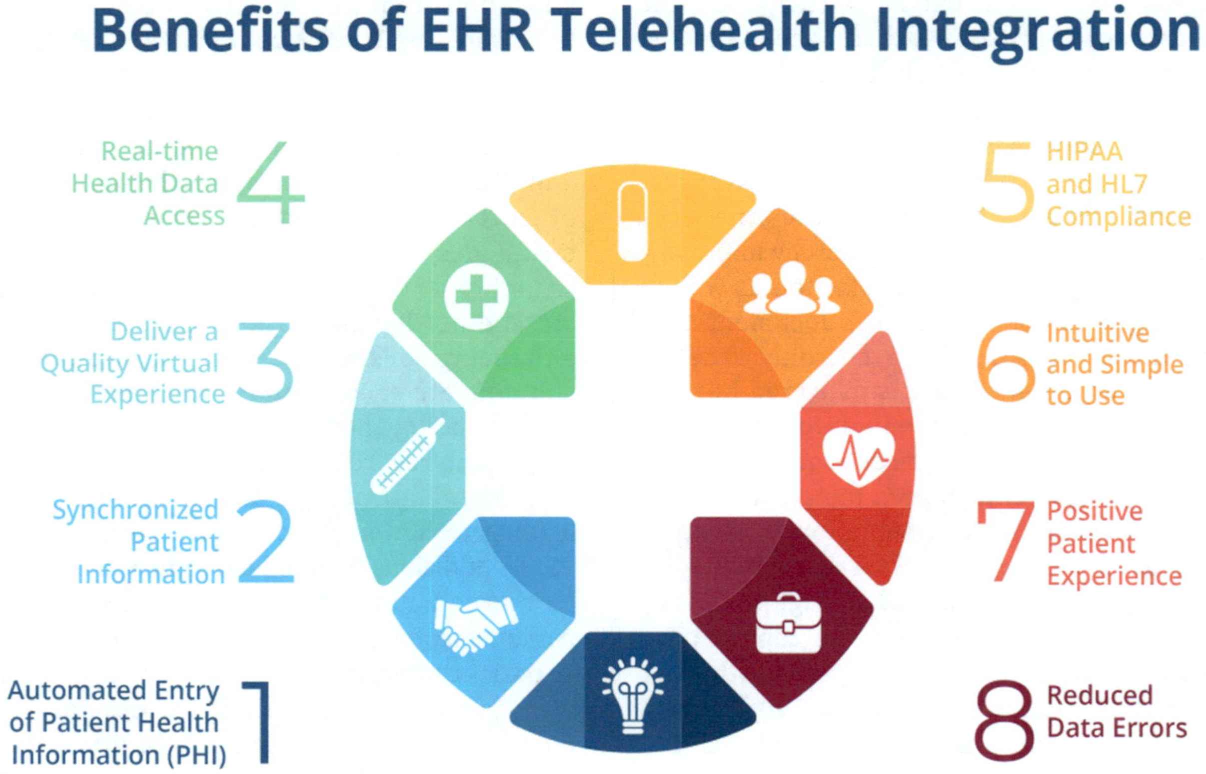

Figure 11.12. Benefits of EHR telehealth integration.

Source: https://i0.wp.com/www.geneca.com/wp-content/uploads/2023/04/3b5a43ce-2d90-4e2d-b6fe-ff854d99374d.png?w=1080&ssl=1.

11.6.3. The Role of Patient Engagement in Record-Keeping

Patient involvement is a critical issue to the quality of clinical recording, impacting the degree of documentation and increasing better health outcomes. When patients are engaged in their own health decisions, they provide valuable information that can be applied to enhance medical records. The co-documentation process, for example, allows for patients and healthcare professionals to work together in recording health information so that the records reflect the patient's voice and experience. The approach not only supports the sustenance of comprehensive and comprehensive documentation but also empowers patients to such an extent that they develop a sense of ownership of their health information. As more patient involvement in healthcare is headed towards more patient-centered models, patient involvement in record-keeping is essential to enable better therapeutic relationships alongside clinical outcomes, in line with the greater emphasis on shared decision-making when delivering healthcare (Maniss et al., 2018). Further, integrating technology within patient engagement activities has been a prominent driving force in transforming record-keeping practices in clinics. EHR systems, with patient access and amendment capability for their health information, are a step towards participatory documentation. They encourage patients to view their records and provide descriptions of their health experiences and preferences, which can be especially useful in clinical decision-making.

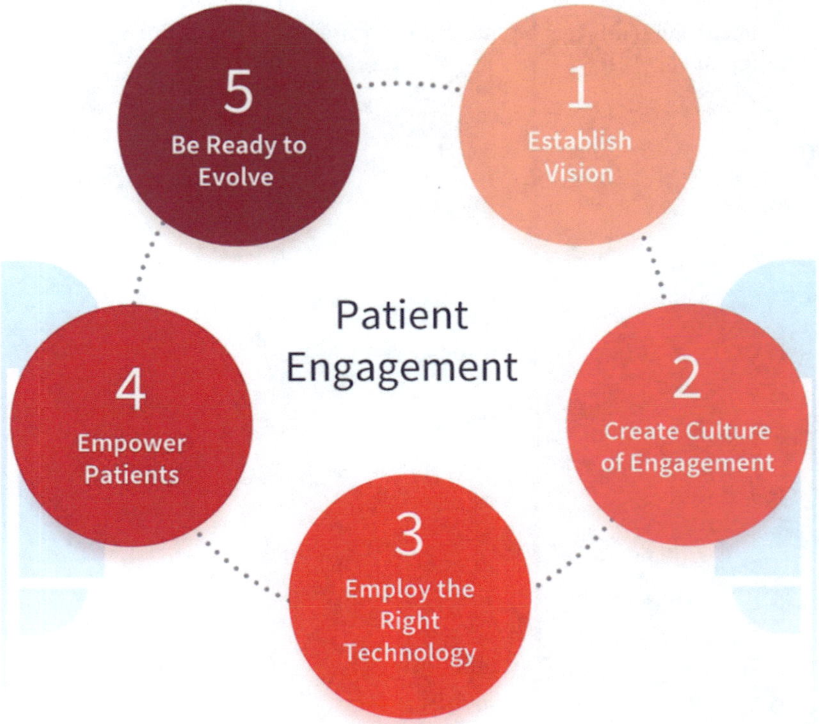

Figure 11.13. Patient engagement.

Source: https://www.tigahealth.com/wp-content/uploads/2021/05/patient-engagement-5.jpg.

However, as noted in a number of criticisms, the use of these electronic systems is likely to have inadequate clinical engagement, thus making it challenging for their success (Gillies & Patel, 2009). Overcoming these challenges through improved information sharing and coordination between patients and their health providers is essential in constructing records that not only satisfy administrative needs but also maximize continuity of care for patients. The ethical implications of patient participation in record-keeping cannot be overstressed, especially confidentiality and data protection. As patients become more directly engaged with their health data, healthcare organizations have an obligation to protect sensitive data and ensure patients are completely informed of their rights to access and contribute. This relationship puts the ethical issues of the healthcare providers in handling patient data in conflict, while promoting openness and empowerment. Consequently, the development of policies facilitating informed patient participation in record-keeping has the potential to produce more ethical clinical documentation. Lastly, the use of patient engagement not only satisfies ethical and legal expectations but also creates a more responsive healthcare environment, positioning health systems to better address the needs of their populations (Gillies & Patel, 2009) (Figure 11.13).

Test Your Knowledge

1. How are artificial intelligence and machine learning expected to transform clinical documentation?
2. In what ways can telemedicine platforms be integrated with electronic health records (EHRs) to ensure seamless documentation of care?

SUMMARY

The importance of clinical documentation and medical records cannot be overemphasized in healthcare. These records not only provide a record of the patients' medical history but also act as an indispensable tool in facilitating effective communication among healthcare professionals. The accuracy and completeness of these records have a direct impact on clinical decision-making and ultimately on patient outcomes. Employers and regulatory bodies also largely rely on psychological tests in making hiring and employment decisions. According to the American Psychological Association (2018), the guidelines provided by the Committee on Professional Practice and Standards (COPPS) are vital in guaranteeing best practices in clinical assessments, ensuring that documentation meets the high standards required in various professional environments. In addition, the increased application of EHRs has transformed the practice of clinical documentation. These computerized systems improve the capacity of healthcare teams to function in an integrated manner, finally leading to enhanced patient-centered care delivery. Yet, as the study on primary care practices emphasizes, the implementation of EHRs holds opportunities and challenges. Practices have found means to address these challenges, which reflects the responsiveness of healthcare professionals to changing technological conditions. EHR capabilities can be enhanced to enable better teamwork that is vital in delivering high-quality care, as suggested by Williams et al. (2007). This flexibility is indicative of the overarching requirement for ongoing improvement of clinical documentation practices. Ultimately, proper clinical documentation and medical records management are important to ensure high-quality patient care. With the continued evolution of the medical practice, the same must apply to documentation and record-keeping requirements. The complementary interaction between precise clinical documentation and enhanced patient results reiterates the necessity of continued education and training for health care professionals. The standards established by organizations such as COPPS and observations derived from research conducted on EHR usage will play a crucial role in delineating future practices and standards. While the healthcare systems struggle to improve accountability and openness, an overarching focus on clinical documentation will continue to be critical to furthering the quality of care provided at all levels of the healthcare continuum.

In clinical documentation and medical records, the impact of systematic methods such as the trigger review method (TRM) takes a pivotal role in enhancing PS. Recent studies have proven that TRM explicitly reveals hidden patient safety incidents (PSIs) in clinical records and thus presents enormous learning and improvement prospects for healthcare workers. As shown in a small study of 25 GP trainees, the implementation of TRM led to the detection of approximately 80 undiagnosed PSIs, and nearly half were deemed preventable (McKay et al.,2013, 2013). This shows that systematic review methods in clinical practice not only enhance the standards of safety but also equip future professionals with skill sets in identifying and managing risks, ultimately enhancing a culture of continuous improvement in the treatment of patients. Moreover, retrospective analysis of records has been found to be an efficient mechanism in the evaluation of the quality of clinical documentation. Around 1184 medical records review in a teaching hospital showed significant improvement in the quality of documentation, thus testifying to its effectiveness in a Clinical Risk Management system (Guzzo et al., 2017). It highlighted strengths and weaknesses in documentation habits to demonstrate that even though overall quality is better, certain critical problems persist. Such analysis promotes responsibility as well as serving as the basis for corrective actions of a particular kind, enhancing the learning environment for healthcare providers. These weaknesses need to be rectified in order to fulfill the global aims of clinical documentation: offering high-quality patient care and achieving maximum organizational efficiency. The crossing of effective training practices with stiff evaluation processes serves to further underscore the necessity of continuous education in clinical documentation processes. The positive reception of TRM training by GP trainees signals growing recognition of the role that systematic documentation plays in optimizing safety results within healthcare settings (McKay et al., 2013). In addition, identification of best and worst practices via a systematic review of medical records provides a feedback loop that will revise both existing practitioners and training programs. As the medical record evolves further with advances in technology and regulatory requirements, it is necessary to build a culture that appreciates accurate documentation, thereby fulfilling the benefits of such practices in terms of improved patient outcomes and greater operational efficiency along the healthcare continuum.

KEY TERMS FROM THIS CHAPTER

- Behavioral healthcare
- Clinical documentation activities
- Compliance guidelines
- EHR systems
- Ethical standards
- Healthcare industry
- Healthcare philosophies
- High-quality patient care
- Integrated care settings
- Medical documentation
- Clinical decision-making
- Collaborative documentation
- Decision-making process
- Electronic medical records (EMRs)
- Healthcare delivery systems
- Healthcare organizations
- Healthcare technology
- HIT integration
- Medical concerns
- Medical history

CRITICAL THINKING QUESTIONS

1. **Which of the following best describes an electronic health record (EHR)?**
   a. Paper records stored in filing cabinets
   b. A digital version of a patient's chart accessible in real time
   c. A transcription of handwritten notes
   d. A personal journal kept by the patient
2. **Which ethical principle is most closely related to maintaining patient confidentiality in medical records?**
   a. Beneficence
   b. Justice
   c. Autonomy
   d. Non-maleficence
3. **What is a key best practice in clinical documentation to ensure legal defensibility?**
   a. Use of non-standard abbreviations
   b. Documenting only abnormal findings
   c. Charting after the fact
   d. Accurate, timely, and complete documentation
4. **Why is the use of standard terminology in documentation important?**
   a. To reduce paper usage
   b. To allow for easier billing only
   c. To improve clarity and interoperability
   d. To discourage use of digital systems
5. **Which of the following is a common challenge in maintaining accurate clinical documentation?**
   a. Overdocumentation due to copy-pasting in EHRs
   b. Excessive use of handwritten records
   c. Limited access to internet in hospitals
   d. Inadequate storage space for paper records

Short Answer Questions

1. How has the practice of clinical documentation evolved from handwritten notes to modern electronic health records (EHRs)?
2. What are the key differences between paper-based records, electronic health records (EHRs), and personal health records (PHRs)?
3. What are the primary legal and ethical obligations healthcare providers must follow when documenting patient information?
4. What are some established best practices for accurate, clear, and timely clinical documentation that ensure quality care and medico-legal protection?
5. What common barriers do healthcare professionals face in maintaining high-quality clinical documentation?
6. How can incomplete, inaccurate, or delayed documentation negatively impact patient outcomes, clinical decision-making, and provider accountability?
7. In what ways is patient involvement in reviewing and contributing to their own health records transforming the healthcare documentation landscape?

Answers to Critical Thinking Questions

1. (b); 2. (c); 3. (d); 4. (c); 5. (a)

REFERENCES

1. Bugeja, M., & Abela, J. C.(2014). Continuity of information and care: A pilot study in a health center. Malta Medical Journal. 2014, Vol.26(2), p. 29-36 https://core.ac.uk/download/46602484.pdf (accessed on 27th June 2025).

2. McKay J, de Wet C, Kelly M, Bowie P. Applying the Trigger Review Method after a brief educational intervention: potential for teaching and improving safety in GP specialty training?. *BMC Med Educ*. 2013;13:117. Published 2013 Aug 30. doi:10.1186/1472-6920-13-117(accessed on 27th June 2025).

3. Lee, W. W., Alkureishi, M. L., Isaacson, J. H., Mayer, M., Frankel, R. M., London, D. A., Wroblewski, K. E., & Arora, V. M. (2018). Impact of a brief faculty training to improve patient-centered communication while using electronic health records. *Patient education and counseling*, *101*(12), 2156–2161. https://doi.org/10.1016/j.pec.2018.06.020(accessed on 27th June 2025).

4. Purkayastha, S., Allam, R., Maity, P., & Gichoya, J. W. (2019). Comparison of Open-Source Electronic Health Record Systems Based on Functional and User Performance Criteria. *Healthcare informatics research*, *25*(2), 89–98. https://doi.org/10.4258/hir.2019.25.2.89(accessed on 27th June 2025).

5. Binobaid S, Fan IS, Almeziny M, Investigation Interoperability Problems in Pharmacy Automation: A Case Study in Saudi Arabia, International Conference on ENTERprise Information Systems/International Conference on Project MANagement/International Conference on Health and Social Care Information Systems and Technologies, CENTERIS/ProjMAN / HCist 2016, Procedia Computer Science, Volume 100, 2016, Pages 329–338.(accessed on 27th June 2025).

6. Ledesma, A., Al-Musawi, M. & Nieminen, H. Health figures: an open source JavaScript library for health data visualization. *BMC Med Inform Decis Mak* **16**, 38 (2016). https://doi.org/10.1186/s12911-016-0275-6(accessed on 27th June 2025).

7. American Psychological Association (2018). Professional practice guidelines for occupationally mandated psychological evaluations. *The American psychologist*, *73*(2), 186–197. https://doi.org/10.1037/amp0000170(accessed on 27th June 2025).

8. Oroviogoicoechea, C., & Watson, R. (2009). A quantitative analysis of the impact of a computerised information system on nurses' clinical practice using a realistic evaluation framework. *International journal of medical informatics*, *78*(12), 839–849. https://doi.org/10.1016/j.ijmedinf.2009.08.008(accessed on 27th June 2025).

9. Guzzo, A. et al (2017). Quality Assessment of medical records as a tool for Clinical Risk Management: A three year experience of a Teaching Hospital Policlinico Umberto I, Rome. Senses and Sciences. https://doi.org/10.14616/SANDS-2017-2-371379(accessed on 27th June 2025).

10. Brown, E. L. (2017). Postpartum depression screening of women veterans in Alaska: Quality improvement project. https://core.ac.uk/download/286607496.pdf (accessed on 27th June 2025).

11. Williams, C. H., Leatherman, S., Christianson, J. B., & Sutherland, K. (2007). Paying for Quality: Understanding and Assessing Physician Pay-for-Performance Initiatives. *The Synthesis project. Research synthesis report*, (13), 24373. (accessed on 27th June 2025).

12. Ryan, Jim; Doster, Barbara; Daily, Sandra; and Lewis, Carmen, "Business Process Redesign in

the Perioperative Process: A Case Perspective for Digital Transformation" (2019). *Transactions of the International Conference on Health Information Technology Advancement*. 67. https://scholarworks.wmich.edu/ichita_transactions/67(accessed on 27th June 2025).

13. Davis, T. S., Reno, R., Guada, J., Swenson, S., Peck, A., Saunders-Adams, S., & Haas-Gehres, L. (2019). Social Worker Integrated Care Competencies Scale (SWICCS): Assessing social worker clinical competencies for health care settings. *Social work in health care*, *58*(1), 75–92. https://doi.org/10.1080/00981389.2018.1547346(accessed on 27th June 2025).

14. Kalenderian, E., Maramaldi, P., Kim, S., Etolue, J., McClellan, L., Simmons, K., Yansane, A., White, J. M., Walji, M. F., & Ramoni, R. B. (2016). Strategic Shift to a Diagnostic Model of Care in a Multi-Site Group Dental Practice. *International journal of dentistry and oral health*, *2*(4), 10.16966/2378-7090.209. https://doi.org/10.16966/2378-7090.209(accessed on 27th June 2025).

15. Fair Labor Association. (2006). Tracking chart 2006 Nike, Indonesia 070033365E. https://core.ac.uk/download/33600570.pdf (accessed on 27th June 2025).

16. Ghabeljoo, J. (2017). End of life care practices for patients who die in intensive care units (ICU). https://core.ac.uk/download/70419827.pdf (accessed on 27th June 2025).

17. Gillies, A. C., & Patel, I. (2009). IT and the NHS: Investigating different perspectives of IT using soft systems methodology. Studies in Ethics, Law, and Technology, 3 (2). ISSN 19416008 https://core.ac.uk/download/9632821.pdf (accessed on 27th June 2025).

18. Khoumbati, K., Themistocleous, M., Irani, Z., & Mantzana, V. (2008). Information Systems and Healthcare XXIV: Factors Affecting the EAI Adoption in the Healthcare Sector. Communications of the Association for Information Systems, 22, pp-pp. https://doi.org/10.17705/1CAIS.02205 (accessed on 27th June 2025).

19. Maryati, W., Ismayani, A., & Rahayuningrum, I. O. (2019). Quality of medical information determine the quality of diagnosis code. https://core.ac.uk/download/480549983.pdf (accessed on 27th June 2025).

20. Johnson, C. W. (2011). Identifying common problems in the acquisition and deployment of large-scale software projects in the US and UK healthcare systems. https://core.ac.uk/download/110438.pdf (accessed on 27th June 2025).

21. Kaye, V., McCormick, K., Ousey, K., Stephenson, J., et al. (2016). Investigating staff knowledge of safeguarding and pressure ulcers in care homes. https://core.ac.uk/download/30734203.pdf (accessed on 27th June 2025).

22. Dossetor PJ, Freeman JM, Thorburn K, et al. Health services for aboriginal and Torres Strait Islander children in remote Australia: A scoping review. *PLOS Glob Public Health*. 2023;3(2):e0001140. Published 2023 Feb 13. doi:10.1371/journal.pgph.0001140(accessed on 27th June 2025).

23. Leamon, A. E. (2016). The electronic health record scorecard: A measure of utilization and communication skills. https://core.ac.uk/download/79664897.pdf (accessed on 27th June 2025).

24. Pezaro, S., & Lilley, L. (2015). Digital voice recorders - A conceptual intervention to facilitate contemporaneous record keeping in midwifery practice. *Women and birth : journal of the Australian College of Midwives*, *28*(4), e171–e176. https://doi.org/10.1016/j.wombi.2015.04.008(accessed on 27th June 2025).

25. Maniss, Suzanne Ph.D., LCDC, NCC and Pruit, Amanda G. LPC (2018) "Collaborative Documentation for Behavioral Healthcare Providers: An Emerging Practice," Journal of Human Services: Training, Research, and Practice: Vol. 3: Iss. 1, Article 2. (accessed on 27th June 2025).
26. Martinez, J., Bloom, D., Azurdia, G., & Miller, C. (2009). The employment retention and advancement project: Results from the substance abuse case management program in New York City. https://core.ac.uk/download/71342549.pdf (accessed on 27th June 2025).
27. Nicholson, S. and Smith, C.A. (2005), Using lessons from health care to protect the privacy of library users: Guidelines for the de-identification of library data based on HIPAA. Proc. Am. Soc. Info. Sci. Tech., 42:. https://doi.org/10.1002/meet.1450420106(accessed on 27th June 2025).
28. Sherman, J. (2018). Double secret protection: Bridging federal and state law to protect privacy rights for telemental and mobile health users. https://core.ac.uk/download/213019827.pdf (accessed on 27th June 2025).
29. Simpson, L., & Struchen-Shellhorn, W. (2008). The promise of health information technology: Ensuring that Florida's children benefit. https://core.ac.uk/download/71342408.pdf (accessed on 27th June 2025).
30. Tran, T. (2018). Speech recognition technology: Improving speed and accuracy of emergency medical services documentation to protect patients. https://core.ac.uk/download/215485167.pdf (accessed on 27th June 2025).

INDEX

D

H

I

N

O

P

R

S

T

U

V

W